Drug Therapy for Infectious Diseases of the Dog and Cat

Drug Therapy for Infectious Diseases of the Dog and Cat

Valerie J. Wiebe

WILEY Blackwell

This edition first published 2015 © 2015 by John Wiley & Sons, Inc.

Editorial Offices

1606 Golden Aspen Drive, Suites 103 and 104, Ames, Iowa 50014-8300, USA

The Atrium, Southern Gate, Chichester, West Sussex, PO19 8SQ, UK

9600 Garsington Road, Oxford, OX4 2DQ, UK

For details of our global editorial offices, for customer services and for information about how to apply for permission to reuse the copyright material in this book please see our website at www.wiley.com/wiley-blackwell.

Library of Congress Cataloging-in-Publication Data

Wiebe, Valerie J., 1958– , author.

    Drug therapy for infectious diseases of the dog and cat / Valerie J Wiebe.

        p. ;   cm.

    Includes bibliographical references and index.

    ISBN 978-1-118-55734-1 (pbk.)

    1. Dogs–Infections–Treatment.   2. Cats–Infections–Treatment.   3. Communicable diseases–Treatment.   4. Veterinary pharmacology.   I. Title.

    [DNLM: 1. Communicable Diseases–veterinary.   2. Dog Diseases–drug therapy.   3. Cat Diseases–drug therapy. SF 981]

    SF991.W5955 2015

    636.089′51–dc23

                                        2015007222

A catalogue record for this book is available from the British Library.

Wiley also publishes its books in a variety of electronic formats. Some content that appears in print may not be available in electronic books.

Cover images: veterinary-blood-test: ©iStock.com/deyangeorgiev; retriever-vaccination: ©iStock.com/mediaphotos; pills-drug: ©iStock.com/RidvanArda

Set in 8.5/10.5pt Meridien by SPi Global, Pondicherry, India

Printed in Singapore by C.O.S. Printers Pte Ltd

1   2015

Contents

Section G: Antiviral Agents

Preface

How to use this information

This aim of *Drug Therapy for Infectious Diseases of the Dog and Cat* is to present, as simply and clearly as possible, the essentials of approaching infectious disease cases to students and practicing clinical veterinarians whose main interests lie elsewhere. Because the scope of infectious diseases in veterinary medicine is so large, this book is limited to coverage of common infectious diseases of dogs and cats. The emphasis throughout is on basic concepts of disease prevention, diagnosis, empiric therapy, and treatment of established infections. The book concentrates on those aspects of drug therapy most relevant to achieve a positive clinical outcome. It is designed to help the practitioner select therapeutic drugs based on rational decisions that incorporate pharmacology, toxicology, pharmacokinetics, and efficacy.

The book is divided into seven sections, including: (1) Pharmacology guidelines, (2) Empiric therapy pending diagnostic results, (3) Therapy of established infections, (4) Antibiotics, (5) Antifungals, (6) Antiparasitics, and (7) Antivirals. The pharmacology section covers interpretation of MICs, cidal versus static drugs, approaches to infectious disease cases, reasons for antibiotic failure, dose adjustments in renal dysfunction, pregnancy risk categories, drugs safe in lactation, safe writing skills, and basic mathematical calculations. The empiric therapy section attempts to list the most common organisms isolated in a range of infectious disease processes and their treatment, while the section on established infections provides the drug of choice in most instances.

Each drug section is alphabetized for easy referencing and features drug use, availability, contraindications, dose, dose adjustments, administration, storage, stability, side effects, potential drug interactions, pharmacokinetics, and use in pregnancy and lactation. In general, specific organisms are listed alphabetically and drugs will be listed under their generic or chemical name unless they are a combination product. In that case, they will be listed according to the trade or brand name of the product.

An attempt has been made to incorporate a variety of important source information that normally can be found in many different locations. The book is designed to be used in clinics and other environments when a brief introduction to a topic is needed and time does not permit consultation of multiple references. This book is written in a concise format that may not cover many details that are found in larger infectious disease textbooks or the primary literature. Readers are referred to those publications for more detailed supplemental information.

While every effort has been made to assure the accuracy, timeliness, and correct interpretation of the information, the reader is advised that the author, editor, reviewers, and publisher cannot be responsible for errors, omissions, application of this information, or continued currency of the information. Due to the ever evolving nature of infectious diseases, the emergence of new organisms, genetic drift, vector emergence in new areas, and increasing resistance patterns, the reader is advised that decisions regarding the diagnosis and treatment of animals must be based on critical thinking and independent clinical judgment by the clinician.

Acknowledgments

I am deeply indebted to Dr. Jane Sykes, DVM for her outstanding contributions, patience and guidance in assisting me to write this manual. Her role as a consultant helped to improve the format and organization of the manual and strengthen the manuals overall quality. Her commitment to excellence, leadership skills, and positive attitude were greatly appreciated. I would also like to thank Dr. James Howard, DVM for his truly remarkable support in the editing of this first edition. His knowledge of private veterinary practice after 25 years helped to shape the practical approach to the manual. To all my Veterinary and Pharmacy students at the University of California, Davis and the University of California, San Francisco, I dedicate this book to you who inspired me to pull this information together from the many infectious disease lectures and discussions we have had. Thank you to Phong Le for his help with production of the enclosed tables. To my husband, Jim, and my children, Sara, Michael, Bradley, and Jennifer, and grandchildren, Cali and Ethan: thank you for your understanding of the importance of this project to me, but mostly for your constant love, support, and encouragement. Lastly, to my ever loving dog, Wally, a Potcake rescue from Turks and Caicos, who served as a foot warmer at night while typing this book.

SECTION A
Pharmacology Guidelines

Chapter 1: Understanding Minimum Inhibitory Concentrations (MICs)

The National Committee on Clinical Laboratory Standards and the Clinical and Laboratory Standards Institute (CLSI) help to determine the susceptibility testing guidelines for most common organisms and antimicrobial agents in each species. Minimum Inhibitory Concentration (MIC) ranges for sensitive organisms are then set for specific antibiotics. To obtain an MIC for a bacteria, antibiotic concentrations are doubled in concentrations between the range of 0.06–512 µg/mL (0.06, 0.12, 0.25, etc.) to determine the susceptibility of bacteria. As antibiotic concentrations are increased, bacteria stop dividing or are killed. Bacteria that continue to proliferate at concentrations that are inhibitory for the same species are considered resistant. Typically, laboratories report susceptibilities as sensitive, intermediately sensitive or resistant to a particular antibiotic. In general, if a bacterium is resistant to an antibiotic *in vitro*, it should not be considered for *in vivo* (clinical) use. If an organism is considered to have "intermediate" sensitivity to an antibiotic the antibiotic may still be efficacious *in vivo* (clinically) in situations where high concentrations can be achieved (urine, topical therapy). If bacteria are susceptible to a particular antibiotic then it may be useful *in vivo* (clinically) if other variables are favorable (pharmacokinetics, toxicity, penetration to the site of action, etc.). When comparing between antibiotics that are both sensitive, the "breakpoint" must be considered. The breakpoint is also set by the National Committee on Clinical Laboratory Standards. The breakpoint is the concentration of antibiotic that cannot be exceeded *in vivo* (clinically) due to its pharmacokinetics and toxicity. The greater the difference between the MIC of the organism and the breakpoint helps to determine which antibiotic may be more efficacious.

Chapter 2: Static versus Cidal Antibiotics

The definitions of "bacteriostatic" and "bactericidal" antibiotics appear to be straightforward. A "bacteriostatic" antibiotic implies that it only produces "static" effects on bacteria versus a "bactericidal" antibiotic that kills the organisms. However, these categories are not absolute and drugs can act as either "static" or "cidal" under different conditions. Their mechanism of action may be influenced by growth conditions, bacterial density, test duration, and extent of reduction in bacterial numbers. Often agents that are "cidal" may fail to kill every organism in a large inoculum within 18–24 h. Furthermore, agents that are "static" may only kill some bacteria over 18–24 h, but may continue to kill organisms after the test period, but not enough to be called "cidal" (>99.9% in 24 h). Clinically, this is even more arbitrary. Most antibacterials are better described as potentially being both bactericidal and bacteriostatic depending on the organism and the concentrations achieved at the site of action. For theoretical purposes the following description of each is presented.

Bacteriostatic

For bacteriostatic antibiotics (those that prevent growth) the percent time that serum antibiotic concentrations are above the MIC of the organism should be >50% for most patients or closer to 100% for severely ill patients with immunosuppression or with debilitated patients. The dose here can remain the same but the dosing

Drug Therapy for Infectious Diseases of the Dog and Cat, First Edition. Valerie J. Wiebe.

frequency can be increased to improve efficacy (i.e., from BID to TID). These are considered time dependent antibiotics. This differs from concentration dependent (or dose dependent) antibiotics that are considered "cidal". Examples of antibiotics categorized primarily as bacteriostatic agents include: Chloramphenicol, macrolides, tetracyclines, clindamycin, linezolide, and rifampin.

Bactericidal

For bactericidal antibiotics, the peak concentrations of antibiotic are important and should approximate 4–8 times the MIC concentrations of the organism. To maximize the clinical efficacy here, the dose must be increased and the frequency can stay the same. Examples of antibiotics that are considered bactericidal include: Aminoglycosides, penicillins, cephalosporins, carbapenems, vancomycin, fluoroquinolones, metronidazole, nitrofurantoin, and co-trimazole.

Chapter 3: *In Vitro* versus *In Vivo* Efficacy

In vitro culture and sensitivity will assist in antibiotic selection but may not always dictate *in vivo* efficacy. Many other factors also play a role in determining the *in vivo* outcome. Poor owner compliance, administration of an unstable compounded product, poor gastrointestinal absorption (altered formulation, drug/drug, drug/food interactions, variable gastrointestinal transit time, malabsorption, etc.) may all affect the ability of a drug to be absorbed. Following absorption, the distribution of drugs to the site of the infection may also be a challenge. Penetration of drugs into some physiological spaces including the eye, CNS, prostate, intracellular spaces, and into abscesses is often very difficult and is dependent on protein binding, lipophilicity, size, and degree of ionization of the drug molecule. A good example of this is the third generation cephalosporins. While all cephalosporins may appear to be effective judged on their MICs, if being used for CNS disease only cephalosporins with low protein binding can penetrate across the blood brain barrier in sufficient quantities to maintain therapeutic levels (Table 3.1). In addition, some organisms such as *Staphylococcus* spp. that appear to be sensitive *in vitro* to trimethoprim/sulfamethoxazole (TMS) combinations are able to circumvent the drug *in vivo* by utilizing the host's folate

rendering the drug inactive. This is also true for *Enterococcus spp.* where both TMS and cephalosporins appear sensitive *in vitro* but should not be used clinically.

Chapter 4: Approaching Infectious Disease Cases

Is this an infection?

Determine if an infection is the problem: does the animal have two or more of the following?
- Fever,
- leukocytosis,
- increased fibrinogen,
- discospondylitis,
- or other evidence of bacterial infection.

Is eosinophilia or other signs of parasitic infection present?

Where is the infection?

Determine the most likely site of infection based on labs, physical evidence, physical exam, radiographic evidence, history, and so on.

What are the most likely pathogens at this site?

Identify the most likely pathogens (enterics, anaerobes, gram positives, fungus, viruses, parasites) and choose an empiric drug therapy to target these.

Empirically, what will cover these pathogens?

Select a drug that targets the most likely pathogens and that can achieve appropriate drug levels at the site of infection.

What other factors must be considered?

Consider local factors that might alter the efficacy of drug therapy (necrotic tissue, purulent material, biofilm on foreign body, poor blood supply, poor oxygen supply,

Table 3.1 Properties of Cephalosporins

Class	Drugs	Route	Dose Adjustment*	CNS penetration	Organisms Covered
First Generation	Cefadroxil (Duricef)	PO	Yes		**Primarily gram positives:** Methacillin sensitive *S. aureus*, *S. pseudintermedius*, *S. intermedius*, Grp A + B *Streptococcus*
	Cefazolin (Ancef, Kefzol)	IM/IV	Yes		**Some gram negatives:** *E. coli*, *Klebsiella*, *P. mirabilis*
	Cephalexin (Keflex, Rilexine)	PO	Yes		**No coverage of**: Methicillin resistant *Staphylococcus*, *Enterococci* or penicillin resistant *Streptococcus*.
					Anaerobic coverage: Poor, no *B. fragilis* coverage.
Second Generation	Cefaclor (Ceclor)	PO	No		**Gram positive coverage:** Similar to first generation
	Cefoxitin (Mefoxin)	IM/IV	Yes		**Gram negative coverage:** Enhanced compared to 1st generation
	Cefuroxime (Ceftin, Zinacef)	PO/IM/IV	Yes		**Anaerobic coverage:** Some coverage with cefoxitin and cefotetan for *B. fragilis*
Third Generation	Cefdinir (Omnicef)	PO	Yes		**Gram positive coverage:** Maintains varying degrees of gram positive coverage
	Cefixime (Suprax)	PO	Yes		**Gram negative coverage:** Enhanced coverage compared to 1st and 2nd generation agents.
	Cefotaxime (Claforan)	IM/IV	Yes	+++	Covers: *Citrobacter, Enterobacter Salmonella, Serratia, E. coli, Klebsiella, Proteus, Pasteurella*, etc.
	Cefovecin (Convenia)	SC	Yes		Ceftazidime covers Pseudomonas, *Enterobacter* is often resistant. Ceftiofur covers *Actinobacillus, Mannheimia*
	Cefpodoxime (Simplicef, Vantin)	PO	Yes		**Anaerobe coverage:** Some anaerobe coverage. Only Ceftiofur covers Bacteroides and
	Ceftazidime (Fortaz)	IM/IV	Yes	+++	Fusobacterium No other agents cover Bacteroides
	Ceftiofur (Naxcel)	IM/SC	Yes		
	Ceftriaxone (Rocephin)	IM/IV	Yes	+++	
Fourth Generation	Cefipime (Maxipime)	IM/IV	Yes	+++	**Gram positive coverage:** Broad spectrum gram positive coverage
					Gram negative coverage: Broad spectrum gram negative coverage. Covers Pseudomonas similar to ceftazidime.
					Anaerobic coverage: Some coverage, no Bacteroides coverage
Fifth Generation	Ceftaroline (Teflaro)	IV	Yes		**Gram positive coverage:** Enhanced coverage of gram positives (methicillin resistant *Staphylococcus*, *E. faecalis*)
					Gram negative coverage: Same gram negative coverage as 3rd and 4th generation generation No Pseudomonas coverage
					Anaerobic coverage: Limited anaerobic coverage

Notes

PO = Oral, IM = Intramuscular, IV = Intravenous, SC = Subcutaneous routes of delivery

*Dose adjustments in renal impairment required

CNS penetration= (+++) can be used in CNS infections for susceptible organisms etc.). Consider drug penetration into difficult sites (CNS, abscesses, eye, prostate).

What patient factors should be considered?

Select a drug that is safe based on patient specific parameters (species, age, breed, contraindications, drug interactions, and underlying medical conditions).

What route of administration should be used?

Select a route to administer the drug based on the severity of the animal's condition, owner's ability to administer the drug, cost of therapy, and compliance.

What dose should be used?

Select a dose and dosing frequency based on the severity of the infection and patient specific parameters (age, renal function, liver function, etc.) to maintain therapeutic concentrations sufficient to cure the infection and prevent relapse. Monitor the animal for side effects and reduce the dose if necessary.

How long should the animal be treated?

Select a length of time and set goals of therapy (reduced fever, fibrinogen, leukocytosis, titers, improvement in physical signs, negative skin scrapings, negative fecals, etc.). Typically treatment should be based on clinical resolution of signs and symptoms. Treatment should continue for 3–5 days past this point. In some cases prolonged therapy is indicated (fungal, *Mycobacterium*, prostatitis, pyothorax, endocarditis, bone infections, pyelonephritis, etc.)

When should I perform culture and sensitivity?

Culture and sensitivity are recommended in all animals with severe bacterial infections or in any animal not responding to empiric therapy. Typically, cultures should be drawn while the animal is not receiving antibiotics or has not taken antibiotics for 2–3 days (although this is dependent on the severity of the infection).

Chapter 5: Why Antibiotics Fail

1 Host factors
   (a) Immune status (immunosuppression, steroids, cyclosporine, cancer, FeLV, etc.)
   (b) Underlying disease (hypothyroidism, allergies, diabetus, incontinence, etc.)
   (c) Foreign bodies (foxtails, urolithiasis, artificial implants, surgical equipment, remaining tooth root, etc.)
2 Antibiotic properties
   (a) Selection (compliance, stability of compounded agents, correct administration, correct length of treatment, etc.)
   (b) Pharmacokinetics/pharmacodynamics (absorption, dose, frequency, route, etc.)
   (c) Metabolism/elimination (increased metabolism/ elimination, drug interactions, etc.)
   (d) Adverse event profile (toxicity, vomiting drug, not adjusting dose in renal/hepatic disease, etc.)
3 Site of infection
   (a) Intracellular organisms (only some achieve adequate intracellular concentrations-chloramphenicol, tetracyclines, fluoroquinolones, macrolides, TMS, rifampin, etc.)
   (b) Chronic prostatitis (only some penetrate in adequate concentrations: clindamycin, macrolides, chloramphenicol, fluoroquinolones, trimethoprim)
   (c) Surgical intervention required (abscesses, necrotic tissue/bone, drainage, poor blood supply, and so on do not permit drug to achieve sufficient concentrations)
   (d) CNS (only some drugs penetrate: chloramphenicol, metronidazole, TMS, doxcycline, carbepenems, linezolide, rifampin, fluoroquinolones, high-dose penicillins, some third generation cephalosporins (ceftriaxone, cefotaxime, ceftazidime, cefixime, cefepime)
4 Pathogens
   (a) Species (lacks the target for the antibiotic, can circumvent the drug and use the hosts nutrients (folate), slow growing-requiring prolonged therapy, etc.)
   (b) Virulence factors (increased virulence by mutation, crossing host species, naïve hosts, etc.)
   (c) Resistance (innate or acquired resistance to antibiotic, can form dormant cysts, forms, are environmentally resistant to heat, dryness, etc.).

Chapter 6: Adjusting Doses in Renal Failure

Staging recommendations for chronic kidney disease (CKD) in animals has been set by the International Renal Interest Society (IRIS) (Table 6.1). These recommendations can be found on their website at www.iris-kidney.com. Staging is based initially on fasting blood creatinine, assessed on at least two occasions in the stable patient. The patient is then substaged based on proteinuria and systemic blood pressure. Patients with CKD often need dose adjustments in antibiotic, antifungal, antiviral and antiparasitic drug therapy or toxicity due to drug accumulation may occur. There are multiple methods for dose adjusting including dose reduction, lengthening the dosing interval or both. Typically, loading doses do not have to be altered in renal disease. Dose reduction involves reducing each dose while maintaining the normal dosing interval. This establishes more constant drug concentrations, but in patients with severe renal disease, drug accumulation and toxicity may still occur. Alternatively, extending the dosing interval may decrease the risks of toxicity but may increase the potential for subtherapeutic drug concentrations. Dosing guidelines for adjustment of drugs in renal failure are set in human medicine based on the stage of renal disease as determined by the Glomerular Filtration Rate (GFR). There are three categories of renal disease (mild, moderate, and severe). Initial dosing starts with these guidelines and is then adjusted to the patient's response and serum concentrations of drug.

Several antibiotic categories require close attention in renal disease. Aminoglycosides are best avoided when possible in renal disease. If necessary, serum drug concentrations should be monitored and adjusted. Penicillins and carbepenems accumulate readily in renal disease and can be associated with neuromuscular toxicity, myoclonus, seizures, and coma. Meropenem has a reduced tendency to cause seizures and is the preferred drug to imipenem in severe renal disease. Tetracyclines are associated with an antianabolic effect that can

Table 6.1 IRIS (International Renal Interest Society). Staging system for chronic kidney disease (CKD)

Step 1: Staging is initially based on fasting blood creatinine assessed on at least two occasions in the stable patient. (Blood creatinine concentration apply to average size dogs: those of extreme size may vary.)	Blood creatinine, μmol/l or mg/dl		
Renal function remaining	**Cat**	**Dog**	**Comments**
100%	<140 <1.6	<125 <1.4	History suggests the animal is *AT RISK* of developing CKD in the future due to a number of factors (e.g., exposure to nephrotoxic drugs, breed, high prevalence of infectious disease in the area)
Stage 1	<140 <1.6	<125 <1.4	**Nonazotemic.** Some other renal abnormality present (e.g., inadequate urinary concentrating ability without identifiable non renal cause, abnormal renal palpation or renal imaging findings, proteinuria of renal origin, abnormal renal biopsy results, increasing blood creatinine concentrations in samples collected serially).
33% Stage 2	140–250 1.6–2.8	125–180 1.4–2.0	**Mild renal azotemia** (lower end of the range lies within reference ranges for many laboratories, but the insensitivity of creatinine concentration as a screening test means that animals with creatinine values close to the upper reference limit often have excretory failure). Clinical sings usually mild of absent.
25% Stage 3	251–440 2.9–5.0	181–440 2.1–5.0	**Moderate renal azotemia.** Many extrarenal clinical sign may be present
<10% Stage 4	>440 >5.0	>440 >5.0	**Severe renal azotemia.** Increasing risk of systemic clinical signs and uremic crises

(Continued)

Table 6.1 (*Continued*)

Step 2: Cases are then sub-staged based on the proteinuria and blood pressure; Note that UP/C and blood pressure vary independently of each other and the stage of CKD

Urine protein/creatinine ratio (Up/C)

Dogs	Cats	Comments
0–0.2	0–0.2	Non-proteinuric
0.2–0.5	0.2–0.4	Borderline proteinuric
0.5–0.6	0.4–0.6	Proteinuric

Risk of target organ damage from hypertension (systolic blood pressure mm/Hg)

Dogs/Cats	Comments
130–150	Minimal risk
150–160	Low risk
160–180	Med risk
>180	High risk

increase the uremic state of patients with severe renal disease. Doxycycline is preferred over other tetracyclines in this situation. Expired or compounded doxycycline that may be readily hydrolyzed to a renal toxic metabolite should also be avoided. Nitrofurantoin also has a toxic metabolite that may accumulate in renal disease and cause peripheral neuritis.

Interval adjustment

In general, as extrapolated from human medicine, the following antibiotics/antifungals should have the dosing interval adjusted (i.e., every 8 h can be given every 12 h in moderate renal disease and every 12 h can be given every 24 h in severe disease): Cefazolin, cefepime, cefotaxime, cefoxitin, cefpodoxime, ceftazidime, ceftizoxime, cefuroxime, cephalexin, meropenem, sulfamethoxazole, trimethoprim, vancomycin, amoxicillin, ampicillin/sulbactam, ticarcillin, piperacillin, enrofloxacin, tetracycline, flucytosine, and valacyclovir. All animals should be monitored closely for response and toxicity.

Dose adjustment

The following antibiotics/antifungals should have the dose adjusted (i.e., 100% of the dose should be decreased to 75% with moderate renal disease and down to 50% with severe renal disease). Cefixime, clarithromycin, amoxicillin/clavulanate, ticarcillin/clavulanate, erythromycin, metronidazole, piperacillin/tazobactam, penicillin G,

ciprofloxacin, enrofloxacin, fluconazole, itraconazole, rifampin, and famciclovir. Although no data is available, if serum proteins are low cefovecin doses should be reduced to avoid toxicity.

No dose adjustment

The following antibiotics/antifungals typically do not require dose adjusting in renal failure; azithromycin, chloramphenicol, clindamycin, dicloxacillin, nafcillin, penicillin VK, doxycycline, linezolid, minocycline, ketoconazole, and pyrimethamine.

Chapter 7: Pregnancy Risk Categories

The FDA has established pregnancy risk factor categories for human patients based mostly on studies in laboratory animals. In order to extrapolate data to canine and feline patients, we have modified the five FDA risk categories (A, B, C, D, or E) to include teratogenic or embryo toxic potential in all species. Due to ethical concerns, most drugs do not undergo controlled studies in pregnant companion animals or humans. The following categories will be used throughout this book to assist the veterinarian in determining the risk:benefit ratio when a drug is used in a pregnant animal.

Categories

A. Controlled studies in pregnant women and animals fail to demonstrate a risk to the fetus in early or late pregnancy. Fetal harm is considered low risk.

B. Animal reproduction studies have not demonstrated fetal risk and/or reproduction studies have shown an adverse effect (other than a decrease in fertility) but results could not be confirmed in controlled studies.

C. Studies in animals have revealed adverse effects to the fetus (teratogenic, embryocidal, or other) but there are no controlled studies available to confirm reports. Drugs should be given only if the potential benefit justifies the risks.

D. There is positive evidence of human and animal fetal risk in pregnancy, but the benefit from use in pregnancy may be acceptable despite the risk (if the drug is needed in a life threatening situation or to treat a serious disease for which safer drugs cannot be used or are ineffective).

E. Studies in animals or humans have demonstrated fetal abnormalities or there is evidence of fetal risk and the risk of use of the drug in pregnancy clearly outweighs any possible benefit. The drug is contraindicated in pregnancy.

Chapter 8: Lactation Guidelines: Penetration of Drugs into Milk

The transport of drugs into milk from the maternal circulation occurs through multiple routes. Drugs traverse biologic membranes by passive diffusion so that the concentration will be dependent on the concentration gradient as well as the lipid solubility of the drug, degree of ionization, and protein binding. The significance of drug penetration into milk is unknown for most species. Although plasma:milk ratios of drugs are well known for food animals, few studies have focused on "safe" concentrations of drugs in canine or feline neonates. Fortunately, most antibiotics do not cross into milk in high levels (<1%). Therefore, the risk following exposure to maternal milk containing low levels of antibiotic should not be considered high. The most common side effects of low concentrations of antibiotic drugs in neonatal animals would be colic and diarrhea. Oral thrush caused by overgrowth of *Candida* yeast may also occur. Although rare, as with adults, allergic reactions (such as skin rashes) may also occur.

Antibiotics considered to be safe in lactating animals include the aminogylcosides (poorly absorbed by the gut), erthromycins, penicillins, and the cephalosporins. Antibiotics that should be avoided in lactating animals would be those categories of drugs that traditionally would be avoided in young animals (fluoroquinolones, chloramphenicol, sulfamides, etc.). Fluoroquinolones have been associated with arthropathy in animal studies and tetracyclines have been shown to cause inhibition of fibula growth and tooth enamel dysplasia. Chloramphenicol has been associated with significant side effects (polychromasia, anisocytoisis, target cells, and basophilic granulation) in 8–12 week-old puppies. Potentiated sulfonamides are generally considered safe in older animals but may be associated with hepatitis, anemia, KCS, or polyarthritis in neonates. Metronidazole is generally considered safe in neonates but due to its mutagenic and carcinogenic properties it is often not considered the drug of choice if a safer drug can be substituted.

Chapter 9: Safe Writing Skills

Veterinarians frequently provide handwritten prescriptions to their clients that may be filled at human pharmacies where pharmacists often lack training in veterinary pharmacology. These prescriptions present a very high possibility for error or misinterpretation. Care must be given as to how drug names, strengths, dosages, and directions for use are expressed to avoid significant errors. The following safe writing skills are suggested as a mechanism to help prevent errors and avoid wasted time in clarification of prescriptions.

1. Never use the abbreviation "SID". Although commonly used in veterinary medicine for "once daily", it is not recognized in human medicine and frequently is misinterpreted as "QID" or four times daily. The abbreviations "Q.D." or "O.D." may also be misinterpreted. Instead, write out "once daily".

2. Never place a decimal after a whole number (5.0 mg). If the decimal is missed it will result in a 10-fold over dose. Instead write "5 mg".

3. For numbers that are less than one (1), always place a zero (0) in front of the decimal (0.8 mL is correct, not .8 mL). This has resulted in 10-fold overdoses.

4. Always place a space between a number and units to make certain it is clear. Write "25 mg" not "25mg".

5. Always write out the word "unit". A handwritten U or u can be misinterpreted as a zero. This has resulted in numerous 10-fold overdoses of insulin.

6. Always write out "international units" instead of IU. Handwritten "IU" has been mistaken for "IV".

7. Do not use chemical names that start with a number, such as 5-FU, instead write their proper names (e.g., Flurouracil) since five-fold overdoses can occur, or it could be interpreted as 5-flucytosine.

8. For drugs that are commonly abbreviated, such as BUT, HCTZ, Pred, or MTX, write out the proper names.

9. Do not use "ug" or "mcg" abbreviations, instead write out "micrograms" for clarification.
10. Always write clearly and provide an indication for use (for pain, for nausea, etc.) for added confirmation.

Chapter 10: Basic Math Skills

Dilutions

When doing dilutions always think in parts. A 1:10 dilution of a drug means that there is one part drug in a total of 10 parts. So a total of 9 parts of diluent must be added to 1 part drug for a total of 10 parts. A 1:10 dilution of ivermectin would be 1 mL of ivermectin to 9 mL of drug. A 1:20 dilution would be 1 mL ivermectin to 19 mL of diluent. A 1:2 dilution of ivermectin is 1 mL of ivermectin to 1 mL of diluent.

Note: This is not to be confused with a 1:1 parts mixture (not a dilution) where 1 part ivermectin is mixed with 1 part of a second vehicle.

Percent solutions

When working with percent fluids the units will always be expressed in mL/100 mL or grams/100 mL. For instance, a 1% ivermectin solution means that there is 1 gram of ivermectin in 100 mL of solution. That is the same as 1000 mgs/100 mLs or 10 mg/mL.

Percent weights

When working with percent weights the units are always expressed in grams/100 grams. For instance, Ponazuril is available in a 127 gram tube that is 15% active drug. That means that there are 15 g of ponazuril per 100 g of paste, or 15,000 mg/100 g of paste. This is 150 mg/gram paste. Note: when further diluting this aqueous paste one cannot assume that it has the same specific gravity as water. In this case, 127 g of paste (1 tube) = 120 mL of paste.

Converting units

When converting units just use their equivalents and remember to line up units so they cancel. If a dose is in micrograms (µg or mcg) convert it to milligrams first, since most drugs are in mg/mL. For instance, a 24 microgram dose of ivermectin is divided by 1000 because 1000 micrograms = 1 milligram. This is a dose of 0.024 mg.

Weight conversions

1 gram (g) = 1000 milligrams (mg)
1 milligram (mg) = 1000 microgram (µg or mcg)
1 microgram (µg) = 1000 nanograms (ng)
1 pound (lb) = 0.454 kg = 454 grams (g) = 16 ounces (oz)
1 kilogram (kg) = 1000 grams (g) = 2.2 pounds (lb)
1 gram (g) = 15.43 grains (gr) = 1000 mg
1 ounce (oz) = 28.4 grams

Liquid conversions

1 gallon = 4 quarts = 8 pints = 3.785 L
1 quart = 2 pints = 32 fl.oz = 946 mL
1 pint = 2 cups = 16 fl.oz = 473 mL
1 cup = 8 fl.oz = 237 mL = 16 tablespoons
1 tablespoon = 15 ml = 3 teaspoons (tsp)
1 teaspoon = 5 ml
1 liter (L) = 1000 mL = 10 deciliters (dL)
1 deciliter = 100 mL
1 milliliter (mL) = 1 cubic centimeter (cc)

Milliequivalents

When trying to calculate milliequivalents, remember that a mEq is 1/1000 of an equivalent. In general this is just the molecular weight of the chemical divided by its valence. Common molecular weights are shown here. For instance, if you want to know how many milligrams are equivalent to 1 mEq of potassium chloride just get the molecular weight of potassium chloride (74.55 g) and divide it by the valence (1). So the equivalent weight is 74.55 g divided by 1 = 74.55 grams. To convert this to mEq it must be divided by 1000, which is 0.07455 g or 74.55 mg. So, 1 mEq of potassium chloride = 74.55 mgs.

Electrolyte	Molecular wt (g)	Valence
Sodium chloride	58.44	1
Sodium bicarbonate	84.0	1
Sodium lactate	112.0	1
Potassium chloride	74.55	1
Potassium gluconate	234.25	1
Calcium gluconate	430.4	2
Calcium chloride (anhydrous)	111.0	2
Magnesium sulfate (anhydrous)	120.4	2
Magnesium chloride anhydrous)	95.21	2

SECTION B
Empiric Therapy Pending Diagnostic Results

Chapter 11: Arthritis, Osteomyelitis

Description: Monoarthritis, polyarthritis, discospondylitis, osteomyelitis

Clinical presentation

Animals with septic arthritis or polyarthritis may show acute signs of fever, inappetence, lethargy, a stiff gait, lameness, and reluctance to move the affected joint(s). The affected joint(s) may be erythematous and/or painful on palpation. Animals with osteomyelitis often have a history of trauma to the area with surrounding cellulitis. The condition may be acute or chronic. Clinical signs include lameness, pain, fever, inappetence, draining skin lesions, and soft tissue swelling. Patients with discospondylitis may show signs of spinal pain, fever, lethargy, inappetence, pelvic limb pain paresis, or paralysis. Discospondylitis is more commonly reported in dogs, while vertebral osteomyelitis secondary to osteomyelitis from penetrating wounds (soft-tissue trauma or fighting) is more common in cats.

Likely pathogens

Organisms causing polyarthritis include gram positive facultative aerobes (*Staphylococcus*, *Streptococcus*), gram negative bacteria such as *E. coli*, vector borne bacteria (*Rickettsia*, *Ehrlichia*, *Anaplasma*, *Borrelia*), fungi (*Blastomyces*, *Coccidioides*), and protozoa (*Leishmania*). Pathogens implicated in osteomyelitis include a variety of gram-positive and gram-negative aerobes and anaerobes, fungi (both yeasts and molds), and atypical bacteria such as *Bartonella*, *Actinomyces*, *Nocardia*, and

Mycobacteria. Discospondylitis can be caused by a variety of typical gram-positive and gram-negative aerobes and anaerobes, *Brucella* spp., and filamentous fungi (especially *Aspergillus*, *Fusarium*, and *Paecilomyces*). Geographic location, concurrent immunosuppressive disease, and history and type of trauma (surgery, bite wounds, plant awn foreign bodies, etc.) influence the organisms isolated.

Diagnosis

Diagnostic tests to be considered include: cytologic examination of aspirates or smears, aerobic and anaerobic blood cultures, fungal antigen testing, serology for detection of antibodies to vector-borne pathogens or *Brucella*, urine bacterial and fungal culture, culture of tissue specimens or aspirates, and radiographs or advanced imaging using CT or MRI. Radiographic changes consistent with discospondylitis may take up to 2–4 weeks following infection to be detected.

Empiric drug therapy

Empiric therapy should be based on the most likely organisms present. Doxycycline is the drug of choice if a vector-borne bacterial pathogen is suspected. In general, osteomyelitis, discospondylitis, and septic arthritis are most commonly caused by *Staphylococcus* spp. and gram negative bacteria. For osteomyelitis or monoarthritis, if the animal is stable, clindamycin is a reasonable initial choice. Addition of enrofloxacin, gentamicin, or amikacin could be considered if a gram-negative pathogen is suspected. For discospondylitis, cephalexin or amoxicillin/clavulanate can be initiated in stable animals. For hospitalized animals, ampicillin-sulbactam or cefazolin can be given. Antibiotic therapy should subsequently be based on the results of culture and susceptibility. Typically

Drug Therapy for Infectious Diseases of the Dog and Cat, First Edition. Valerie J. Wiebe.
© 2015 John Wiley & Sons, Inc. Published 2015 by John Wiley & Sons, Inc.

long term (>6 weeks) of therapy is required. It is essential that attention also be given to drainage (septic arthritis), removing associated foreign bodies, and reversing concurrent immunosuppression. Antifungal therapy should await the results of antigen testing and/or fungal culture, but itraconazole is a good initial choice for fungal osteomyelitis. Fluconazole is not active against molds so is a poor initial choice for fungal discospondylitis.

Further reading

Burkert, B.A., Kerwin, S.C., Hosgood, G.L., *et al.* (2005) Signalment and clinical features of discospondylitis in dogs: 513 cases (1980–2001). *J Am Vet Med Assoc.*, **227**, 268–275.

Clements, D.N., Owen, M.R., Mosley J.R., *et al.* (2005) Retrospective study of bacterial infective arthritis in 31 dogs. *J Small Anim Pract.*, **46**, 171–176.

Sykes, J.E. and Kapatkin, A.S. (2013) Osteomyelitis, discospondylitis, and infectious arthritis. Ch. 85. In: *Canine and Feline Infectious Diseases*. Sykes, J.E. (ed.), Elsevier, St. Louis, MO, pp. 814–829.

Chapter 12: Bacteremia and Sepsis

Description: Bacterial infection of the bloodstream with an associated host systemic inflammatory response

Clinical presentation

Septic animals may show fever, hypothermia/hyperthermia, tachycardia, tachypnea, brick red mucous membranes, altered mental status, oliguria, or signs of coagulopathy.

Likely pathogens

Typically bacteremia as a result of cutaneous sources of infection is gram positive while organisms that enter the bloodstream from the gastrointestinal, urinary tract, or respiratory tract are more likely to be gram negative. The most common isolates are gram negative bacilli (*E. coli, Klebsiella, Pasteurella, Pseudomonas*), or gram positive cocci (*Staphylococcus* spp., *Streptococcus, Enterococcus)*. Anaerobes are common in cats, but less so in dogs. Other organisms have been isolated including *Erysipelothrix* spp., *Brucella, Citrobacter, Acinetobacter,* *Salmonella, Mycobacterium, Campylobacter, Burkholderia,* and *Ralstonia.*

Diagnosis

Aerobic and anaerobic blood culture, urine culture, and if available, CT and abdominal studies. Organisms found in the urine may not represent those found in the bloodstream.

Empiric drug therapy

Fluid resuscitation, other supportive care, and attempts to locate the nidus or source of infection are required. Broad-spectrum antibiotics should be administered empirically and as soon as possible (ideally within 1 h of initial evaluation). Typically high dose, intravenous combination therapy is advised. Ampicillin in combination with an aminoglycoside could be used if the source of infection is suspected as the urinary tract or abdomen. Ampicillin or clindamycin could be combined with a fluoroquinolone (improved lung penetration) if the lung or a pyothorax may be involved or the patient cannot tolerate aminoglycoside therapy. If penicillinase-producing anaerobes are likely (gastrointestinal compromise, plant foreign body, abscesses, etc.), ampicillin may be substituted with either ampicillin/sulbactam or metronidazole.

Resistant organisms

Broad-spectrum empiric combination therapy targeting likely resistant organisms can be achieved with a variety of drug combinations and should be based on local resistance patterns. For example, if a resistant gram-negative pathogen is suspected, an extended spectrum penicillin (such as ticarcillin/clavulanate) or a carbapenem (such as meropenem) may be used in place of an aminoglycoside. If a resistant *Staphylococcus* or *Enterococcus* infection is suspected, vancomycin may be used in combination with a carbepenem for severe, life threatening sepsis. Treatment should subsequently be rapidly de-escalated based on the results of culture and susceptibility test results to reduce cost and the likelihood of selection for resistant bacteria.

Further reading

Greiner, M., Wolf, G., and Hartmann, K. (2008) A retrospective study of the clinical presentation of 140 dogs and 39 cats with bacteraemia. *J Small Anim Pract.*, **49**, 378–383.

Lewis, D.H., Chan, D.L., Pinheiro, D., *et al.* (2012) The immunopathology of sepsis: pathogen recognition, systemic inflammation, the compensatory anti-inflammatory response, and regulatory T cells. *J Vet Intern Med.,* **234**, 457–482.

Sykes, J.E. and Epstein, S. (2013) Infections of the cardiovascular system. Ch. 86. In: *Canine and Feline Infectious Diseases.* Sykes, J.E. (ed.), Elsevier, St. Louis, MO, pp. 830–846.

Chapter 13: Central Nervous System Infections (Meningitis)

Description: Inflammation of the meninges of the brain or spinal cord secondary to the presence of an infectious agent

Clinical presentation

Affected animals may have a stiff gait, reluctance to move, twitching, neck extension, and hyperesthesia. Fever may or may not be present. Other neurologic deficits (paresis, delayed placing reactions) may also be present. Seizures, behavioral abnormalities, and abnormal mentation may occur. There may be a history of trauma, surgery, signs of upper respiratory tract disease, or otitis externa.

Likely pathogens

Meningitis in dogs can be due to viruses (especially canine distemper virus), typical bacteria (gram negative or gram positive aerobes and anaerobes), vector-borne bacteria (*Ehrlichia canis, Neorickettsia helminthoeca, Rickettsia rickettsii, Anaplasma*), fungi (especially *Cryptococcus*, but also other endemic mycoses and filamentous fungi), protozoa (such as *Toxoplasma* and *Neospora*), and algae (*Prototheca*). In cats, important pathogens include feline infectious peritonitis virus, and a variety of bacteria (especially *Streptococcus, Pasteurella, Mycoplasma*, anaerobes), *Cryptococcus*, and *Toxoplasma*

Diagnosis

Cytologic examination of cerebrospinal fluid and determination of CSF protein concentration; aerobic, anaerobic, and fungal culture of blood or cerebrospinal fluid; and advanced imaging using CT and/or MRI should be considered. Appropriate serologic assays for viral, protozoal and fungal pathogens should be considered (e.g., *Toxoplasma* IgG and IgM; antigen testing for *Cryptococcus* on blood and CSF). Polymerase chain reaction assays for specific pathogens can also be performed on blood and CSF (e.g., for detection of canine distemper virus RNA). At least 0.5 mL of CSF is required for culture and organisms may not grow.

Empiric drug therapy

Bacterial meningitis is rare and empiric treatment should be based on a high suspicion of infection based on the history and results of initial diagnostic testing (such as cytologic evaluation of spinal fluid). Drugs must be selected based on the pathogen suspected and the drug's ability to penetrate the blood/brain barrier. Antibiotics that readily penetrate into the blood/brain barrier include chloramphenicol, metronidazole, trimethoprim-sulfamethoxazole, doxycycline, meropenem, fluoroquinolones, and some third-generation cephalosporins (such as ceftriaxone). If bacterial meningitis is suspected, trimethoprim-sulfamethoxazole, or chloramphenicol are reasonable choices for empiric therapy due to their broad spectrum of activity. If a rickettsial cause of meningitis is suspected, intravenous oxytetracycline or doxycycline are the drugs of choice. Antifungal agents that readily penetrate into the CNS include fluconazole, voriconazole, posaconazole, and flucytosine. Conventional amphotericin B has poor penetration into the CNS but is enhanced with the use of the liposome encapsulated preparation. Furthermore, the minimal concentrations that are achieved are cidal against most susceptible organisms. Acute cryptococcal meningitis is generally treated with a combination of fluconazole and amphotericin B in dogs or flucytosine and amphotericin B in cats. Maintenance oral therapy with fluconazole can then be given.

Further reading

Bradshaw, J.M., Pearson, G.R., and Gruffydd-Jones, T.J. (2004) A retrospective study of 286 cases of neurologic disorders of the cat. *J Comp Path.,* **131**, 112–120.

Greene, C.E. (2013) Infections of the cardiovascular system. Ch. 90. In: *Canine and Feline Infectious Diseases.* Sykes, J.E. (ed.), Elsevier, St. Louis, MO, 886–892.

Griffin, J.F., Levine, J.M., Levine, G.J., *et al.* (2008) Meningomyelitis in dogs; a retrospective review of 28 cases (1999–2007). *J Small Anim Pract.,* **(49)**, 509–517.

Nau, R., Sorgel, F., and Eiffert, H. (2010) Penetration of drugs through the blood-cerebrospinal fluid/blood brain barrier for treatment of central nervous system infections. *Clin Microbiol Rev.,* **23(4)**, 858–883.

Sullins, A.K. and Abdel-Rahman, S.M. (2013) Pharmacokinetics of antibacterial agents in the CSF of children and adolescents. *Paediatr.*, **15(2)**, 93–117.

Chapter 14: Endocarditis (Bacterial)

Description: Infection of the cardiac valves

Clinical presentation

Dogs that appear to be at increased risk are middle aged to older, male, and large breed dogs. Endocarditis is rare in cats. Some patients have pre-existing cardiac lesions (e.g., congenital heart disease such as subaortic stenosis). In dogs, the mitral valve and aortic valve are most often affected. Vegetations can be mobile or sessile and may dislodge resulting in thromboemboli that can lodge in other organs (kidneys, spleen, brain, etc.). Clinical signs can be highly variable depending on organs involved in thromboembolic sequelae. Animals often have fever, inappetence, lethargy, and tachycardia. Diarrhea and vomiting may also be present. Bacterial thromboemboli may cause neurologic signs, lameness, and signs of poly-arthritis or renal failure. Left-sided congestive heart failure with associated respiratory distress may occur in dogs with aortic valve endocarditis.

Likely pathogens

In dogs, the most common causes of endocarditis are streptococci and staphylococci. Gram-negative rods and enterococci can also be involved. *Bartonella* should be considered in dogs with culture-negative endocarditis, especially if the aortic valve is involved. *Bartonella* should also be considered in cats with endocarditis. Rarely, gram positive rods, anaerobes, mycobacteria, and fungi have also been isolated.

Diagnosis

Diagnosis is based on clinical suspicion together with suggestive lesions on echocardiography. Identification of the etiologic agent is based on aerobic and (if suspected) anaerobic blood cultures and *Bartonella* serology and culture. Two major criteria of the following four must be met:
1. positive blood culture for *Streptococci, Staphylococci* or *E. coli*;
2. all three, or most of four, separate blood cultures are positive with the first and last cultures taken over 1 h apart;

3. two positive blood cultures for any organism, when specimens for cultures are drawn more than 12 h apart; and
4. consistent findings on echocardiography.

A diagnosis of possible endocarditis can be made if all of five minor criteria are met, or if one minor criterion is noted in conjunction with positive echocardiography, or if one major and three minor criteria are met. Possible endocarditis is established if a total of five minor criteria are met. Minor criteria include:
1. fever (>103°F);
2. new or worsening heart murmur;
3. existing predisposing heart condition;
4. presence of vascular/embolic phenomena; and
5. positive blood culture not meeting major criteria, or serologic or PCR evidence of a typical organism.

Serology combined with *Bartonella* enrichment culture-PCR is more sensitive than blood culture for detection of *Bartonella* (Galaxy Diagnostic Laboratories).

Obtaining blood cultures

Obtain blood prior to administration of antibiotics or if already on antibiotics just prior to the next dose. Obtain samples from separate venipuncture sites using sterile technique (clip hair and perform aseptic surgical preparation of each site, wear sterile gloves for blood collection). For severely ill patients, draw samples every 15 min over 1 h prior to initiating antibiotics. Inoculate one blood culture bottle for each blood draw (or one aerobic and one anaerobic blood culture bottle if anaerobic blood cultures are being performed). Typically 2 mL is collected from cats and small dogs and 10 mL is collected from large dogs. Gently invert bottles to mix blood with culture media. Do not refrigerate blood culture bottles after inoculation, protect from light and temperature extremes and send or ship to lab immediately.

Empiric drug therapy

A combination of ampicillin with an aminoglycoside or ampicillin with a fluoroquinolone is often effective empiric treatments until culture and susceptibility results are reported. Treatment should be de-escalated according to blood culture results as soon as possible. Antimicrobials should initially be administered intravenously for as long as possible (ideally a minimum of 7–10 days), after which they can be given orally provided the animal is stable. At least 4–6 weeks of therapy are recommended or until underlying disease has resolved and valvular lesions have resolved. Echocardiography should be repeated every 4 weeks. A combination of doxycycline and rifampin or an aminoglycoside and ampicillin could be used to treat *Bartonella* endocarditis, but prognosis is guarded and in humans, *Bartonella* endocarditis generally requires valve replacement.

Further reading

Greiner, M., Wolf, G., and Hartmann, K. (2008) A retrospective study of the clinical presentation of 140 dogs and 39 cats with bacteraemia. *J Small Anim Pract.*, **49**, 378–383.

MacDonald, K.A., *et al.* (2004) A prospective study of canine infective endocarditis in Northern California (199–2001): Emergence of *Bartonella* as a prevalent etiologic agent. *J Vet Intern Med.*, **18**, 56.

Pennisi, M.G., Marsilio, F., Hartmann, K., *et al.* (2013) *Bartonella species* infection in cats. ABCD guidelines on prevention and management. *J Feline Med Surg.*, **15(7)**, 563–569.

Sykes, J.E. and Epstein, S. (2013) Infections of the cardiovascular system. Ch. 86. In: *Canine and Feline Infectious Diseases.* Sykes, J.E. (ed.), Elsevier, St. Louis, MO, pp. 830–846.

Sykes, J.E., Kittleson, M.D., Pesavento, P.A., *et al.* (2006) Evaluation of the relationship between causative organisms and clinical characteristics of infective endocarditis in dogs: 71 cases (1992–2005). *J Am Vet Med Assoc.*, **228**, 1723–1734.

Varnat, M., Broadhurst, J., Linder, K.E., *et al.* (2012) Identification of *Bartonella henselae* in 2 cats with pyogranulomatous myocarditis and diaphragmatic myositis. *Vet Pathol.*, **49(4)**, 608–611.

Chapter 15: Intra-Abdominal Infections

Description: Bacterial peritonitis, hepatobiliary infections, hepatic abscesses

Clinical presentation

Intra-abdominal infections in dogs and cats include bacterial peritonitis, hepatobiliary infections, and hepatic abscesses. Bacterial peritonitis in dogs and cats usually follows a loss of integrity of the gastrointestinal tract (due to gastrointestinal foreign bodies, neoplasia, surgery, trauma, etc.). Clinical signs include lethargy, anorexia, vomiting, diarrhea, abdominal pain, weakness, dehydration, fever, mucosal pallor, abdominal pain, thin body condition, abdominal enlargement, tachypnea, tachycardia, and weak pulses. Cats can show signs of hypothermia and bradycardia. Biliary tree

infections are uncommon. Animals with hepatobiliary tract infections may show similar signs; signs of septic shock typically follow necrosis of the gall bladder wall or rupture of hepatic abscesses. Hepatic abscesses are rare, but dogs with hepatobiliary neoplasia, chronic cholecystitis, colonic surgery, cholelithiasis, or migrating foxtails appear to be at risk.

Likely pathogens

Organisms isolated in dogs and cats with bacterial peritonitis reflect the normal flora of the gastrointestinal tract. Mixed aerobic-anaerobic infections with *E. coli*, *Enterococcus*, and *Clostridium* spp. are common. Other bacterial species include *Staphylococcus*, *Streptococcus*, *Pseudomonas*, *Acinetobacter*, anaerobes, and other enteric gram-negative bacteria (*Proteus*, *Citrobacter*, *Serratia*, *Klebsiella*, and *Enterobacter*). In cats, *Actinomyces* as well as *Pasteurella* are common. Isolates from hepatic abscesses include *E. coli*, *Klebsiella pneumoniae*, *Staphylococcus*, and *Clostridium* in dogs and *Bacteriodes*, *Enterococcus*, and *Staphylococcus* in cats. Chronic cholangitis in cats may be associated with liver fluke (*Platynosomum fastosum*) infestations in tropical areas.

Diagnosis

For patients with intra-abdominal infections, diagnosis can be obtained through abdominal imaging (radiography and ultrasound), laboratory analysis and cytologic examination of abdominal fluid or bile (obtained using cholecystocentesis), and aerobic and anaerobic bacterial culture and susceptibility testing of fluids.

Empiric drug therapy

Management of peritonitis requires aggressive supportive care and addressing the need for resolution of leakage from the source of infection (gastrointestinal, biliary, or genitourinary), usually through a surgical approach. Drainage of abdominal fluid is also required. Ultrasound guided, open drainage, suction drainage, or vacuum-assisted peritoneal drainage have all been attempted with varying degrees of success. Animals with bacterial cholangitis and cholecystitis are treated with supportive care and antimicrobial drugs. Cholecystectomy is indicated for animals with necrotizing cholecystitis. Empiric antibiotics with activity against both gram negative enteric and anaerobes should be administered intravenously. Combination therapy is typically required, a fluoroquinolone with ampicillin/sulbactam, metronidazole with a fluoroquinolone, or ticarcillin/clavulanate with a carbapenem are reasonable choices initially until culture results are available. Hepatic abscesses typically have a poor prognosis and require aggressive surgical management (liver lobectomy, abscess drainage, and omentalization) together with broad spectrum antibiotic therapy.

Further reading

Carreira, V.S., Vieira, R.F., Machado, G.F., *et al.* (2008) Feline cholangitis/chonlangiohepatitis complex secondary to *Platynosomum fastosum* infection in a cat. *Rev Bras Parasitol Vet.*, **17(1)**, 184–187.

Sykes, J.E. (2013) Intra-abdominal infections. Ch. 88. In: *Canine and Feline Infectious Diseases*. Sykes, J.E. (ed.), Elsevier, St. Louis, MO, pp. 859–870.

Chapter 16: Neonatal Infections

Description: Infections occurring in newborns within 21 days after birth

Clinical presentation

Death during gestation or neonatal death (within the first 3 weeks after birth) may be the result of infection by viruses, bacteria, and protozoa (e.g., *Toxoplasma* or *Neospora*). Infection during gestation may result in resorption, abortion, mummification, or retention. Infection during the neonatal period can result in fading puppy or kitten syndrome. Identification and management of a possible underlying infectious cause is critical since it may affect subsequent litters from the same animal or multiple litters in large breeding operations.

Likely pathogens

Viral causes of abortion and neonatal death in dogs include canine herpesvirus, canine parvovirus 2, canine distemper, and canine adenovirus. Bacterial causes include *Brucella canis* and *Streptococcus canis* (which can contribute to neonatal sepsis secondary to ascending umbilical infections), with rare descriptions of infections by *Leptospira*, *Salmonella*, and *Campylobacter*. *Neospora* is an important protozoal cause of *in-utero* and neonatal

infections in dogs, and in both dogs and cats, *Toxoplasma gondii* should also be considered. In cats, viruses include feline leukemia virus, feline immunodeficiency virus, feline panleukopenia virus, feline herpesvirus, and feline calicivirus. Streptococci can also cause umbilical infections in kittens. Of the fungi, *Candida* can rarely cause opportunistic infections of the gastrointestinal tract in puppies and kittens that are co-infected with parvoviruses.

Diagnosis

Diagnosis should be based on histopathology of deceased neonates, aborted fetus, and the placenta. Fresh tissues should also be submitted for culture and PCR testing for specific infectious agents. Collection of serum from the dam should also be considered to allow testing for antibodies to pathogens such as *Brucella*.

Empiric drug therapy

Supportive care of littermates is critical if viral infections are suspected. Maintaining body warmth of neonates with exogenous heat (to a rectal temperature just above 100°F or 37.8°C) is recommended if canine herpesvirus infection is suspected, but is often unsuccessful. Administration of acyclovir (20 mg/kg PO q6 h × 7 days) may also be considered if canine herpesvirus infection is suspected. Streptococcal infections are treated with penicillin or ampicillin. See sections in this book on other pathogens for recommended treatment.

Further reading

Dubey, J.P., Lappin, M.R., and Thulliez, P. (1995) Diagnosis of induced toxoplasmosis in neonatal cats. *J Am Vet Med Assoc.*, **207(2)**, 19–185.

Lamm, C.G., Ferguson, A.C., Lehenbauer, T.W., *et al.* (2010) Streptococcal infection in dogs. *Vet Pathol.*, **47**, 387–395.

Lamm, C.G. and Njaa, B.L. (2012) Clinical approach to abortion, stillbirth and neonatal death in dogs and cats. *Vet Clin North Amer Small Anim Pract.*, **42(3)**, 501–513.

Powell, C.C. and Lappin, M.R. (2001) Clinical ocular toxoplasmosis in neonatal kittens. *Vet Ophthalmol.*, **4(2)**, 87–92.

Smith, K.C. (1997) Herpesviral abortion in domestic animals. *Vet J.*, **15(3)**, 253–268.

Vela, A., Falsen, E., Simarro, I., *et al.* (2006) Neonatal mortality in puppies due to bacteremia by *Streptococcus dysgalactiae subsp. Dysgalactiae*. *J Clin Microbiol.*, **44(2)**, 666–668.

Chapter 17: Infections Associated with Neutropenia

Description: Febrile neutropenia

Clinical presentation

Infections associated with neutropenia are not uncommon in animals treated with chemotherapy. Patients may present with neutropenia and fever without obvious clinical evidence of a source either by history or physical examination. Animals typically have lethargy, fever, and a neutrophil count of < 1000 cells/μL. Nadirs to doxorubicin, mitoxantrone, or cyclophosphamide occur 7–10 days after administration, vinca alkaloids 5–7 days, cisplatin and carboplatin 7–14 days, and lomustine 21 days (dogs)/28 days (cats) after administration. Sources of infection often include the gastrointestinal tract, urinary tract, cutaneous lesions, or catheters. Gastrointestinal toxicities from chemotherapy drugs occur at the same time as the nadir, which increases the likelihood of bacterial translocation across the gastrointestinal barrier.

Likely pathogens

Gram negative facultative aerobes, particularly enterics (*Klebseilla, E. coli, Pseudomonas*) from gastrointestinal sources are common isolates. Gram positive bacteria (*Staphylococcus, Streptococcus, Enterococcus*) are also common isolates. *Candida* infections are rare but should be considered.

Diagnosis

Aerobic and anaerobic blood and fungal cultures should be considered. A CBC should be obtained at the start of chemotherapy as a baseline and then should be monitored one week after treatment or at the expected nadir time. If the neutrophil count is <1500 cells/μL after treatment in the absence of clinical signs of bacteremia, antibiotics should be initiated to prevent infection. If the animal is ill or febrile, bacteremia should be suspected.

Empiric drug therapy

Oral antimicrobial prophylaxis with amoxicillin-clavulanic acid plus a fluoroquinolone, clindamycin plus a fluoroquinolone, or trimethoprim-sulfa are recommended for animals that develop severe neutropenia. For animals with signs of sepsis, broad-spectrum bactericidal antibiotics should be used with activity against gram negative bacteria that may be nosocomial (such as *Pseudomonas aeruginosa*) and/or multidrug resistant, pending the results of culture and susceptibility testing. Suitable choices include a combination of ampicillin and an aminoglycoside; a combination of ampicillin and a fluoroquinolone; ticarcillin-clavulanic acid; a third-generation cephalosporin such as cefepime; or meropenem. If fever persists and there is likelihood of methicillin resistant *Staphylococcus* spp. or a drug-resistant enterococcal infection, then a combination of vancomycin and amikacin should be considered. In animals with prolonged neutropenia the use of filgrastim (recombinant human granulocyte colony stimulating factor) (5 μg/kg SQ q24 h) can be given to help stimulate granulopoiesis.

Further reading

Anasari, S.H., Nasim, S., Ahmed, A., *et al.* (2006) Febrile neutropenia in pediatric peripheral blood stem cell transplantation, in-vitro sensitivity data and clinical response to empiric antibiotic therapy. *J Coll Physicians Surg Pak.*, **16(11)**, 704–708.

Britton, B.M., Kelleher, M.E., Gregor, T.P., *et al.* (2012) Evaluation of factors associated with prolonged hospital stay and outcome of febrile neutropenic patients receiving chemotherapy; 70 cases. *Vet Comp Oncol.*, **10**, 1111.

Dhaliwal, R.S. (2010) Managing oncologic emergencies. Ch. 13. In: *Cancer Management in Small Animal Practice*, Henry, C.J. (ed.), Saunders, Elsevier, Maryland Heights, MO, pp. 122–135.

Chapter 18: Otitis Externa and Otitis Media

Description: Inflammation/infection of the ear canal or middle ear

Clinical presentation

Otitis externa is common in dogs and rare in cats. Dogs present with erythema involving the pinnae, external meatus, and lining of the ear canal. Pruritis, head shaking, swelling, discharge, foul odor, ulcerative lesions, pain, and aural hematomas may be present. Long-term stenosis, occlusion, fibrosis, and mineralization of the canal may occur. The tympanic membrane may be ruptured. Underlying allergic dermatitis is present in 90% of affected dogs, but other underlying problems include plant awn foreign bodies or neoplasia. In kittens, otitis externa is most frequently associated with ear mites. In animals presenting with otitis media, the tympanic membrane may be distorted, discolored, or ruptured. The ear canal may contain pus or blood and the animal may show vestibular signs, facial paralysis, or deafness.

Likely pathogens

Staphylococcus pseudintermedius is a common isolate. Others include *S. schleiferi*, *S. aureus*, *Proteus*, *E. coli*, *Corynebacterium*, *Klebsiella*, *Enterococcus*, and *Streptococcus*. Chronic long-term antibiotic treatment may select for infection with *Pseudomonas aeruginosa* (often multidrug resistant). Fungal infections are also common with *Malassezia pachydermatis* being the most common isolate. Other fungal causes of otitis externa include *Candida*, *Aspergillus*, and dermatophytes. The parasites *Otodectes cynotis* (ear mites), *Otobius megnini*, and *Demodex* also cause otitis externa. Otitis media can result from extension of bacterial or fungal infection from the external ear canal after rupture of the tympanic membrane, or via hematogenous spread or extension of infection along the eustachian tubes as a result of chronic rhinosinusitis.

Diagnosis

Diagnosis is based on otoscopic exam, cytologic examination of material collected using ear swabs, aerobic bacterial culture, with or without imaging (radiographs, CT). Myringotomy may be required to collect material from the middle ear for cytologic examination and culture.

Empiric drug therapy

Identification and treatment of underlying predisposing conditions (allergic dermatitis, hypothyroidism, foreign bodies, neoplasia, parasitic infections) is critical. Clients should be taught how to properly flush the ear canal and instill topical antimicrobial drugs and/or glucocorticoids (orally or topically). Flushing may not be possible until several days of topical antimicrobial drugs and glucocorticoids have been administered to reduce pain. Once tolerated, cleaning is performed every 12–24 hours for 5–7 days, then every second or third day until clinical signs resolve. Subsequently, weekly maintenance cleaning may be required to prevent reinfection. Isotonic saline or Tris-EDTA may be used as a flush once to twice daily, either before topical antimicrobials are instilled, or as a solution that contains antimicrobials. Oral glucocorticoids (prednisolone, 0.5 mg/kg q12–24 h) may help reduce pain and inflammation and should be considered for 1–2 weeks with a tapering dose over

another 4 weeks. Several topical otic combination preparations are available (e.g., Synotic, Baytril otic, Posatex, Surolan, Mometamax, Otomax). Compounded alternatives have included a 1:2 mixture of enrofloxacin (22.7 mg/mL) and dexamethasone sodium phosphate (4 mg/mL), or a 1:2 solution of enrofloxacin (22.7 mg/mL) and Tris EDTA. These may be preferred when the integrity of the tympanic membrane is in question. Systemic antibiotic therapy is often not required but is indicated in animals with otitis media or ulcerations of the pinna. Suitable choices include cephalexin (if cocci are present on cytologic examination), marbofloxacin (if rods are present), with or without an antifungal such as fluconazole or itraconazole (if *Malassezia* yeasts are present). Antiparasitics such as ivermectin, selemectin, or moxidectin/imidacloprid can be used empirically if parasites are identified. Gentle ear flushing with warm isotonic saline under anesthesia may be required to remove purulent material if owner-administered treatment fails, but clients should be warned of the possibility of vestibular complications, which may be transient or permanent. Animals with severe chronic otitis externa that is not responsive to medical therapy may be candidates for salvage therapy with total ear canal ablation with or without bulla osteotomy.

Further reading

Gotthelf, L.N. (2004) Diagnosis and treatment of otitis media in dogs and cats. *Vet Clin North Am Small Anim Pract.*, **34(2)**, 469–487.

Matousek, J.L. (2004) Ear disease. *Vet Clin North Am Small Anim Pract.*, **34(2)**, 21–22.

Sykes, J.E., Nagle, T.M., and White, S.D. (2013) Pyoderma, otitis externa, and otitis media. Ch. 84. In: *Canine and Feline Infectious Diseases*. Sykes, J.E. (ed.), Elsevier, St. Louis, MO, pp. 800–813.

Chapter 19: Pancreatitis

Description: Inflammation of the pancreas due to pancreatic enzyme tissue irritation, destruction with or without secondary bacterial infection, abscesses

Clinical presentation

Dogs with acute pancreatitis present with anorexia, vomiting, abdominal pain, diarrhea, fever, and lethargy. Overweight dogs, small breed dogs such as miniature schnauzers, older dogs, and those with a history of consumption of fatty meals are predisposed. Dogs may develop secondary ileus, hepatic disease, biliary obstruction, coagulopathies, disseminated intravascular coagulation, and cardiac arrhythmias. Vomiting or abdominal pain are less common in cats when compared with dogs. Cats may show signs of lethargy, poor appetite, dehydration, tachypnea, and hypothermia. Dietary fat, trauma, chemicals (azathioprine, organophosphates), *Herpes*, or FIP have also been associated with pancreatitis in cats.

Likely pathogens

Pancreatitis in dogs and cats is typically a sterile process that does not involve infectious agents. Rarely, bacteria such as gram negative facultative aerobes, anaerobes, and *Enterococci* can spread hematogenously to the pancreas. Other organisms associated with pancreatitis include *Leptospira* spp., *Toxoplasma gondii*, and fungi (*Cryptococcus neoformans*). Liver fluke (*Eurytrema procyonis*) infestation in cats has also been associated with pancreatitis.

Diagnosis

Abdominal ultrasound, CBC, feline trypsinlike immunoreactivity, and pancreatic lipase immunoreactivity should be performed. Ultrasound is diagnostic in dogs. The pancreas is visible and appears nonhomogeneous. It may have cysts or abscesses. A pancreatic biopsy is diagnostic in cats, but severely ill cats are anesthetic risks. Serum amylase and lipase are of little value. Leukocytosis and hyponatremia are generally present.

Empiric drug therapy

Pancreatitis is a sterile process that does not require antibiotics unless severe disease is present or an abscess or concurrent infection exists. Food and liquids should be withheld for at least 4–5 days. Fluid therapy, pain control, antiemetics, and proton pump inhibitors should be given for 7–10 days. Surgical intervention may be required in some cases. Antibiotics that have demonstrated efficacy in humans with severe pancreatitis include intravenous imipenem and cefuroxime. For cats with liver flukes, prazaquantel/pyrantyl/febantel can be given orally.

Further reading

Son, T.T., Thompson, L., Serro, S., *et al.* (2010) Surgical intervention in the management of severe acute pancreatitis in cats: 8 cases (2003–2007). *J Vet Emerg Crit Care*, **20(4)**, 426–435.

Steiner, J.M. and Williams, D.A. (1999) Feline exocrine pancreatic disorders. *Vet Clin North Am Small Anim Pract.*, **29(2)**, 551–575.

Vyhnal, K.K., Barr, S.C., Hornbuckle, W.E., *et al.* (2008) *Eurytrema procyonis* and pancreatitis in a cat. *J Fel Med Surg.*, **10(4)**, 384–387.

Chapter 20: Peritonitis and Abscesses

Description: Inflammation of the peritoneum from a bacterial infection

Clinical presentation

Cats with peritonitis typically have feline infectious peritonitis (FIP), which is a fatal viral disease. They may present with a lack of appetite, fever, weight loss, jaundice, diarrhea, and difficulty breathing from fluid that has accumulated in the abdomen. Non-effusive forms of FIP may also have loss of vision and ataxia. In dogs and cats, bacterial peritonitis, typically presents with severe vomiting, bloating, progressive lethargy, fever, tachycardia, abdominal pain/rigidity, and inappetence. This may be due to a secondary infection from gastrointestinal perforation (post-surgery, trauma, ulcers from steroids, or NSAIDs, foreign bodies, neoplasia, torsion, intussusception), rupture of the genitourinary tract (post-surgery, ruptured prostatic abscess, ruptured pyometra, necrotizing cystitis), rupture of an intra-abdominal abscess (gallbladder, hepatic abscess), or ascending infection of the umbilicus in neonates.

Likely pathogens

Organisms isolated from patients with secondary peritonitis reflect the normal flora of the gastrointestinal tract. Mixed aerobic-anaerobic infections are involved with *E. coli*, *Enterococcus*, and *Clostridium* spp. Other isolates include *Staphylococcus*, *Streptococcus*, *Pseudomonas*, *Actinobacter*, *Anaerobes*, Enterobacteriacae (*Proteus*, *Citrobacter*, *Serratia*, *Klebseilla*, and *Enterobacter*), *Actinomyces* as well as *Pasteurella* in cats.

Diagnosis

Peritonitis is diagnosed by abdominal imaging, and cytology of peritoneal fluids. Aerobic and anaerobic bacterial culture and sensitivity as well as CBC should be performed. Fluid analysis from dogs and cats with peritonitis reveals a high protein concentration (increased erythrocytes and total nucleated cell counts), degenerative neutrophils, and intracellular bacteria. A blood-to-fluid glucose difference of 20 mg/dL is 100% sensitive and specific for the diagnosis of bacterial peritonitis in cats and dogs.

Treatment

Management of peritonitis is early control of the septic source either via non-operative or operative means. Ultrasound and CT guided percutaneous drainage of the abdomen/extraperitoneal abscesses is a safe alternative to surgery in select patients, but open drainage, suction drains and vacuum-assisted peritoneal drainage remain controversial. Empiric therapy using a fluoroquinolone plus ampicillin/sulbactam or metronidazole, or a fluoroquinolone with an extended spectrum penicillin with a betalactamase inhibitor (ticarcillin/clavulanate, piperacillin/tazobactam), or a carbepenem may be necessary to cover all potential aerobes and anaerobes.

Further reading

Culp, W.T., Zeldis, T.E., Reese, M.S., *et al.* (2009) Primary bacterial peritonitis in dogs and cats: 24 cases (1990–2006). *J Am Vet Med Assoc.*, **234**, 906–913.

Hosgood, G. and Salisbury, S.K. (1988) Generalized peritonitis in dogs: 50 cases (1975–1986). *J Am Vet Med Assoc.*, **193**, 1448–1450.

Ragetly, G.R., Bennett, R.A., and Ragetly, C.A. (2011) Septic peritonitis: treatment and prognosis. *Compend Contin Educ Vet.*, **33(10)**, 1–5.

Sykes, J.E. (2013) Intra-abdominal infections. Ch. 88. In: *Canine and Feline Infectious Diseases.* Sykes, J.E. (ed.), Elsevier, St. Louis, MO, pp. 859–870.

Chapter 21: Pneumonia/ Bronchitis

Description: Inflammation of the bronchi or lung affecting the alveoli

Clinical presentation

Pneumonia and bronchitis may be the result of viral, bacterial, parasitic, or fungal infections. Dogs with bacterial bronchitis may be asymptomatic or present with cough, fever, lethargy, inappetence, lower pulmonary involvement, weakness, dehydration, weight loss, nasal discharge, tachypnea, tachycardia, respiratory distress, wheezes, crackles, and reduced lung sounds. With severe cases, hemoptysis, vomiting, regurgitation, neurologic signs, and septic shock may be involved. Cats typically present with fever, lethargy, and/or inappetence. Aspiration pneumonia is common in adult dogs and rare in cats. Conditions that predispose dogs to aspiration pneumonia include; brachycephalic breeds, obstructive syndrome, laryngeal paralysis, surgery, foreign bodies, esophageal disorders, seizures, vomiting, swallowing disorders, anesthesia, and so on. Cats may rarely develop pneumonia following viral infections or hematogenous spread.

Likely pathogens

The most prevalent organism isolated in dogs with aspiration pneumonia is *E. coli*. Other isolates include: *Mycoplasma* spp., *Pasteurella* spp., *Staphylococcus* spp., *Klebseilla* spp., *Enterococcus* spp., *Pseudomonas*, *Acinetobacter*, and *Corynebacterium. Pseudomonas* is common in dogs with tracheal collapse but rare with opportunistic respiratory infections. Most infections are mixed infections with gram negative aerobes and anaerobes. In dogs with foreign bodies (foxtails), anaerobes, *Pasteurella, Actinomyces,* and gram positive cocci are common. Lower respiratory infection isolates in cats may include *Mycoplasma, Pasteurella* spp., *E. coli* spp., *S. canis, S. zooepidemicus, Enterobacter* spp., as well as anaerobes and other gram-positives (*Enterococcus, Corynebacterium, Staphylococcus*) and gram negatives (*Pseudomonas, Acineto bacter, Klebsiella, Proteus, Bordetella* spp., *Moreaxella*, etc.).

Diagnosis

Bacterial bronchitis or bronchopneumonia is based on radiographs, clinical signs, and underlying predisposing factors. Transtracheal wash, endotracheal wash, BAL, or fine needle aspirates of consolidated lung tissue can be used to obtain samples for histopathology, culture, and sensitivity.

Empiric drug therapy

Empirically dogs with bacterial tracheobronchitis can be given doxycycline or amoxicillin/clavulanate for 7 days. For cats and dogs with bronchopneumonia empiric systemic therapy should initially be broad spectrum with coverage of gram negative, anaerobes, and gram positives. Clindamycin provides anaerobic and gram positive coverage, alternatively ampicillin or ampicillin/sulbactam can be used. These should be combined with a fluoroquinolone. If fluoroquinolone resistance is likely, a third generation cephalosporin (cefotaxime, ceftriaxone), a carbapenem (meropenem, imipenem), an aminoglycoside (gentamycin, amikacin), or ticarcillin/clavulanate may be substituted.

Further reading

Dear, J.D. (2014) Bacterial pneumonia in dogs and cats. *Vet Clin North Am Small Anim Prac.*, **44(1)**, 143–159.

Priestnall, S.L., Mitchell, J.A., Walker, C.A., *et al.* (2014) New and emerging pathogens in canine infectious respiratory disease. *Vet Path.*, **51(2)**, 492–504.

Sykes, J.E. (2013) Bacterial bronchopneumonia and pyothorax. Ch. 87. In: *Canine and Feline Infectious Diseases.* Sykes, J.E. (ed.), Elsevier, St. Louis, MO, pp. 847–858.

Tart, K.M., Babski, D.M., and Lee, J.A. (2010) Potential risks, prognostic indicators, and diagnostic and treatment modalities affecting survival in dogs with presumptive aspiration pneumonia: 125 cases (2005–2008). *J Vet Emerg Crit Care* (San Antonio), **20**, 319–329.

Chapter 22: Prostatitis

Description: Acute or chronic inflammatory disease of the prostate gland

Clinical presentation

Acute prostatitis typically occurs in young male dogs, although catheterized animals may also be predisposed. Dogs may present with fever, depression, anorexia, urethral discharge, dysuria, and painful prostate on palpation. Stiff gait, constipation, and vomiting may also be present. Chronic prostatitis may present with a normal prostate that is not painful and recurrent urinary tract infections or asymptomatic bacteriuria. Animals may have symptoms of frequency, urgency, infertility, and dysuria. With prostatic abscess formation, fever, depression, lethargy, enlarged prostate, tenesmus, constipation, dysuria, hemorrhagic or purulent urethral discharge, septic shock, and abdominal pain may be present. Cats rarely develop prostatitis with most cases presenting with chronic disease.

Likely pathogens

E. coli, Enterococcus, Enterobacter, Staphylococcus spp., *Streptococcus, Klebseilla, Proteus,* and *Pseudomonas* are the most common bacterial isolates. *Brucella* has also been isolated in canine patients. Other organisms including Leismaniasis and *Blastomyces* have been reported.

Diagnosis

Prostatic palpitation, CBC, urinalysis, urine culture, prostatic fluid evaluation, ultrasound-guided prostatic aspiration, and biopsy should be performed.

Empiric drug therapy

For acute prostatitis, empiric antibiotic therapy can target organisms in the urine since they are frequently the same organism. Antibiotics easily penetrate into an acutely inflamed prostate, so most antibiotics will reach therapeutic concentrations. Treatment should be given for up to 28 days. Reculture prostatic fluid prior to discontinuation and 3–5 days after stopping antibiotics. TMS should be avoided due to the incidence of aplastic anemia and other side effects with prolonged TMS therapy in dogs. In chronic prostitis, there is difficulty in drug penetration across the blood-prostate fluid barrier. Canine prostatic fluid is usually acidic so only basic antibiotics (clindamycin, macrolides) and lipophilic drugs (chloramphenicol, macrolides, enrofloxacin, and trimethoprim) can cross the barrier effectively. Tetracyclines, penicillin, ampicillin, cephalosporins, and aminoglycosides have poor penetration. For gram-positive organisms, erythromycin, clindamycin, or trimethoprim can be given. For gram-negative organisms, trimethoprim, or a fluroquinolone may be given. At least 6–12 weeks of therapy are suggested. Castration is recommended as adjuvant therapy in all cases to prevent recurrences. Surgical drainage or prostatic omentalization may be required in severe cases or those with abscess involvement.

Further reading

Barsanti, J.A. (1996) Genitourinary infections. Ch. 91. *Infectious Diseases of the Dog and Cat.* Greene, C.E. (ed.), Saunders, Elsevier, St. Louis, MO, pp. 935–961.

Fox, L.E., Fords, S., Alleman, A.R., *et al.* (1993) Aplastic anemia associated with prolonged high-dose trimethoprim-sulfadiazine administration in two dogs. *Vet Clin Pathol.*, **22(3)**, 89–92.

Mir, F., Fontaine, E., Reyes-Gomez, E., *et al.* (2012) Subclinical leismaniasis associated with infertility and chronic prostatitis in a dog. *J Small Am Pract.*, **53(7)**, 419–422.

Pointer, E. and Murray, L. (2011) Chronic prostatitis, cystitis, pyelonephritis, and balanoposthitis in a cat. *J Am Anim Hosp Assoc.*, **47(4)**, 258–261.

Chapter 23: Pyothorax Infections

Description: Pleural empyema, purulent pleuritis

Clinical presentation

Pyothorax in dogs and cats is typically the result of a penetrating injury (bite wounds, grass awns, trauma), esophageal perforation, or spread of infection from the lung space. In cats, pyothorax is a common cause of pleural effusion. Migrating parasites (*Cuterebra, Aelurostrongylus, Toxocara*), upper respiratory infections, and bronchopneumonia may be underlying causes of pyothorax in cats. In dogs, pyothorax develops secondary to foreign bodies, esophageal perforation, bite wounds, or other trauma to the thoracic wall.

Likely pathogens

Common organisms isolated in cats include *Pasteurella* and anaerobes, with >40% being mixed anaerobes and facultative bacteria. *Actinomyces, Streptococcus* spp., and *Mycoplasma* spp., have also been isolated. In dogs, isolates include obligate anaerobes, gram negative enterics (*E. coli, Klebseilla* spp.) or mixed anaerobes/aerobic infections. Both *Actinomyces* spp. and *Streptococcus canis* should be considered with foxtail or grass awn related infections.

Diagnosis

Is based on radiographs and cytology of pleural fluid. Culture and sensitivity of pleural fluid should be performed to identify organisms and dictate treatment.

Empiric drug therapy

Treatment involves thoracocentesis, lavage and antibiotics. Antimicrobial therapy alone is not sufficient to facilitate drug penetration. Indwelling thoracostomy tubes with suction from days up to 3 weeks may be required. Warm isotonic lavage with saline every 5–24 h may be beneficial. Antibiotics targeting *Pasteurella, Actinomyces,* and anaerobes should be selected. Penicillins, aminopenicillins (ampicillin, amoxicillin), clindamycin, metronidazole, and ampicillin/sulbactam all cover anaerobic bacteria. Penicillin, amoxicillin/clavulanate, and ampicillin/sulbactam are effective against *Pasteurella*. Ampicillin/sulbactam alone is typically effective in cats. In dogs, ampicillin in combination with metronidazole for 6 weeks has been curative. If gram negative organisms are present, a fluoroquinolone or ceftriaxone can be added. Switching to oral antibiotics can be considered upon clinical and objective improvement (adequate drainage and removal of chest tube, temperature normalization). Oral antibiotic treatment based on culture results (amoxicillin/clavulanate, fluoroquinolone, metronidazole, etc.) should be continued for another 1–4 weeks, again based on clinical, biochemical, and radiological response. In cats, antiparasitics should be considered if appropriate.

Further reading

Barrs, V.R. and Beatty, J.A. (2009) Feline pyothorax: new insights into an old problem. *Vet J.*, **179 (2)**, 163–178.

Johnson, M.S. and Martin, M.W. (2007) Successful medical treatment of 15 dogs with pyothorax. *J Sm Anim Prac.*, **48(1)**, 12–16.

Sykes, J.E. (2013) Bacterial bronchopneumonia and pyothorax. Ch. 87. In: *Canine and Feline Infectious Diseases*. Sykes, J.E. (ed.), Elsevier, St. Louis, MO, pp. 847–858.

Waddell, L.S., Brady, C.A., and Drobatz, K.J. (2002) Risk factors, prognosis, prognostic indicators, and outcome of pyothorax in cats: 80 cases (1986–1999). *J Am Vet Med Assoc.*, **221**, 819–824.

Chapter 24: Sinus Infections

Description: Sinusitis, acute or chronic inflammation, swelling and infection of the sinuses.

Clinical presentation

Sinus infections in dogs and cats are caused by a variety of organisms (viruses, parasites, bacteria, and fungus). Bacterial/fungal rhinitis is believed to occur post-inflammation and mucosal injury, followed by secondary invasion of bacteria or fungus. Animals present with sneezing, mucopurulent nasal discharge, ocular discharge, cough, gagging or retching, epistaxis, pawing at the face or nose, ulceration of the external nares, crusted exudates, and depigmentation. With chronic infections, osteomyelitis and stenotic nares may be seen. If animals present with unilateral infection a fungal infection, neoplasia, tooth root abscess, or foreign body (foxtail) may be involved. With nasal discharge that occurs in both nasal passages a viral or bacterial cause should be considered.

Likely pathogens

Fungal infections including *Cryptococcus*, *Aspergillus*, and *Penicillium* should be ruled out. Bacterial isolates in dogs have included gram positives (*Staphylococcus* spp., *Streptococcus* spp.), gram negatives (*E. coli*, *Pasteurella*, *Proteus*, *Pseudomonas*, *Bordetella*), and anaerobes (*Clostridium*). In cats, viral infections are common (Feline herpesvirus-1 and *Calicivirus*) or bacterial infections (*Chlamydophila felis*, *Mycoplasma* spp., *Bordetella bronchiseptica*). Other isolates include: gram positives (*Staphylococcus* spp., *Streptococcus*, *Corynebacterium*), gram negatives (*Pasteurella*, *E. coli*, *Pseudomonas*, *Klebseilla*), and anaerobes (*Capnocytophaga* spp.). Parasitic infections of the sinus also occur, including *Pneumonyssoides caninum* mite infections in dogs.

Diagnosis

Nasal radiographs, rhinoscopy, histopathology on nasal biopsies, tissue culture, and serum antigen titers for Cryptococcus.

Empiric drug therapy

Supportive care (fluids, nutrition, saline nebulization, analgesics) is typically required in all animals. In cats, *Herpesvirus* (FHV-1) is one of the most common isolates. Famciclovir and L-lysine may be beneficial for cats with FHV-1. Kittens are often infected with *Calicivirus* or *Chlamydia*. If *Mycoplasma*, *Chlamydophila*, or *Bordetella* species are suspected, doxycycline is the treatment of choice. Fluoroquinolones (pradofloxacin, enrofloxacin) or azithromycin may also be given. *Cryptococcus* spp. is the primary fungal isolate in cats where empiric therapy with fluconazole is the drug of choice. In dogs, unilateral discharge is most commonly seen from foxtails and tooth root abscesses. The nidus of infection needs to be identified and removed. Empiric antibiotics should cover gram positives and anaerobes as well as *Actinomyces*

spp. High dose amoxicillin or amoxicillin/clavulanate may be effective empiric therapy. Nasal *Aspergillus* spp. infections are primarily reported in dogs and are typically unilateral. Oral itraconazole would be the best empiric therapy until surgical debridement, biopsy, culture and sensitivity are performed. Topical clotrimazole installation is an alternative. Bilateral infection with purulent discharge in dogs with other systemic signs of infection (fever, lethargy, cough, etc.) is more commonly associated with bacterial infections, which may be treated initially with amoxicillin/clavulanate. Other drugs that have good penetration into sinus secretions include clindamycin, chloramphenicol, fluoroquinolones, macrolides, and doxycycline. Treatment should be switched to the appropriate antibiotic once culture and sensitivity are performed. Cancer should be ruled out in adult animals and may be missed due to secondary invasion by bacteria or fungal infections.

Further reading

Barrs, V.R., VanDoom, T.M., Houbraken, J., *et al.* (2013) *Aspergillus felis* sp. nov., an emerging agent of invasive aspergillosis in humans, cats and dogs. *PLoS One.*, **8(6)**, e64871.

Bowles, D.B. and Fry, D.R. (2009) Nasal *Cryptococcus* in two dogs in New Zealand. *NZ Vet J.*, **57(1)**, 53–57.

Bredal, W.P. (1998) The prevalence of nasal mite (*Pneumonyssoides caninum*) infection in Norwegian dogs. *Vet Parasitol.*, **76(3)**, 233–237.

Frey, E., Pressler, B., Guy, J., *et al.* (2003) *Capnocytophaga* sp. isolated from a cat with chronic sinusitis and rhinitis. *J Clin Microbiol.*, **41(11)**, 5321–5324.

Chapter 25: Skin and Soft Tissue Infections

Description: Pyoderma, cellulitis, fasciitis

Clinical presentation

Animals with pyoderma may present with erythema, edema, pruritus, epidermal collarettes, papules, pustules, and alopecia. Cellulitis, deep nodules, fistulous tracts may develop with deep pyoderma. Deeper systemic infections should be ruled out. Chronic cases may result in pigmentation and lichenification. Pyoderma may be on the surface, superficial, or deep.

Necrotizing fasciitis is a medical emergency and requires surgical intervention. Immunosuppressed dogs (young, cushinoid, hypothyroidism, cancer, chemotherapy) may have demodicosis of the head, forelegs, groin, trunk, paws, or ears that develops secondary pyoderma. Acute onset of intense pruritus on the ventral chest, abdomen, lateral elbows, and pinnae in dogs with a history of recent exposure to other dogs may also be indicative of sarcoptic mange. Animals present with erythematous maculopapular rash, alopecia and crusting, and lesions due to self trauma. Due to poor recovery of mites on skin scrapings (30%) these are often misdiagnosed as atopy or allergies.

Likely pathogens

In dogs, *S. pseudintermedius*, *S. intermedius*, *S. aureus*, *Clostridium perfrigens*, *Streptococcus* spp., *Pseudomonas* spp., *E. coli*, *Proteus* spp., and obligate anaerobes are the most common organisms isolated. Demodex and sarcoptic mange are common and should be ruled out prior to other treatment. In cats, *Pasteurella*, *E. coli*, *Proteus*, and obligate anaerobes are common.

Diagnosis

Biopsy culture of pustules, aerobic and anaerobic culture, blood culture, gram stain, skin scraping (Demodex), and cytology with modified Wright's stain should be performed.

Empiric drug therapy

Management of underlying atopic skin disease is essential for chronic skin disease. Acutely, antibacterial shampoos (ethyl lactate, chlorhexidine, triclosan) may be used alone (twice weekly for 10 min or daily for deep pyoderma). Benzoyl peroxide is effective for greasy dermatitis but may be too drying for others. Topical antibiotics (neomycin, gentamycin, polymyxin B, bacitracin, silver sulfadiazine, acetic acid solutions, mupirocin) may be useful for localized pyoderma. Oral antibiotics given for deep pyoderma in dogs include: Cephalexin, clindamycin, doxycycline, and amoxicillin/clavulanic acid. These should be administered for a minimum of 8 weeks. Superficial pyoderma may be treated for 4 weeks and at least 7 days post resolution of lesions. Both fluoroquinolones and third generation cephalosporins may increase the risk of resistance. If underlying demodectic mange or sarcoptic is identified or suspected, oral ivermectin or milbemycin, benzoyl peroxide shampoo, rotenone ointment, antihistamines, and antibiotics may be indicated.

Further reading

Sykes, J.E., Nagle, T.M., and White, S.D. (2013) Pyoderma, otitis externa, and otitis media. Ch. 84. In: *Canine and Feline Infectious Diseases*. Sykes, J.E. (ed.), Elsevier, St. Louis, MO, pp. 800–813.
Weese, J.S. and van Duijkeren, E. (2010) Methacillin-resistant *Staphylococcus aureus* and *Stapylococcus pseudintermedius* in veterinary medicine. *Vet Microbiol.*, **140(3–4)**, 418–429.

Chapter 26: Urinary Tract Infections

Description: Uncomplicated lower urinary tract infections, complicated UTI, pyelonephritis

Clinical presentation

Clinical signs are based on bacterial virulence, site of infection, immune status of host, and duration of infection. Uncomplicated bladder infections (cystitis) are typically present with pollakiuria, stranguria, dysuria, hematuria, inappropriate urination, or incontinence. Females may have a higher incidence of UTIs due to anatomic differences. Animals with lower and upper urinary tract infections (pyelonephritis, prostatitis, metritis) may present with cystitis, fever, pain, lethargy, anorexia, and inflammatory leukograms. Pyuria with or without hematuria may be present. If the animal has immunosuppression, diabetes, chronic prostatitis, or pyelonephritis, they may be asymptomatic or symptoms of other systemic diseases may predominate. In asymptomatic animals, polyuria/polydipsia may still be present.

Diagnosis

Diagnosis is based on clinical history, physical examination, urinalysis, and urine culture and sensitivity. Typically, cystocentesis is the preferred method. Urethral catheterization is used secondarily in situations where pyoderma of the ventral abdomen may exist or if transitional cell carcinoma is suspected. Free catch samples are not recommended for culture and sensitivity. Urinalysis and culture should be interpreted with the method of collection and clinical signs. Urine specific gravity, glucosuria, crystalluria, uroliths, and bladder neoplasias may be contributing factors. Hematuria, pyuria, bacteriuria, and proteinuria are typically present in urine. Immunosuppression, hyperadrenocorticism, and steroids may significantly alter the ability to detect bacteriuria and pyuria. Urine sediment allowed to air dry and stained with modified Wright's stain will help to identify bacteria, but definitive diagnosis should be based on culture and sensitivity. At least 3–5 days after completion of antibiotics is typically suggested prior to repeat urine culture although many bacteria, particularly those that are resistant may grow during therapy. Samples should be stored in a closed sterile container and refrigerated. Ideally samples should be cultured immediately but can be stored refrigerated for up to 6 h.

Interpretation of MICs

Culture and sensitivity results should be used as a guideline only and may not always reflect *in vivo* efficacy. Reference drugs may not always reflect *in vivo* efficacy. Reference drugs may be indicators of drug sensitivity to a particular class of drugs but differences between drugs (ciprofloxacin vs enrofloxacin) may still exist due to altered absorption, dosing frequency, and pharmacokinetics. Organisms such as methacillin resistant *Staphylococcus* spp. (MRSP) may appear sensitive *in vitro* to TMS, but are not often effective *in vivo* due to the fact that MRSP can utilize the host's folate and circumvent the antibiotic. Susceptibilities for *Enterococcus* spp. are similar. These often appear sensitive *in vitro* to cephalosporins, TMS, clindamycin, and aminoglycosides, but these are not effective clinically. In most cases, if the *in vitro* results suggest resistance, the antibiotic should not be used. If intermediate sensitivity is obtained, high doses of an antibiotic that can concentrate in urine may still be used to achieve a response. If all antibiotic alternatives demonstrate resistance an expended antibiotic sensitivity profile should be requested (carbapenems, third generation cephalosporins).

Organisms

E. coli is traditionally the most common isolate from the urine of feline and canine patients. It is common (54% isolates) in female dogs, older dogs, and neutered dogs. *Enterococcus faecalis*, *Pseudomonas aeruginosa*, *Proteus*, *Klebseilla*, and *Staphylococcus* spp. are also common and may be associated with significant resistance. In rare cases, fungi (*Candida* spp.) or *Corynebacterium* spp. may be isolated.

Empiric treatment

Treatment should be based on culture and sensitivity results whenever possible and tailored to each specific patient. Underlying disease (diabetes, stones, prostatitis, immune suppression, etc.) must all be factored into therapy. For uncomplicated initial infections amoxicillin or cephelexin alone may be sufficient. TMS has been recommended but has a higher incidence of side effects (keratoconjunctivitis, hypersensitivity, and immune-mediated effects). For animals with a higher potential for resistance, potentiated beta-lactams (amoxicillin/clavulanate), fluoroquinolones, or extended release cephalosporins (cefovecin) may be useful. Treatment of uncomplicated infections should be given for 7–14 days. Shorter courses (3 days) may be effective but further studies are required. For pyelonephritis, 6–8 weeks of antibiotics are indicated with regular ultrasound monitoring. Ideally cultures should be repeated 3–5 days following completion of antibiotics. If economic constraints are an issue, urine sediment (gram+/−, cocci/rods) may be a somewhat useful guide to therapy. Gram negative rods may indicate *E. coli*, *Enterobacter* spp., or *Klebsiella* spp. suggesting sensitivity to TMS or cephalosporins. Identification of gram negative bacillus (*Proteus* spp.) or a gram positive cocci (*Staphylococcus* spp., *Streptococcus* spp.) would suggest a cephalosporin or amoxicillin as good options. If animals are not responding after 48 h of treatment, drug therapy should be reassessed.

Resistant organisms

Treatment failure suggests either failure to eradicate the current infection or a relapse (reinfection). Multidrug resistance (MDR) urinary tract infections are becoming more common in veterinary medicine. *E. coli*, *Enterobacter*, *Enterococcus*, and resistant *Staphylococcus* are all expressing increased levels of drug resistance. Drug therapy here must be based on culture and sensitivity and elimination of underlying etiologic conditions. Radiographs, ultrasound, assessment for neoplasms, prostatitis, stones, incontinence, diabetes, structural anomalies, compromised host defenses, as well as other predisposing factors, should be assessed. For recurrent bladder infections where the underlying problems cannot be corrected, prophylactic antibiotics, cranberry extract, and urinary antiseptics may be attempted.

Further reading

Hall, J.L., Holmes, M.A., and Baines, S.J. (2013) Prevalence and antimicrobial resistance of canine urinary tract pathogens. *Vet Rec.*, **173(22)**, 549.

Olin, S.J., Bartges, J.W., Jones, R.D., *et al.* (2013) Diagnostic accuracy of a point of care urine bacteriologic culture test in dogs. *J Am Vet Med Assoc.*, **243(12)**, 1719–1725.

Smee, N., Loyd, K., and Grauer, G.F. (2013) UTIs in small animal patients: Part 2: Diagnosis, Treatment, and Complications. *J Amer Anim Hosp Assoc.*, **49(2)**, 83–94.

SECTION C
Therapy of Established Infections

Chapter 27: *Acanthamoeba*

Description: Non-parasitic amoeba, free living, active trophozoites, dormant cyst
Zoonotic Potential: Environmental, not a zoonotic

Microbiology/epidemiology

Acanthamoeba are found worldwide in soil and water. Environmental exposure to *Acanthamoeba* is common and typically does not result in infection. Immunosuppressed or debilitated patients may be predisposed. Routes of infection include inhalation of cysts from the air, nasal exposure during swimming in contaminated water, or direct corneal contamination. Organisms are believed to migrate up the olfactory nerves to the brain or spread hematogenously from the lungs or wounds to the brain. *A. castellanii, A. culbertsoni,* and *A.* sp. *genotype* T1 have been isolated from dogs. Although rare in cats and dogs, it is likely under reported. It has been reported in greyhounds, German shepherds, boxers, Labrador mixes and an Akita. Young dogs (4–13 months) appear to be predisposed. Recent reports have isolated *A. castellani* strains and *Parachlamydia Acanthamoeba* (an endosymbiont of *Acanthamoeba*) from corneal samples of cats with refractory conjunctivitis and keratitis.

Clinical disease

Dogs may present with clinical signs similar to distemper. Mild ocular discharge, anorexia, lethargy, and fever may occur early. Pneumonia and neurologic signs (head tilt, seizures, etc.), incoordination, decreased righting, peripheral edema, high serum sodium, and hypoosmolality have been reported. Leukopenia and CSF pleocytosis are common. Cats may present with conjunctivitis or keratitis. Symptoms are very similar to herpes or fungal infections so that *Acanthamoeba* ocular infections may be vastly underdiagnosed.

Diagnosis

Acanthamoeba can be diagnosed by routine cytology and histology sections. The microbiology laboratory should be alerted if *Acanthamoeba* are being suspected. Typically tissue specimens should not be placed in fixative or frozen following collection. Special stains and culture media may be required to increase the sensitivity and confirm the diagnosis. Corneal scrapings should be submitted for wet mount, cytology, and histologic staining. For diagnostic assistance, specimen collection guidance and shipping instructions, contact your diagnostic laboratory.

Treatment

Successful treatment of disseminated *Acanthamoeba* infections has not been reported in cats or dogs. Multidrug regimens have met with mixed results in humans. Ketoconazole with rifampin and trimethroprim-sulfamethoxazole therapy was used successfully for treatment of two immunocompetent pediatric patients with CNS infection. Use of a combination of amphotericin B, rifampin, and 5-flucytosine initially followed by oral itraconazole, 5-flucytosine, and rifampin has been effective short term in a number of patients. The use of 5-flucytosine is contraindicated in dogs. The CDC currently is recommending miltefosine for human cases of *Acanthamoeba*, which must be obtained from the CDC (770–488–7100). For keratitis, chlorhexidine (0.006%) and hexamidine solutions have been used with some success. Recent evidence

Drug Therapy for Infectious Diseases of the Dog and Cat, First Edition. Valerie J. Wiebe.
© 2015 John Wiley & Sons, Inc. Published 2015 by John Wiley & Sons, Inc.

demonstrates that either compounded topical voriconazole (1%) solution (q2 h × 6 months) or oral voriconazole may be a safe and efficacious alternative. Treatment is prolonged for up to 6 months in most cases and topical therapy must be initiated at hourly intervals.

Drug therapy

Disseminated disease
- 5-flucytosine with rifampin and either itraconazole or ketoconazole (cats)
- Ketoconazole, rifampin, and TMS (dogs)
- Miltefosine

Keratitis
- Compounded voriconazole (1%) ophthalmic solution
- Oral voriconazole

Drug therapy alternatives

- Topical chlorhexidine (0.006%) ophthalmic solution
- Topical chlorhexidine (0.006%) ophthalmic solution plus 0.1% propamidine isethionate (Brolene)

Further reading

Bang, S., Edell, E., Eghrari, A.O., et al. (2010) Treatment with voriconazole in 3 eyes with resistant *Acanthamoeba* keratitis. *Am J Ophthalmol.*, **149(1)**, 66–69.

Bauer, R.W., Harrison, L.R., Watson, C.W., et al. (1993) Isolation of *Acanthamoeba sp.* from a greyhound with pneumonia and granulomatous amebic encephalitis. *J Vet Diagn Invest.*, **5**, 386–391.

Greene, C.E., Howerth, E.W., and Kent, M. (2013) Nonenteric amebiasis: acanthamebiasis, hartmannelliasis and balamuthiasis. In: *Infectious Diseases of the Dog and Cat.* 4th Edn. Greene, C.E. (ed.), Elsevier Health Science, pp. 802–805.

Ithoi, I., Mahmud, R., Abdul Basher, M.H., et al. (2013) *Acanthamoeba* genotype T4 detected in naturally-infected feline corneas found to be in homology with those causing human keratitis. *Trop Biomed.*, **30(1)**, 131–140.

Richter, M., Matheis, F., Gonczi, E., et al. (2010) *Parachlamydia acanthamoebae* in domestic cats with and without corneal disease. *Vet Ophthalmol.*, **13(4)**, 235–237.

Tu, E.T., Joslin, C.E., and Shoff, M.E. (2010) Successful treatment of chronic stromal *Acanthamoeba* keratitis with oral voriconazole monotherapy. *Cornea*, **29(9)**, 1066–1068.

Yoder, J.S., Verani, J., Heidman, N., et al. (2012) *Acanthamoeba* keratitis: The persistence of cases following a multistate outbreak. *Ophthalmic Epidemiol.*, **19(4)**, 221–225.

Chapter 28: *Acinetobacter*

Description: Aerobic, short, nonmotile, gram negative rod
Zoonotic Potential: Zoonotic transmission possible via colonization of susceptible hosts

Microbiology/epidemiology

Acinetobacter is a gram negative coccobacillus. It can be recovered from soil and water and is a commensal on skin and mucous membranes. *Acinetobacter* often contaminates wet surfaces including kennels, sinks, feeding tubes, humidifiers, and ventilator tubing. In human hospitals, it is one of the most common bacterial species cultured from the hands of health care workers. Nosocomial infections are common in human hospitals and have been reported in veterinary hospitals. *Acinetobacter* is known for its ability to rapidly acquire and transfer multiple antimicrobial drug resistance genes.

Clinical disease

Acinetobacter may be isolated from the respiratory tract of animals with pneumonia, although care should be taken to distinguish contamination from infection in this situation. Catheter-related urinary tract infections and life-threatening systemic infections may also occur (e.g., peritonitis, bacteremia) in debilitated animals.

Diagnosis

Diagnosis of *Acinetobacter* infection requires aerobic bacterial culture in association with cytologic evidence of inflammation and consistent clinical abnormalities. Susceptibility testing should also be requested due to the tendency of *Acinetobacter* to be resistant to multiple antimicrobial drugs.

Treatment

Treatment should be based on culture and susceptibility results. Antimicrobials with activity against *Acinetobacter* include extended-spectrum penicillins, third generation cephalosporins, and carbapenems. However, drug selection should be based on susceptibility results due to the high incidence of multidrug resistance.

Further reading

Boerlin, P., Eugster, S., Gaschen, F., *et al.* (2001) Transmission of opportunistic pathogens in a veterinary teaching hospital. *Vet Microbiol.*, **82(4)**, 347–359.

Francey, T., Gaschen, F., Nicolet, J., *et al.* (2000) The role of *Acinetobacter baumannii* as a nosocomial pathogen for dogs and cats in an intensive care unit. *J Vet Intern Med.*, **14(2)**, 177–183.

Zordan, S., Prenger-Berninghoff, E., Weiss, R., *et al.* (2011) Multidrug resistant *Acinetobacter baumannii* in veterinary clinics, Germany. *Emerg Infect Dis.*, **17(9)**, 1751–1754.

Chapter 29: *Actinomyces*

Description: Facultative to strictly anaerobic, thin, filamentous, branched, gram positive bacterial rod
Zoonotic Potential: Environmental, not considered a zoonotic

Microbiology/epidemiology

Actinomyces are related to *Nocardia* and can be difficult to distinguish from *Nocardia*. *Actinomyces* spp. often form sulfur granules (large aggregates of bacteria) in tissues. Multiple species have been identified in dogs (e.g., *A. bowdenii*, *A. canis*, *A. hordeovulneris*, *A. odontolyticus*). Most infections in dogs and cats are caused by *A. viscosus* and *Arcanobacterium pyogenes* (formerly *Actinomyces pyogenes*). *Actinomyces* spp. are commensal organisms found in association with mucous membranes of the oral cavity, gastrointestinal tract and female genital tract. *Actinomyces* cause disease when inoculated into tissues together with other facultative and obligate anaerobes. Young to middle-aged hunting dog breeds may be at increased risk due to exposure to foreign bodies such as plant awns. Infection may follow bite wounds, trauma to the oral cavity, or dental procedures that result in retained tooth fragments.

Clinical disease

Pulmonary *Actinomycosis* and pyothorax
Pulmonary actinomycosis may result from an aspiration event, or inhalation or migration of a foxtail into the lungs. Direct introduction of *Actinomyces* into the pleural space through the thoracic wall (in association with foreign bodies or bite wounds) can also result in pyothorax.

Thoracic radiographs may show lobar consolidation, interstitial to alveolar infiltrates, pleural effusion, and/or mass lesions.

Soft tissue infections
Actinomyces soft tissue infections are characterized by focal or multifocal abscesses with draining tracts and fistulas. Discharge may contain sulfur granules. In dogs, soft tissue infections may result in mass lesions of the head, neck, or body wall that can resemble tumors.

Abdominal and retroperitoneal Actinomycosis
Abdominal actinomycosis can follow abdominal surgery, penetration of abdominal organs, or uterus by migrating foxtails. Retroperitoneal infections occur when plant awns migrate through the crura of the diaphragm and can result in persistent fever, spinal pain, and/or pelvic limb paresis or paralysis.

Brain abscess and meningitis
Actinomyces brain abscesses and meningitis have rarely been described in dogs. These may be the result of a migrating foxtail, extension of a cervicofacial site infection, hematogenous spread, or trauma.

Diagnosis

Diagnosis of actinomycosis should be based on history and consistent clinical signs. The presence of sulfur granules in affected tissues or purulent material strongly suggests infection by *Actinomyces*. Submission of multiple specimens or biopsies for aerobic and anaerobic bacterial culture may be required to confirm the diagnosis. The laboratory should be alerted to the possibility of *Actinomycosis* to ensure that specimens are processed appropriately.

Treatment

Broad spectrum antibiotics may be required during the initial treatment period due to the polymicrobial nature (anaerobic, enteric, gram positive) of *Actinomyces* infections. Cefoxitin, ticarcillin/clavulanate, amoxicillin/clavulanate, or ampicillin/sulbactam with a fluoroquinolone may be effective. High dose intravenous penicillin G or ampicillin, followed by a prolonged course of oral therapy (typically weeks to months) is required. Surgical debridement/drainage is often required. The nidus of infection (foxtail, foreign body, tooth root) must be removed to prevent recurrence. If this is not possible, long-term antimicrobial therapy with a beta-lactam may be required to prevent recurrence.

Drug therapy

- Penicillin G, parenteral
- Ampicillin, parenteral

Drug therapy alternatives

- Amoxicillin
- Doxycycline
- Clindamycin

Further reading

Anvik, J.O. and Lewis, R. (1976) *Actinomyces* encephalitis associated with hydrocephalus in a dog. *Can Vet J.,* **17(2)**, 42–44.

Barnes, L.D. and Grahn, B.H. (2007) *Actinomyces* endophthalmitis and pneumonia in a dog. *Can Vet J.,* **48(11)**, 1155–1158.

Clarridge, III J.E. and Zhang, Q. (2002) Genotypic diversity of clinical *Actinomyces* species: phenotype, source, and disease correlation among genospecies. *J Clin Microbiol.,* **40**, 3442–3448.

Doyle, R.S., Bellinger, C.R., Campay, L., and McAllister, H. (2005) Pyothorax in a cat managed by intrathoracic debridement and postoperative ventilatory support. *Ir Vet J.,* **58(4)**, 211–215.

Russo, T.A. (1995) Agents of *Actinomyces*; In: *Principles and Practice of Infectious Diseases*. 4th edn, Mandell, G.L., Bennett, J.E., and Dolin, R. (eds). Churchill, New York, pp. 2280–2288.

Walker, A.L., Jang, S.S., and Hirsch, D.C. (2000) Bacteria associated with pyothorax of dogs and cats; 98 cases. *J Am Vet Med Assoc.,* **216**, 359–363.

Chapter 30: Adenovirus (Infectious Canine Hepatitis)

Description: Canine DNA adenovirus-1, non-enveloped, double stranded DNA virus
Zoonotic Potential: Host specific, not considered a zoonotic

Microbiology/epidemiology

Canine adenovirus-1 is found worldwide and is less common then canine adenovirus-2 that is a noted cause of respiratory disease in dogs. Canine adenovirus-1 is the cause of infectious canine hepatitis (ICH). ICH is an infectious disease causing acute liver failure in domestic dogs and other mammals. The virus is spread via feces, urine, blood, saliva, and nasal discharge. Dogs acquire the infection through oral or nasal inoculation. Dogs <1 year of age, those that are not vaccinated, and animals that are in overcrowded conditions (shelters, pet stores, kennels) are at highest risk. The incubation period is approximately 4–9 days. The virus spreads in the tonsils and then to the lymph nodes, liver, kidneys, spleen, lungs, and eyes. Dogs with acute disease may either recover or die within 2 weeks. The disease is uncommon since the advent of the vaccine, but may still be problematic in populations that are not vaccinated.

Clinical disease

Three disease syndromes exist;
1. Peracute disease with circulatory collapse, coma and death after a brief illness that lasts 24–48 h,
2. Acute disease with high morbidity/mortality (10–30%) with recovery or death in a two-week period, and
3. Chronic disease with death due to hepatic failure weeks or months after initial infection.

Symptoms may include fever, lethargy, inappetence, vomiting, hemorrhagic diarrhea, abdominal pain, dehydration, conjunctivitis, petechial hemorrhages, tachypnea, cough, corneal edema (blue eye), icterus, and rarely, neurologic signs.

Diagnosis

Diagnosis is made by recognizing the combination of symptoms and abnormal blood tests that occur in ICH. Diagnosis is challenging since most dogs are unable to mount sufficient antibodies to the virus before they die making serologic tests inconclusive. Postmortem diagnosis is easily achieved from tissue samples that demonstrate characteristic intranuclear inclusion bodies on impression smears of liver biopsies. Diagnosis can be confirmed using histopathology, PCR, and viral isolation, but these are typically not widely available.

Treatment

Treatment is supportive with fluids, electrolytes, dextrose, and blood products. Lactulose and oral ampicillin may be required for hepatic encephalopathy. Heparin can be given for DIC. For severe corneal edema and uveitis, topical glucocorticoids, and atropine may be used to prevent glaucoma. Prevention using vaccines has almost eliminated the disease. Attenuated live CAV-1 vaccines, starting at 6 weeks of age, given every 3–4 weeks with the last vaccine no earlier than 16 weeks, protects most puppies from acquiring the infections.

Drug therapy

Supportive (fluid, blood products, antacids, enteral feeding).

Further reading

Abdelmagid, O., Larson, L., Payne, L., *et al.* (2004) Evaluation of the efficacy and duration of immunity of a canine combination vaccine against virulent parvovirus, infectious canine hepatitis virus, and distemper virus experimental challenges. *Vet Ther.,* **5(3)**, 173–186.

Decaro, N., Campolo, M., Elia, G., *et al.* (2007) Infectious canine hepatitis: an "old" disease reemerging in Italy. *Res Vet Sci.,* **83**, 269–273.

Sykes, J. (2013) Infectious canine hepatitis. Ch. 18. In: *Canine and Feline Infectious Diseases.* Sykes, J.E. (ed.), Elsevier, St. Louis, MO, pp. 182–186.

Chapter 31: *Aelurostrongylus Abstrusus* (Feline Lungworm)

Description: Nematodes, small worms with undulating tail, <400 µm long
Zoonotic Potential: Host specific, not considered a zoonotic

Microbiology/epidemiology

Aelorostrongylus abstrusus is the most common lungworm of cats and is found worldwide. The parasite is common in cats that are allowed to hunt. The life cycle includes snails or slugs as intermediate hosts, and frogs, lizards, birds, or rodents as transport hosts of encysted larvae. Following ingestion of the transport host, the larvae migrate from the stomach to the lungs via the peritoneal and thoracic cavities. They reach the lungs within 24 h and become embedded in the terminal bronchioles 8–9 days after infection. Eggs are laid into alveolar ducts and alveoli about 4 weeks after infection, where they form nodules and hatch. The mature larvae escape, get coughed up, swallowed, and passed in the feces. First-stage larvae are found in the feces about 6 weeks after the infection.

Adults can live up to 9 months or longer. The prevalence varies between 1.9 and 18.5% among stray cats.

Clinical disease

Cats may be asymptomatic if only a mild infection is present. With heavy infections, cats develop a chronic cough accompanied by progressive dyspnea, anorexia, diarrhea, and emaciation. Chronic wasting and pulmonary wheezes may be seen. The lungs usually have solidified, gray, raised nodules. Generalized alveolar disease has been seen in chronic cases.

Diagnosis

Diagnosis of *A. abstrusus* should be considered in any cats with respiratory signs, particularly outdoor cats that hunt. Infection can be confirmed by the demonstration of the first-stage larvae (L-1) in the feces. Eggs or first-stage larvae can also be found in tracheal washes or sputum. The limitations to fecal evaluation include;
1. no larvae are passed during the prepatent period,
2. larvae may be intermittently shed, and
3. adult worms can persist in the lungs after the end of the patent period, which is typically 2–3 months.

Treatment

Treatment is difficult and not always required. The treatment of choice is fenbendazole or ivermectin may be effective. Moxidectin (1%)/imidacloprid (10%) (Advantage Multi), and Emodepside/praziquantel (Profender) have recently been shown to be effective against *A. abstrusus*.

Drug therapy

- Fenbendazole
- Ivermectin

Drug therapy alternatives

- Moxidectin (1%)/imidacloprid (10%) (Advantage Multi)
- Emodepside /Praziquantel (Profender)

Further reading

Kirkpatrick, C.E. and Megella, C. (1987) Use of ivermectin in treatment of *Aelurostrongylus abstrusus* and *Toxocara cati* infection in a cat. *J Amer Vet Med Assoc.,* **190(10)**, 1309–1310.

Traversa, D., Cesare, A. di, Milillo, P., *et al.* (2009) Efficacy and safety of imidacloprid 10%/moxidectin 1% spot-on formulation in the treatment of feline aelurostrongylosis. *Parasitology Research*, **105(Suppl. 1)**, 55–62.

Traversa, D., DiCesare, A., and Conboy, G. (2010) Canine and feline cardiopulmonary parasitic nematodes in Europe: emerging and underestimated. *Parasit and Vectors*, **3**, 62.

Traversa, D., Milillo, P., Cesare, A., *et al.* (2009) Efficacy and safety of emodepside 2.1%/praziquantel 8.6% spot-on formulation in the treatment of feline aelurostrongylosis. *Parasitology Research*, **105(Suppl. 1)**, 83–90.

Chapter 32: Anaerobic Species (*Bacteroides* and *Provotella*)

Description: Anaerobic bacteria, pleomorphic rods
Zoonotic Potential: Not considered a zoonotic

Microbiology/epidemiology

Anaerobes are the predominant species colonizing the colon. *Provotella* spp. are common colonizers of mouth flora and other mucosal membranes. *Provotella* spp. are often associated with dental and lung abscesses, while *Bacteriodes* are more commonly associated with abdominal infections (liver and abdominal abscesses, surgical procedures, trauma, etc.). *B. fragilis* is the medically important species reported in cats and dogs due to its relative resistance to a number of antibiotics. Nosocomial strains may be extremely virulent and can colonize otherwise healthy animals.

Clinical disease

Animals may present with a variety of symptoms including intra-abdominal, lung, orbital or brain abscesses, endocarditis, bacteremia, and skin infections. Anaerobic infections of the skin are common and may result in cellulitis, necrotizing fasciitis, and crepitant cellulitis.

Diagnosis

Anaerobic culture and gram stain.

Treatment

Surgical intervention to lance and drain abscesses as well as supportive care is recommended. CT or ultrasound guided drainage may be indicated for some abscesses. *Bacteriodes* spp. typically produce beta-lactamases, so that penicillins are typically not effective. Abscesses may also contain mixed aerobic/anaerobic flora so combination antibiotics may be required. Antibiotics with beta-lactam inhibitors (amoxicillin/clavulanate, piperacillin/tazobactam) are effective in treating polymicrobial abscesses. Both metronidazole and clindamycin have good activity and penetration for *B. fragilis* infections. Pradofloxacin may be useful for anaerobes in cats.

Drug therapy

* Metronidazole
* Clindamycin

Drug therapy alternatives

* Cefoxitin
* Pradofloxacin
* Ampicillin/Sulbactam
* Imipenem
* Meropenem
* Amoxicillin/Clavulanate

Further reading

Jang, S.S., *et al.* (1997) Organisms isolated from dogs and cats with anaerobic infections and susceptibility to selected antimicrobial agents. *J Am Vet Med Assoc.*, **210(11)**, 1610–1614.

Radaelli, S.T. and Platt, S.R. (2002) Bacterial meningoencephalomyelitis in dogs: a retrospective study of 23 cases (1990–1999). *J Vet Intern Med.*, **16(2)**, 159–163.

Silley, P., Stephan, B., Greife, H.A., *et al.* (2012) Bactericidal properties of pradofloxacin against veterinary pathogens. *Vet Microbiol.*, **157(1–2)**, 106–111.

Wagner, K.A., *et al.* (2007) Bacterial culture results from liver, gallbladder, or bile in 248 dogs and cats evaluated for hepatobiliary disease: 1998–2003. *J Vet Intern Med.*, **21(3)**, 417–424.

Wang, A.L., Ledbetter, E.C., and Kern, T.J. (2009) Orbital abscess bacterial isolates and *in vitro* antimicrobial susceptibility patterns in dogs and cats. *Vet Ophthalmol.*, **12(2)**, 91–96.

Chapter 33: *Anaplasma* Species

Description: Tick-borne, obligate, intracellular, gram negative bacteria
Zoonotic Potential: A zoonotic, vector (tick-borne) transmission to humans

Microbiology/epidemiology

Anaplasma was formally known as *Ehrlichia phagocytophilum* or human granulocytic ehrlichiosis. The primary *Anaplasma* species infecting dogs and cats are *A. platys* (which causes cyclic thrombocytopenia) and *A. phagocytophilum* (granulocytic anaplasmosis). *A. platys* is thought to be transmitted by the brown dog tick (*R. sanguineus*), and *A. phagocytophilum* is transmitted by ticks that belong to the *Ixodes ricinus-persulcatus* complex. A variety of wildlife species, especially small rodents, are believed to be reservoirs of *A. phagocytophilum* infection. In the US, the disease follows the distribution of the tick vectors, and is most prevalent in the upper midwest and the northeastern USA. Dogs that have been exposed to *A. phagocytophilum* may be co-infected with other vector-borne pathogens, especially *Borrelia burgdorferi*, which is transmitted by the same tick species.

Clinical disease

Most infections are subclinical. Dogs infected with *A. platys* may have thrombocytopenia without any other clinical signs, although some may show signs such as fever, lethargy, lymphadenopathy, and mucosal hemorrhages. Dogs with granulocytic anaplasmosis typically show non-specific signs of fever, lethargy, and inappetence. Other signs include variable lameness or reluctance to move due to polyarthritis, vomiting, cough, scleral injection, polydipsia, peripheral lymphadenopathy, splenomegaly, petechial hemorrhages, and neurologic signs such as cervical pain and placing deficits. Thrombocytopenia is the most consistent finding on bloodwork. Disease has been less commonly described in cats.

Diagnosis

Diagnosis of *A. phagocytophilum* infection requires detection of bacterial morulae within granulocytes together with positive *Anaplasma* IFA serology (to differentiate it from *Ehrlichia ewingii* in endemic regions, which also infects granulocytes); a four-fold rise in titer using acute and convalescent phase serology; and/or PCR on whole blood. Serologic cross-reactions occur among *Anaplasma* species, so serology alone is not diagnostic for *A. phagocytophilum* infection. *A. platys* infections are diagnosed by finding morulae within platelets on blood smears or via PCR of whole blood, buffy coat, splenic, or bone marrow aspirates. A positive in-clinic ELISA assay (such as the SNAP 4Dx Plus, IDEXX Laboratories) indicates previous exposure to an *Anaplasma* spp. and when used alone is not diagnostic for active infection.

Treatment

Treatment should include vector control and supportive care for severely ill patients. Intravenous fluid therapy (crystalloids) and antiemetics may be required. Most animals respond rapidly (1–2 days) to tetracyclines, which should be continued for 2 weeks.

Drug therapy

Doxycycline.

Drug therapy alternatives

- Oxytetracycline
- Tetracycline
- Minocycline

Further reading

Adaszek, L., Gorna, M., Skrzypczak, M., *et al.* (2013) Three clinical cases of *Anaplasma phagocytophilum* infection in cats in Poland. *J Feline Med Surg.*, **15(4)**, 333–337.

Carrade, D.D., Foley, J.E., Borjesson, D.L., *et al.* (2009) Canine granulocytic anaplasmosis: a review. *J Vet Intern Med.*, **23(6)**, 1129–1141.

Heikkila, H.M., Bondarenko, A., Mihalkov, A., *et al.* (2010) *Anaplasma phagocytophilum* infection in a domestic cat in Finland: case report. *Acta Vet Scand.*, **52**, 62.

Sykes, J. and Foley, J.E. (2013) Anaplasmosis. Ch. 29. In: *Canine and Feline Infectious Diseases*. Sykes, J.E. (ed.), Elsevier, St. Louis, MO, pp. 290–299.

Woldehiwet, Z. (2010) *In-vitro* studies on the susceptibility of ovine strains of *Anaplasma phagocytophilum* to antimicrobial agents and to immune serum. *J Comp Pathol.*, **143(2–3)**, 94–100.

Chapter 34: *Ancylostoma* Species (Hookworms)

Description: Nematode hookworms, adults 1 cm in length

Zoonotic Potential: Zoonotic transmission to humans is common (larval migrains)

Microbiology/epidemiology

Ancylostoma caninum and *Ancylostoma tubaeforme* are species specific for dogs and cats, respectively. *A. braziliense*, *A. ceylanicum*, and *Uncinaria stenocephala* can affect both species.

The life cycle is complex with the infective stage (filariform larvae) present in the soil. The filariform larvae penetrate the skin and/or enter via the oral route. Nursing is the most common form of transmission in neonates. Transplacental transmission remains controversial. Paratenic hosts (rodents) are important in transmission of ancylostomosis in cats and dogs. After infective larvae (L3) penetrate the skin or mucous membranes, larvae migrate via capillaries and lymphatics into the right heart and cross through the pulmonary alveolus. Larvae are coughed up and swallowed, or deposited into skeletal muscle and tissues. Dormant L3 larvae may re-activate prior to the onset of warm, wet seasons. Adult worms can remain present for many years and over that time shed millions of eggs resulting in high levels of environmental contamination. Eggs are hardy and can survive for years, even in extreme environmental conditions. Hookworms are most prevalent in tropical humid environments (southeast USA). Poor husbandry, hygiene, and sanitation increase the incidence of transmission and auto-infection.

Clinical disease

Abdominal infections
Most serious hookworm infections occur during the first two months of the animal's life and are acquired from the mother's milk. Most animals present with weight loss, diarrhea, malabsorption, and abdominal discomfort. Puppies can present acutely with dark tarry stools or bloody watery diarrhea (that can clinically mimic Parvovirus).

Pulmonary
Animals may develop pneumonitis from migration of larvae through pulmonary tissues. Animals may present with wheezing or coughing. Diffuse pulmonary infiltrate may be observed on radiographs. Eosinophillia may be noted on CBC.

Dermal
Local reactions to migrating hookworm larvae may be manifested by puritus, erythema, and popular rashes.

Diagnosis

Direct visualization of characteristic hookworm eggs in fecal flotation.

Treatment

Treatment should be repeated 1–2 weeks following initial treatment because dormant somatic larvae may activate with new adults present in 10–12 days. For severe infections, blood transfusion, supplemental iron, and a high-protein diet may be indicated. Attention to environmental sanitation is critical (e.g., move dog pens off of dirt or gravel and onto less porous surfaces such as concrete that can be washed twice weekly). Concrete runways should be washed at least twice a week. Sunlit clay or sandy runways can be decontaminated with sodium borate (1 kg/2 m²). Perinatal transmission of infection can be greatly reduced by treating bitches with daily doses of fenbendazole from day 40 of gestation to day 14 postpartum. Pups should be treated as early as possible; ideally, treatment should be given 2 weeks after birth and repeated at two-week intervals up to 2 months of age, and then monthly to 6 months of age. Nursing bitches should be treated at the same time as puppies. Kittens should be treated at 3, 5, 7, and 9 weeks of age, and then monthly to 6 months of age. Nursing queens should be treated at the same time as kittens.

Drug therapy

- Pyrantel pamoate
- Fenbendazole

Drug therapy alternatives

- Milbemycin
- Moxidectin
- Selemectin

Many combination products (Heartgard Plus, Advantage Multi, Drontal plus, Milbemax, Iverhart Plus, Profender, Procox, Safe-Guard, Trifexis) contain drugs that will effectively treat hookworms.

Further reading

Epe, C. (2009) Intestinal nematodes: biology and control. *Vet Clin North Am Small Anim Pract.*, **39(6)**, 1091–1097.
Nolan, T.J. and Lok, T.B. (2012) Macrocyclic lactones in the treatment and control of parasitism in small companion animals. *Current Pharm Biotechnol.*, **13(6)**, 1078–1094.

Chapter 35: *Ascaris* Species (Roundworms)

Description: Nematodes, roundworms, adults are large (15 cm)
Zoonotic Potential: Common zoonotic infection in humans

Microbiology/epidemiology

Ascaris species pass through three developmental stages (eggs, larva, and adult). Eggs are found in contaminated soil or food. Eggs are resistant to cold and heat and are most prevalent in tropical climates. Animals become infected by ingestion of contaminated food, soil, or an intermediate host (mouse, rat). Many animals are infected via prenatal infection where the larvae migrate through the placenta *in utero*. Lactating animals may also acquire the infection via mother's milk. Following ingestion, eggs reach the small intestine where hatched larvae penetrate through the intestine mucosa and migrate into the venous circulation. The larvae then migrate into the pulmonary vessels. The larvae grow and pass up the trachea where they are coughed up and swallowed. The worms return to the jejunum where they become adults. Eggs are passed in the feces and then into the environment. There are two species that commonly infect dogs: *Toxocara canis* and *Toxascaris leonina*. In cats, most infections are due to *Toxocara cati*, but may also be caused by *T. leonina*.

Clinical disease

Ascarids rarely cause symptoms in adult animals. In young animals (<2 months), there may be intermittent vomiting and diarrhea. Worms can be found in the vomitus or passed in the stool. Heavy infestation in very young animals can result in a pot-bellied appearance, abdominal pain, anorexia, weakness, scant feces, coughing, and pneumonitis due to migrating larvae, bronchospasms, eosinophilia, jaundice, bile duct obstruction, anemia, stunted growth, a dull hair coat, and with severe infestation, sudden death.

Diagnosis

Worms can be seen in rare cases if passed in the feces. Stool samples are typically abundant with eggs. Gastrointestinal radiographs with contrast may demonstrate an outline of worms.

Treatment

A variety of drugs are effective against *Ascaris* spp. In heavy infections with multiple parasites, *Ascaris* spp. should be treated first prior to other parasites. Ineffective drugs may irritate adult *Ascaris*, potentially penetrating the bowel. Older animals (>6 months) may develop an acquired resistance to ascarids. Larvae may encyst in tissues to avoid the animal's immune system and rarely complete the life cycle. In the encysted stage they also avoid the effects of most dewormers. Pregnancy is believed to activate encysted larvae where activated larvae then migrate to the placenta and into mammary glands.

Pyrantel pamoate is the drug of choice in young animals. Start at 2 weeks of age and repeat q2 weeks × 4 doses. Do not use in heavy worm burdens or partial intestinal obstruction since paralyzed worms may necessitate or complicate surgery. Deworming before pregnancy reduces the burden of migrating larvae but does not eliminate the encysted larvae in the mother's body. Fenbendazole (50 mg/kg PO q24 h starting at 40 days gestation and given through Day 14 postpartum) results in 89% fewer roundworms in pups. Pulmonary symptoms may be ameliorated with inhaled bronchodilator therapy or corticosteroids, if necessary. Vitamin A supplementation may improve growth development. In endemic areas most animals will become re-infected within 3–6 months, so repeat stool samples should be evaluated and retreatment if stool ova persist.

Drug therapy

- Fenbendazole
- Febantel

Drug therapy alternatives

- Albendazole
- Selamectin
- Emodepside – may be effective in vertical transmission of *T. cati*.
- Nitazoxanide

Further reading

Mehlhom, H., Hanser, E., Harder, A., *et al.* (2003) Synergistic effects of pyrantel and the febantel metabolite fenbendazole on adult *Toxocara canis*. *Parasitol Res.*, **90(Suppl 3)**, 151–153.

Wolken, S., Schaper, R., Mencke, N., *et al.* (2009) Treatment and prevention of vertical transmission of *Toxocara cati* in cats with an emodepside/praziquantel spot-on formulation. *Parasitol Res.*, **105**, S75–81.

Chapter 36: *Aspergillus* Species

Description: Fungus mold, ubiquitous soil saprophyte, branching septate hyphae, acute angle branching with spores

Zoonotic Potential: Environmental, not considered a zoonotic

Microbiology/epidemiology

Infection is typically via inhalation of large inoculums of airborne spores (conidia). *Aspergillus* spp. are considered opportunistic pathogens that grow worldwide, but are more common in hot, dry environments. *Aspergillus* spp. concentrate in soil, potted plants, hay, compost, food, and manure. *Aspergillus* spp. are common isolates of the respiratory tract where they may colonize mucus membranes. The majority of disseminated aspergillosis cases in dogs are caused by *A. terrus*, but *A. deflectus*, *A. flavis*, and *A. fumigates* have also been reported. In canine and feline sino-nasal aspergillosis, the most common species isolated is *A. fumigates*. Dolichocephalic and German shepherd breeds, as well as brachycephalic cats (Persians, Himalayans), appear predisposed. Direct transmission between animals and zoonotic transmission generally does not occur. Animals with immunosuppression, neutropenia, cancer, panleukopenic, feline leukemia, feline infectious peritonitis, uncontrolled diabetes, severe endoparasitic disease, or those receiving immunosuppressive drugs (cytotoxic, high-dose steroids) appear to be at highest risk. An increased incidence of *Aspergillus* spp. fungal otitis following widespread use of topical fluoroquinolones in humans suggests that elimination of normal flora may select for *Aspergillus* over growth.

Clinical disease

Chronic *Aspergillus* spp. infections of the skin, soft tissue or mucus membranes (otomycosis, sino-orbital, sino-nasal) are not uncommon in dogs and cats, particularly in atopic or allergic animals. Disseminated *Aspergillus* infections (diskospondylitis, pulmonary, osteomyelitis, and pyelonephritis) are rare and typically only seen in animals with predisposing factors. Isolation of *Aspergillus* spp. from skin, mucus membranes, or hair may only represent transient contamination unless associated with histological or cytological evidence of disease.

Sino-nasal

Clinical presentation in canine patients involves chronic, serous, mucopurulent, or sanguinopurulent nasal discharge. Affected dogs are generally systemically healthy with no clear evidence of immune suppression. The infection may start unilaterally and become bilateral after destruction of the nasal septum. Dogs may have regional pain, episodic epistaxes, stridor, open-mouthed breathing, facial deformity, ocular involvement, ulceration, and hyperkeratosis of the nasal planum. Cats present with similar symptomology but may have extensive extranasal or orbital tissue involvement as well as mandibular lymphadenomegaly. The most common etiologic agents are *A. fumigates* followed by *A. flavus* and *A. niger*. A new *Aspergillus* spp., *A. felis*, is reported to cause rhinosinusitis in cats.

Otomycosis/keratomycosis

Otomycosis and keratomycosis occur rarely in dogs and cats. Dogs with chronic skin infections and a history of oral and topical antibiotic/steroid use are prone to otomycosis with *A. niger*, *A. versicolor*, and *A. ochraceus*. Cats typically have keratomycosis associated with *A. flavus* or *A. fumigatus*. A history of diabetes or feline herpesvirus may be a predisposing factor.

Disseminated

Disseminated aspergillosis is a rare and often fatal disease in dogs. *A. terreus* and *A. deflectus* are the primary etiologic agents. The majority of cases involve young to middle age females. An IgA and IgM deficiency has been suggested. Clinical presentation may include discospondylitis, osteomyelitis, spinal hyperpathia, vestibular abnormalities, uveitis, ataxia, paraparesis, weight loss, anorexia, lameness, or renal failure.

Diagnosis

There is no single diagnostic test that has 100% sensitivity and specificity. *Aspergillus* spp. infections must be diagnosed via biopsy and/or appropriate fluid analysis. Biopsy must demonstrate local tissue invasion. Fungal culture, speciation, and antifungal sensitivity may also be warranted. Serum EIA, serum or urine antigen, and PCR may be sent to Miravista Labs if local labs cannot run assays. Confirmation of sino-nasal *Aspergillus* spp. infection requires at least two of the following to be positive:
1. Detection of serum antibody (false negatives are high),
2. Diagnostic imaging (radiographs, CT, or MRI showing cavitary destruction of turbinates, thickening of mucosa or inner surface of frontal sinus, thick reactive bone, maxillary recess), and
3. Isolation of the organism from brush samples or squash preparation of mucosal biopsy tissue obtained by endoscopic exam.

Treatment

Treatment must be targeted at reducing/decolonizing the fungal masses (fungal balls). Surgical excision, debridement, local irrigation, and removal of any nidus of infection are critical prior to drug therapy.

Drug therapy

Sino-nasal

Treatment is dependent on the extent of the infection. Topical therapy can be utilized if the cribriform plate is intact. Localized debridement and irrigation of the sinuses under anesthesia is recommended prior to instillation of topical clotrimazole (1% in PEG) or enilconazole (2%). Ideally, localized infusions should be performed by a specialist. Clotrimazole is reported to have the most favorable outcome if infused over one hour (30 mL for small dogs and 60 mL for large dogs). Repeat infusions can be attempted if there is no improvement after 2 weeks. Enilconazole may be attempted in cases where there is no response to clotrimazole therapy, but availability is often in question. Concurrent oral therapy with itraconazole or voriconazole is recommended for patients with invasive infections into soft tissues or those that fail topical therapy. Once resolved, dogs are also predisposed to secondary bacterial infections. Less information is available for the treatment of cats with sino-nasal aspergillosis. Topical clotrimazole and sinusotomy have been attempted, but oral itraconazole (10 mg/kg/day) appears to be the most effective long term treatment.

Otomycosis/keratomycosis

Treatment of otomycosis can be done with the commercially available Posatex Otic Solution which contains posaconazole. Keratomycosis can be treated with a 1% topical voriconazole solution. This must be compounded by a sterile compounding pharmacy and applied every 2–4 h.

Disseminated aspergillus

Treatment of disseminated *Aspergillus* in canine and feline patients often results in an unfavorable outcome. Retrospective studies indicate that the infection is typically refractory to amphotericin-B, particularly if the infection is due to *A. terreus*. Long term treatment with oral itraconazole, posaconazole or voriconazole may prolong survival, but are very expensive. Voriconazole and posaconazole are the treatments of choice with or without amphotericin-B. Voriconazole should be given orally due to reports of toxicosis in dogs receiving the intravenous formulation.

Drug therapy alternatives

Intravenous Liposomal amphotericin B or caspofungin used in combination with voriconazole may be attempted in severe disseminated disease, but the overall success of these expensive combinations is currently unknown in canine and feline patients.

Further reading

Peeters, D. and Clercx, C. (2007) Update on canine sinonasal aspergillosis. *Vet Clin North Amer Small Anim Pract.*, **37(5)**, 901–916.

Schultz, R.M., Johnson, E.G., Wisner, E.R., *et al.* (2008) Clinicopathologic and diagnostic imaging characteristics of systemic aspergillosis in 30 dogs. *J Vet Intern Med.*, **22**, 851–859.

Sykes, J.E. (2013) Aspergillosis. Ch. 65. In: *Canine and Feline Infectious Diseases.* Sykes, J.E. (ed.), Elsevier, St. Louis, MO, pp. 633–648.

Chapter 37: *Babesia* Species

Description: Protozoan parasite, intraerythrocytic, multiple species
Zoonotic Potential: Considered a significant zoonotic to humans

Microbiology/epidemiology

Babesia species that infect dogs are *B. canis* and *B. gibsoni*. *B. canis* consist of three subspecies (*B. canis vogeli*, *B. canis canis*, and *B. canis rossi*). *B. canis canis* is primarily found in Europe and Africa and is transmitted by the cow tick (*D. reticulates*), while *B. canis rossi* is primarily found in Africa and is transmitted by the yellow dog tick (*Haemaphysalis*). *B. canis vogeli* is transmitted by the brown dog tick (*R. sanguineus*). *B. canis vogeli* infections are found throughout the world with the most common diagnosed in warm, humid areas such as the Southern USA. Seroprevalence in adult dogs is between 3.8–59%. This may be even higher in greyhounds kept in kennels with poor tick control, or following exposure to wild canids (100%). *B. gibsoni* occurs throughout the world, is transmitted by a variety of ticks, and is prevalent in American pit bull terriers. It is believed to be transmitted by dog fights and perinatal transmission. Many other species have been identified including *B. conradae* in dogs from Southern California and *B. microti* from Spain and North America. Feline *Babesia* is less common but has been reported in cats from Africa, Sudan, Brazil, Spain, Portugal, and Israel.

Clinical disease

Clinical signs are dependent on the species of *Babesia*, the age of the host and the immunologic response of the host. Dogs may often have subclinical infections unless they are infected with a more virulent species. *B. canis vogeli* may only be associated with fever and no other overt hematologic signs. Clinical signs include lethargy, pallor, splenomegaly, fever, thrombocytopenia, hemolytic anemia, anorexia, and weakness. Dogs may have jaundice, bilirubinuria, and hemoglobinuria. *B. canis rossi* may be associated with neurologic signs, thrombocytopenia, hyperbilirubinemia, tachypnea, anuria, and leukocytosis. Cats with *B. felis* may present with lethargy, anorexia, weakness, unkempt haircoat, and diarrhea. Elevated ALT, total bilirubin, and hyperglobulinemia may also be present.

Diagnosis

There are no exact tests for the diagnosis of *Babesia*. Cytology using whole blood, buffy-coat smears, and tissue aspirates are diagnostic but may be less sensitive than PCR. PCR of whole blood or splenic aspirates must be interpreted based on clinical signs. Serial samples 2–4 weeks apart will increase sensitivity. Serum immunofluorescent antibody serology may produce false negatives and positives so acute and convalescent serology may be required for diagnosis. A positive Comb's test, spherocytosis, and autoagglutination may be present. Hyperbilirubinemia may be present with acute infections from *B. canis canis* and *B. canis rossi*. Dogs with *B. canis rossi* may have elevated liver and renal parameters as well as hemoglobinemia, hypoalbuminemia, hypoglycemia, and metabolic acidosis.

Treatment

Animals may require significant supportive care including packed red blood cell transfusions or intravenous crystalloid fluid therapy. Azithromycin (10 mg/kg PO q24 h × 10 days) and atovaquone suspension (13.3 mg/kg PO q8 h × 10 days) is the drug combination of choice for *B. canis*, *B. gibsoni*, and *B. conradae*. Imidocarb dipropionate (5–6.6 mg/kg IM × 1; repeat in 14 days) is active against *B. canis*. It does not clear *B. gibsoni* or *B. conradae* infections but may reduce morbidity and mortality. Diminazene aceturate (3.5–5.0 mg/kg IM × 1 (*B. canis*); repeat dose in 24 h for *B. gibsoni*. This can be followed with a single dose of imidocarb (6–7.5 mg/kg IM) to clear *B. canis* infections. Clindamycin (25 mg/kg PO q12 h × 90 days) plus doxycycline (5 mg/kg PO q12 h × 90 days) plus metronidazole 15 mg/kg PO q12 h × 90 days) may be effective (further documentation needed) for *B. canis* and *B. gibsoni* that fail azithromycin and atovaquone therapy. Glucocorticoids (2–3 weeks) may be required in dogs with significant immune-mediated complications from *B. canis rossi*. Cats infected with *B. felis* may be given primaquine phosphate (0.5 mg/kg PO q24 h × 1–3 days). Preventative measures are very important due to the fact that animals may become re-infected in endemic areas. Amitraz-impregnated collars significantly reduce infections in dogs. Owners should avoid having their animals interact with other aggressive dogs or wild canids and the kenneling of animals where tick control is not adequate.

Drug therapy

- Azithromycin and atovaquone
- Imidocarb dipropionate
- Diminazene aceturate

Drug therapy alternatives

Clindamycin plus doxycycline plus metronidazole.

Further reading

Birkenheuer, A.J. (2013) Babesiosis. Ch. 75. In: *Canine and Feline Infectious Diseases*. Sykes, J.E. (ed.), Elsevier, St. Louis, MO, pp. 727–736.

Birkenheuer, A.J., Correa, M.T., Levy, M.G., *et al.* (2005) Geographic distribution of babesiosis amung dogs in the United States and association with dog bites: 150 cases (2000–2003). *J Am Vet Med Assoc.*, **227**, 942–947.

Birkenheuer, A.J., Levy, M.G., and Breitschwerdt, E.B. (2004) Efficacy of combined atovaquone and azithromycin for therapy of chronic *Babesia gibsoni* (Asian genotype) infections in dogs. *J Vet Intern Med.*, **18**, 494–498.

Penzhorn, B.L., Lewis, B.D., deWaal, D.T., *et al.* (1995) Sterilization of *Babesia canis* infections by imidocarb alone or in combination with diminazene. *J S Afr Vet Assoc.*, **66**, 157–159.

Chapter 38: *Bartonella* Species (Cat Scratch Disease)

Description: Gram negative bacilli, pleomorphic, intraerythrocytic
Zoonotic Potential: Considered a significant zoonotic in immunosuppressed humans

Microbiology/epidemiology

At least 10 *Bartonella species* are reported from dogs and cats. *B. hensalae* was first isolated in 1992 in human patients with HIV. The organism is frequently isolated from cats and can occasionally infect humans with immunosuppression. It is the primary cause of cat scratch disease. Fleas, ticks, lice, and biting flies are believed responsible for transmission as well as cat claws contaminated with flea feces. Cats that are young, feral, and live in warm, humid climates are predisposed. Dogs with tick exposure, from rural environments or have outdoor exposure, and those that roam are considered high risk.

Clinical disease

Cats may present with a small papule at the site of inoculation, caudal stomatitis, uveitis, fever, lymphadenopathy, neurologic signs, or reproductive disorders. Rarely, endocarditis, myocarditis, and/or osteomyelitis can occur. In dogs, endocarditis, lethargy, fever, cardiac murmur, arrhythmias, cough, tachypnea, inappetence, joint effusions, and lameness are reported. Dogs may also present without fever and negative blood culture endocarditis. Complications may include thromboembolitic disease, epistaxis, neutrophilic polyarthritis, peripheral edema, splenomegaly, lesions of the nasal cavity, skin nodules, and hepatitis.

Diagnosis

Blood or tissue culture are useful, but may have false positives. PCR of whole blood or tissues may confirm active infection more rapidly than culture. Positive results must be correlated to clinical signs since healthy animals may be bacteremic. Serology (IFA Elisa) may be useful in dogs with endocarditis when cultures and PCR are negative.

Treatment

Treatment of bartonellosis should include vector control. *Bartonella* spp. are typically sensitive to a variety of antibiotics. Tetracyclines (doxycycline) and macrolides have been considered the agents of choice historically. However, aminoglycosides, fluroquinolones, amoxicillin/clavulanate, and ampicillin have also been administered with success. Drug therapy is recommended for 2 weeks in immunocompetent patients and for 6 weeks in immuno-compromised patients or those with endocarditis. High dose doxycycline may be effective in clearing feline patients with *B. hensele*. For patients with endocarditis, ampicillin (10–20 mg/kg IV q6–8 h) with gentamycin (dogs: 9–14 mg/kg or cats: 5–8 mg/kg IV, IM, SC q24 h) can be administered.

Drug therapy

Doxycycline

Drug therapy alternatives

- Amoxicillin/clavulanate
- Ampicillin with gentamycin (acute endocarditis)
- Doxycycline with rifampin (stable endocarditis)
- Azithromycin with amoxicillin (stable endocarditis)
- Fluoroquinolones with amoxicillin (stable endocarditis)

Further reading

Balakrishnan, N., Cherry, N.A., Linder, K.E., *et al.* (2013) Experimental infection of dogs with *Bartonella vinsonii subsp. Berkhoffii. Vet Immunol Immunopathol.*, **156(1–2)**, 153–158.

Brunt, J., Guptill, L., Kordick, D., *et al.* (2006) American Association of feline practitioners 2006, Panel report on diagnosis, treatment, and prevention of *Bartonella* spp. Infections. *J Feline Med Surg.*, **8**, 213–226.

Chomel, B.B., Boulouis, H.J., Maruyama, S., *et al.* (2006) *Bartonella* spp. in pets and effect on human health. *Emerg Infect Dis.*, **12(3)**, 389–394.

Sykes, J.E. and Chomel, B.B. (2013) Bartonellosis. Ch. 52. In: *Canine and Feline Infectious Diseases*. Sykes, J.E. (ed.), Elsevier, St. Louis, MO, pp. 498–511.

Chapter 39: Blastomycosis

Description: Dimorphic fungus, soil hyphae with tissue budding yeasts
Zoonotic Potential: Can be transmitted to humans but not a significant zoonotic

Microbiology/epidemiology

Blastomycosis is common in dogs and humans in North America, particularly in the South Central and the upper Midwest states. The fungus exists in the environment as hyphae, which produce airborne conidia. Mammals acquire the infection by inhalation of conidia, which are transformed to yeasts in the lungs. Young dogs, large dogs (>15 kg), hunting breeds, and those with outdoor exposure to disturbed soil, woodpiles, and bodies of water appear to be at increased risk. Blastomycosis is reported rarely in cats and often not in association with environmental exposure, since exclusively indoor cats have also been reported to acquire the disease.

Clinical disease

Animals may present with subclinical, acute, or chronic infections. Dogs may develop either localized pulmonary infections or disseminated infection. Dogs typically present with fever, lethargy, weakness, thin body condition, dehydration, and respiratory findings (cough, harsh lung sounds). Physical findings may demonstrate firm cutaneous masses, skin lesions, peripheral lymphadenopathy, and lesions on mucosal membranes (tongue, gingiva, mucosal junctions). Multiple other extrapulmonary sites may be involved including: ocular (chorioretinitis, anterior uveitis, retinal detachment, glaucoma), gastrointestinal (vomiting, diarrhea, hematemesis, melena), bone (bony masses, osteomyelitis, arthritis, hypertrophic osteopathy), reproductive tissues (mammary and testicular masses, orchitis, prostatomegaly), intranasal (retrobulbar, CNS involvement), and cardiac (myocardium, endocardium, pericardium). Cats may present with similar symptoms but typically with more gastrointestinal and neurologic signs (ataxia, pelvic limb paresis, circling, blindness, hyperesthesia, and decreased placing reactions).

Diagnosis

Diagnosis is based on identification of organisms (yeasts) on cytology of fine needle aspirates of infected tissues. Yeasts may also be found on impression smears of skin lesions, respiratory lavage specimens, and bodily fluids (CSF, urine, ocular, synovial). Antigen assays (ELISA) of serum or urine may also be used with >90% sensitivity, but may cross react with *Histoplasma*. Serum or urine antigen, antibody or PCR can be sent into MiraVista Laboratories (www.Miravistalabs.com) if local diagnostic laboratories do not perform these tests. Histopathology, fungal culture, and antibody serology may also be useful but culture results are slower and may have a higher risk of false negatives.

Treatment

The treatment of choice is typically itraconazole until resolution of clinical signs and symptoms. Urine *Blastomyces* galactomannan antigen concentrations may also decline with effective treatment. Treatment may take up to 3–6 months or greater than a year in some animals. Initial treatment with amphotericin-B is recommended for animals with severe infection, followed by oral therapy with itraconazole. For patients with CNS or ocular disease, liposomal amphotericin-B followed by voriconazole is recommended due to better drug penetration. Fluconazole and ketoconazole have significantly less efficacy and more toxicity than itraconazole.

Drug therapy

- Amphotericin-B
- Itraconazole

Drug therapy alternatives

- Liposomal amphotericin B
- Voriconazole
- Posaconazole
- Fluconazole

Further reading

Arceneaux, K.A., Taboada, J., and Hosgood, G. (1998) Blastomycosis in dogs: 115 cases (1980–1995). *J Am Vet Med Assoc.*, **213**, 658–664.

Breider, M.A., Walker, T.L., Legendre, A.M., *et al.* (1988) Blastomycosis in cats: five cases (1979–1986). *J Am Vet Med Assoc.*, **193**, 570–572.

Legendre, A.M., Rohrbach, B.W., Toal, R.L., *et al.* (1996) Treatment of blastomycosis with itraconazole in 112 dogs. *J Vet Intern Med.*, **10**, 365–371.

Sykes, J.E. and Merkel, L.K. (2013) Blastomycosis. Ch. 60. In: *Canine and Feline Infectious Diseases.* Sykes, J.E. (ed.), Elsevier, St. Louis, MO, pp. 574–586.

Chapter 40: *Bordetella Bronchiseptica* (Kennel Cough)

Description: Gram negative aerobic bacteria, small pleomorphic coccobacillus, flagella
Zoonotic Potential: A zoonotic organism in immunocompromised patients

Microbiology/epidemiology

Bordetella species are found worldwide. There are at least nine species, but only *B. bronchiseptica* is noted to cause respiratory disease in dogs and cats. The infection is readily transmitted via aerosolization between animals housed in stressful conditions (shelters, pet stores, boarding kennels, etc.). *Bordetella* spp. only survive for a few hours in respiratory secretions but can survive in soil for 45 days and in lake water for 24 weeks.

Incubation is 2–10 days and shedding may last for up to 2 months. Young animals (<8 weeks) may develop severe bronchopneumonia rapidly so that treatment in this age group should be initiated as soon as possible. Although rare, *B. broniseptica* has caused infections in immunosuppressed human patients and these individuals should avoid contact with infected animals.

Clinical disease

Clinical signs are highly variable and are dependent on the animals underlying immunity, bacterial strain, and the presence of co-infections. Dogs often present with serous to mucopurulent nasal discharge, sneezing, harsh cough, and stertor. Infection may progress into bronchopneumonia with fever, lethargy, productive cough, and anorexia. Cats typically develop sneezing but frequently lack the harsh cough noted in dogs. They may also have a fever, ocular discharge, and lymphadenopathy. Pneumonia in kittens may develop rapidly with tachypnea, cyanosis, and death. Bronchopneumonia may be a result of co-infection with other bacteria or viruses. Rarely, animals may inadvertently be injected systemically with the intranasal vaccine which may cause local reactions, hepatic necrosis and even death (see Treatment section).

Diagnosis

Diagnosis is by culture and sensitivity as well as PCR. Bacterial culture may be done on nasal and oropharyngeal swabs, transtracheal, and bronchoalveolar lavage specimens or tissue specimens. False negatives may occur with low numbers and prior antibiotic treatment. PCR results may have false positives and negatives due to recent intranasal vaccination or low bacterial numbers.

Treatment

Animals should be isolated to avoid further transmission. Vaccination should provide protection within 3 days. Antibiotics should be reserved for animals that are at high risk (age <8 weeks, immunosuppressed, etc.) or those that have persistent clinical signs (>7–10 days). Animals with severe infection should be treated with intravenous fluids, nutrition, and supplemental oxygen. Antibiotic therapy should be based on culture and sensitivity if possible due to the fact that some strains have demonstrated resistance to penicillins and sulfa drugs. Doxycycline is typically considered the drug of choice empirically due to tissue penetration. However, bactericidal antibiotics may be required for severe or persistent bronchopneumonia

or tracheobronchitis. Nebulized aminoglycosides may be effective in some cases of refractory bronchopneumonia. Susceptibility to TMS, penicillins, and quinolones is variable. Treatment should continue for 2–4 weeks although may require up to 6 months in some animals. Treatment of inadvertent systemic administration of the intranasal vaccine should consist of subcutaneous fluids at the site of injection along with gentamicin (2–4 mg/kg in 10–30 mL of saline). Oral doxycycline may then be administered for 5–7 days.

Drug therapy

Doxycycline

Drug therapy alternatives

- Chloramphenicol
- TMS
- Fluoroquinolones
- Aminoglycosides
- Extended spectrum third generation penicillins

Further reading

Egberink, H., Addie, D., Belak, S., *et al.* (2009) *Bordetella bronchiseptica* in cats. ABCD guidelines on prevention and management. *J Feline Med Surg.*, **11(7)**, 610–614.

Foley, J.E., Rand, C., Bannasch, M.J., *et al.* (2002;Molecular epidemiology of feline bordetellosis in two animal shelters in California, USA. *Prev Vet Med.*, **54(2)**, 141–156.

Speakman, A.J., Dawson, S., Corkill J.E., *et al.* (2000;Antibiotic susceptibility of canine *Bordetella bronchiseptica* isolates. *Vet Microbiol.*, **71(3–4)**, 193–200.

Chapter 41: *Borrelia Burgdorferi* (Lyme Disease)

Description: Spirochete, intracellular parasite, cork screw shaped
Zoonotic Potential: Vector borne (tick) zoonotic in humans

Microbiology/epidemiology

Borrelia burgdorferi is the most common vector-borne disease in the USA. Lyme disease is endemic in the Northeast, Northwest, and Midwest. The spirochete is transmitted primarily by *Ixodes scapularis* ticks in the East and upper Midwest and *Ixodes pacificus* ticks in the West. The disease is most common in animals with exposure to wooded areas abundant with deer. Peak season is typically between May to September. Some strains of *B. burgdoriferi* have increased virulence (Osp C type A). Cats can be infected, but are relatively resistant. Ticks have three stages. Eggs hatch into larvae in spring and ingest a blood meal from white-footed mice, birds, squirrels, shrews, or lizards that harbor the infection. The larvae detach and then develop into nymphal ticks that feed on cats, dogs, humans, mice, and eventually deer.

Clinical disease

More than 95% of naturally infected dogs are asymptomatic. Many animals may be subclinical and have titers present for months to years. It may be difficult to distinguish infection versus exposure. Symptoms in dogs may not occur until 2–5 months after infection. Dogs may present with fever, arthritis, malaise, inappetence, thrombocytopenia, lameness, or renal disease (1–2%). Joints may be swollen, warm, and tender. Latent effects may involve the large joints and arthritis may develop early or late (2 years). Dogs with Lyme nephritis may be dehydrated, have edema, pleural effusion, ascites, hypertension, neurologic complications, and retinal detachment. Complications include thromboembolic events and oliguric/anuric renal failure.

Diagnosis

Diagnosis must be based on clinical signs, exposure history and positive antibody response. A new diagnostic method (C6 peptide test for Lyme), serology and PCR testing for *Ehrlichia* can be performed. A CBC may demonstrate mild to moderate thrombocytopenia and leukocytosis. Dogs with renal disease may have azotemia, mild to marked hypoalbuminemia, metabolic acidosis, electrolyte changes, hyperphosphatemia, hypochloremia, mild hyperkalemia, or hypokalemia. Urinalysis may show isosthenuria, proteinuria, pyuria, hematuria, and urine protein to creatinine ratios are often >5. Renal biopsy is advocated early to prove if immune-complex disease exists. Seropositive dogs should be screened and monitored for proteinuria. Lyme nephritis (LN) mimics other forms of protein-losing nephropathy and sometimes *Leptospirosis*. Renal biopsy helps show if immune-complex disease exists, but may not prove LN specifically.

Treatment

Seropositive dogs with clinical abnormalities thought to arise from Lyme disease generally are treated with doxycycline (10 mg/kg PO q24 h for 30–60 days). Proteinuric

dogs may require standard therapy for protein-losing nephropathy, long-term antimicrobials, and perhaps immunosuppressive therapy. Cefuroxime axetil is effective oral treatment for early Lyme disease if animals do not tolerate doxycycline. For severe disease, intravenous ceftriaxone or penicillin can be given. Corticosteroids or acetazolamide may be necessary for animals with CNS involvement and cranial nerve palsy. Tick control should be recommended and should include a product that repels or protects against tick attachment. The use of the Lyme vaccine remains controversial.

Drug therapy

- Oxytetracycline
- Doxycycline
- Cefuroxime

Drug therapy alternatives

- Penicillin
- Cetriaxone
- Cefotaxime

Further reading

Ktimer, P.M., Miller, A.D., Li, Q., *et al.* (2011) Molecular and pathological investigations of the central nervous system in *Borrelia burdorferi*-infected dogs. *J Vet Diagn Invest.*, **23(4)**, 757–763.

Littman, M.P. (2003) Canine borreliosis. *Vet Clin North Am Small Anim Pract.*, **33(4)**, 827–862.

Littman, M.P., Goldstein, R.E., Labato, M.A., *et al.* (2006) ACVIM small animal consensus statement on Lyme disease in dogs: diagnosis, treatment, and prevention. *J Vet Intern Med.*, **20(2)**, 422–434.

Skotarczak, B. (2002) Canine borreliosis-epidemiology and diagnostics. *Ann Agric Environ Med.*, **9(2)**, 137–140.

Susta, L., Uhl, E.W., Grosenbaugh D.A., *et al.* (2012) Synovial lesions in experimental canine Lyme borreliosis. *Vet Pathol.*, **49(3)**, 453–461.

Chapter 42: Brucella (Canine Brucellosis)

Description: Aerobic gram negative bacteria, small intracellular, slow growing coccobacilli
Zoonotic Potential: Highly infectious zoonotic

Microbiology/epidemiology

Seroprevalence studies indicate that canine brucellosis is widespread in the Southern USA, Central and Southern America, and Asia. Dogs can be infected with *B. abortus*, *B. melitensis*, and *B. suis*. In cats, *B. suis* is the common isolate. Infection is acquired by inhalation, ingestion, insemination, transmission *in utero*, and/or nursing. *B. abortus* can survive in water and soil for up to 4 months, and *B. canis* remains viable in semen for up to 48 h. The disease appears to becoming more prevalent in breeding kennels where the incidence may be as high as 13%. Animals may also acquire the disease by ingestion of fomites in water, food bowls, equipment, and bedding or contact with infected fetal membranes, aborted fetuses, vulvar discharge or urine from infected dogs. *B. canis* is the leading cause of infertility, abortion, and early death in puppies. Strays and feral dogs are considered reservoirs in some countries.

Clinical disease

Infected animals are rarely systemically ill and fever is uncommon. The most common sign of *B. canis* is infertility. Bitches typically present with late term abortion (45–55 days) resulting in the birth of stillborn puppies that appear to have autolyzed tissues. Subcutaneous edema, congestion, and hemorrhage of the abdominal area, lesions in the liver, spleen, kidneys, and intestines. Abortion is usually accompanied by a vaginal discharge lasting up to 6 weeks. If puppies survive, they may die within hours or weeks. Some litters contain both live and dead pups, although most live pups die shortly thereafter. Those that survive suffer generalized lymphadenopathy and persistent hyperglobulinemia. Typically, they develop clinical disease on reaching sexual maturity. Scrotal distention, and epididymis enlargement, orchitis, scrotal dermatitis, prostatitis, and testicular atrophy may also be present. Sperm abnormalities may also be evident with 90% being abnormal by week 20. Extrareproductive tract sites such as the eye, intervertebral disc space, and reticuloendothelial system may also be sites of infection.

Diagnosis

Isolation and identification of *B. canis* is diagnostic. Placenta, lymph nodes, prostate, and spleen are suitable samples for culture. Compared to blood culture, the diagnostic sensitivity of whole blood PCR is 100% in naturally infected dogs. The rapid slide agglutination test (RSAT) is a rapid and sensitive test designed to detect antibodies to *Brucella* LPS antigen. This is most accurate as a screening test from 8 to 12 weeks after infection. Blood is the sample of choice because of the lack of contaminating organisms and prolonged bacteremia. Following infection, bacteremia starts at 2 weeks and persists for at least 6 months post-infection and can be detected for up to 64 months. The laboratory should be notified of suspected *Brucella* cases if culture is requested.

Treatment

No antimicrobial therapy has shown consistent long term cures of *B. canis*. Due to the intracellular nature of the organism and pharmacologically difficult areas for drugs to penetrate (prostate), neutering and at least a month of therapy (enrofloxacin) is advised. Animals should be followed closely and seropositive animals should be treated further. Combination therapy with multiple drugs appears to have the best efficacy. An aminoglycoside (1–2 weeks) plus doxycycline (6 weeks) or a fluoroquinolone are often used. In humans, optimal therapy has used an aminoglycoside for 1–2 weeks in addition to oral doxycycline with rifampin for 6–8 weeks. In breeding kennels, new animals should be isolated and testing should be done on all animals prior to breeding. At least two seronegative tests should be performed one month apart.

Drug therapy

- Aminoglycoside plus enrofloxacin
- Aminoglycoside plus doxycycline

Drug therapy alternatives

- Aminoglycoside plus minocycline
- Aminoglycoside plus ciprofloxacin
- Aminoglycoside plus doxycycline plus rifampin

Further reading

Graham, E.M. and Taylor, D.J. (2012) Bacterial reproductive pathogens of cats and dogs. *Vet Clin North Am Small Anim Pract.*, **42(3)**, 561–582.

Henderson, R.A., Hoerlein, B.F., Kramer, T.T., *et al.* (1974) Discospondylitis in three dogs infected with *Brucella canis*. *J Am Vet Med Assoc.*, **165(5)**, 451–455.

Makloski, CL. (2011) Canine brucellosis management. *Vet Clin North Am Small Anima Pract.*, **41(6)**, 1209–1219.

Patil, M.Y., Antin, S.M., and Gupta, A. (2011) Skeletal brucellosis. *J Indian Med Assoc.*, **109(3)**, 171–173.

Chapter 43: Calicivirus

Description: Single stranded RNA virus, non-enveloped, spherical capsid
Zoonotic Potential: Host specific, not considered a zoonotic

Microbiology/epidemiology

Feline calicivirus (FCV) is a primary component (10–50%) of feline upper respiratory infection in cats. Cats in multicat households are at highest risk of infection. Infected cats may develop persistent oropharyngeal infections and act as carriers of the infection. Carrier cats may shed the virus for weeks to months, but it can last a lifetime in some cats. Transmission is via direct contact with respiratory secretions, aerosolization, via flea feces, or ingestion of fleas. Kittens and mildly affected cats are particularly likely to shed calicivirus, and may shed virulent virus without showing overt signs. Highly virulent strains have been isolated in older cats that were vaccinated from shelters or clinics with outbreaks in the USA and Europe. A high mortality rate is associated with infection of this virulent systemic disease (VSD). FCV has also been evaluated as a possible cause of feline interstitial cystitis and enteritis in cats.

Clinical disease

FCV typically presents with erosive or ulcerative lesions on the nasal planum, tongue, lips, and conjunctiva. Lesions may last for 2–3 weeks or result in persistent infection. Ulceroproliferative or lymphoplasmacytic stomatitis and hyperemia of the buccal mucosa are common. Pyrexia with transient lameness due to synovitis has been described within days to weeks of the initial signs or in some cases after vaccination. Cats with VSD show severe signs of anorexia, high fever, weight loss, nasal/ocular discharge, footpad ulceration, head and limb edema, and crusting of the nose, lips, pinnae, periocular regions, and distal limbs. Pulmonary edema, pleural effusion, icterus, hepatic necrosis, pancreatitis, vomiting, diarrhea, and coagulopathy have been reported. Cats may die suddenly of cardiac arrest.

Diagnosis

FCV infection can be diagnosed by viral isolation from swabs, or transtracheal and bronchoalveolar wash specimens. False negatives may occur, but this is more sensitive than other tests. PCR and serology may also be useful although results may be complicated by prior vaccines, low level shedding, and subclinical shedding. Acute and convalescent titers may be useful for outbreaks of virulent strains.

Treatment

Treatment is support for most cases. All cats should be isolated and if VSD-FCV is being considered, gloves, gowns, and shoe covers should be used by everyone in contact with the animal. Fomites have been carried home on the clothing of visitors and technicians resulting in further spread of infection. Subcutaneous fluid administration, supplemental oxygen, antimicrobial drugs for secondary bacterial infections, nebulization, as well as enteral nutrition for severe cases may be required. There is no identified antiviral treatment for FCV. Therapy is preventative and supportive. Sodium hypochlorite (5% bleach diluted at 1:32), potassium peroxymonosulfate (Trifectant, Virkon-S), and chlorine dioxide have been proven effective against FCV and should be used on any surface where an infected cat has had contact. Potassium peroxymonosulfate can be used to clean carpeted areas.

Drug therapy

Vaccinations (inactivated and attenuated live) for FCV are available and should be administered according to vaccine guidelines. Inactivated vaccines should be reserved for immunosuppressed or pregnant animals. Vaccination of queen cats prior to pregnancy is preferred. Exposure of kittens to the virus prior to full vaccination is a common cause of infection. In shelters or catteries where FCV may be in high prevalence, vaccination as early as 4 weeks may be considered.

Drug therapy alternatives

Supportive care (fluid therapy, systemic antibiotics, nebulized saline/antibiotics, enteral feeding).

Further reading

Radford, A.D. (2009) Feline calicivirus infection. ABCD guidelines on prevention and management. *J Feline Med and Surg.,* **11(7)**, 556–564.

Rohayem, J., Bergmann, M., Gebhardt, J., *et al.* (2010) Antiviral strategies to control calicivirus infections. *Antiviral Res.,* **87(2)**, 162–178.

Sykes, J.E. (2013) Feline respiratory viral infections. Ch. 23. In: *Canine and Feline Infectious Diseases*. Sykes, J.E. (ed.), Elsevier, St. Louis, MO, pp. 239–251.

Chapter 44: *Campylobacter* Species

> **Description:** Gram negative bacillus, comma shaped, seagull wing appearance
> **Zoonotic Potential:** Considered a zoonotic to humans

Microbiology/epidemiology

Most *Campylobacter species* are nonpathogenic but can cause disease in companion animals. *Campylobacter* commonly colonizes the gastrointestinal tract of wild and domestic animals and can be isolated from both healthy and diarrheic dogs and cats. Both *C. jejuni* and *C. upsaliensis* have been reported in association with puppies with diarrhea that are <1 year of age. Other isolates identified include *C. coli*, *C. lari*, and *C. helveticus*. In cats, *C. upsaliensis*, *C. helveticus*, and *C. jejuni* are commonly reported. Animals at risk are those from kennels that come into contact with contaminated feces, water, or food. Although it is self-limiting in many animals, young animals with under-developed immune systems may be at the highest risk. Although the exact risk of zoonotic infection is not known, multiple studies now indicate that owners of dogs shedding *Campylobacter* are at higher risk of infection.

Clinical disease

Puppies and kittens less than 6 months of age may present with fever, vomiting, anorexia, lymphadenitis, and severe diarrhea.

Diagnosis

The diagnosis of campylobacteriosis is a challenge due to the fact that it can be present in high numbers in healthy animals. Diagnosis is based on isolation of the organism from stool or blood. Fecal leucocytes and occult blood are suggestive of *Campylobacter* or other enteroinvasive bacteria (*Salmonella*, *E. coli*, etc.). Culture of *C. jejuni* and *C. coli* in an animal with diarrhea should be considered as a presumptive diagnosis with the consideration that it could just represent colonization.

Treatment

Campylobacter is often self-limiting. Supportive care may be all that is required. Antimicrobials are recommended in cases where the patient has a high fever, bloody or severe diarrhea, or in patients with persistent infection. Antibiotics should be administered early in very young animals with moderate infections. A variety of antibiotics are effective including macrolides, tetracyclines, fluoroquinolones, and chloramphenicol.

Drug therapy

- Erythromycin
- Azithromycin
- Doxycycline

Drug therapy alternatives

- Fluoroquinolones
- Chloramphenicol

Further reading

Amar, C., Kittl, S., Spreng, D., *et al.* (2014) Genotypes and antibiotic resistance of canine *Campylobacter jejuni* isolates. *Vet Microbiol.*, **168(1)**,124–130.

Gras, L.M., Smid, J.H., Wagenaar, J.A., *et al.* (2013) Increased risk for *Campylobacter jejunia* and *C. coli* infection of pet origin in dog owners and evidence for genetic association between strains causing infection in humans and their pets. *Epidemiol Infect.*, **141(12)**, 2526–2535.

Weese, J.S. (2011) Bacterial enteritis in dogs and cats: diagnosis, therapy, and zoonotic potential. *Vet Clin North Am Small Anim Pract.*, **41(2)**, 287–309.

Chapter 45: *Candida* Species

> **Description:** Saprophytic yeast, gram positive, small, oval, thin walled, budding cells
> **Zoonotic Potential:** Environmental, not considered zoonotic

Microbiology/epidemiology

Candida species are normal inhabitants of the gastrointestinal tract, oropharynx, and genitourinary tract. The species is found worldwide and is a very common cause of nosocomial infection in humans. In animals, *Candida* infections are found less commonly. Animals with uncontrolled diabetes, immunosuppression, malignancy, parvovirus infection, gastrointestinal surgery, or those on broad spectrum antibiotics may be at higher risk. Animals with indwelling catheters or feeding tubes that disrupt the epithelial barrier are at increased risk. *C. albicans* is the primary species associated with disease in cats and dogs. Other species causing infection including *C. glabrata, C. krusei, C. guilliermondii, C. para psilosis, C. tropicalis,* and *C. rugosa* have also been reported.

Clinical disease

Animals with caniduria may present with urinary frequency, dysuria, stranguria, hematuria, lethargy, inappetence, and weight loss. This may be associated with urethritis, cystitis, or pyelonephritis. Disseminated *Candida* is rare in animals, but may occur in immunocompromised animals. Patients with fungemia may present with endophthalmitis, cutaneous infections, osteomyelitis, septic arthritis, phlebitis, pericarditis, or abscesses. Patients may also present with cutaneous *Candida* infections causing erosions, crusting, or alopecia. Animals with vulvovaginitis may have vaginal erythema, swelling, and discharge. Small papules and pustules may be noted. Overgrowth of *Candida* in the intestinal tract may also occur in puppies following parvoenteritis, animals on broad spectrum antibiotics or immunosuppressives. These animals may have persistent vomiting, diarrhea, or death despite aggressive fluids and antibiotics.

Diagnosis

Isolation of the organism in conjunction with clinical symptoms is diagnostic. KOH preparations or wet mounts typically demonstrate budding yeasts with or without pseudohyphae. If negative, the organism is easily grown on culture. Fungal endophthalmitis may be noted by indirect fundoscopic exam or anterior chamber aspiration. Speciation is important for severe infections due to the fact that some species (*C. glabrata, C. krusei*) are innately resistant to some antifungals.

Treatment

Underlying conditions that are predisposing factors should be corrected (diabetes, steroid taper, etc.). Catheters or other tubing should be removed or changed. Debridement or drainage of any accessible sites should be performed. Minor skin infections may be treated with topical therapy including antiseptic wipes, azole shampoos, creams, or ointments. Candiduria may be treated with fluconazole with or without

5-flucyctosine (cats). If resistant, clotrimazole 1% bladder irrigation has been performed under anesthesia. Otic infections can be treated with miconazole 1% solution or clotrimazole (Mometamax). Severe resistant otic infections may be treated with posaconazole containing solutions (Posatex). Systemic infections typically can be treated with oral ketoconazole or fluconazole. For more severe infections itraconazole, voriconazole, posaconazole, or amphotericin-B are alternatives, depending on the sensitivity. Some organisms such as *C. glabrata* may be innately resistant to fluconazole as well as other medications.

Drug therapy

- Fluconazole
- Itraconazole

Drug therapy alternatives

- Ketoconazole
- Amphotericin B
- Voriconazole
- Posaconazole
- 5-flucytosine (cats only)

Further reading

Mora-Duarte, J., Betts, R., Rotstein, C., *et al.* (2002) Comparison of caspofungin and amphotericin B for invasive candidiasis. *N Engl J Med.,* **347**, 220–2029.

Pressler, B.M., Vaden, S.L., Lane, I.F., *et al.* (2003) *Candida spp.* Urinary tract infection in 13 dogs and seven cats: predisposing factors, treatment and outcome. *J Am Anim Hosp Assoc.,* **39**, 263–270.

Sykes, J.E. (2013) Candidiasis. Ch. 67. In: *Canine and Feline Infectious Diseases.* Sykes, J.E. (ed.), Elsevier, St. Louis, MO, pp. 653–657.

Toll, J., Ashe, C.M., and Trepanier, L.A. (2003) Intravesicular administration of clotrimazole for treatment of candiduria in a cat with diabetes mellitus. *J Am Vet Med Assoc.,* **223**, 1156–1158.

Chapter 46: Canine Influenza Virus (CIV)

Description: Type A influenza virus, enveloped, negative sense, single-stranded RNA virus
Zoonotic Potential: Host specific, not considered a zoonotic

Microbiology/epidemiology

The "Canine influenza virus (CIV)" is an influenza A H3N8 virus. Genetic analysis has shown that H3N8 was transferred from race horses in Florida to racing greyhounds and then adapted to dogs through point mutations. This is now considered a new dog-specific lineage of H3N8. In 2005, the virus was identified as a newly emerging pathogen in the dog population in the USA, although serology demonstrates it may go back to 1999. H3N8 virus is spread by direct contact with aerosolized respiratory secretions from infected dogs, contaminated objects and individuals. The incubation period is 2–5 days. Viral shedding occurs for 7–10 days following the onset of symptoms. It does not induce a persistent carrier state. The disease is rapidly transmitted between dogs. Although there is high morbidity, the mortality appears low. CIV has currently been reported in 38 states and is considered endemic in New York, South Florida, Northern Colorado, and Southern Wyoming. Dogs at highest risk are in kennels, shelters, and dog daycare centers.

Clinical disease

Dogs may be asymptomatic (20%), have mild disease, or have severe symptoms. Dogs with mild disease typically have a fever, soft/moist or dry cough (10–30 days), and runny nose (thick, purulent, bloody, or greenish discharge). Approximately 80% have mild symptoms. Severe illness is characterized by the onset of high fever and pneumonia in 10–20%. Fatality rates of dogs that develop pneumonia secondary to canine influenza can reach up to 50% without proper treatment. Animals with severe infections typically die from severe hemorrhagic pneumonia and vasculitis.

Diagnosis

Dogs developing upper respiratory infections that have not been vaccinated should be evaluated for CIV. Diagnosis can be made from blood samples or nasal secretions. PCR tests as well as ELISA titers can be performed. Methods to detect current infection include an in-house flu antigen ELISA kit (Becton-Dickinson Flu-A kit) and PCR (reference laboratories). Serology of acute and convalescent samples (1 week after onset of symptoms and after 2–3 weeks) can be collected, but cannot be used acutely. A four-fold rise in titer is diagnostic. Prior vaccination can complicate interpretation.

Treatment

Treatment is primarily supportive. Fluid therapy and antibiotics to cover secondary bacterial infections may be required. Ideally, a transtracheal wash and culture and sensitivity testing should be performed to choose an antibiotic for treatment of severely ill dogs. If an empirical treatment choice must be made, good choices should include a combination of broad spectrum antibiotics such as a fluoroquinolone and a beta-lactam. *Pasteurella*, *Staphylococcus*, *Streptococcus*, and *Mycoplasma* pneumonias should all be considered. Antibiotics including doxycycline, enrofloxacin, and amoxicillin/clavulanate are frequently less effective for CIV. Cough suppressants such as hydrocodone can be given for a non-productive cough but should not be given to dogs with a productive cough. Vaccines are available for the prevention of H3N8 and should be administered to dogs at high risk. The inactivated vaccine should be administered starting as early as 6 weeks with a second booster 3–4 weeks later. Immunity does not occur until 1 week after the first vaccine, so that shelter animals will not be protected unless isolated for the first week after intake and vaccination. Tamiflu is not recommended since it is the primary line of defense against human influenza pandemics and should be reserved for this purpose. The drug is also only effective if started early after infection (48 h), which is rarely in a timeframe that is recognized in dogs.

Drug therapy

- Fluids
- Antibiotics (base on culture results)

Further reading

Rosenthal, M. (2007) CIV may have started circulating earlier than originally thought. *Veterin Forum.*, **24(7)**, 12.

Tremayne, J. (2006) Canine flu confirmed in 22 states. *DVM*, **1**, 66–67.

Yin, S. (2007) Managing canine influenza virus. *Veterin Forum.*, **24(9)**, 40–41.

Yoon, K., Cooper, V., Schwartz, K., *et al.* (2005) Influenza virus infection in racing greyhounds. *Emerging Infect. Dis.*, **11(12)**, 1974–1976.

Chapter 47: *Capillaria Aerophila* (Lungworm)

Description: Nematode parasites of the respiratory tract, 62–105 μm length
Zoonotic Potential: Not considered a zoonotic, has been reported rarely in humans

Microbiology/epidemiology

C. aerophila is a respiratory tract parasitic infection that is found in dogs, foxes, cats, and other wild mammals. The parasite is found worldwide and causes pulmonary or bronchial "capillariasis". The life cycle has a single host and is acquired from other infected carnivores. Adult worms lay eggs in the lungs. Eggs are coughed up and swallowed and then passed in feces. Earthworms may act as intermediate hosts. After ingestion, the larvae hatch in the intestines and migrate to the lungs. They mature into adults about 40 days post-infection.

Clinical disease

Clinical disease is typically minor with animals presenting with mild irritation of the respiratory tract, coughing, dyspnea, rhinitis, tracheitis, or bronchitis. Eosinophilia may be present. Infected animals may have a whistling sound when breathing, frequent sneezing, or a deep, wheezing cough. Severe infections may involve secondary bacterial pneumonia and sinus infections.

Diagnosis

Capillaria is typically diagnosed by the presence of *C. aerophila* eggs in the nasal or tracheal lavage, or the feces.

Treatment

Treatment with anthelmintics, such as fenbendazole or ivermectin, is highly effective. Alternatively, albendazole or mebendazole are also effective. Environmental decontamination is also recommended. Eggs and larva live in the soil. Sunlight and drying of outdoor kennels may help to minimize re-infestation.

Drug therapy

- Fenbendazole
- Ivermectin

Drug therapy alternatives

- Albendazole
- Mebendazole

Further reading

Banzon, T. (1982) Capillariasis. In: *Handbook Series in Parasitic Zoonoses, Section C. Parasitic Zoonoses, Vol. II*, Schultz, M.G. (ed.), CRC Press, Boca Raton, FL, pp. 63–65.

Cross, J.H. (1998) *Capillaria aerophila*. In: *Zoonoses: Biology, Clinical Practice and Public Health Control*, Palmer, S.R., Lord Soulsby, and Simpson, D.I.H. (eds). Oxford University Press, pp. 767–769.

Lalosević, D., Lalosević, V., Klem, I., *et al.* (2008) *Pulmonary capillariasis* miming bronchial carcinoma. *Am J Trop Med Hyg.*, **78(1)**, 14–16.

Saeed, I., Maddox-Hyttel, C., Monrad, J., *et al.* (2006) Helminths of red foxes (*Vulpes vulpes*) in Denmark. *Vet. Parasitol.*, **139(1–3)**, 168–179.

Soulsby, E.J. (1982) *Helminths, Arthropods and Protozoa of Domesticated Animals*. 7th edn. Lea & Febiger, Philadelphia, pp. 340–341.

Chapter 48: *Cestode* Species (Tapeworms)

Description: Tapeworms, segmented, intestinal or tissue parasites, cyst forming
Zoonotic Potential: Considered a significant zoonotic to humans

Microbiology/epidemiology

Cestodes are common parasites of domestic and wild animals worldwide. The life cycle is complex and typically involves an intermediate and definitive host. Species that most commonly affect dogs and cats are *Dipylidium caninum*. The animal becomes infected after ingesting the crushed, infected flea, its larvae, or its eggs. Stomach acid releases the larvae from the eggs. Larvae can then mature into adult worms and attach themselves to the intestinal mucosa. Eggs from cestodes are passed out in the feces. Lice may also be intermediate hosts. Tapeworm infections in dogs and cats can also be caused by several members of the *Taenia* genus. Dogs may acquire *T. hydatigena* by consuming infected raw venison or livestock, *T. ovis* and *T. multiceps* may be acquired by eating undercooked lamb or sheep, *T. crassiceps* may infect dogs after eating rats or mice, and *T. serialis* and *T. pisiformis* may be acquired if a dog consumes dead rabbits. Cats may acquire *T. taeniaeformis* following consumption of mice and rats. Dogs and cats may also harbor *Echinococcus multilocularis* (fox tapeworm). The worm eggs are shed with the feces of dogs, foxes, and other canids, and can contaminate food and drinking water. These are infective for humans and other animals. Contact with contaminated dogs can also be contagious to humans, because their haircoat can carry the eggs. The life cycle of both *Taenia* and *Echinococcus* species involves a tissue stage where the tapeworm escapes into the blood and then into the liver. It may then migrate into the abdominal cavity where it can form cysts. Cysticercus or hydrated cysts may form in tissues and cause significant tissue damage. Poor hygiene, ingestion of raw infected meat, and lack of flea control are risk factors for the development cestode infections. Although dogs and cats are not heavily affected by *Taenia* infections, they can easily transmit the disease to livestock and humans.

Clinical disease

Most animals are asymptomatic. Animals with heavy infections may present with abdominal discomfort and frequently proglotids may be found around the anus. Owners may note that the dog is "scooting" due to irritation. In puppies, heavy infestations may cause anemia, lethargy, restlessness, delayed growth, vomiting and diarrhea, or constipation. Occasionally, the entire worm may be coughed up or passed into the feces.

Diagnosis

Clinical diagnosis is usually made by observing the white mobile tapeworm segments in the feces or crawling around the anus. Tapeworm segments are passed infrequently and may not be noted on routine fecal examination. Diagnosis of *Taenia* versus *Echinococcus* species cannot be performed on eggs but can be based of morphology differences of gravid segments.

Treatment

Flea control is critical in the management and prevention of *D. caninum*. Animals may be re-infected within two weeks of treatment in a flea infested household. Flea collars and other flea control products as well as treatment of the household and yard are important preventative measures. In areas that are rural and endemic for *Taenia*, keep animals away from carcasses and from hunting and eating of wild animals. Meat from wild animals must be frozen at −20°C for 10 days or thoroughly cooked prior to eating. Efforts to reduce the number of stray animals and rodents are advised.

Drug therapy

Praziquantel is the drug of choice for *Echinococcus*, *Dipylidium*, and *Taenia*. Alternatives are active against *Taenia* species, but may not cover all *Echinococcus* or *Dipylidium* species.

Drug therapy alternatives

- Albendazole
- Mebendazole
- Fenbendazole

Further reading

Conboy, G. (2009) Cestodes of dogs and cats in North America. *Vet Clin North Am Small Anim Pract.*, **39(6)**, 1075–1090.
Fourie, J.J., Crafford, D., Horak, I.G., *et al.* (2013) Prophylactic treatment of flea-infested dogs with an imidacloprid/flumethrin collar (Seresto, Bayer) to preempt infection with *Dipylidium caninum. Parasitol Res.*, **112(Suppl. 1)**, 22–46.
Georgi, J.R. (1987) Tapeworms. *Vet Clin North Am Small Animal Pract.*, **17(6)**, 1285–1305.
Schroeder, I., Altreuther, G., Schimmel, A., *et al.* (2009) Efficacy of emodepside plus praziquantel tablets (Profender tablets for dogs) against mature and immature Cestode infections in dogs. *Parasitol Res.*, **105(Suppl. 1)**, S31–38.
Tuzer, E., Bilgin, Z., Oter, K., *et al.* (2010) Efficacy of praziquantel injectable solution against feline and canine tapeworms. *Turkiye Parazitol Derg.*, **34(1)**, 17–20.

Chapter 49: *Cheyletiella* Species (Walking Dandruff)

Description: Arthrod mite, ectoparasite, large, claw-like mouth parts
Zoonotic Potential: Can occasionally infect humans

Microbiology/epidemiology

Cheyletiella is the genus of mites that live on the skin of dogs, cats, and occasionally, humans. *C. yasguri* and *C. blakei* are the common species on cats and dogs and both can transiently affect humans. The adult mites have eight legs and hooks at the end of their palpi. Adults do not borrow under the skin but live in keratin. The mites cause a mild form of dermatitis and are often noticed by owners who report "walking dandruff", which is the mite carrying skin scales. Occasionally mites have been isolated from the nasal cavities. Adults live on the host for up to 21 days (their entire life cycle) and are only viable in the environment for 10 days. Animals acquire the infection by direct contact with another affected animal. Cheyletiellosis is highly contagious. Animals at highest risk are typically from environments where flea control is not prevalent since most flea control products eliminate the mite.

Clinical disease

Animals may present with variable symptoms. They may be asymptomatic or present with scratching, severe itching, scaling, flaky dandruff, reddened skin, small bumps, scabs, and hair loss. Nasal mites cause sneezing and scratching of the face. Lesions are typically worse on the lower back. Owners may be symptomatic as well with red, itchy bumps on the arms, trunk, or buttocks. The mites do not live on humans so symptoms typically resolve within weeks.

Diagnosis

Cheyletiella may be strongly suspected based on the signs and symptoms. Diagnosis is typically by skin scrapping of affected lesions. Combing, plucking hair or acetate tape applied to the skin can also be useful to obtain samples. Diagnosis via vacuum samples has demonstrated significant sensitivity. Mites or eggs can be seen microscopically. Eggs may also be found in stools due to self-grooming.

Treatment

Weekly use of topical pesticides or monthly spot-on therapies work well. Fipronil containing products are safe for use in cats. Due to the contagious nature of the mite, all animals in the household or kennel should be treated at the same time and environmental flea sprays should be used to decontaminate the area. In practice, treatment lasts 6–8 weeks and should continue for 2 weeks beyond clinical cure.

Drug therapy

- Fipronil
- Selamectin
- Milbemycin
- Moxidectin
- Ivermectin

Drug therapy alternatives

- Pyrethrin-based products
- Lyme sulfur

Further reading

Curtis, C.F. (2004) Current trends in the treatment of *Sarcoptes*, *Cheyletiella* and *Otodectes* mite infestations in dogs and cats. *Vet Dermatol.*, **15(2)**, 108–114.

Fisher, M.A. and Shanks D.J. (2008) A review of the off-label use of selamectin (Stronghold/Revolution) in dogs and cats. *Acta Vet Scand.*, **25**, 46.

Nolan, T.J. and Lok, J.B. (2012) Macrocyclic lactones in the treatment and control of parasitism in small companion animals. *Curr Pharm Biotechnol.*, **13(6)**, 1078–1094.

Paradis, M. and Villeneuve A. (1988) Efficacy of ivermectin against *Cheyletiella yasguri* infestation in dogs. *Can. Vet. J.*, **29(8)**, 633–635.

Saevik, B.K., Bredal, W., and Ulstein, T.L. (2004) *Cheyletiella* infestation in dogs: observations on diagnostic methods and clinical signs. *J Small Anim Pract.*, **45(10)**, 495–500.

Scarampella, F., Pollmeier, M., Visser, M., *et al.* (2005) Efficacy of fipronil in the treatment of feline *cheyletiellosis*. *Vet Parasitol.*, **129(3–4)**, 333–339.

Chapter 50: *Chlamydia* Species

Description: Gram negative, obligate intracellular bacteria, extracellular elementary body
Zoonotic Potential: Host specific, not considered a zoonotic

Microbiology/epidemiology

Chlamydia infections are found worldwide and cause infections of the ocular, respiratory, gastrointestinal, and genitourinary tract in a variety of host species. In feline patients, *C. felis* and *C. pneumonia* are primary causes of ocular disease. In dogs, *C. psittaci* and *C. abortus* have been reported in association with ocular and respiratory disease. *Chlamydia* are believed to be transmitted by direct contact with respiratory secretions and possibly by vaginal secretions and feces. Cats aged 2–12 months appear to be at highest risk. Recent reports have also found *Parachlamydia acanthamoebia* (an endosymbiont of *Acanthamoeba*) from corneal samples of cats with conjunctivitis and keratitis.

Clinical disease

Cats may present with acute or chronic conjunctivitis, chemosis, blepharospasm, serous to mucopurulent ocular discharge. Nasal discharge and sneezing may or may not be present. It may also cause reproductive disease in cats and is believed to be associated with arthritis.

Diagnosis

Diagnosis is based on culture, serology, and PCR. Culture of *Chlamydia* is difficult and may result in false negatives. Acute and convalescent titers are not widely used and may have false positives due to vaccines. PCR of conjunctival swabs, scrapings, or biopsies confirm active infection in combination with clinical signs. False positives may occur with attenuated live *Chlamydia* vaccines.

Treatment

Doxycycline is the drug of choice. At least 4 weeks of therapy are recommended. Treatment of cat colonies should be done at one time and may require longer therapy 6–8 weeks. Treatment must continue until clinical resolution for 2 weeks. For cats intolerate to doxycycline, amoxicillin/clavulanate or pradofloxacin may be given. Attenuated live vaccines for *C. felis* may be given to cats at high risk of infection (catteries). Vaccination shortens the disease course and reduces severity but does not entirely prevent infection or shedding. Fever, anorexia, lethargy, and lameness may be noted following vaccination in some cats.

Drug therapy

Doxycycline.

Drug therapy alternatives

- Amoxicillin/clavulanate
- Pradofloxacin
- Enrofloxacin

Further reading

Gruffydd-Jones, T., Addie, D., Belak, S., *et al.* (2009) *Chlamydophila felis* infection. ABCD guidelines on prevention and management. *J Feline Med Surg.*, **11**, 605–609.

Sibitz, C., Rudnay, E.C., Wabnegger, L., *et al.* (2011) Detection of *Chlamydophila* pneumonia in cats with conjunctivitis. *Vet Ophthalmol.*, **14**, 67–74.

Sprague, L.D., Schubert, E., Hotzel, H., *et al.* (2009) The detection of *Chlamydophila psittaci* genotype C infection in dogs. *Vet J.*, **181**, 274–279.

Sykes, J.E. (2013) Chlamydial infections. Ch. 33. In: *Canine and Feline Infectious Diseases*. Sykes, J.E. (ed.), Elsevier, St. Louis, MO, pp. 326–333.

Chapter 51: *Citrobacter* Species

Description: Gram negative aerobic bacteria, rod shaped *Enterobacter*
Zoonotic Potential: Colonized animals may be a source for zoonotic infection

Microbiology/epidemiology

Citrobacter primarily inhabit the gastrointestinal tract of animals and people and are ubiquitous in the environment. They are important causes of nosocomial infections in hospital patients, but rarely cause disease in otherwise healthy animals. Neonatal and immunosuppressed animals may develop enteritis with bacteremia. Puppies with parvovirus are noted to have catheter related infections due to *Citrobacter* that may result in septicemia. Cats may develop vaginitis and salpingitis. Systemic infections typically can cause multi-organ damage. A variety of species have been isolated that are pathogenic but most have similar virulence factors so that speciation is typically not required. *C. freundii, C diversus*, and *C. koseri* have all been isolated from cats and dogs. *Citrobacter* share virulence factors with other Enterobacteriacease including endotoxins. In hospitalized patients, the bacteria can colonize the urine, respiratory tract, abdominal wounds, and ulcers.

Clinical disease

Animals developing *Citrobacter* infections may develop interstitial pneumonitis, hepatitis, peritonitis, meningitis, and sepsis. Puppies may have weakness, mucohemorragic diarrhea, septicemia, myocarditis, suppurative myocarditis, and/or a diffuse, moderate, histiocytic meningitis. Immunosuppressed adults may present with focal necrotic hepatitis, fibrinous peritonitis, interstitial pneumonia, and hemorrhagic gastrointestinal disease.

Diagnosis

Asymptomatic colonization of the respiratory and urinary tract with *Citrobacter* is not uncommon. Therefore, culture results should be interpreted with clinical signs and symptoms. Culture and sensitivity are recommended due to the potential for a high level of resistance in nosocomial infections.

Treatment

Treatment is based on culture results. Empirically, third generation cephalosporins and extended spectrum penicillins may be effective, but resistance to these has also been seen clinically. Both carbapenums and fluoroquinolones may also be used.

Drug therapy

- Cephalosporins third generation
- Penicillins, Extended Spectrum

Drug therapy alternatives

- Imipenem
- Meropenem
- Fluoroquinolones

Further reading

Cassidy, J.P., Callanan, J.J., McCarthy, G., *et al.* (2002) Myocarditis in sibling boxer puppies associated with *Citrobacter koseri* infection. *Vet Pathol.*, **39(3)**, 393–395.

Ewers, C., Bethe, A., Wieler, L.H., *et al.* (2011) Companion animals: a relevant source of extended-spectrum B-lactamase-producing fluoroquinolone-resistant *Citrobacter freundii*. *Int J Antimicrob Agents.*, **37(1)**, 86–87.

Galarneau, J.R., Fortin, M., Lapointe, J.M., *et al.* (2003) *Citrobacter freundii* septicemia in two dogs. *J Vet Diagn Invest.*, **15(3)**, 297–299

Lobetti, R.G., Joubert, K.E., Picard, J., *et al.* (2002) Bacterial colonization of intravenous catheters in young dogs suspected to have parvoviral enteritis. *J Am Vet Med Assoc.*, **220(9)**, 1321–1324.

Stafford Johnson, J.M., Martin, M.W., and Stidworthy, M.F. (2003) Septic fibrinous pericarditis in a cocker spaniel. *J Small Anim Pract.*, **44(3)**, 117–120.

Chapter 52: *Clostridium Difficile*

Description: Gram positive anaerobe, spore forming organism
Zoonotic Potential: Colonization may represent a reservoir for human infection

Microbiology/epidemiology

Clostridium difficile is recognized as the most common cause of antibiotic associated colitis in the human world. In dogs, antibiotics or immunosuppressive therapy prior to hospitalization are risk factors for hospital acquired colonization. *C. difficile* can be isolated from the feces of normal and diarrheic dogs, with reported carriage rates of 0–10% in healthy dogs and 18–40% of veterinary inpatients. A carriage rate of 58% has been reported in therapy dogs that visit human hospitals. Colonization rates of 2–9% are reported in cats with a much higher rate of 9–38% being reported in veterinary inpatients. Isolates from 69% of dogs are reported as toxigenic, with genes encoding for toxins A (an enterotoxin) and B (a cytopathic toxin). Toxins cause necrosis and inflammation of intestinal cells. Despite colonization with toxin producing strains, most patients colonized with *C. difficile* do not develop diarrhea.

Clinical disease

Animals contracting *C. difficile* have a wide range of clinical signs ranging from asymptomatic carriage to fulminant colitis. Hospitalized animals receiving antibiotic therapy typically become symptomatic several days after initiating antibiotics. The most common clinical sign associated with *C. difficile* is a mild watery diarrhea. Cats typically have acute onset of watery diarrhea and anorexia. Dogs and cats may also present with vomiting, fever, and abdominal discomfort. More severe cases present with a large volume of watery diarrhea with traces of blood. These patients may also have general malaise, leukocytosis, and severe diarrhea. Severe bloody diarrhea with elevated total white blood cell count can be a clue to the diagnosis of *C. difficile*. In some cases, severe sepsis with hypotension and abdominal distention secondary to bowel perforation may be seen.

Diagnosis

A stool culture with isolation of *C. difficile* is helpful, but may be confusing since many asymptomatic carriers exist. A cytotoxin assay is the most sensitive method for detection of toxin B, but is labor intensive and expensive. An enzyme immunoassay specific for toxin B can be performed that has both high specificity and sensitivity. A thickened bowel wall and edema of the colon wall may be appreciated on radiographs, CT, or ultrasound exam. Pseudomembranous colitis or yellow inflammatory plaques may be seen endoscopically.

Treatment

C. difficile infections are typically treated by discontinuation of the offending antibiotic and initiation of either metronidazole or oral tylosin. A 10 day course of metronidazole or tylosin is typically sufficient to treat most infections. Metronidazole can also be administered rectally if needed. For non-responsive cases tylosin plus rifampin, cholestyramine, probiotics, or even enemas to lavage the bowel may be of benefit. The use of vancomycin should be reserved for metronidazole resistant organisms. Vancomycin capsules or the IV solution may be given orally. Fecal transplantation may also be curative.

Drug therapy

Metronidazole

Drug therapy alternatives

- Vancomycin
- Tylosin

Further reading

Clooten, J., Kruth, S., Arroyo, L., *et al.* (2008) Prevalence and risk factors for *Clostridium difficile* colonization in dogs and cats hospitalized in an intensive care unit. *Vet Microbiol.*, **129**, 209–214.

Marks, S.L., Kather, E.J., Kass, P.H., *et al.* (2002) Genotypic and phenotypic characterization of *Clostridium difficile* in diarrheic and healthy dogs. *J Veter Intern Med.*, **16**, 533–540.

McGowan, K.L. and Vader, H.A. (1999) *Clostridium difficile* in children. *Clin Microbio Newsletter*, **21(7)**, 49–53.

Johnson, S. and Gerding, D.N. (1998) *Clostridium difficile* associated diarrhea. *Clinical Infectious Disease*, **26(5)**, 1027–1036.

Chapter 53: *Clostridium Tetani/Botulinum*

Description: Gram positive anaerobic bacteria, sluggish motile, spore forming bacilli
Zoonotic Potential: Not considered a zoonotic

Microbiology/epidemiology

Clostridium is found worldwide and affects both dogs and cats. *C. botulinum* is rarely reported in cats and dogs and is typically only reported following ingestion of waterfowl that is infected. Botulism is typically from ingestion of type C toxin in dogs and cats. *C. tetani* is found in the soil and animal feces. It rarely causes disease in cats and only occasionally in dogs. Infection is primarily via spore contamination of wounds. Young dogs of large breeds, active, and intact male dogs are predisposed. Young, outdoor cats are also predisposed.

Clinical disease

Dogs and cats with botulism may present with ataxia, pelvic limb paresis, or quadriplegic with absent voluntary motor activity and inability to rise. Neurologic exam may show decreased cranial nerve function, decreased gag reflex, ptyalism, weak blink reflex, mucopurulent ocular discharge, and mydriasis. Segmental reflexes may be intact or absent and pain sensation remains intact. Tachypenia, tachycardia, and pneumonia may be present. Hyperthermia/hypothermia, lethargy, dehydration, and anorexia may be present. In animals with tetanus, a wound may or may not be present. Dogs typically have generalized disease, with wrinkled forehead, erect ears, retracted lips, prolapsed third eyelids, anxiety, trembling, bradycardia/tachycardia, bradyarrhythmias, stiff gait, laryngeal spasm, hypersalivation, hyperthermia, and muscle stiffness. Dogs with localized disease of the forelimb have caudal retraction of the limb and extension of the elbow and carpus. Cats may have extensor rigidity of a single limb where a wound may be identified.

Diagnosis

Diagnosis is based on clinical signs and symptoms in conjunction with history and laboratory diagnostics. *C. botulinum* toxin may be isolated in patients stool, serum, or suspected food. The toxin in feces, vomit, serum, or foodstuff can be performed by the mouse inoculation bioassay that is confirmative, but has a slow turn around. A more rapid ELISA toxin test can also be run on serum but has a low sensitivity. Electromyography (EMG) and electroneurography can help support a diagnosis of botulism. *C. tetani* is primarily diagnosed by clinical judgment and patient history. Lockjaw and weakness may be an early sign. Culture of specimens is not productive. Strychnine poisoning and rabies are differential diagnosis.

Treatment

Supportive care is the treatment for patients with botulism. Removal of contaminated food stuff by induction of vomiting or enemas may be indicated if early in the disease course. There is no specific canine or feline treatment. Equine tetanus antitoxin (100–1000 units/kg IV or IM or 500 units SC near wound site) or human tetanus immunoglobulin (500 units IM-near wound if found) may be administered after an initial intradermal test dose. Animals that react should receive diphenhydramine and/or dexamethasone prior to administration. A reduction in the infusion rate may reduce vomiting, retching and tachypnea. This is also indicated for *C. tetani* infections. Antimicrobial therapy (metronidazole) should be given for tetanus, but is not indicated for botulism. Following stabilization, wounds should be washed, debrided, and flushed with hydrogen peroxide.

Drug therapy

- Equine tetanus antitoxin (Tetanus)
- Human tetanus immune globulin (Tetanus)
- Metronidazole (Tetanus)

Drug therapy alternatives

Penicillin G (tetanus).

Further reading

Burkitt, J.M., Sturges, B.K., Jandrey, K.E., *et al.* (2007) Risk factors associated with outcome in dogs with tetanus: 38 cases (1987–2005). *J Am Vet Med Assoc.*, **230**, 76–83.

Sykes, J.E. (2013) Tetanus and botulism. Ch. 54. In: *Canine and Feline Infectious Diseases.* Sykes, J.E. (ed.), Elsevier, St. Louis, MO, pp. 520–530.

Tomek, A., Kathmann, I., Faissler, D., *et al.* (2004) Tetanus in cats: Three case descriptions. *Schweiz Arch Tierheilkd.*, **146**, 295–302.

Chapter 54: Coccidiomycosis

Description: Dimorphic fungus, branching septate hyphae
Zoonotic Potential: Considered a potential zoonotic

Microbiology/epidemiology

Coccidioides species are normal inhabitants of sandy, salty, and dry soil. It is found in both the Western hemisphere and in South and Central America. Epidemics are typically associated with physical disruption of soil (construction, dust storms, earthquakes, etc.) in endemic areas that have had a cycle of moist conditions followed by drought. *C. immitis* is typically reported in patients in the California Central Valley and *C. posadasii* is typically noted in other areas. Animals typically acquire the infection by inhalation of arthroconidia from the environment. Large breeds, young dogs, and those with outdoor exposure may have an increased risk of infection. Cats may also acquire the infection, but are typically more resistant than dogs and appear to be more predisposed to *C. posadasii*.

Clinical disease

Most infections are subclinical. Mild clinical signs with lethargy, inappetence, weight loss, and intermittent fever may be noted. Chronic cases may be associated with gagging, retching, and enlarged tracheobronchial lymph nodes. Pneumonia and septic shock may develop. Dissemination to multiple other areas may occur including the CNS, skin, peripheral lymph nodes, eyes, testes, prostate, pericardium, liver, spleen, gastrointestinal tract, urinary system, or bone.

Diagnosis

Diagnosis is based on travel history to endemic areas and consistent clinical and radiographic findings. Confirmation can be via cytologic examination of aspirates or body fluid, serology assays that detect antibodies, histopathology, and /or fungal culture.

Treatment

Treatment is typically successful with an azole. Fluconazole is the treatment of choice, particularly for CNS involvement and is typically less expensive. Itraconazole and ketoconazole have been used successfully, but are alternatives due to the cost of itraconazole and the side effects of ketoconazole. Itraconazole failures may be due to compounded drug which is typically poorly absorbed. Therapeutic monitoring is recommended here. Itraconazole commercial capsules must be given with an acidic food and the commercial solution must be given on an empty stomach. Amphotericin B, voriconazole, and posaconazole can be used for refractory disease.

Drug therapy

- Fluconazole
- Itraconazole

Drug therapy alternatives

- Ketoconazole
- Amphotericin B
- Voriconazole
- Posaconazole

Further reading

Greene, R.T. and Troy, G.C. (1995) Coccidioidomycosis in 48 cats: a retrospective study (1984–1993). *J Vet Intern Med.*, **9**, 86–91.

Shubitz, L.E., Burkiewicz, C.D., Dial, S.M., *et al.* (2005) Incidence of *Coccidioides* infection among dogs residing in a region in which the organism is endemic. *J Am Vet Med Assoc.*, **226**, 1846–1850.

Sykes, J.E. (2013) Coccidioidomycosis. Ch. 63. In: *Canine and Feline Infectious Diseases.* Sykes, J.E. (ed.), Elsevier, St. Louis, MO, pp. 613–623.

Chapter 55: *Corynebacterium* Species

Description: Gram positive aerobic or facultative anaerobic bacteria, pleomorphic bacilli or coccobacilli
Zoonotic Potential: Considered a zoonotic, reservoir for human infections

Microbiology/epidemiology

Corynebacterium are normal inhabitants of the skin, nasopharynx, gastrointestinal, and genital tract of animals. *Corynebacterium* are not considered virulent organisms and rarely invade issues. The virulence of *C.*

diphtheriae is due to its exotoxin, which acts as a potent cardiotoxin, a neurotoxin, and can produce multi-organ damage. *C. diphtheria* biotypes (nontoxin producing) have been isolated from cats with otitis media, but there has been no obvious evidence of zoonotic transmission. However, many cats have been demonstrated to harbor a toxogenic *C. ulcerans*, which has been associated with zoonotic disease in immunosuppressed humans. Cats are believed to be a reservoir of *C. ulcerans* in the UK. *C. urealyticum* is also associated with bladder infections in dogs and cats. Animals at high risk appear to be those with recurrent bladder infections from neurologic dysfunction and pelvic trauma, urological procedures, foreign bodies, bladder mucosa abnormalities, immunosuppressed states, and prior antibiotic treatment.

Clinical disease

Isolation of *Corynebacterium* does not suggest infection and may only represent colonization. Most infections in dogs and cats with *Corynebacterium* involve bladder infections. Although rare, these infections are often difficult to treat. Animals typically present with hematuria, stranguria, pollakiuria, and urinary incontinence. The urine is alkaline >8.0 with struvite crystals, pyuria, and bacteriuria. *C. ulcerans* has been reported to cause pneumonia, systemic infections, and intracranial abscesses in dogs.

Diagnosis

Culture and sensitivity are diagnostic. Persistent bacteria with alkaline urine and struvite crystalluria in the face of antimicrobial administration should raise the suspicion for *Corynebacterium* infection. Ultrasound may demonstrate encrusting cystitis with variable echotexture and shape during ultrasonography, appearing as sediment along the mucosal surface that does not move as the patient is rotated. The bladder may also have adherent bladder mucosal plaques.

Treatment

C. urealyticum infections are often resistant to penicillins, amoxicillin/clavulanate, and fluoroquinolones. Tetracyclines, macrolides, or glycopeptide antimicrobials have been used successfully in humans for *C. urealyticum* bladder infections but treatment should be based primarily on sensitivity reports. Debridement of plaques surgically and acidification of urine along with antimicrobials is recommended. Isolates from ear infections have also shown sensitivity to chloramphenicol, doxycycline, and amikacin with moderate susceptibility to aminoglycosides and enrofloxacin.

Drug therapy

- Doxycycline
- Chloramphenicol

Drug therapy alternatives

- Vancomycin IV
- Gentamicin Otic
- Enrofloxacin Otic

Further reading

Bailiff, N.L., Westropp, J.L., Jang, S.S., *et al.* (2005) *Corynebacterium urealyticum* urinary tract infection in dogs and cats: 7 cases (1996–2003). *J Am Vet Med Assoc.*, **15:226(10)**, 1676–1680.

Bilderback, A.L. and Faissler D. (2009) Surgical management of a canine intracranial abscess due to a bite wound. *J Vet Emerg Crit Care.*, **19(5)**, 507–512.

Cavana, P., Zanatta, R., Nebbia, P., *et al.* (2008) *Corynebacterium urealyticum* urinary tract infection in a cat with urethral obstruction. *J Feline Med Surg.*, **10(3)**, 269–273.

Henneveld, K., Rosychuk, R.A., Olea-Popelka, F.J., *et al.* (2012) *Corynebacterium* spp. In dogs and cats with otitis externa and/or media: a retrospective study. *J Am Anim Hosp Assoc.*, **48(5)**, 320–326.

Sykes, J.E., Mapes, S., Lindsay, L.L., *et al.* (2010) *Corynebacterium ulcerans* bronchopneumonia in a dog. *J Vet Intern Med.*, **24(4)**, 973–976.

Chapter 56: *Coxiellosis* Species (Q Fever)

Description: Gram negative coccobacillus, obligate intracellular, spore forms
Zoonotic Potential: Considered a significant zoonotic reservoir to humans

Microbiology/epidemiology

Coxiellosis burnrtii is the organism responsible for Q fever in humans. Although not a significant disease in cats and dogs, its zoonotic potential to veterinarians and other animal handlers is extreme. The bacteria are found worldwide with reservoirs noted in cattle, goats, sheep, ticks, and potentially cats. Transmission is typically via inhalation of organisms or contact with infected tissues or fluids (predation, unpasteurized milk, exposure to infected animals). High bacterial loads may be found in vaginal secretions, milk, saliva, urine, and feces. Animals in rural areas are pre-disposed. Animals or humans with exposure to placental contents (C-sections, necropsies, etc.), particularly from cats or cattle are at extremely high risk. Incubation post-exposure is from 9 days to 4 weeks.

Clinical disease

The infection is typically subclinical in cats and dogs, although they may demonstrate reproductive disorders (premature birth, abortion, stillbirths, prolonged vaginal bleeding). Humans are the only mammals that develop significant disease (fever, pneumonia, hepatitis, endocarditis, neurologic signs, osteomyelitis).

Diagnosis

Cell culture, histopathology, serology and PCR are all diagnostic. Cell culture requires specialized facilities. Placental materials may be submitted for immunohistochemistry and fluorescence *in situ* hybridization. Serology (acute and convalescent) may be performed but seroconversion may not occur for up to one month. PCR can be performed on whole blood, tissue, vaginal swabs, milk, and feces in acute infections.

Treatment

Doxycycline is the drug of choice (2–3 weeks). Azithromycin for 3–5 days or fluoroquinolones have also been used. For endocarditis, combination therapy is recommended (doxycycline, ciprofloxacin, and rifampin) for prolonged periods (up to 2 years).

Drug therapy

- Doxycycline
- Azithromycin
- Fluoroquinolones

Drug therapy alternatives

- Chloramphenicol
- Rifampin

Further reading

Angelakis, E. and Raoult, D. (2010) Q fever. *Vet Microbiol.*, **140**, 297–309.

Cairn, K., Brewer, M., and Lappin, M.R. (2007) Prevalence of *Coxiella burnetti* DNA in vaginal and uterine samples from healthy cats of north central Colorado. *J Feline Med Surg.*, **9**, 201.

Komiya, T., Sudamasu, K., Kang, M.I., *et al.* (2003) Seroprevalence of *Coxiella burnetii* infections among cats in different living environments. *J Vet Med Sci.*, **65**, 1047–1048.

Sykes, J.E. and Norris, J.M. (2013) Coxiellosis and Q fever. Ch. 32. In: *Canine and Feline Infectious Diseases.* Sykes, J.E. (ed.), Elsevier, St. Louis, MO, pp. 320–325.

Chapter 57: *Cryptococcus* Species

Description: Dimorphic, round, oval, encapsulated yeast
Zoonotic Potential: Environmental, not considered a zoonotic

Microbiology/epidemiology

Cryptococcus is found worldwide and may concentrate in soil under Eucalyptus trees or areas contaminated with bird feces. Endemic areas include tropical and subtropical environments. Animals acquire the infection by inhalation of the basidiospores producing colonization of the airways. There are 19 different species of *Cryptococcus*. Only a few cause disease in cats and dogs (*C. neoformans, C. gatti*). Young adult cats and dogs appear to have the highest incidence. Animals with immune suppression, malignancy, or on immunosuppressive drugs may have increased risk of infection. Disseminated infections typically occur in immunosuppressed people and most likely in animals with underlying immunodeficiency.

Clinical disease

Animals may not develop symptoms until 2–13 months after exposure. Cats may present with significant lethargy, inappetence, low grade fever, and upper respiratory signs (sneezing, mucopurulent or hemorrhagic nasal discharge, subcutaneous swelling over the bridge of the nose). Single or multiple ulcerated or non-ulcerative cutaneous lesions of the buccal mucosa may be present. With severe disease, lymphadenopathy, tachypnea, bilateral mydriasis, optic neuritis, chorioretinitis, retinal detachment, skin lesions, osteomyelitis, arthritis, swollen digits, and neurologic signs (ataxia, seizures, head tilt, nystagmus, etc.) may be present. In dogs, weight loss, lethargy, inappetence, and neurologic signs are very common. Dogs may also show signs of gastrointestinal or pancreatic involvement and often present with severe disease.

Diagnosis

Diagnosis is based on cytology, culture, or histopathology with or without cryptococcal antigen detection in body fluids. CSF fluid typically has an elevated protein concentration and visible yeasts. However, CSF taps carry a risk of cerebellar herniation. Serum antigen testing or samples from other sites are preferred. CT, MRI, and ultrasound may demonstrate mass lesions and osteomyelitis.

Treatment

Cats may demonstrate improvement in 1–2 weeks after starting therapy. For localized disease, oral fluconazole may be given until antigen titers are negative. This may take 2–12 months. With severe disease, supportive care (steroids, fluids, tube feeding, anticonvulsant medications) may be required. Cats with severe disease may have induction therapy with amphotericin B and flucytosine and then maintenance therapy with fluconazole. Dogs should not receive 5-flucytosine but can be given amphotericin B with fluconazole or terbinafine for disseminated disease. If CNS disease is present liposomal amphotericin B or voriconazole can be given due to increased drug penetration into the CNS. Fluconazole penetrates into the CNS but itraconazole penetrates poorly.

Drug therapy

- Fluconazole
- Amphotericin B
- 5-Flucytosine (cats only)

Drug therapy alternatives

- Itraconazole
- Voriconazole

Further reading

Datta, K., Bartlett, K.H., Baer, R., *et al.* (2009) Spread of *Cryptococcus gatti* into Pacific Northwest region of the United States. *Emerg Infect Dis.*, **15**, 1185–1191.

Sykes, J.E. and Malik, R. (2013) Cryptococcosis. Ch. 62. In: *Canine and Feline Infectious Diseases*. Sykes, J.E. (ed.), Elsevier, St. Louis, MO, pp. 599–612.

Trivedi, S.R., Malik, R., Meyer, W., *et al.* (2011) Feline *Cryptococcus* impact of current research on management. *J Feline Med Surg.*, **13**, 163–172.

Chapter 58: *Cryptosporidium* Species

Description: Coccidian protozoan parasite, small yeast-like, four spore oocysts, merozoites
Zoonotic Potential: Potential for zoonosis in immunosuppressed patients

Microbiology/epidemiology

Cryptosporidium are found worldwide and are primarily found in the gastrointestinal tract. *C. felis* is reported in cats and *C. canis* has been isolated in dogs. Other species have also been identified in dogs and cats (*C. parvum, C. muris*). The incidence is as high as 29.4% of cats and 15.1 % of dogs with diarrhea. Animals acquire the infection via oral–fecal routes. Oocysts are passed in feces and are ingested via grooming, shared litter boxes, hunting, or contaminated food or water. Once ingested, oocycts develop in the intestine with release of sporozoites. Colonization does not imply illness and many animals shedding *Cryptospordium* do not have diarrhea. Animals at risk of developing diarrhea are typically those that are young or immunosuppressed due to lymphoma, FeLV, parvovirus, or distemper virus.

Clinical disease

Diarrhea is typically watery, without mucus or blood, and is typically described as small bowel diarrhea. Clinical signs are typically more severe in cats. Small intestines may be slightly thickened. Co-infection with Giardia or *T. foetus* may worsen symptoms.

Diagnosis

Diagnosis is based on fecal examination, either cytologic-modified acid-fast staining of a thin fecal smear or flotation. Immunofluorescent antibody assays (IFA) on feces and PCR are also available. IFA is considered the gold standard if available.

Treatment

Treatment may not be required for asymptomatic animals since the disease may be self-limiting. A highly digestible diet and probiotics may be beneficial in some animals. For more severe infections a variety of drugs have been used, but no large trials have been performed for this disease state. Azithromycin (10 mg/kg PO q24 h × 5–7 days), nitazoxanide (10–25 mg/kg PO q12 h × 7 days with food), and tylosin (10–15 mg/kg PO q12 h × 14 days in capsules for cats) have all been shown to be effective treatment. The goal of therapy is resolution of diarrhea since no treatment has consistently eliminated the organisms.

Drug therapy

- Azithromycin
- Nitazoxanide
- Tylosin

Drug therapy alternatives

- Probiotics
- Highly digestible diet

Further reading

Fayer, R., Trout, J., Xiao, L., *et al.* (2001) *Cryptosporidium canis. sp.* from domestic dogs. *J Parasit.*, **87**, 1415–1422.

Lappin, M.R. (2013) Cryptosporidiosis. Ch. 81. In: *Canine and Feline Infectious Diseases*. Sykes, J.E. (ed.), Elsevier, St. Louis, MO, pp. 785–792.

Scorza, V. and Tangtrongsup, S. (2010) Update on the diagnosis and management of *Cryptosporidium spp.* infections in dogs and cats. *Top Compan Anim Med.*, **25**, 163–169.

Chapter 59: *Ctenocephalides* Species (Fleas)

Description: Arthropod insects, ectoparasites, wingless, hard, flat bodies
Zoonotic Potential: May bite humans and are vectors of human disease

Microbiology/epidemiology

The dog flea (*C. canis*) and the cat flea (*C. felis*) are ectoparasites found worldwide. *C. felis* is typically more prevalent than *C. canis*. *Ctenocephalides* adult females live and feed on the blood of mammals. In the process they transmit a variety of important disease causing agents including *D. caninum*, *B. henselae*, and *Rickettsia* as well as others. Fleas can live without food for up to 60 days but must feed prior to laying eggs. Many eggs are laid (4000) onto the hosts fur where they develop over 2–3 weeks through four stages (embryo, larva, pupa, and adult).

Clinical disease

Flea infestations in cats and dogs may present as slight to severe itching. Animals may bite, scratch, and lick areas that are infested. Flea infestation in dogs typically results in chewing of the abdomen/medial surface of the thigh and radius/carpus/tibia and tarsus while flea bite hypersensitivity results in chewing of the tail and back/dorsolumber area. This differs from atopic dermatitis where dogs typically chew and lick their paws and rub areas of their face and neck. Heavy flea infestations may cause anemia, particularly in young animals. Flea bite allergy due to the fleas' saliva may present as compulsive itching, skin irritation, hair loss, and secondary skin infections.

Diagnosis

Adult fleas can easily be seen on the animal's skin. Flea combs can also be used to demonstrate adults. The fur can also be parted in areas where fleas concentrate (base of the ears, above the tail). Small black specks of "flea dirt" (feces) may be noted. If these are placed onto a damp white tissue a red halo will be noted to discriminate "flea dirt" from dirt.

Treatment

Drugs therapies can target the adult flea, the eggs, or the larvae. Multiple agents are available. Flea-control products are available in an oral tablet, once-a-month topical spot-ons, dog collars, sprays, dips, powders, shampoos, and injectables. A combination of these is preferred as well as environmental control of fleas. Effective flea control must target the fleas in both indoor and outdoor environments. Powders, sprays, foggers containing insecticides or growth promoters are effective. For single animal households with animals with indoor/outdoor exposure an adulticide with a larvidal and ovicidal activity is recommended (examples: selamectin, fipronil, imidacloprid). For allergic animals, nitenpyram or spinosad with a growth inhibitor (lufenuron, etc.) are recommended. This reduces the flea feeding time and rapidly kills fleas.

Drug therapy

- Nitenpyram
- Imidacloprid/Moxidectin
- Imidacloprid/pyriproxyfen
- Selamectin
- Fipronil/S-methoprene
- Spinosad
- Spinosad/Milbemycin

Drug therapy alternatives

- Amitraz Collar (Not cats)
- Permethrin (Not cats)

Further reading

Bruet, V., Bourdeau, P.J., Roussel, A., *et al.* (2012) Characterization of pruritus in canine atopic dermatitis, flea bite hypersensitivity and flea infestation and its role in diagnosis. *Vet Dermatol.*, **23(6)**, 487–491.

Foil, L., Andress, E., Freeland, R.L., *et al.* (1998) Experimental infection of domestic cats with *Bartonella henselae* by inoculation of *Ctenocephalides felis* (*Siphonaptera: Pulicidae*) feces. *J Med Entomol.*, **35**, 625–628.

Hirunkanokpun, S., Thepparit, C., Foil, L.D., *et al.* (2011) Horizontal transmission of *Rickettsia felis* between cat fleas: *Ctenocephalides felis. Mol Ecol.*, **20**, 4577–4586.

Marchiondo, A.A., Holdsworth, P.A., Fourie, L.J., *et al.* (2013) World Association for the Advancement of Veterinary Parasitology (WAAVP) 2nd edn. Guidelines for evaluating the efficacy of parasiticides for the treatment, prevention and control of flea and tick infestations on dogs and cats. *Vet Parasitol.*, **194(1)**, 84–97.

Chapter 60: *Cuterebra* Species (Botfly Larvae)

Description: Parasitic fly larvae "bots"
Zoonotic Potential: Does not pose a health risk to humans

Microbiology/epidemiology

There are at least 34 species of *Cuterebra* in North America alone. The subgenus *Cuterebra* and *Trypoderma* comprise the species that have obligatory parasitic larvae in rodents and lagomorphs but may accidentally infect cats and dogs. Adult flies live only a few weeks, during which they mate and lay eggs. Eggs are laid along trails where rodents or rabbits pass. Eggs hatch with increases in temperature and first star larvae move onto the animals fur finding entry through any natural opening (nose, mouth, eyes, anus, vulva). They then migrate through the tissues (soft palate, trachea, abdominal cavity) and deposit into subcutaneous tissues. The larvae grow and form a pore from which they will hatch within 3–6 weeks. The mature bot larva emerges and burrows into the soil where it becomes an adult fly. Cats and dogs with access to outdoor areas where infected rodents and rabbits are present are at risk.

Clinical disease

Cats and dogs may demonstrate a variety of clinical symptoms depending on where the larvae migrate (skin, eyes, nose, respiratory tract, brain, etc.). The most common presentation in cats and dogs are subcutaneous cysts (2–4 mm) that may form around the face or neck. These typically have an opening that is well defined with serous drainage. Localized larvae typically do not cause significant disease in animals. Larvae that migrate into deeper tissues may cause respiratory distress and neurologic signs. Respiratory symptoms (sneezing, nasal discharge, unilateral facial swellings, dyspnea, bloody nasal discharge, soft palate/pharyngeal swelling) are often noted 1–2 weeks prior to CNS disease in cats. Cats may be more predisposed to larval migration into the CNS where it can cause feline ischemic encephalopathy. Clinical signs may vary from acute onset of status epilepticus to multiple signs including head tilt, unilateral, or bilateral central blindness, head pressing, cognitive dysfunction, continuous vocalization, proprioceptive deficits, circling, or severely depressed mentation. Animals demonstrating acute disease typically have rapidly progressive disease, which is often fatal. Rarely larvae have entered into the anterior chamber of the eye or the globe resulting in chemosis, blepharospasm, ocular discharge, uveitis, and blindness.

Diagnosis

Localized infections are easily diagnosed due to the distinctive subcutaneous cysts containing a developing bot. Respiratory and neurologic infections are more difficult to diagnose. Acute symptoms of respiratory disease (unilateral nasal discharge, nasal/facial swelling) or acute onset of neurologic signs following respiratory symptoms (1–2 weeks) along with eosinophilia may be suggestive. MRI and CAT scans may be diagnostic of CNS disease. Evaluation of the pharynx, larynx, and nasal passages under anesthesia may demonstrate larvae. An enzyme-linked immunosorbent assay has been developed but may not be accurate in acute CNS disease where IgG may not be present in sufficient quantities.

Treatment

Local subcutaneous bots can be removed by surgical excision or by expanding the cyst opening with forceps and carefully removing the bot without crushing it. Surgical excision of anterior chamber larva has also been accomplished with preservation of vision. Ivermectin (0.1–0.3 mg/kg) has been used to treat migrating larvae. The prognosis for cats with CNS disease is poor, but treatment of respiratory disease with ivermectin and steroids may be effective. CNS disease has been treated successfully in a dog with ivermectin, anticonvusants, antihistamines, and a tapering dose of steroids. Topical insecticides (fipronil, imidacloprid) may be of some value as a preventative.

Drug therapy

Ivermectin.

Drug therapy alternatives

- Steroids
- Antihistamines
- Anticonvulsants (CNS disease)

Further reading

Crumley, W.R., Rankin, A.J., and Dryden, M.W. (2011) Ophthalmomyiasis externa in a puppy due to *Cuterebra* infestation. *J Am Anim Hosp Assoc.*, **47(6)**, 150–155.

Glass, E.N., Cornetta, A.M., DeLahunta, A., *et al.* (1998) Clinical and clinicopathologic features in 11 cats with *Cuterebra* larvae myiasis of the central nervous system. *J Vet Int Med.*, **2**, 365–368.

Stiles, J. and Rankin, A. (2006) Ophthalmomyiasis interna anterior in a canine: surgical resolution. *Vet Ophthalmol.*, **9(3)**, 165–168.

Thawley, V.J., Suran, J.N., and Boller, E.M. (2013) Presumptive central nervous system cuterebriasis and concurrent protein-losing nephropathy in a dog. *J Vet Emerg Crit Care.*, **23(3)**, 335–339.

Tieber, L.M., Axlund, T.W., Simpson, S.T., *et al.* (2006) Survival of a suspected case of central nervous system cuterebrosis in a dog: clinical and magnetic resonance imaging findings. *J Am Anim Hosp Assoc.*, **42**, 238–242.

Williams, K.J., Summers, B.A., and de Lahunta, A. (1998) Cerebrospinal cuterebriasis in cats and its association with feline ischemic encephalopathy. *Vet Pathol.*, **35**, 330–343.

Chapter 61: *Cytauxzoon Felis*

Description: Apicomplexan, hemoprotozoan, erythrocytic piroplasma and non-erythrocytic schizont forms
Zoonotic Potential: Host specific, not known to infect humans

Microbiology/epidemiology

Cytauxzoon felis is a tick borne life threatening infection of wild and domestic cats. It is not believed to infect dogs or other mammals. The disease is transmitted by *A. americanum* (Lone star tick) and *D. variabilis* (American dog tick). Symptoms occur approximately 2 weeks after initial infection. Outdoor cats that have exposure to wooded or rural areas are predisposed. Bobcats are reported to be the primary reservoir. Infections have primarily been reported throughout the South Central, South East, and Mid-Atlantic States of the USA. The prognosis is typically poor in symptomatic cats with only 60% surviving after aggressive treatment. Asymptomatic carriers have also been reported.

Clinical disease

Cats typically present acutely with lethargy, anorexia, vocalization, elevated nictitans, anemia, dyspnea, tachypenia, icterus, and fever. Fevers of >104° F (40°C) are common. As the infection progresses, pallor, tachycardia, tachypnea, cardiac murmurs, and hypothermia may occur. Schizont-distended mononuclear cells may also occlude small veins of the liver, lung, spleen, and lymph node. Tissue hypoxia, inflammation, DTIC, splenomegaly, hepatomegaly, lymphadenomegaly, pleural effusion, sepsis, hemolysis, hemolytic anemia, and seizures may occur.

Diagnosis

Whole blood PCR is the most sensitive diagnostic test for Cytauxzoonosis. A CBC may demonstrate pancytopenia, bicytopenia, and a characteristic signet ring intraerythrocytic inclusion. Neutropenia, lymphopenia, thrombocytopenia, and non-regenerative anemia are also observed.

Treatment

Cats are typically extremely ill and require significant supportive care. Cats often die within a day of presentation unless aggressive anti-protozoal and supportive therapy is initiated. Crystalloid fluids, antipyretics, and analgesics (buprenorphine) are typically administered. Whole blood or packed RBC transfusion may be required. Subcutaneous heparin (200 u/kg q8 h) is recommended by some. Placement of a feeding tube allows for easy administration of oral drugs and nutrients. Atovaquone (15 mg/kg PO q8 h × 10 days) with azithromycin (10 mg/kg PO q24 h × 10 days) results in 60% survival rates. Atovaquone is expensive but may be purchased via compounding pharmacies. Successfully treated cats should wear flumethrin-impregnated collars and be kept indoors to avoid tick exposure. Reinfection and transmission to other cats via ticks by carrier cats should be avoided.

Drug therapy

Atovaquone with azithromycin.

Further reading

Brown, H.M., Berghaus, R.D., Latimer, K.S., *et al.* (2010) Identification and genetic characterization of *Cytauxzoon felis* in asymptomatic domestic cats and bobcats. *Vet Parasit.*, **172**, 311–316.

Cohn, L.A. (2013) Cytauxzoonosis. Ch. 76. In: *Canine and Feline Infectious Diseases*. Sykes, J.E. (ed.), Elsevier, St. Louis, MO, pp. 739–746.

Cohn, L.A, Birkenheuer, A.J., Brunker, J.D., *et al.* (2011) Efficacy of atovaquone and azithromycin or imidocarb dipropionate in cats with acute *cytauxzoonosis. J Vet Intern Med.*, **25**, 55–60.

Chapter 62: Dematiaceous Fungi (*Phaeohypomycosis, Chromoblastomycosis*)

Description: Darkly pigmented, brown/black molds
Zoonotic Potential: Not documented, but may have potential for transmission in immunosuppressed humans

Microbiology/epidemiology

Dematiaceous molds are found throughout the environment in soil, wood, and decomposing vegetation. Soils from indoor plants may serve as reservoirs of conidia. This large group of molds is responsible for a wide range of diseases including Phaeohyphomycosis, Chromoblastomycosis, and eumycotic mycetoma. Chromoblastomycosis is typically a cutaneous or subcutaneous infection characterized by epidermal hyperplasia, microabscesses, and granulomatous inflammation. Phaeohyphomycosis in veterinary patients have been reported from a variety of Genera (*Alternaria, Bipolaris, Cladophialophora, Curvularia, Exophiala, Moniliella, Phialophora, Cladophialophora*, etc.). Most animals acquire infection via inoculation by traumatic implantation or inhalation causing invasive or allergic sinusitis. Disseminated infections are uncommon but may occur in immunosuppressed animals. Animals on long term immunosuppressive drugs (cyclosporine) may be at increased risk.

Clinical disease

Cats and dogs that are immunocompetent typically present with local lesions. Lesions may be on the digits, pinnae, nasal planum or nasal cavity. Lesions may progress locally or may disseminate to local lymph nodes or the respiratory tract. Lesions may appear as solitary cysts, with well-encapsulated subcutaneous granuloma with necrosis. Nasal lesions may appear as dark masses that may be confused for melanomas. Animals with CNS disease may present with obtundation, seizures, abnormal placing reactions, circling, tremors, ataxia, and abnormal cranial nerve function.

Diagnosis

Histopathology samples must be stained with melanin-specific stains (Fontanna–Masson). Culture of tissue or fine needle aspirates with identification of the mold is the gold standard for diagnosis.

Treatment

Aggressive surgical resection with wide margins is the treatment of choice for local infections. Digit amputation may be required for lesions of the distal phalanx. Medical therapy with itraconazole, voriconazole, or posaconazole is recommended post-surgically for up to 6 months (due to the high rate of recurrences) or for 10–12 months for peritonitis or intracranial disease.

Amphotericin B lipid complex with flucytosine and an azole may be effective therapy. Dogs should not receive flucytosine. Discontinuation of immunosuppressive drugs is necessary to achieve clinical response.

Drug therapy

- Itraconazole
- Posaconazole
- Voriconazole

Drug therapy alternatives

- Amphotericin B lipid complex
- Flucytosine (cats only)
- Fluconazole

Further reading

Grooters, A.M. (2013) Miscellaneous fungal diseases. Ch. 68. In: *Canine and Feline Infectious Diseases*. Sykes, J.E. (ed.), Elsevier, St. Louis, MO, pp. 660–667.

Grooters, A.M. and Foil, C.S. (2012) Miscellaneous fungal infections. Ch. 65. In: *Infectious Diseases of the Dog and Cat*. Greene, C.E. (ed.), 4th edn. WB Saunders, Philadelphia, PA, pp. 675–688.

Naggie, S. and Perfect, J.R. (2009) Molds: *Hyalohyphomycosis, Phaeohyphomycosis* and *Zygomycosis*. *Clin Chest Med.*, **30**, 337–353.

Chapter 63: *Demodex Canis/Felis* (Red Mange)

Description: Demodicidae mites
Zoonotic Potential: No zoonotic potential due to host specificity

Microbiology/epidemiology

Demodicosis is caused by overpopulation of *Demodex* mites when the animal's immune system is unable to keep the mites under control. *D. canis* is found in dogs and *D. felis* or *D. gatoi* is associated with feline demodectic mange. Mites are transmitted to puppies or kittens from their mothers after birth during nursing. Mites live normally in the hair follicles and are typically found on the face and other areas of the body. Animals with a weakened immune system from underdevelopment, stress, malnutrition, or breed disposition are more susceptible to mite overgrowth and symptoms. Young puppies are at highest risk and may have mild symptoms of irritation to severe widespread inflammation with secondary bacterial infections. Feline demodicosis is a rare skin infection. *D. gatoi* is a contagious, transmissible, superficial demodicosis that is typically pruritic and can be generalized. The generalized form is often associated with an underlying immunosuppressive or metabolic disease such as feline leukemia virus infection, feline immunodeficiency virus infection, diabetes mellitus, or neoplasia.

Clinical disease

Animals may present with localized or generalized disease. Dogs <2 years of age typically have focal alopecia, erythema, redness, scaling, hair loss, comedones, and/or hyperpigmentation. Focal lesions are typically around the eyes, corners of the mouth, forelimbs, and paws. A small percentage of these cases may advance to a more diffuse or generalized form of disease. Secondary bacterial infections, fever, lethargy, generalized lymphadenopathy, deep folliculitis, furunculosis, or cellulitis may occur. Pododermatitis is common. In feline demodectosis, there are one or several areas of focal alopecia (head, neck, face). In generalized disease, alopecia, crusting, ceruminous otitis externa, and secondary pyoderma of the whole body may be noted.

Diagnosis

Diagnosis is typically accomplished by deep skin scrapings or hair plucking, which reveals mites, eggs, and larval forms. Acetate tape impression has recently been found to be a more sensitive method. This may be more challenging in feline demodectosis where mites and eggs are in smaller numbers. Dermatophyte cultures are also recommended, because dermatophytosis and demodicosis can be concomitant conditions.

Treatment

Small localized areas of demodicosis may resolve without treatment as the animal's immune system matures, although treatment is still recommended. Goodwinol, a rotenone-based insecticide ointment can be administered. Treatment is required in cases of diffuse localized demodicosis. For generalized demodicosis, the prognosis is often guarded. Hair clipping and body cleansing with shampoo (benzoyl peroxide) may be helpful. Whole-body amitraz dips (0.025%) applied every 2 weeks along with a systemic macrocyclic lactone is advised. Milbemycin (0.5–1 mg/kg PO q24 h)

and moxidectin/imidacloprid (topically 2–4 times every 4 weeks) are considered effective and safe. For refractory cases, ivermectin or moxidectin with slowly escalating doses and monitoring for toxicities is recommended. This is contraindicated in a number of breeds including collies and other herding breeds. Antiparasitics should be given until clinical signs resolve and two negative skin scrapings are obtained 1 month apart (typically 4–6 months). Antibacterials should be administered to animals with pyoderma. In cats, weekly lime-sulfur dips (2% or 4oz:1 Gallon) for 4–6 weeks are safe and usually effective. Imidacloprid/moxidectin applied topically every 2 weeks for 3–4 months is also effective. Amitraz (0.0125–0.025%) has been used, but can cause anorexia, depression, and diarrhea in cats. Dogs and cats should be spayed or neutered to prevent stress that may cause disease recurrence and lessen the chance of passing on inherited immunodeficiency traits.

Drug therapy

- Goodwinol (topical)
- Amitraz dip
- Milbemycin
- Moxidectin
- Moxidectin/Imidacloprid
- Ivermectin

Drug therapy alternatives

- Hydrogen peroxide shampoo
- Lyme sulfur dip 2% (cats)

Further reading

Baima, B. and Sticherling, M. (2002) Demodicidosis revisited. *Acta Dermato-Venereol.*, **82(1)**, 3–6.

Beale, K. (2012) Feline demodicosis: a consideration in the itchy or overgrooming cat. *J Fel Med Surg.*, **14(3)**, 209–213.

Hsu, C.K., Hsu, M.L., Lee, J.Y., *et al.* (2009) Demodicosis: A clinicopathological study. *J Amer Acad Dermatol.*, **60(3)**, 453–462.

Mueller, R.S. (2012) An update on the therapy of canine demodicosis. *Comp. Contin Educ Vet.*, **34(4)**, 1–4.

Chapter 64: Dermatophytosis

Description: Keratophilic fungi, zoophilic
Zoonotic Potential: Zoonotic potential for young and immunocompromised humans

Microbiology/epidemiology

Superficial cutaneous infections caused by dermatophytes are typically due to *Microsporum*, *Trichophyton*, and *Epidermophyton* species. Animals typically become infected via contact with other infected animals or through contact with contaminated fomites. *M. gypseum* is a geophilic dermatophyte grown in warm, humid environments. *Microsporum canis* is a zoophilic dermatophyte that is responsible for the majority (90%) of feline and canine (60%) dermatophyte infections. *Trichophyton mentgrophytes* are zoophilic dermatophytes adapted to rodents and hedgehogs but also infect cats and dogs. Young or immunosuppressed animals and shelter animals have a higher predisposition. Persian and Himalayan cats as well as Yorkshire and Jack Russell terriers appear predisposed.

Clinical disease

The disease severity is based on the fungal strain and host response. Pathogenic dermatophytes typically invade traumatized tissues. Incubation typically is 1–3 weeks. Lesions may be single or multiple with circular regions of alopecia and an erythematous margin. Scaling, crusting, follicular papules, pustules, and hyperpigmentation may occur. *T. mentagrophytes* may present with progressive alopecia. Longhaired cats and dogs may develop a poor hair coat, increased shedding and mycetomas with draining purulent fluid. Dogs have lesions on the face, limbs, tail, or erythematous areas of the ungula fold, deformity and friability of the claw or footpad. Cats may present with alopecia lesions with scale and crust of the pinnae, nose, limbs, or tail. They may also have mycetomas that are nodular or ulcerative on the dorsum or neck.

Diagnosis

Diagnosis is via Wood's lamp, cytology, culture, or histopathology. Culture of plucked hair is the preferred diagnostic technique. Wood's lamp has low sensitivity and false positives and negatives.

Treatment

Healthy animals may clear the infection without treatment in 2–3 months. Treatment is recommended in multi-animal households or in animals with immunocompromised household members. Multiple antifungals may be used. All animals with positive cultures should be treated with systemic and topical therapy. Culture negative animals in an infected household should be treated with topical therapy (lime sulfur 237 mL in 3.6 L water). Miconazole/chlorhexidine shampoos are also an alternative. Clipping (disinfected clippers, 10% bleach) of long haired animals may improve treatment outcome. All surfaces, bedding, bowls, blankets, leashes, collars, carpet must be washed, steam dried, and so on, otherwise they will be a source of recontamination. Bleach solution (1:10), 0.2% enilconazole solution, or accelerated hydrogen peroxide solutions can be used for environmental decontamination. Two to three months of treatment are typically required. Treatment should continue until two successive cultures are negative.

Drug therapy

- Lime sulfur (1:16) topical wash
- Itraconazole

Drug therapy alternatives

- Miconazole/chlorhexidine shampoo
- Fluconazole
- Ketoconazole
- Terbinafine
- Griseofulvin

Further reading

Chermette, R., Ferreiro, L., and Guillot, J. (2008) Dermatophtosis in animals. *Mycopathologia.*, **166**, 385–405.

Moriello, K.A. (2004) Treatment of dermatophytosis in dogs and cats: review of published studies. *Vet Dermatol.*, **15**, 99–107.

Sykes, J.E. and Outerbridge, C.A. (2013) Dermatophytosis. Ch. 58. In: *Canine and Feline Infectious Diseases.* Sykes, J.E. (ed.), Elsevier, St. Louis, MO, pp. 558–569.

Chapter 65: *Dipylidium Caninum* (Flea Tapeworm)

Description: Cyclophyllid cestode endoparasite, gravid proglottids, adult worms are 45 cm/18 inches
Zoonotic Potential: Can infect humans, especially young children and infants

Microbiology/epidemiology

The flea tapeworm is found worldwide and infects animals afflicted by fleas or chewing lice. Dogs, cats, and other mammals including humans may become infected. The adult worms live in the intestine of animals and pass gravid proglottids containing the eggs into the feces. Flea larvae are the intermediate host that ingests the eggs. They pupate and transform into adult fleas that are then ingested by dogs or cats during grooming. These may also be inadvertently swallowed by children in flea infested environments resulting in restlessness and diarrhea.

Clinical disease

Tapeworm infection usually does not cause pathology in the dog or cat. However, this may depend on the degree of infection, breed of host, age, and other underlying conditions. Animals with heavy burdens may present with lethargy, malaise, irritability, poor appetite, poor hair coat, diarrhea, colic, weight loss, and rarely seizures.

Diagnosis

Diagnosis is based on stool examination for proglottids or eggs. Small white-tan colored "rice-like" grains (proglottids) can be seen on fresh stool samples or sometimes around the anus. Fecal flotation may have false negatives due to the fact that the eggs are heavy and do not float.

Treatment

The best way to prevent infection is to treat animals regularly for fleas and lice. Flea collars containing imidacloprid/flumethrin have been demonstrated to be highly effective at reducing flea and *D. canuinum* infestations. As with most tapeworm infections, the drugs of choice are praziquantel or epsiprantel. Most products are highly effective so that 1–2 treatments are typically effective. Prazaquantel is approved for *D. caninum* in both dogs and cats.

Drug therapy

• Prazaquantel
• Emodepside/praziquantel topical

Drug therapy alternatives

Imidacloprid/flumethrin flea collar.

Further reading

Charles, S.D., Altreuther, G., Reinemeyer, C.R., *et al.* (2005) Evaluation of the efficacy of emodepside/praziquantel topical solution against cestode (*Dipylidium caninum, Taenia taeniaeformis,* and *Echinococcus multicularis*) infections in cats. *Parasit Res.,* **97(1)**, 33–40.

Dantas-Torres, F. and Otranto, D. (2014) Dogs, cats, parasites, and humans in Brazil: Opening the black box. *Parasit Vectors,* **14(7)**, 22–25.

Fourie, J.J., Crafford, D., Horak, I.G., *et al.* (2012) Prophylactic treatment of flea-infested dogs with an imidacloprid/flumethrin collar (Seresto, Bayer) to preempt infection with *Dipylidium caninum. Parasit Vectors,* **5**, 151.

Tuzer, E., Bilgin, Z., Oter, K., *et al.* (2010) Efficacy of praziquantel injectable solution against feline and canine tapeworms. *Turkiye Prazitol Derg.,* **34(1)**, 17–20.

Chapter 66: *Dirofilaria Immitis* (Heartworm)

Description: Parasitic roundworm, mosquito vector
Zoonotic Potential: Can be transmitted to humans by mosquitoes but not considered a zoonotic

Microbiology/epidemiology

Dirofilaria immitis infections are found worldwide and are carried by at least 70 mosquito species. Infections are common in dogs and other mammals, but are rare in cats and humans. Microfilariae are ingested by female mosquitoes that feed on infected blood. After two molts (2 weeks), infective third-stage larvae (L3s) are present in mosquito mouth parts. The L3 larvae molt to L4 larvae in subcutaneous tissues of a newly infected dog. These migrate through tissues until a final molt to a sexually immature adult (2 months). Adults enter the vascular system and deposit in the heart and pulmonary arteries. Mature adult females may reach 25–30 cm in length 6 months after infection. Microfilaremia occurs at 6–7 months after infection in dogs. Worms may live for up to 5–7 years. Chronic heartworm infection in dogs leads to congestive heart failure and pulmonary disease. While dogs are a natural host for *D. immitis*, cats are an atypical host. The majority of larvae do not survive in cats, they typically do not have circulating microfilariae and the numbers are lower (2–5). More recent evidence suggests that an intracellular endosymbiont bacterium (*Wolbachia pipientis*) of *D. immitis* may be responsible for the significant inflammatory reactions of worm and larval die off so that the bacterium is treated concomitantly.

Clinical disease

Dogs show no signs of infection in the 6 month prepatent period and diagnostic tests cannot detect infection at this time. With mature worm infections animals may be asymptomatic or present with a variety of symptoms. Animals with heavy infections that are active typically have a cough and exercise intolerance. As the infection progresses, dogs may have weight loss, fainting, coughing up blood, dyspnea, ascites, arrhythmias, jugular venous distension, and congestive heart failure. Cardiac output is reduced, pulmonary hypertension, compensatory right heart enlargement, glomerulonephritis, proteinuria, DIC, caval syndrome, and right heart failure may occur. Migrating larvae may rarely have aberrant migration into the eye, brain, or arteries of the leg resulting in seizures, blindness, or lameness. Cats with acute heartworm disease may have shock, vomiting, diarrhea, fainting, and sudden death. The signs of heartworm-associated respiratory disease (HARD) can persist even after complete elimination of the heartworm infection. Pulmonary emboli from dying worms are more likely to be fatal in cats than dogs because of less collateral circulation and fewer vessels.

Diagnosis

Antigen tests (enzyme-linked immunosorbent assay (ELISA) tests, solid substratum ELISA tests, immunochromatograhic (immunomigratory) tests, and colloidal gold agglutination tests) can be used to detect the glycoprotein in the reproductive tract of the female worm. Immature worms, low worm burdens (<2 females), or only male infections may not be detected. These have 98–100% specificity. Antibody tests may be more specific in cats than antigen tests but false positives may occur for up to 3 months after the infection is cleared. Microfilariae may also be identified microscopically by direct examination of fresh blood, blood treated with an anticoagulant, or examination of the buffy coat in a microhematocrit tube.

Treatment

Animals need complete evaluation of the heart, liver and kidney function prior to treating. Treatment guidelines are regularly updated by the American Heartworm Society. To evaluate the most current recommendations for treating adult heartworm infection see (www.heartwormsociety.org). No treatments are approved for use in cats. Surgery, monthly heartworm preventative, doxycycline, and short course steroids have been used. Melarsomine dihydrochloride (Immiticide) remains the drug of choice for adult heartworm disease in dogs. Dogs should be stabilized prior to treatment. For dogs with *Class 1–3 stage disease:* Give 2.5 mg/kg deep IM injection × 1 dose as directed by the Manufacturer with cage rest and exercise restrictions. After one month, give 2.5 mg/kg deep IM injection q24 h × 2 doses. Other

supportive therapies should be considered on a case-by-case basis. Doxycycline is also indicated due to the *Wolbachia pipientis* endosymbiont. Surgical removal of the adult heartworms may be indicated, especially in advanced cases with substantial heart involvement. Monthly administration of ivermectin at three times the dose for at least 18 months will also eventually kill the adult worms but is not considered the treatment of choice for dogs with a heavy infection. Daily doxycycline with ivermectin has shown efficacy in patients with early disease. Multiple heartworm preventatives are available that contain: ivermectin, milbemycin, selamectin, and moxidectin and are considered 99% effective.

Drug therapy

Melarsomine plus doxycycline.

Drug therapy alternatives

Ivermectin plus doxycycline.

Further reading

Berdoulay, P., Levy, J.K., Snyder, P.S., *et al.* (2004) Comparison of serological tests for the detection of natural heartworm infection in cats. *J Amer Anim Hosp Assoc.*, **40(5)**, 376–84.
Nelson, C.T., McCall, J.W., Rubin, S.B., *et al.* (2005) Guidelines for the diagnosis, prevention and management of management of heartworm (*Dirofilaria immitis*) infection in dogs. *Vet Parasitol.*, **133(2–3)**, 255–266.
Nelson, C.T., McCall, J.W., Rubin, S.B., *et al.* (2005) Guidelines for the diagnosis, prevention and management of management of heartworm (*Dirofilaria immitis*) infection in cats. *Vet Parasitol.*, **133(2–3)**, 267–275.
Todd-Jenkins, K. (2007) The role of Wolbachia in heartworm disease. *Vet Forum* (Veterinary Learning Systems), **24(10)**, 28–30.
Vezzani, D. and Carbajo, A. (2006) Spatial and temporal transmission risk of *Dirofilaria immitis* in Argentina. *Int J Parasitol.*, **36(14)**, 1463–1472.

Chapter 67: Distemper (Canine)

Description: RNA virus, enveloped, pleomorphic Morbillivirus
Zoonotic Potential: Not a zoonotic in humans

Microbiology/epidemiology

Canine distemper virus (CDV) affects a variety of animal species (dogs, ferrets, raccoons, and large wild felines). The virus is found worldwide with at least eight lineages. Dogs in the USA acquire the America-1 linage. Although the vaccine has eliminated many cases, puppies, particularly in kennels and shelter environments with inadequate immunity, continue to be a major source of infection. Older dogs in areas that vaccinations may not be given or are not appropriately given may also contract distemper. Transmission is typically by direct contact with aerosols or oronasal secretions from an affected animal. CDV is shed in all secretions starting day 5 after infection up until 3–4 months. The virus does not survive in the environment for any length of time (<1 day).

Clinical disease

Clinical disease in dogs usually presents as a severe, multisystemic disease that primarily affects the gastrointestinal tract, respiratory tract, and nervous system. Dogs may present with kennel cough, or parvovirus enteritis type of symptoms. Fever, lethargy, inappetence, vomiting, diarrhea, dehydration, tachypnea, cough, conjunctivitis, neurologic signs, and hyperkeratosis of the footpad and nasal planum may be present. Dogs with severe neurologic signs have a poor prognosis.

Diagnosis

Diagnosis is often based on clinical judgment when animals present with full spectrum disease. Laboratory diagnosis may involve multiple tests (virus isolation, direct immunostaining, Distemper ELISA antigen, RT-PCR, serology, histopathology). ELIZA may be the most inexpensive and rapid, but multiple samples and tests are required for a confirmation.

Treatment

Supportive care is the mainstay of therapy. For severe infections, intravenous fluids, enteral nutrition, antiemetics, antimicrobials, oxygen, nebulization, and coupage may be required. Animals should be isolated if possible. Doxycycline is recommended for respiratory complications. For severe bronchopneumonia, intravenous broad spectrum antimicrobials (ampicillin or Unisyn with a fluoroquinolone) are recommended. Vitamin A and ascorbic acid supplementation have been advocated. Diazepam, phenobarbital, or potassium bromide can be used for seizures. Steroids (dexamethasone IV single dose or tapered dosing) may reduce the severity of progressive CNS signs. Botulinum toxin has recently been suggested. Euthanasia is recommended for dogs with neurologic signs that are rapidly progressive.

Drug therapy

- Doxycycline
- Ampicillin/fluoroquinolone
- Unisyn/fluoroquinolone

Drug therapy alternatives

- Vitamin A
- Vitamin C

Further reading

Beineke, A., Puff, C., Seehusen, F., *et al.* (2009) Pathogenesis and immunopathology of systemic and nervous canine distemper. *Vet Immunopathol.*, **127**, 1–18.

Newbury, S., Larson, L.J., and Schulz, R.D. (2009) Canine distemper virus. In: *Infectious Disease Management in Animal Shelters*, Miller, L. and Hurley, K. (eds). Wiley-Blackwell, Ames, IA, pp. 161–172.

Schubert, T., Clemmons, R., Miles, S., and Draper, W. (2013) The use of botulinum toxin for the treatment of generalized myoclonus in a dog. *J Am Anim Hosp Assoc.*, **49(2)**, 122–127.

Chapter 68: *Ehrlichia* Species

Description: Gram negative aerobic rickettsial bacteria, intracellular
Zoonotic Potential: Tick borne zoonotic disease in humans and animals

Microbiology/epidemiology

Erhlichia species are found worldwide. The primary species infecting cats and dogs include *E. canis*, *E. ewingii*, *E. chaffeenis*, and rarely, an *E. muris*-like agent. *E. canis* is the most common infection reported in dogs and is the cause of canine monocytic ehrlichiosis (CME). *E. ewingii* causes canine granulocytic ehrlichiosis and *E. chaffeenis* causes monocytic ehrlichiosis in people with dogs being the primary reservoir. *E. canis* is primarily reported in tropical environments, *E. ewingii* is found in South-Central/South-Eastern USA, *E. chaffeensis* is found in Southern USA and *E. muris*-like agents are in the Midwest USA. *Ehrlichia* are spread by the bite of a tick (*Rhipicephalus sanguineus*, *Dermacentor variabilis*, *Amblyomma americanum*). Cats may be infected with *E. canis* but clinical disease is rare.

Clinical disease

Clinical disease in dogs with CME may be acute, sub-clinical, or chronic. Signs may occur 8–20 days following infection. Clinical signs are variable but typically include lethargy, inappetence, fever, and weight loss. Ocular, nasal discharge, peripheral edema, petechia, ecchymotic hemorrhages, and bleeding may also occur. Neurologic symptoms (seizures, ataxia, twitching, vestibular signs) may develop. Acute disease may last 2–4 weeks with spontaneous recovery or development of a subclinical phase that may persist for months to years. In chronic CME, pancytopenia, lethargy, inappetence, bleeding, mucosal pallor, muscle atrophy, fever, lymphadenopathy, splenomegaly, dyspnea, anterior uveitis, retinal hemorrhage and detachment, polyuria/polydipsia, edema, polymyositis, granular lymphocytosis, and secondary opportunistic infections may occur. Dogs with *E. ewingii* infection may present with no signs, fever, lethargy, anorexia, neutrophilic polyarthritis, vomiting, diarrhea, joint effusions, stiff gait, head tilt, anisocoria, and tremors. With *E. chaffeensis* infections, dogs may present with lymphadenopathy, anterior uveitis, and epistaxis.

Diagnosis

Diagnosis is based on clinical signs in combination with laboratory results. Cell culture, morule detection, IFA serology, ELISA serology, Western immunoblotting, and PCR are all available. IFA serology is typically the gold standard. Both acute and convalescent serology is required for confirmation.

Treatment

Supportive care and antibiotics is the mainstay of therapy. Intravenous fluids and blood products may be required. Treatment for a minimum of 2 weeks is suggested for *E. ewingii* and 4 weeks is required for *E. canis*. Intravenous doxycycline or oxytetracycline should be given initially until oral therapy is tolerated. Erythropoietin and granulocyte colony-stimulating factor with prednisone may be of value in cases of severe chronic ehrlichiosis. DDAVP (1 µg/kg SC q24 h × 3 days) may be given for bleeding. Tick control

(flumethrin collars for cats and pyrethroid or amitraz collars for dogs) to prevent recurrence is also recommended.

Drug therapy

- Doxycycline
- Oxytetracycline

Drug therapy alternatives

Chloramphenicol.

Further reading

Kommenou, A.A., Mylonakis, M.E., Kouti, V., *et al.* (2007) Ocular manifestations of natural canine monocytic ehrlichiosis (*Ehrlichia canis*): a retrospective study of 90 cases. *Vet Ophthalmol.*, **10**, 137–142.

Mylonakis, M.E., Koutinas, A.F., Breitschwerdt, E.B., *et al.* (2004) Chronic canine erlichiosis (*ehrlichia canis*): a retrospective study of 19 natural cases. *J Am Anim Hosp Assoc.*, **40**, 174–184.

Sykes, J.E. (2013) Erhlichiosis. Ch. 28. In: *Canine and Feline Infectious Diseases.* Sykes, J.E. (ed.), Elsevier, St. Louis, MO, pp. 278–289.

Chapter 69: *Entamoeba Histolytica*

Description: Enteric protozoan, trophozoites, cyst stages
Zoonotic Potential: Considered a zoonotic infection

Microbiology/epidemiology

Entamoeba species are found throughout the world. *E. histolytica* and *E. dispar* have been reported in dogs. It is endemic in Mexico, India, Africa, and Central and South America. Animals acquire the infection by ingestion of cysts in contaminated food and water or via oral–fecal contamination. Cysts exist in the ileum and multiply. Local tissue invasion may occur in the colon or spread hematogenously. Young and immunosuppressed animals may have increased risk of disseminated infections. Animals do not excrete cysts and the trophozoites are very fragile in the environment. *Entamoeba* typically have a single host life cycle. In dogs, autochonous infections are common, primarily in densely housed kennels and pet shops. Mixed intestinal infections with *E. histolytica*, *E. dispar*, *Giardia* spp. and enteropathogenic bacteria (*Salmonella* spp.) may occur. Cross-infection in cats is possible by mutual grooming.

Clinical disease

Most animals are asymptomatic. Dogs may present with acute colitis with explosive, profuse bloody diarrhea. Fever, abdominal pain, lethargy, and anorexia may also be noted. Few or no leukocytes may be evident in stool. Erosion or ulceration of the colon with classical "flask-shaped" ulcers may be noted. Disseminated infections may occur, resulting in hepatic abscesses and pleuropulmonary, peritoneal, and CNS infections. Cats may develop diarrhea, hematochezia, septicemia, and necrotic colitis.

Diagnosis

Stool examination and/or tissue biopsy for parasite trophozoites are diagnostic. Microscopic identification of trophozoites in stool samples must be done soon after collection. Trophozoites die rapidly so stools must be examined within 20 min. Direct smears of fresh feces reveal sluggish, amoeboid motility. Methylene blue staining or trichromeor iron-hematoxylin stains are ideal for diagnosis. ELIZA-based antigen tests and immunostaining may also be of benefit.

Treatment

Treatment is supportive and includes fluid therapy and antibiotics. Treatment depends on the severity of infection. Historically metronidazole (at doses used for giardia) has been the drug of choice, followed by an agent (such as paromomycin, diiodohydroxyquin, or diloxanide furoate) that acts on the organism in the lumen. Metronidazole should be administered for at least 10 days. Recent evidence in humans suggests that nitazoxanide may be the drug of choice due to its efficacy against both luminal and invasive parasite forms, although it remains to be studied in veterinary species.

Drug therapy

Metronidazole plus a luminal amoebicide.

Drug therapy alternatives

Nitazoxanide.

Further reading

Chacin-Bonilla, M.L. (2012) Current pharmacotherapy of amebiasis, advances in new drugs, and design of a vaccine. *Invest Clin.*, **53(3)**, 301–314.

Itoh, N., *et al.* (2011) *Giardia* and other intestinal parasites in dogs from veterinary clinics in Japan. *Parasitol Res.*, **109(1)**, 253–256.

Itoh, N., Muraoka, N., Aoki, M., and Itagaki, T. (2011) Prevalence of intestinal parasites and genotyping of *Giardia intestinalis* in pet shop puppies in east Japan. *Vet Parasitol.*, **176(1)**, 74–78.

Lappin, M.R. (2005) Enteric protozoal diseases. *Vet Clin North Am Small Anim Pract.*, **35(1)**, 81–88.

Little, S.E., Johnson, E.M., Lewis, D., *et al.* (2009) Prevalence of intestinal parasites in pet dogs in the United States. *Vet Parasitol.*, **166**, 144–152.

Shimada, A., Muraki, Y., Awakura, T., *et al.* (1992) Necrotic colitis associated with *Entamoeba histolytica* infection in a cat. *J Comp Pathol.*, **106(2)**, 195–199.

Tupler, T., Levy, J.K., Sanshin, S.J., *et al.* (2012) Enteropathogens identified in dogs entering a Florida animal shelter with normal feces or diarrhea. *J Am Vet Med Assoc.*, **241(3)**, 338–343.

Chapter 70: Enterobacter Species

Description: Gram negative aerobic rod
Zoonotic Potential: Multidrug resistant strains may colonize or be transmitted to humans

Microbiology/epidemiology

Enterobacter commonly inhabit the gastrointestinal tract and are one of many "enteric bacteria" that make up the group Enterobacteriaceae. A variety of species are pathogenic in animals including *E. cloacae*, *E. aerogenes*, and *E. agglomerans*. *Enterobacter* species are opportunistic and typically are involved in nosacomial infections involving hospitalized patients (trauma, urinary tract infections, abdominal wounds, bacteremia, respiratory infections). Zoonotic infections in humans have been attributed to *Enterobacter* infections in dogs.

Clinical disease

Enterobacter are rarely a cause of disease in dogs and cats, but have been associated with nosocomial infections (cystitis associated with urinary catheterization, post-operative empyemas, and pancreaticobiliary duct infections). Animals are typically hospitalized patients with a history of broad spectrum antibiotic use. Infections have occurred in animals on respirators, and in burn patients.

Diagnosis

Aerobic culture and sensitivity in combination with clinical signs and symptoms are diagnostic.

Treatment

Enterobacter species are often multidrug resistant and can present a therapeutic challenge. Treatment must be based on culture and sensitivity results. Empiric therapy may include amoxicillin/clavulanate or chloramphenicol. With severe infections, multidrug therapy is required due to the high level of resistance with this organism.

Drug therapy

- Extended spectrum penicillins
- Third generation cephalosporins

Drug therapy alternatives

- Imipenem
- Meropenem
- Fluoroquinolones
- Chloramphenicol

Further reading

Bubenik, L. and Hosgood, G. (2007) Frequency of urinary tract infection in catheterized dogs and comparison of bacterial culture and susceptibility testing results for catheterized and noncatheterized dogs with urinary tract infections. *J Am Vet Med Assoc.*, **231(6)**, 893–899.

Gibson, J.S., Morton, R.N, Cubbold, H.E., *et al.* (2008) Multidrug-resistant *E. coli* and *Enterobacter* extraintestinal infection in 37 dogs. *J Vet Intern Med.*, **22(4)**, 844–850.

Marsh-Ng, M.L., Burney, D.P., and Garcia, J. (2007) Surveillance of infections associated with intravenous catheters in dogs and cats in an intensive care unit. *J Am Anim Hosp Assoc.*, **43(1)**, 13–20.

Sidjabat, H.E., Hanson, N., Smith-Moland, E., *et al.* (2007) Identification of plasmid-mediated extended-spectrum and Amp C beta-lactamases in *Enterobacter spp.* isolated from dogs. *J Med Microbiol.*, **56(3)**, 426–434.

Weese, J.S. (2008) Investigation of *Enterobacter cloacae* infections at a small animal veterinary teaching hospital. *Vet Microbiol.*, **130(3–4)**, 426–428.

Chapter 71: *Enterococcus*

Description: Gram positive aerobic, nonhemolytic, *Streptococci* in pairs or short chains
Zoonotic Potential: Animals may serve as reservoirs for drug resistant organisms

Microbiology/epidemiology

Enterococcus species live in the intestinal tract, oral cavity, urethra, and vagina. *E. faecalis* and *E. faecium* are the primary species reported in dogs and cats. *Enterococcus* are part of the normal flora of animals but with the widespread use of broad spectrum antibiotics, overgrowth of this species has resulted in a significant increase in infections due to their relative innate resistance to most antibiotics. Nosocomial infections are now common with these organisms that can become highly multidrug resistant and survive in very harsh external environments. The organisms can be found on almost all hospital surfaces including doorknobs, stethoscopes, computer keys, phones, personal clothing, devices, equipment, and so on. Virulent strains have been identified that enable them to invade tissues. Diabetic patients, neonates, recent surgery, trauma, catheterization, burn patients, or those with a history of antimicrobial therapy or hospitalization have an increased risk of infection.

Clinical disease

Enterococcus species produce a variety of infections in small animals including urinary tract infections, bacteremia, endocarditis, intra-abdominal infections, and osteomyelitis. Wound colonization may occur with superinfection in compromised hosts and those on antimicrobial therapy. *Enterococcus* is a common cause of endocarditis. Dogs may present with fever, lethargy, tachycardia, joint pain, swelling, systolic heart murmurs, and signs of embolic complications.

Diagnosis

Diagnosis is based on gram stain, aerobic culture, and sensitivity.

Treatment

Species identification and antibiotic sensitivities should always be performed due to the high potential for resistance. Antibiotic therapy should be based on the severity of the infection and culture results. Uncomplicated urinary tract infections may respond to high doses of beta-lactams (amoxicillin), doxycycline, nitrofurantoin, or chloramphenicol monotherapy (1–2 weeks). For serious infections, bactericidal combinations of a beta-lactam (ampicillin, penicillin) with an aminoglycoside are recommended for synergy. Trough and peak aminoglycoside levels should be monitored to ascertain therapeutic concentrations are being achieved. Endocarditis should be treated for at least 4–6 weeks. *E. faecalis* may have very high level resistance to aminoglycosides. Ceftriaxone and ampicillin have been used in human endocarditis cases with high aminoglycoside resistance. Linezolide may be effective but should not be used long term and is expensive. Vancomycin should be reserved for human patients but may be the only effective drug in some high level resistance cases. If used, therapeutic monitoring is required to prevent the further development of vancomycin resistant enterococcus infections. Although in vitro susceptibilities may suggest susceptibility to cephalosporins and sulfamethoxazole these are not effective *in vivo*.

Drug therapy

For severe infections
- Ampicillin sodium plus gentamycin sulfate
- Vancomycin

For mild-moderate infections
- Amoxicillin
- Chloramphenicol
- Nitrofurantoin (bladder infections only)

Drug therapy alternatives

- Linezolide
- Ceftriaxone with ampicillin

Further reading

Damborg, P., Top, J., Hendrickx, A.P., *et al.* (2009) Dogs are a reservoir of ampicillin-resistant *Enterococcus faecium* linages associated with human infections. *Appl Environ Microbiol.*, **75**, 2360–2365.

Sykes, J.E. (2013) Streptoccal and enterococcal infections. Ch. 34. In: *Canine and Feline Infectious Diseases*. Sykes, J.E. (ed.), Elsevier, St. Louis, MO, pp. 334–346.

Thompson, M.F., Litster, A.L., Platell, J.L., *et al.* (2011) Canine bacterial urinary tract infections: new developments in old pathogens. *Vet J.*, **190(1)**, 22–27.

Chapter 72: *Erysipelothrix* Species

Description: Anaerobic gram positive bacillus
Zoonotic Potential: Considered a zoonotic in animal and meat handlers

Microbiology/epidemiology

Erysipelothrix species are found worldwide. The organisms live in decomposing nitrogenous substances with reservoirs in swine, turkeys, ducks, fish, and mice. Occupational exposure (meat cutters, trappers, food handlers, veterinarians, slaughterhouse workers) has resulted in cutaneous and systemic infections in humans. *E. rhusiopathiae* causes disease in swine while *E. tonsillarum* (serovar 7) is a pathogen in dogs. It is an uncommon pathogen and is believed to be transmitted from direct contact with other infected animals, fish or carcasses. Immunosuppressed animals may have an increased risk of infection. Localized cellulitis is common in humans after inoculation via a cut or abrasion. Severe swelling, pain, and purplish erythema may develop.

Clinical disease

Dogs may present with fever, shifting-leg lameness, and heart murmurs. Erythematous cutaneous lesions, lethargy, and anorexia have also been reported. *E. rhusiopathiae* causes endocarditis (aortic valve), arthritis, discospondylitis, and septicemia in dogs.

Diagnosis

Deep tissue biopsy should be submitted for histopathology and culture. Aerobic and anaerobic cultures should be performed. Blood cultures should be performed for suspected bacteremia or endocarditis but are negative in localized skin disease.

Treatment

Erysipelthrix is highly susceptible to penicillins. Amoxicillin (2 weeks) can be used for localized infections. Alternatively imipenem and cephalosporins may be effective for more severe infections. Endocarditis should be treated for prolonged periods (6–8 weeks) and mortality may be high. Immunosuppressive drugs should be discontinued if possible.

Drug therapy

- Amoxicillin
- Penicillin G parenteral

Drug therapy alternatives

- Cefazolin
- Imipenem

Further reading

Foster, J.D., Hartman, F.A., and Moriello, K.A. (2012) A case of apparent canine erysipeloid associated with *Erysipelothrix rhusiopathiae* bacteraemia. *Vet Derm.*, **23**, 528.

Goudswaard, J., Hartman, E.G., Janmaat, A., and Huisman, G.H. (1973) *Erysipelothrix rhusiopathiae* strain 7, a causative agent of endocarditis and arthritis in the dogs. *Tijdschr Diergeneesk.*, **98**, 416–423.

Schrauwen, E., Devriese, L.A., Hoorens, J., *et al.* (1993) *Erysipelothrix tonsillarum* endocarditis in a dog. *Vlaams Diergeneeskd Tijdschr.*, **62**, 160–161.

Takahashi, T., Takagi, M., Yamaoka, R., *et al.* (1994) Comparison of the pathogenicity for chickens of *Erysipelothrix rhusiopathiae* and *Erysipelothrix tonsillarum*. *Avian Pathol.*, **23**, 237–245.

Takahashi, T., Fujisawa, T., Yamamoto, K., *et al.* (2000) Taxonomic evidence that serovar 7 of *Erysipelothrix* strains isolated from dogs with endocarditis are *Erysipelothrix tonsillarum*. *J Vet Med B.*, **47**, 311–313.

Chapter 73: *Escherichia Coli* (Enterotoxigenic/ Enterohemorrhagic)

Description: Gram negative aerobic bacteria, facultative enteric bacillus
Zoonotic Potential: Animals may serve as reservoirs for drug resistant organisms

Microbiology/epidemiology

Enterotoxigenic and enterohemorrhagic *E. coli* consist of multiple strains that cause enteric infections. There are at least seven strains recognized:
1. Enteropathogenic *E. coli* (EPEC),
2. Enterotoxigenic *E. coli* (ETEC),
3. Enterohemmorrhagic *E. coli* (EHEC),
4. Necrotoxigenic *E. coli* (NTEC),
5. Enteroinvasive *E. coli* (EIEC),

6. Enteroaggregative *E. coli* (EAEC), and
7. Adherent-invasive *E. coli* (AIEC).
ETEC pathovars are responsible for up to 31% of canine diarrheas. Diarrheagenic *E. coli* are common in the agricultural environment (cattle feces, slaughter houses, contaminated water, fresh fruits, and vegetables). Animals ingesting contaminated food or water may acquire the infection. Raw meat and unpasteurized milk have been sources of infection in humans. In dogs that eat raw meat, EHEC strains may result in cutaneous and renal glomerular vasculopathy. AIEC strains have been identified with granulomatous colitis in young Boxers, French bulldogs, and Border collies.

Clinical disease

Some strains can cause severe life threatening diarrhea. Patients typically present with fever, lethargy, inappetence, diarrhea, and vomiting. In patients that present with hemorrhagic colitis without fever, enterohemorrhagic *E. coli* should be considered. Hemolytic uremic syndrome characterized by bloody diarrhea, acute renal failure, thrombocytopenia, and hemolysis may result from infections with enterohemorrhagic *E. coli*. Boxers may present with severe colitis, colonic thickening and ulceration, weight loss, and hypoalbuminemia.

Diagnosis

Stool culture of dogs and cats with *E. coli* infections is non-diagnostic due to the fact that even healthy animals shed *E. coli*. However, culture and sensitivity are encouraged for dogs with potential granulomatous colitis due to the emergence of AIEC fluoroquinolone resistant strains. Immunoassay for Shiga toxin, ST, and LT are available. PCR tests are available through some laboratories to differentiate pathogenic from non-pathogenic strains. Ultrasound in boxers may demonstrate mild to moderate mesenteric or sublumbar lymphadenomegaly and thickened colonic wall. Histopathology of cutaneous lesions from EHEC may demonstrate fibrinoid vascular necrosis, dermal thrombosis, and leukocytoclastic vasculitis. Histopathology lesions from Boxers and French bull dogs with granulomatous colitis from AIEC strains may demonstrate neutrophilic inflammation, epithelial ulceration, crypt hyperplasia, and distortion and abundant macrophages that stain positive.

Treatment

Enterotoxigenic and hemorrhagic strains of *E. coli* are sensitive to most common antibiotics. However, studies in human medicine suggest that antibiotics may increase the risk for development of hemolytic uremic syndrome. Antimotility agents (loperamide) are also contraindicated since they may prolong the duration of infection. Treatment is typically supportive with fluids and electrolytes. Most patients will recover without antibiotic treatment in 5–10 days with supportive care and a bland diet. Antibiotic treatment (fluoroquinolone for 8 weeks) is recommended for dogs with AIEC granulomatous colitis.

Drug therapy

Enrofloxacin (Granulomatous colitis).

Drug therapy alternatives

Supportive care (antihypertensives, fluid therapy, red blood cell transfusion, probiotics, dialysis).

Further reading

Cowan, L.A., Hertzke, D.M., Fenwick, B.W., *et al.* (2010) Clinical and clinicopathologic abnormalities in greyhounds with cutaneous and renal glomerular vasculopathy;18 cases (1992–1994). *J Am Vet Med Assoc.*, **6**, 789–793.

Gouveia, E.M., Silva, I.S., Nakazato, G., *et al.* (2013) Action of phosphorylated mannanoligosaccharides on immune and hematological responses and fecal consistency of dogs experimentally infected with enteropathogenic *Escherichia coli* strains. *Braz J Microbiol.*, **44(2)**, 499–504.

Mansfield, C.S., James, F.E., Craven, M., *et al.* (2009) Remission of histiocytic ulcerative colitis in Boxer dogs correlates with eradication of invasive intramucosal *Escherichia coli*. *J Vet Intern Med.*, **23(5)**, 964–969.

Oswald, E., Schmidt, H., Morabito, S., *et al.* (2000) Typing of intimin genes in human and animal enterohemorrhagic and enteropathogenic *Escherichia coli*: Characterization of a new intimin variant. *Infect Immun.*, **68(1)**, 64–71.

Sykes, J. and Marks, S.L. (2013) Enteric *Escherichia coli* infections. Ch. 46. In: *Canine and Feline Infectious Diseases*. Sykes, J.E. (ed.), Elsevier, St. Louis, MO, pp. 445–451.

Chapter 74: *Eschericha Coli* (Nonenterohemorrhagic)

Description: Gram negative aerobic bacteria, facultative enteric bacillus
Zoonotic Potential: Animals may serve as reservoirs for drug resistant organisms

Microbiology/epidemiology

E. coli are normal bacteria that colonize the gastrointestinal tract of animals. Nondiarrheagenic *E. coli* are the most common bacteria isolates in microbiology laboratories and are responsible for numerous extraintestinal infections. They are considered opportunistic pathogens in hospitalized or debilitated animals. They are the most common isolates from both canine and feline urinary tract infections. Animals may be at increased risk of urinary tract infections if they are incontinent, diabetic, obstructed, catheterized, have prostatitis, cancer, or other underlying disorders.

Clinical disease

Dogs and cats may present with a variety of clinical symptoms due to *E. coli* infection. Most present with typical signs of urinary tract infection. Patients that are hospitalized or on ventilators may develop colonization of the respiratory tract with resulting *E. coli* pneumonia or bronchitis. Peritonitis from *E. coli* is common post surgery or following other abdominal trauma. It is a very common cause of sepsis, pyometra, cellulitis, and neonatal infections.

Diagnosis

Diagnosis is by gram stain and aerobic culture in patients with relevant clinical syndromes.

Treatment

Although most *E. coli* are still very sensitive to amoxicillin, ampicillin, and first generation cephalosporins, treatment should be based on sensitivity reports due to increasing resistance. Mild, uncomplicated urinary tract infections can still be treated with amoxicillin, amoxicillin/clavulanate or TMS until susceptibility is confirmed. In more serious infections or those with a recent history of antibiotic use, third generation cephalosporins may be indicated until culture and sensitivity is available. For simple bladder infections due to *E. coli* the use of cefovecin or short course enrofloxicin has been evaluated as a means to improve owner compliance and reduce resistance. For more serious infections fluoroquinolones, aminoglycosides, third generation cephalosporines, ampicillin/sulbactam, or carbapenems may be required.

Drug therapy

- Amoxicillin
- Amoxicillin/clavulanate

- TMS
- Cephalexin

Drug therapy alternatives

- Fluoroquinolones
- Third generation cephalosporins
- Ampicillin/sulbactam
- Imipenem/Meropenem
- Aminoglycosides

Further reading

Boothe, D., Smaha, T., Carpenter, D.M., *et al.* (2012) Antimicrobial resistance and pharmacodynamics of canine and feline pathogenic *E. coli* in the United States. *J Am Anima Hosp Assoc.*, **48(6)**, 379–389.

Cooke, C.L., Singer, R.S., Jang, S.S., *et al.* (2002) Enrofloxacin resistance in *Escherichia coli* isolated from dogs with urinary tract infections. *J Am Vet Med Assoc.*, **220(2)**, 190–192.

Hagman, R. and Greko, C. (2005) Antimicrobial resistance in *Escherichia coli* isolated from bitches with pyometra and from urine samples from other dogs. *Vet Rec.*, **157(7)**, 193–196.

Hall, J.L., Holmes, M.A., and Baines, S.J. (2013) Prevalence and antimicrobial resistance of canine urinary tract pathogens. *Vet Rec.*, **173(22)**, 549.

Ogeer-Gyles, J., Mathews, K., Weese, J.S., *et al.* (2006) Evaluation of catheter-associated urinary tract infectons and multi-drug-resistant *Escherichia coli* isolates from the urine of dogs with indwelling urinary catheters. *J Am Vet Med Assoc.*, **229(10)**, 1584–1590.

Shaheen, B.W., Boothe, D.M., Oyarzabal, O.A., *et al.* (2010) Antimicrobial resistance profiles and clonal relatedness of canine and feline *Escherichia coli* pathogens expressing multi-drug resistance in the United States. *J Vet Intern Med.*, **24(2)**, 323–330.

Westropp, J.L., Sykes, J.E., Irom, S., *et al.* (2012) Evaluation of the efficacy and safety of high dose short duration enrofloxacin treatment regimens for uncomplicated urinary tract infections in dogs. *J Vet Intern Med.*, **26(3)**, 506–512.

Chapter 75: Feline Coronavirus (Feline Infectious Peritonitis: FIP)

Description: Feline RNA virus, single stranded, large, enveloped
Zoonotic Potential: Host specific, not a zoonotic

Microbiology/epidemiology

Feline coronavirus (FCoVs) causes enteric disease and feline infectious peritonitis (FIP) in cats. The virus is found worldwide. The virus affects young cats, particularly those in shelters and catteries. Cats developing FIP may have progressive disease over weeks to months that are typically fatal. Cats may acquire the infection from fecal-oral transmission. Cats are pre-disposed to infection in households with >6 cats (50–100% seroprevalence), but <10% actually develop FIP. Cats may be exposed to the feline enteric coronavirus first which then mutates to the more virulent FIP virus or co-infection with both the enteric and the virulent strain may occur.

Clinical disease

Cats may present with tachypnea, pleural effusion (yellow appearance), rapid, shallow breathing, muffled heart and lung sounds, pyrexia, dehydration, mucosal pallor, icterus, thin body condition, ascites, hepatomegaly, mesenteric lymphadenopathy, intestinal pyogranulomas, testicular enlargement, neurologic signs, and ocular signs.

Diagnosis

Diagnosis is by immunohistochemical or immunocytochemistry of fluid from body cavities. Fluorescent or immunoperoxidase antibody staining done on effusion specimens or tissues is the most sensitive assay, but can still have false negatives. Most cats also have a regenerative anemia, lymphopenia, eosiniphilia, hyperproteinemia, hyperglobulinemia, serum albumin: globulin ratio of >0.8, hyponatremia, hypokalemia, hypochloremia, hyperglycemia, elevated liver enzymes, azotemia, hyperbilirubinemia, and hypocholesterolemia. Serum concentrations of alpha-1-acid glycoprotein of >1500 μg/mL is also suggestive of FIP. Serology and PCR tests may not be accurate and may have false positives.

Treatment

Treatment is supportive and typically the prognosis is poor. Fluid therapy and nutritional support are required. Temporary remission has occurred in some cats with prednisolone therapy (1–2 mg/kg PO q12–24 h). Glucocorticoids, feline IFN, human IFN, chlorambucil, ribavirin, cyclophosphamide, pentoxifylline, and other medications have been attempted with limited success.

Drug therapy

- Prednisolone
- Feline interferon

Further reading

Addie, D., Belak, S., Boucraut-Baralon, C., *et al.* (2009) Feline infectious peritonitis. ABCD guidelines on prevention and management. *J Feline Med Surg.*, **11**, 594–604.

Pedersen, N.C. (2009) A review of feline infectious peritonitis virus infection: 1963–2008. *J Feline Med Surg.*, **11**, 225–258.

Sykes, J.E. (2013) Feline coronavirus. Ch. 20. In: *Canine and Feline Infectious Diseases*. Sykes, J.E. (ed.), Elsevier, St. Louis, MO, pp. 195–208.

Chapter 76: Feline Immunodeficiency Virus (FIV)

Description: RNA Lentivirus, enveloped retroviridae
Zoonotic Potential: Host specific not considered a zoonotic

Microbiology/epidemiology

Feline immunodeficiency virus (FIV) infects both wild and domesticated cats worldwide. Similar to HIV infections in humans, the virus results in a chronic persistent infection that causes immunodeficiency. The virus is found in high concentrations in saliva and is believed to be transmitted primarily via bites from infected animals. Transmission may also occur through venereal spread, transplacental transmission, parturition, lactation, or blood transfusions. Animals at highest risk are older animals, males, outdoor cats, cats with a history of bite wounds, and those with other illnesses. Progression and severity of disease are based on host immunity, and the viral strain. Neonatal and geriatric cats may progress to terminal disease much more rapidly.

Clinical disease

Cats typically have three stages of disease; acute, subclinical, and terminal. Acute disease may not be obvious to owners. The virus replicates and is found in high concentrations 8–12 weeks following infection. There is a decline in CD4+ and CD8+ T cells over 3–6 months. Cats may develop lethargy, fever, anorexia, diarrhea, stomatitis, weight loss, lymphadenopathy, and neutropenia. Subclinical infection may last for months to years. Hyperglobulinemia and progression of CNS disease may occur. The terminal phase of FIV typically is associated with periodontal disease, gingivitis, lymphoplasmacytic stomatitis, feline odotoclastic resorptive lesions, bacterial skin and ear infections, upper respiratory infections, dermatophytosis, mycobacterial infections, fungal infections, demodecosis, and parasitic infections. A variety of cancers (lymphoma, squamous cell, leukemia, mast cell, and others) may also be present.

Diagnosis

All animals should be tested for FIV. Serology on whole blood or serum using ELISA, Western blotting and IFA are the gold standard. PCR can be performed on blood but the sensitivity and specificity are variable.

Treatment

Cats in the terminal phase of FIV should be provided supportive care. Fluid therapy, nutritional support, dental extractions, and antimicrobials (amoxicillin/clavulanate) for stomatitis are recommended. Chlorhexidine based mouth washes and topical lactoferrin (200 mg chemical powder q24 h) are helpful for mouth ulcers. In severe cases, oral prednisolone can be given but can cause an increased viremia. Topical prednisolone acetate and atropine may be given for anterior uveitis. Appropriate opportunistic therapy should be given but may need to be lifelong. Darbepoetin or erythromycin may be useful for nonregenerative anemia. Human granulocytic colony stimulating factor (G-CSF) should not be administered systemically but can be given orally (1–50 Units/cat q24 h) for stomatitis. Antiviral therapy and interferons remain experimental but may be of benefit. Zidovudine (5–15 mg/kg PO q12 h) can be beneficial but can cause marrow suppression, so CBCs must be monitored weekly. Fosivudine (45 mg/kg PO q12 h) has also been used experimentally and may have fewer side effects.

Drug therapy

- Zidovudine (AZT)
- Fosivudine

Drug therapy alternatives

- Human recombinant alpha interferon (IFN-alpha)
- Prednisolone
- Topical lactoferrin powder

Further reading

Goldkamp, C.E., Levy, J.K., Edinboro, Ch., *et al.* (2008) Seroprevalences of feline leukemia virus and feline immunodeficiency virus in cats with abscesses or bite wounds and rate of veterinarian compliance with current guidelines for retrovirus testing. *J Am Vet Med Assoc.*, **232**, 1152–1158.

Hosie, M.J., Addie, D., Belak, S., *et al.* (2009) Feline immunodeficiency. ABCD guidelines on prevention and management. *J Feline Med Surg.*, **11**, 575–584.

Sykes, J.E. (2013) Feline Immunodeficiency virus infection. Ch. 21. In: *Canine and Feline Infectious Diseases.* Sykes, J.E. (ed.), Elsevier, St. Louis, MO, pp. 209–223.

Chapter 77: Feline Leukemia Virus (FeLV)

Description: RNA Gammaretrovirus, enveloped
Zoonotic Potential: Host specific, not considered a zoonotic

Microbiology/epidemiology

Feline leukemia virus remains a significant feline disease despite vaccines that now prevent most infections. It affects both wild and domestic cats worldwide and causes immune suppression, bone marrow disorders, and hematopoietic neoplasia. FeLV progresses rapidly to immunosuppression, but unlike FIV, cats may regress to a state of permanent viral latency. Some may even eliminate the virus. Positive tests may therefore not imply disease or increased mortality in an otherwise healthy cat. Transmission is believed to occur through salivary secretions by licking, mutual grooming, and sharing of food and water dishes. Bites, blood transfusions, fleas, and lactation may also transmit the virus. Outdoor cats, adults, aggressive or intact cats, and cats from multicat households are more likely to become infected. Many infected cats may live for up to several years with a good quality of life.

Clinical disease

Early disease can present as fever, lethargy, and/or lymphadenopathy. Infection may then occur and persist for life. Some cats may have reactivated disease with immunosuppression (pregnancy, immunosuppressive drugs). With progressive infection, cats develop a variety of clinical diseases including; neoplasias, opportunistic infections, pure red cell aplasia, aplastic anemia, myelodysplasia, myelofibrosis, immune mediated diseases, peripheral lymphadenopathy, neurologic disease, gastrointestinal disease as well as osteochondromatosis.

Diagnosis

Screening should be performed using ELISA or related immunochromatographic in-house assays for free FeLV antigen in serum. A complete CBC with blood smear should also be done to evaluate for the presence of FeLV related disorders. A reticulocyte count, Coomb's test, and PCR assay for hemoplasmas should also be performed on cats that are infected.

Treatment

Treatment is supportive and includes the same medications that would be given otherwise for cancer or opportunistic infections. Immunosuppressives should be avoided. Antivirals such as zidovudine (AZT) have shown minor benefits. Feline recombinant interferon omega (1 million U/kg SC q24 h × 5 consecutive doses starting on days 0, 14, and 60) or human recombinant interferon alpha (1 to 50 U/cat PO q24 h) may have short term benefits (2 months). Prevention with early vaccination of kittens and maintenance of kittens indoors is recommended. Two doses of vaccine (3–4 weeks apart) given in the left pelvic distal limb from 8–9 weeks of age followed by a booster at one year and then every 1–3 years is currently recommended.

Drug therapy

Zidovudine.

Drug therapy alternatives

- Feline recombinant interferon omega
- Human recombinant interferon alpha

Further reading

Hartmann, K. (2011) Clinical aspects of feline immunodeficiency and feline leukemia virus infection. *Vet Immunol Immunopathol.*, **143**, 190–201.

Lutz, H., Addie, D., Belak, S., *et al.* (2009) Feline leukemia. ABCD guidelines on prevention and management. *J Feline Med Surg.*, **11**, 565–574.

Sykes, J.E. and Hartmann, K. (2013) Feline leukemia virus infection. Ch. 22. In: *Canine and Feline Infectious Diseases.* Sykes, J.E. (ed.), Elsevier, St. Louis, MO, pp. 224–238.

Chapter 78: Feline Panleukopenia Virus

Description: Single stranded non-enveloped DNA parvovirus
Zoonotic Potential: Host specific, not known to infect humans

Microbiology/epidemiology

Feline panleukopenia virus (FPV) is noted to cause enteritis and panleukopenia worldwide in domestic and wild cats, foxes, mink, and raccoons. It has been described as cat plague, feline infectious enteritis, feline distemper, and feline ataxia. FPV is similar to canine parvovirus (CPV-2) and can survive long periods in the environment (>1 year). Young cats (<1 year) or improperly/unvaccinated cats are at highest risk. Cats acquire the disease via direct contact with virus in feces, vomit, saliva, fleas, or contaminated surfaces with fomites (bedding, food dishes, clothing, and shoes of handlers of infected animals). Ferrets and mink may also transmit the infection. FPV is highly contagious and can be fatal to the affected cats often causing severe panleukopenia.

Clinical disease

Cats typically present with fever, lethargy, inappetence, vomiting, bloody diarrhea, anemia, self-biting of the tail, lower back/legs, decreased hematocrit, platelets, severe dehydration, neurologic signs, and rarely sudden death. The virus attacks the gastrointestinal tract causing ulceration, malnutrition, and severe panleukopenia. Hypothermia, septic shock, DIC, and secondary bacterial infection carry a poor prognosis. Exposure during pregnancy can result in cerebellar hypoplasia in offspring. Late complications can also include cardiomyopathy and myocarditis.

Diagnosis

Clinical diagnosis is based on characteristic gastroenteric illness and severe pancytopenia in a susceptible cat. Fecal analysis and blood culture is required to rule out other illnesses. Diagnosis is made by fecal ELISA, tissue histopathology, fecal or tissue PCR, electron microscopy of virus in feces, or virus isolation.

Treatment

Vaccination to prevent infection is highly effective and widely available. Active infections in young kittens (<2 months) is most often fatal. In older cats, mortality rates are still high (10–30%) even if treated. Supportive care is the mainstay of treatment. Blood transfusions are required to improve pancytopenia. Intravenous crystalloids, correction of electrolyte abnormalities (sodium), and parenteral antimicrobials (gram negative/anaerobic coverage) may be of benefit. Dextrose supplementation, antiemetics, vitamins A, B, and C, and enteral nutrition may also be required. Cats with low white cell counts (<1000/μL) have a poor prognosis. Pregnant cats should not be given modified live vaccines.

Drug therapy

- Supportive care (blood transfusions, intravenous fluids, electrolytes, dextrose)
- Antibiotics (ampicillin, metronidazole, amoxicillin/clavulanate, fluoroquinolones, carbapenems, clindamycin)
- Vitamins A, B, and C

Further reading

Jakel, V., Cussler, K., Hanschmann, K.M., *et al.* (2012) Vaccination against feline panleukopenia: implications from a field study in kittens. *BMC Vet Res.*, **8**, 62–65.

Mostl, K., Egberink, H., Addie, D., *et al.* (2013) Prevention of infectious diseases in cat shelters: ABCD guidelines. *J Feline Med Surg.*, **15(7)**, 546–554.

Sykes, J.E. (2013) Feline panleukopenia virus infection and other viral enteritides. Ch. 19. In: *Canine and Feline Infectious Diseases.* Sykes, J.E. (ed.), Elsevier, St. Louis, MO, pp. 187–194.

Chapter 79: *Francisella Tularensis* (Tularemia)

Description: Aerobic gram negative bacteria, pleomorphic, coccobacillus
Zoonotic Potential: Significant zoonotic potential in meat, animal handlers

Microbiology/epidemiology

Francisella species exist in two biotypes with four subspecies (Biotype A in North America and Type B in Europe and Asia). *F. tularensis*, subsp. *tularensis* (Type A) is endemic in Missouri, Kansas, Arkansas, and Oklahoma and carriers a much higher mortality rate compared to Type B. Cases have also been reported from Montana, Massachusetts, Oregon, and central Virginia. The bacterium is carried in hundreds of wild animal species and household pets that act as hosts. It is transmitted between animals by ectoparasites (ticks, biting flies) and contaminated environmental conditions. The bacteria can be spread by inhalation, ingestion, or via direct skin contact. Typically young animals are more susceptible, with cats being at higher risk. Cats and dogs may acquire the disease from hunting infected rabbits or rodents. Humans may acquire the bacterium via ectoparasites, by handling animal hides or carcasses, or by ingesting contaminated lake or stream water. Veterinarians, meat handlers, trappers, hunters, and laboratory workers may be at increased risk.

Clinical disease

Incubation may take 2–10 days. The animal may become lethargic, febrile, have anorexia, and peripheral lymphadenopathy. A non-healing ulcer at the point of entry is often noted. Cats may present with vomiting, dehydration, icterus, hepatomegaly, thin body condition, abdominal lymphadenomegaly, splenomegaly, and oral and/or lingual ulcers. Hypothermia, bradycardia, and seizures have also been reported. Dogs may also have mucoid ocular discharge and tonsillitis. Plague is the primary differential diagnosis. The disease rapidly progresses to death in many animals and diagnosis is often at necropsy.

Diagnosis

The diagnosis must be confirmed by culture, PCR, and/or serologic testing. PCR can be performed easily, but culture and sensitivity must be performed in approved laboratories. Public health agencies should be notified of suspected cases and where samples can be submitted.

Treatment

Few animals have been diagnosed with tularemia so little information is available on efficacy of drug treatment. Aminoglycosides, fluoroquinolones, and tetracyclines have been used in humans successfully. Antibiotics (2–3 weeks), supportive care, and isolation of suspected cases are required. Animals should remain in isolation for a minimum of 3 days following initiation of antibiotics. Proper biohazard regulations with regard to personnel protective gear (gowns, gloves, glasses, and a high density surgical mask), biohazardous waste, and environmental decontamination should be adhered to.

Drug therapy

Aminoglycosides with or without chloramphenicol (for CNS disease),

Drug therapy alternatives

- Fluoroquinolones
- Tetracyclines

Further reading

Kugeler, K.J., Mead, P.S., Janusz, A.M., *et al.* (2009) Molecular epidemiology of *Francisella tularensis* in the United States. *Clin Infect Dis.*, **48**, 863–870.

Spagnoli, S.T., Kuroki, K., Schommer, S.K., *et al.* (2011) Pathology in practice. *Francisella tularensis. J Am Vet Med Assoc.*, **238**, 1271–1273.

Sykes, J.E. and Chomel, B.B. (2013) Tularemia. Ch. 56. In: *Canine and Feline Infectious Diseases*. Sykes, J.E. (ed.), Elsevier, St. Louis, MO, pp. 537–545.

Chapter 80: *Fusarium* Species

Description: Halohyphomycosis mold, branched/unbranched hyphae
Zoonotic Potential: Not considered a zoonotic

Microbiology/epidemiology

Fusarium species grow in soil and are typically pathogenic to plants. Animals may acquire the infection via traumatic inoculation of contaminated material. Typically *F. sporothrichioides* and *F. solani* are the species identified in dogs. Neutropenic or immunosuppressed animals may develop disseminated disease. The main active mycotoxin is zearalenone an estrogenic metabolite that can result in ovarian atrophy.

Clinical disease

Lesions or mycetoma may develop at the point of entry. Lesions may have a necrotic center with induration or may appear as cellulitis, onchomycosis, or keratitis.

Pulmonary lesions, sinusitis, allergic bronchopulmonary, and fungal balls similar to those seen with *Aspergillus* infections may occur. Ingestion of *Fusarium* mycotoxin contaminated food may also result in nausea, vomiting, diarrhea, and fever, as well as systemic disease (dermatitis, bone marrow suppression, kidney lesions, anemia, and hemorrhaging). Dogs fed *Fusarium* contaminated feed showed decreased food intake, a reduction in blood pressure, heart rate, serum concentrations of total protein, globulin, fibrinogen, and increased monocyte count. Catheter related infections, cystitis, endophthalmitis, and CNS disease may also occur.

Diagnosis

Tissue or blood culture isolation of organisms.

Treatment

Surgical excision and topical antifungals (compounded amphotericin-B) may be effective for minor localized infections. Catheters should be removed. For more severe soft tissue infections or osteomyelitis, long term antifungal therapy with amphotericin-B, voraconazole, or posaconazole is indicated. Itraconazole has been suggested but may not be effective in many cases. *F. solani* is not responsive to azoles. Keratitis can be treated with topical and oral voriconazole. Disseminated disease in neutropenic patients typically has a poor prognosis, regardless of antifungal therapy.

Drug therapy

- Amphotericin-B
- Voriconazole
- Posaconazole

Further reading

Evans, J., Levesque, D., Delahunta, A., *et al.* (2004) Intracranial fusariosis: A novel cause of fungal meningoencephalitis in a dog. *Vet Pathol.*, **41**, 510–514.

Kano, R., Maruyama, H., Kubota, M., *et al.* (2011) Chronic ulcerative dermatitis caused by *Fusarium sporotrichioides*. *Med Mycol.*, **49(3)**, 303–305.

Maxwell, C., Leung, K., Smith, T., *et al.* (2007) Effects of foodborne *Fusarium* mycotoxins with and without a polymeric glucomannan mycotoxin adsorbent on food intake and nutrient digestibility, body weight, and physical and clinicopathologic variables of mature dogs. *Amer J Veter Res.*, **68**, 1122–1129.

Chapter 81: *Giardia* Species

Description: Enteric Protozoa, flagellate trophozoite and cyst forms
Zoonotic Potential: Animals are reservoirs for human infection

Microbiology/epidemiology

Giardia is an important and common intestinal parasite affecting cats and dogs. It is found worldwide in rivers, streams, and lakes. Wild animals (beavers, muskrats, etc.) serve as reservoirs. *Giardia* exist as trophozoites and cysts that get excreted into stools. The cyst form is the infective form and is highly resistant to environmental conditions as long as it does not get desiccated. Transmission is typically by ingestion of contaminated food or water. Puppies and kittens in kennels or shelters have increased shedding rates (up to 50%) and act to further contaminate other animals.

Clinical disease

Animals may be asymptomatic carriers or present with acute or chronic diarrhea. Diarrhea is often watery and may be associated with malaise, flatulence, greasy stools, steatorrhea, rancid foul odor, nausea, vomiting, and dehydration. Chronic diarrhea can progress to soft, semiformed stools, weight loss, and failure to absorb fat, lactose, vitamin A, and vitamin B12. In young animals delayed development may occur.

Diagnosis

Giardia can be diagnosed by repeat stool samples looking for trophozoites or cysts. The trophozoites appear under a light microscope as "smiling faces". Stool samples may not always show trophozoites due to intermittent excretion. Immunoassays are the most sensitive and are a rapid means of detecting *Giardia*. IDEXX snap tests report 92% sensitivity and 99% specificity.

Treatment

No single therapy has been shown to be 100% effective. Drug resistance may develop to any of the drugs used. Environmental controls should be instituted to prevent reinfection. Fenbendazole (50 mg/kg PO q24 h × 3 days) or metronidazole (10–25 mg/kg PO q12 h × 7 days) is typically effective. Ronidazole (30–50 mg/kg PO BID × 7 days) in combination with chlorhexidine shampooing and environmental decontamination (4-chlorine-M-cresol) has been noted to be effective in outbreaks in dog kennels.

Drug therapy

- Metronidazole
- Fenbendazole

Drug therapy alternatives

- Drontal-Plus
- Tinidazole
- Ronidazole

Further reading

Covacin, C., Aucoin, D.P., Elliot, A., *et al.* (2011) Genotypic characterization of *Giardia* from domestic dogs in the USA. *Vet Parasitol.*, **177**, 28–32.

Fiechter, R., Deplazes, P., and Schnyder, M. (2012) Control of *Giardia* infections with ronidazole and intensive hygiene management in a dog kennel. *Vet Parasit.*, **187(1–2)**, 93–98.

Gruffydd-Jones, T., Addie, D., Belak, S., *et al.* (2013) Giardiasis in cats: ABCD guidelines on prevention and management. *J Feline Med Surg.*, **15(7)**, 650–652.

Keith, C.L., Radecki, S.V., and Lappin, M.R. (2003) Evaluation of fenbendazole for treatment of *Giardia* infection in cats concurrently infected with *Cryptosporidium parvum*. *Am J Vet Res.*, **64(8)**, 1027–1029.

Scorza, A.V. and Lappin, M.R. (2004) Metronidazole for the treatment of feline Giardiasis. *J Feline Med Surg.*, **6(3)**, 157–160.

Tangtrongsup, S. and Scorza, V. (2010) Update on the diagnosis and management of *Giardia* spp. infections in dogs and cats. *Top Companion Animal Med.*, **25(3)**, 155–162.

Chapter 82: *Helicobacter* Species

Description: Flagellate, gram negative, spiral shaped motile bacteria
Zoonotic Potential: May serve as a reservoir of non-*H. pylori* helicobacters in immunosuppressed humans

Microbiology/epidemiology

Cats and dogs are typically colonized with non-*H. pylori* helicobacter-like organisms. These are isolated from both healthy and vomiting animals. *H. felis* has been associated with disease in a number of studies in dogs. Animals may acquire the infection via oral–fecal or oral–oral transmission or by contact with infected water supplies or vomitus. Animals housed together may be at greater risk of infection. Sheep may serve as a reservoir for *H. canis* zoonotic infection.

Clinical disease

Helicobacter infections are often asymptomatic. Theoretical symptoms are intermittent vomiting, inappetence, pica, belching, weight loss, fever, and polyphagia. Infection with non-*H. pylori* Helicobacters has been associated with chronic lymphoplasma gastritis and lymphoid follicular hyperplasia. Although an association exists, no direct correlation can be made with the degree of colonization and disease severity. More severe gastritis with marked hyperplasia and neutrophilic infiltrates has been reported in cats and puppies.

Diagnosis

Clinical diagnosis is most commonly based on histopathology, cytology, rapid urease testing, and tissue PCR.

Treatment

Treatment of *Helicobacter* infections should be reserved for those that are symptomatic. Treatment has been derived from human medicine and has included clarithromycin plus amoxicillin in combination with bismuth subsalicylate (0.22 mL/kg PO q6–8 h in dogs only) for 14–21 days. Metronidazole can be substituted for clarithromycin. Proton pump inhibitors such as omeprazole and H2 antagonists such as famotidine may also be effective symptomatically.

Drug therapy

- Amoxicillin
- Clarithromycin
- Bismuth subsalicylate (dogs only)

Drug therapy alternatives

Metronidazole

Further reading

Haesebrouck, F., Pasmans, F., Flahou, B., *et al.* (2009) Gastric *Helicobacters* in domestic animals and nonhuman primates and their significance for human health. *Clin Microbiol Rev.*, **22(2)**, 202–223.

Neiger, R. and Simpson, K.W. (2000) *Helicobacter* infection in dogs and cats:facts and fiction. *J Vet Intern Med.*, **14(2)**, 125–133.

Swennes, A.G., Turk, M.L., Trowel, E.M., *et al.* (2014) *Helicobacter canis* colonization in sheep; a zoonotic link. *Helicobacter.*, **19(1)**, 65–68.

Sykes, J.E. and Marks, S.L. (2013) Gastric *Helicobacter*-like infections. Ch. 49. In: *Canine and Feline Infectious Diseases.* Sykes, J.E. (ed.), Elsevier, St. Louis, MO, pp. 465–473.

Chapter 83: *Hepatozoon Americanum/Canis* (Hepatozoonosis)

Description: Protozoal parasite, Apicomplexan, tick borne pathogen
Zoonotic Potential: Species specific, not a known zoonotic

Microbiology/epidemiology

Canine hepatozoonosis is caused by one of two species, *Hepatozoon canis* and *H. americanum*. *H. canis* infects canine species in Asia, Africa, Europe, the Middle East, and North and South America. *H. americanum* primarily infects dogs in the South Eastern and South Central USA. Domestic cats may also be infected with *H. felis*. *H. americanum* is transmitted by the Gulf Coast tick (*A. maculatum*) and *H. canis* is transmitted by the brown dog tick (*R. sanguineus*). Other tick species have been implicated in Japan and South America. The life cycle is completed in the tick (gamonts, oocysts, sporocysts) that eventually are acquired via oral ingestion (grooming, tick-infected prey). Sporozoites migrate across the intestine and travel to skeletal muscle where they form "onion-skin cysts". Pyogranulomas may develop following merogony with infection of the bone marrow, lymph nodes, liver, kidney, and lungs.

Clinical disease

Most animals are asymptomatic. Dogs with *H. americanum* may develop immunosuppression and co-infections with *Ehrlichia*, *Babesia*, *Anaplasma*, *Leishmania*, parvovirus, or distemper. Dogs typically present with mucopurulent ocular discharge, lethargy, fever, weight loss, muscle atrophy, joint pain, stiffness, weakness, pelvic limb paresis, ataxia, inability to rise, anorexia, and pale mucus membranes. Leukocytosis, elevated ALP, hypoglycemia, hypoalbuminemia, periosteal proliferation, anemia, and hypocalcemia are often present. Cats typically are asymptomatic unless immunosuppressed with FIV or FeLV. They may present with anorexia, weight loss, fever, lymphadenopathy, ulcerative glossitis, hypersalivation, anemia, serous ocular discharge, and icterus.

Diagnosis

Muscle biopsy is the most reliable diagnostic test. Cysts, meronts and pyogranulomas can be seen on histopathology. PCR of whole blood is useful but may have false positive results in early disease. Antibody serology (ELISA) and whole blood smears are useful but may have false positives (ELISA) or false negatives (cytology). Buffy coat examination is twice as sensitive as blood smears for *H. canis*.

Treatment

H. americanum may be treated with a combination of trimethoprim-sulfa (15 mg/kg PO q12 h), clindamycin (10 mg/kg PO q8 h) and pyrimethamine (0.25 mg/kg PO q24 h) for 14 days. Response typically occurs in 48–72 h, but does not eliminate the disease. Long-term treatment (2 years) with decoquinate (10–20 mg/kg PO q12 h) is required to prevent relapse. Alternatively, ponazuril (10 mg/kg PO q12 h × 14 d) followed by decoquinate may also be useful. PCR can be used to monitor every 3–6 months and treatment discontinued after PCR becomes negative. *H. canis* infections may be treated with imidocarb dipropionate (5–6 mg/kg SC or IM q14 d) in combination with doxycycline (10 mg/kg PO q21–28 d) until blood smears are negative (1–8 weeks). Cats may be treated with doxycycline (5 mg/kg PO q24 h × 10 d).

Drug therapy

- Clindamycin plus TMS plus pyrimethamine plus decoquinate *(H. americanum)*
- Imidocarb dipropionate plus doxycycline *(H. canis)*

Drug therapy alternatives

- Ponazuril plus decoquinote *(H. americanum)*
- Doxycycline alone (cats)

Further reading

Baneth, G. (2011) Perspectives on canine and feline hepatozoonosis. *Vet Parasitol.*, **181**, 3–11.
Vincent-Johnson, N. (2013) Canine and feline hepatozoonosis.
   Ch. 77. In: *Canine and Feline Infectious Diseases*. Sykes, J.E.
   (ed.), Elsevier, St. Louis, MO, pp. 747–759.

Chapter 84: Herpes Virus (Canine)

Description: Herpesviridae, Enveloped virus
Zoonotic Potential: Host specific, does not infect humans

Microbiology/epidemiology

Canine herpesvirus (CHV-1) is found worldwide in domestic and wild canine species. It is associated with acute neonatal death or "fading puppy syndrome". The virus is temperature sensitive (replicates at <37°C) and sensitive to disinfectants. The virus remains dormant in the neural ganglia and may be reactivated in stressful conditions or pregnancy. Dogs acquire the infection via direct oronasal contact or transplacental transmission. The incubation period is 6–10 days. Neonates with low body temperatures of <38°C are at high risk. Puppies >3–5 weeks may develop subclinical infection.

Clinical disease

Symptoms are non-specific and may include vocalization, anorexia, dyspnea, abdominal pain, incoordination, diarrhea, serous to hemorrhagic nasal discharge, mucous membrane petechiation, and death. Surviving older neonates develop blindness, ataxia, deafness, and/or complete recovery. Adults may develop upper respiratory signs (sneezing, serous oculonasal discharge, keratitis).

Diagnosis

Typically diagnosis is confirmed on necropsy of deceased littermates.

Treatment

Untreated neonates have 100% mortality and treatment is rarely effective. Supportive care including appropriate fluids, anticonvulsants, respiratory support, tube feeding, correction of clotting abnormalities, maintenance of body temperature and broad spectrum antibiotics to cover secondary bacterial infections is often required. The antibiotic drug of choice is ceftiofur, which may be preferred due to its limited effects on gastrointestinal bacterial flora. Antiviral therapy for CHV-1 is not well established. Acyclovir (20 mg/kg IV, PO q8 h × 21 days) has been used in humans. Famciclovir may also be effective. Herpetic keratoconjunctivitis requires concomitant therapy with trifluridine or iododeoxyuridine.

Drug therapy

- Acyclovir
- Ceftiofur

Drug therapy alternatives

Famciclovir.

Further reading

Carmichael, L.E and Greene, C.E. (1990) Canine herpesvirus
   infection. In: *Clinical Microbiology and Infectious Diseases of the
   Dog and Cat*. Greene, C.E. (ed.), W.B. Saunders, Philadelphia,
   PA, pp. 252–258.
Davidson, A.P. (2013) Canine herpesvirus infection. Ch. 16. In:
   Canine and Feline Infectious Diseases. Sykes, J.E. (ed.), Elsevier,
   St. Louis, MO, pp. 166–169.
Verstegen, J., Dhaliwal, G., and Verstegen-Onclin, K. (2008)
   Canine and feline pregnancy loss due to viral and non-
   infectious causes: a review. *Theriogen.*, **70(3)**, 304–319.

Chapter 85: *Histoplasma Capsulatum*

Description: Dimorphic fungus, microconidia/ macroconidia mold
Zoonotic Potential: Direct transmission from dogs/ cats typically does not occur

Microbiology/epidemiology

Histoplasma capsulatum is found in the mold form in soil. It grows best in humid, shady areas at modest temperature. *H. capsulatum* is endemic in the Mississippi and Ohio River valley and Central America. Bird and bat droppings promote growth. It is common in caves, bird roosts, chicken coops, schools, prisons, wood piles, dead trees, and old buildings. Animals become exposed when contaminated soil or materials are disturbed so that the spores become airborne. *Hisoplasma* is low in pathogenicity and primarily invades the reticuloendothelial system (lymph nodes, bone marrow, liver, spleen, and adrenal glands). Most cases are asymptomatic. Cats appear to be more susceptible than dogs. Cats with FeLV, lymphoma, FIP, or a history of glucocorticoid use may have an increased risk. Working dogs (Weimaraners, Brittany spaniels, Pointers), dogs with cancer, and those with heartworm disease may be at a higher risk.

Clinical disease

Cats may present with nonspecific signs such as weight loss, inappetence, dehydration, dyspnea, tachypnea, and fever. Cough and nasal discharge may also be present. Chorioretinitis, anterior uveitis, skeletal involvement, nodular or ulcerative draining skin lesions, peripheral lymphadenopathy, vomiting, diarrhea, oral ulceration, myelopathy, and hematuria have all been reported in cats. In dogs, diarrhea, weight loss, lethargy, fever, mucosal pallor, hilar lymphadenopathy, melena, tenesmus, hematochezia, dyschezia, and increased frequency of defecation are commonly reported. Other signs including respiratory difficulty, icterus, vomiting, hepatomegaly, lymphadenomegaly, nasal discharge, ocular signs, polyuria, polydipsia, lameness, neurological signs such as seizures, paralysis/paresis, chronic cutaneous or gingival lesions, and skin nodules have also been reported.

Diagnosis

Fungal serology, cytological exam, culture and *H. capsulatum* antigen assay may be used. Antigen assays may be the most accurate on cat urine. Urine or serum sensitivity and specificity need further study in cats and dogs and false positives may occur with other fungal agents. Cytology of fine-needle aspirates of the liver, spleen, lymph node, lung, bone marrow, rectal scrapings, CSF, synovial fluid, ascites, or pleural fluid show pyogranulomatous inflammation with *H. capsulatum* yeasts both extracellularly and intracellularly. Organisms can be found in up to 20% of cases using cytology with Diff-Quik or Wright stain. Fungal cultures take 2–6 weeks so may not always be useful. Serology may only demonstrate exposure and false negatives are common. Chest radiographs may demonstrate diffuse, linear, nodular or military interstitial patterns, mixed interstitial-alveolar-bronchial patterns, and pleural effusions in cats. In dogs, alveolar, interstitial, bronchial patterns, tracheobronchial lymphadenopathy, lung lobe consolidation, and pleural effusion may be present. Mineralization of lesions may be present in dogs, but are not reported in cats.

Treatment

Treatment is effective with a variety of antifungal therapies but is dependent on the severity of the disease and the immune status of the animal. At least 6 months of therapy is required and often antifungal therapy may be required for 1–2 years. The length of therapy should be based on lesion resolution and on serial monitoring of urine *H. capsulatum* antigenuria. Supportive care including crystalloid fluids, oxygen, blood transfusions, nutritional support, antiemetics and medications for hepatic encephalopathy (lactulose, etc.) may be required. Topical atropine, glucocorticoids or even enucleation may be necessary for severe ocular involvement.

Drug therapy

- Amphotericin-B
- Itraconazole

Drug therapy alternatives

- Fluconazole
- Voriconazole (resistant cases)
- Posaconazole (resistant cases)

Further reading

Aulakh, H.K., Aulakh, K.S., and Troy G.C. (2012) Feline histoplasmosis: a retrospective study of 22 cases (1986–2009). *J Am Anim Hosp Assoc.*, **48**, 182–187.

Cook, A.K., Cunningham, L.Y., Cowell, A.K., *et al.* (2012) Clinical evaluation of urine *Histoplasma capsulatum* antigen measurement in cats with suspected disseminated histoplasmosis. *J Feline Med Surg.*, **14**, 512–117.

Sykes, J.E. and Toboada, J. (2013) Histoplasmosis. Ch. 61. In: *Canine and Feline Infectious Diseases*. Sykes, J.E. (ed.), Elsevier, St. Louis, MO, pp. 587–598.

Chapter 86: Hyalohyphomycosis (*Paecilomyces/Scedosporium*)

Description: Nonpigmented, hyaline, transparent fungi

Zoonotic Potential: No direct transmission reported from animals, saprophytic organism typically not transmitted between hosts

Microbiology/epidemiology

Hyalohyphomycosis is caused by nonpigmented fungi (*Fusarium*, *Acremonium*, *Paecilomyces*, *Pseudallescheria* (*Scedosporium*), *Sagenomella*, *Phialosimplex*, *Geosmithia*, *Geomycs*) that are found worldwide and primarily invade tissues. Animals acquire the infection primarily via cutaneous inoculation from trauma. The disease appears to occur more commonly in dogs than cats. Immunosuppressed animals or those receiving immunosuppressive therapy are more likely to develop disseminated disease.

Clinical disease

Dogs typically present with local infections of the skin, nasal mucosa, or cornea. Disseminated infections may involve the respiratory tract, kidneys, bone marrow, lymph nodes, liver, spleen, bones, and CNS. Animals with local skin or bone lesions should be evaluated for lesions in the chest or abdomen.

Diagnosis

Tissue or fine needle aspirate culture along with cytologic or histologic evidence of fungal infection is diagnostic. Species identification is required due to differences in prognosis and antifungal drug efficacy between species. Antifungal drug sensitivities may be performed by specialized labs (University of Texas Health Science Center).

Treatment

Treatment outcome in veterinary patients is often poor due to the high rate of dissemination and the innate resistance of some species to antifungal therapy. Drug therapy should be based on antifungal culture and sensitivity. Cutaneous lesions that have not disseminated have been treated with surgical excision and itraconazole for at least 6 months. Itraconazole and amphotericin B have been utilized in animals with limited success. In humans, treatment of *P. variotti* and *P. lilacinus* disseminated infections has been successful with caspofungin and itraconazole combination therapy. Oculomycosis due to *P. lilacinus* has been successfully treated with surgical debridement and voriconazole. Ketoconazole in combination with terbinafine has been successful in some human cases refractory to amphotericin B. Tapering animals off of any immunosuppressive drugs is required for a successful outcome.

Drug therapy

- Itraconazole (local disease)
- Amphotericin B with itraconazole
- Caspofungin with itraconazole

Drug therapy alternatives

- Ketoconazole with terbinafine
- Voriconazole
- Posaconazole

Further reading

Chamilos, G. and Kontoyiannis, D.P. (2005) Voriconazole resistant disseminated *Paecilomyces variotti* infection in a neutropenic patient with leukemia on voriconazole prophylaxsis. *J Infection.*, **51**, 225–228.

Grooters, A.M. and Foil, C.S. (2012) Miscellaneous fungal infections. Ch. 65. In: *Infectious Diseases of the Dog and Cat.* 4th edn, Greene, C.E. (ed.), W.B. Saunders, Philadelphia, PA, pp. 675–688.

Letscher-Bru, V. and Herbrecht, R. (2003) Caspofungin: The first representative of a new antifungal class. *J. Antimicrob Chemother.*, **51**, 513–521.

Naggie, S. and Perfect, J.R. (2009) Molds: Hyalohyphomycosis, phaeohyphomycosis and zygomycosis. *Clin Chest Med.*, **30**, 337–353.

Pastor, F.J. and Guarro, J. (2006) Clinical manifestations, treatment and outcome of *Paecilomyces lilacinus* infections. *Clin Micro Infect.*, **12(10)**, 948–960.

Scott, I.U., Flynn, H.W., Miller, D., *et al.* (2001) Exogenous endophthalmitis caused by amphotericin B-resistant *Paecilomyces lilacinus*: treatment options and visual outcomes. *Arch Ophthalmol.*, **119**, 916–919.

Chapter 87: *Isospora* Species

Description: Coccidian, protozoa, oocysts
Zoonotic Potential: Host specific, not considered a zoonotic

Microbiology/epidemiology

Isospora is a host specific intestinal coccidian. Cats are the host of *I. felis* and *I. rivolta* while dogs are the hosts of *I. canis*, *I. obioensis*, *I. neorivolta*, and *I. burrowsi*. The parasite lives in the small intestine and oocysts pass out with the feces. Animals acquire the infection through ingestion of contaminated food, water, tissues, or ingestion of sporulated oocycts that are carried on flies, cockroaches, beetles, and so on. Puppies and kittens in shelter environments may have a much higher incidence of infection. Most infections are asymptomatic in adult animals.

Clinical disease

Infected puppies and kittens may present with watery diarrhea, vomiting, inappetence, weight loss, and abdominal discomfort. In severe infections animals may present with dehydration, fever, and diarrhea that may contain blood. Subclinical infections may also occur with clinical signs only occurring during periods of stress. Anemia and electrolyte abnormalities may result from the diarrhea.

Diagnosis

Oocysts can be noted on wet mounts or with acid-fast stains of fecal material. Small intestine histopathology demonstrates hypertrophic cysts, shortened villi, hyperplasia of lymph nodes, inflammation, and eosinophils.

Treatment

Isospora infections are generally self-limiting without treatment. However, treatment can speed recovery and prevent further environmental contamination. Animals with depressed immunity may not clear infections and may require prolonged courses of treatment.

Drug therapy

- Ponazuril
- Toltrazuril
- Sulfadimethoxine

Drug therapy alternatives

Trimethoprim-sulfonamide.

Further reading

Dubey, J.P. (2009) The evolution of knowledge of cat and dog coccidian. *Parasitology*, **136**, 1469–1475.

Lappin, M.R. (2010) Update on the diagnosis and management of *Isospora* spp. infections in dogs and cats. *Top Companion Animal Med.*, **25**, 133–135.

Lappin, M.R. (2013) Isosporiasis. Ch. 82. In: *Canine and Feline Infectious Diseases*. Sykes, J.E. (ed.), Elsevier, St. Louis, MO, pp. 793–799.

Chapter 88: *Klebsiella* Species

Description: Aerobic gram negative bacilli, polysaccharide capsule, produces endotoxins
Zoonotic Potential: Animals may serve as reservoirs for resistant bacteria

Microbiology/epidemiology

Klebsiella belong to the family Enterobacteriaceae. Similar to other Enterobacteriaceae, *Klebsiella* produce endotoxins that may be responsible for sepsis. *Klebsiella* infections are primarily considered nosocomial infections in cats and dogs with the exception of bladder infections and occasional pneumonias. Nosocomial pneumonias may also develop in animals that are hospitalized and on respirators. Airways may be colonized with bacteria so culture of airways without other signs of pneumonia may be insignificant. *Klebsiella* infections have also been noted in neonatal animals that succumb to sepsis as well as septicemia and multi-organ failure of adult dogs. Occasional outbreaks of severe enteritis and septicemia have occurred in healthy animals in kennels where contaminated feed may have been responsible.

Clinical disease

Pneumonia is typically not seen in healthy animals but may be an opportunistic organism in debilitated or immune suppressed animals. Animals may present with dyspnea, fever, and progressive signs of pneumonia. Animals may also present with signs of urinary tract infection. Rarely, animals may acquire surgical wound infections, neonatal sepsis, peritonitis, enteritis, and multi-organ failure (cardiovascular, respiratory, gastrointestinal, pancreatic, renal, and hepatic) due to *Klebsiella* infections.

Diagnosis

Aerobic culture and gram stain of blood, urine, and tracheal wash in combination with signs and symptoms of infection.

Treatment

Klebsiella is typically sensitive to a variety of antibiotics including first through third generation cephalosporins. However, nosocomial pathogens may be multidrug resistant and very difficult to treat. Culture and sensitivity should be performed in all animals with severe infections. Even carbapenemase-producing strains have been reported in companion animals.

Drug therapy

Cephalosporins (first through third).

Drug therapy alternatives

- Fluoroquinolones
- Extended spectrum penicillins
- Imipenem
- Meropenem
- Aminoglycosides

Further reading

Cavana, P., Tomesello, A., Ripanti, D., *et al.* (2009) Multiple organ dysfunction síndrome in a dog with *Klebsiella* pneumonia septicemia. *Schweiz Arch Tierheilkd.*, **151(2)**, 69–74.

Grobbel, M., Lubke-Becker, A., Alesik, E., *et al.* (2007) Antimicrobial susceptibility of *Klebsiella spp.* and *Proteus* spp. from various organ systems of horses, dogs and cats as determined in the BfT-GermVet monitoring program 2004–2006. *Berl Munch Tierarztl Wochenschr.*, **120(9–10)**, 402–411.

Roberts, D.E., McClain, H.M., Hansen, D.S., *et al.* (2000) An outbreak of *Klebsiella* pneumonia infection in dogs with severe enteritis and septicemia. *J Vet Diagn Invest.*, **12(2)**, 168–173.

Schafer-Somi, S., Spergser, J., Breitenfellner, J., *et al.* (2003) Bacteriological status of canine milk and septicemia in neonatal puppies–a retrospective study. *J Vet Med B Infect Dis Vet Public Health.*, **50(7)**, 343–346.

Stolle, I., Prenger-Berninghoff, E., Stamm, I., *et al.* (2013) Emergence of OXA-48 carbapenemase-producing *Escherichia coli* and *Klebseilla* pneumonia in dogs. *J Antimicrob Chemother.*, **68(12)**, 2802–2808.

Chapter 89: Leishmaniosis

Description: *Leishmania* protozoa, Trypanosomatidae family
Zoonotic Potential: Zoonotic vector borne parasite

Microbiology/epidemiology

Leishmania are vector borne protozoa primarily transmitted by female sandflies (*Phlebotomus, Lutzomyia*). *Leishmania* species are found worldwide and comprise at least 30 species. Canine and feline visceral leishmaniosis is caused by *L. infantum*. Cats appear relatively resistant to infection. Localized disease is typically caused by *L. braziliensis*. Dogs and rodents are reservoirs for human infection. Transmission may also occur by vertical transmission, venereal or via blood transfusion. Risk factors for infection in dogs includes >2 years of age, prolonged outdoor exposure, short haircoat, lack of insecticide control, and poor sanitation conditions. Most cases of visceral leishmaniosis are reported from Europe and Latin America with sporadic cases reported in the USA. In the USA, most case reports are from dogs with a history of travel to endemic areas. Occasional cases from the Midwest and East coast have occurred without a travel history. American tegumentary leishmaniasis is a localized cutaneous form of disease that is endemic in parts of South America with expansion into the USA.

Clinical disease

Symptoms are highly variable. Animals may develop subclinical infection or acute life threatening infections. Clinical disease may not occur for years after infection and may show mild popular or severe exfoliative dermatitis. Cutaneous lesions may appear as scaling, ulcerative, nodular, or popular with alopecia. Dogs may have long, brittle toe nails. Systemic disease follows cutaneous signs and includes fever, weight loss, muscle atrophy, inappetence, lethargy, oral ulcers, progressive splenomegaly, lymphadenomegaly, mucosal pallor, diarrhea, vomiting, polydipsia, hepatomegaly, epistaxis, melena, lameness, joint swelling, polyarthritis, myositis, blepharitis, uveitis, keratoconjunctivitis, prostatitis, vasculitis, anemia, and glomerulonephritis.

Diagnosis

Diagnosis can be made by cytologic examination, leishmania culture, antibody serology, PCR, or histopathology. Impression smears of affected tissues may demonstrate organisms making diagnosis simple. Serum serology with IFA or ELISA is sensitive (>90%) but may also be positive in healthy animals, so must be interpreted with clinical signs. Cats may have lower antibody titers.

Treatment

Multiple drugs have activity against leishmaniosis. However, parasitic cure is rare and relapses are frequent. The treatment of choice is meglumine antimoniate (100 mg/kg SC q24 h or 50 mg/kg SC q12 h × 4 weeks) with allopurinol (10 mg/kg PO q12 h) until clinical signs resolve and serology becomes negative (6–12 months). Miltefosine (2 mg/kg PO q24 h × 28 days) with allopurinol may be used as an alternative to meglumine but cure rates are lower and relapses occur more frequently. Allopurinol alone or combined with surgery may be effective for localized disease and in some cats. Liposomal amphotericin-B is considered the drug of choice in humans with leishmaniosis. Due to the likelihood of reinfection of dogs with leishmaniosis, the World Health Organisation does not recommend the use of drug protocols used in humans for dogs. In severe cases, or in areas where the disease is not endemic and the likelihood of recurrence is minimal, Liposomal amphotericin-B (3 mg/kg IV q48 h on Mondays, Wednesdays, and Fridays to a total dose of 21 mg/kg) may be considered. Prevention of re-infection by the use of spot-on repellants with permethrin, indoor housing of animals at night, neutering of animals to decrease transplacental transmission, and screening of donor blood products may help reduce infection rates.

Drug therapy

- Meglumine antimoniate plus allopurinol
- Miltefosine plus allopurinol

Drug therapy alternatives

- Liposomal amphotericin-B
- Allopurinol alone

Further reading

Maroli, M., Gradoni, L., Oliva, G., *et al.* (2010) Guidelines for prevention of leishmaniosis in dogs. *J Am Vet Med Assoc.*, **236**, 1200–1206.

Oliva, G., Roura, X., Crotti, A., *et al.* (2010) Guidelines for treatment of leishmaniasis in dogs. *J Am Vet Med Assoc.*, **236**, 1192–1198.

Paltrinieri, S., Solano-Gallego, L., Fondati, A., *et al.* (2010) Guidelines for diagnosis and clinical classification of leishmaniasis in dogs. *J Am Vet Med Assoc.*, **236**, 1184–1191.

Sykes, J.E., Baneth, G., and Petersen, C.A. (2013) Leishmaniosis. Ch. 74. In: *Canine and Feline Infectious Diseases.* Sykes, J.E. (ed.), Elsevier, St. Louis, MO, pp. 713–726.

Chapter 90: *Leptospira* Species

Description: Aerobic spirochete bacteria
Zoonotic Potential: Zoonotic, mobile, hook-shaped end

Microbiology/epidemiology

Leptospira bacteria are primarily excreted in the urine of wild and domestic mammals. Infected animals excrete the organisms into water and soil where they can remain viable for months. Humans are accidental hosts via direct contact with infected animals or contaminated soil or water. Veterinarians, farmers, sewer workers, and abattoir workers are at increased risk of infection. *L. interrogans* and *L. kirschneri* are the most common isolates in dogs. Outbreaks of disease often occur 3 months after wet weather. Transmission occurs via mucous membranes, cuts, abrasions, or inhalation of aerosolized infected water. Both dogs and cats can become infected, but cats appear to be more resistant to infection. Dogs that drink, swim, or wade in contaminated water sources, or those exposed to farm animals or rodent urine, can become infected. Large breed, outdoor, intact male dogs, urban cats, cats that hunt, or animals exposed to rat, mouse, or raccoon urine, may be at increased risk.

Clinical disease

The organism can penetrate intact mucus membranes or abraded skin and rapidly disseminate to the blood, eye, and even spinal fluid. Incubation is believed to be about 7 days in dogs. Clinical infection is dependent on the strain virulence, dose and host's immunity. Animals may show a mild, transient fever that may go unrecognized. The bacteria may persist in renal tubules without producing disease. Signs of kidney disease may show up months to a year after infection. In severe acute infections, animals may develop a biphasic fever, shivering, malaise, muscle tenderness, and ocular symptoms. This may be followed by an afebrile period with nausea, vomiting, diarrhea, lethargy, polyuria, polydipsia, hepatic dysfunction, jaundice, impaired renal function, myocardial damage, hemorrhage, vascular collapse, severe pulmonary hemorrhage syndrome, and CNS inflammation. Pregnant animals may have abortions, still births, and neonatal deaths.

Diagnosis

Diagnosis is often difficult due to the variability of the disease. Multiple assays have been used including Darkfield microscopy on urine, culture of blood and urine, serology of serum, histopathology of kidney tissue, and PCR of blood, urine, and tissue. The gold standard is currently serologic diagnosis using microscopic agglutination tests (MAT). A four-fold or greater increase in titer to at least one serovar over time is usually required for diagnosis in early disease or a four-fold decrease in late disease.

Treatment

Antibiotic treatment is highly effective and should be instituted early in the disease. The drug of choice is doxycycline. This is believed to be better at clearing the infection from the kidney. Parenteral ampicillin or penicillin G can be used as an alternative, but these are less effective at clearing organisms from the kidney. More recent studies evaluating multiple senovars *in vitro* demonstrated similar efficacy to doxycycline for azithromycin, cefotaxime, ceftriaxone, and fluoroquinolones. *In vivo* studies have further demonstrated the efficacy of minocycline and tigecycline. Survival benefits were comparable to that of doxycycline. Supportive care, dialysis if available, and immunization of animals at risk are recommended.

Drug therapy

Doxycycline PO, IV.

Drug therapy alternatives

- Ampicillin IV
- Penicillin IV
- Minocycline PO

Further reading

Hospenthal, D. and Murray, C.K. (2003) *In vitro* susceptibilities of seven *Leptospira* species to traditional and newer antibiotics. *Antimicrob Agents Chemother.*, **47(8)**, 2646–2657.

Sykes, J.E. (2013) Leptospirosis. Ch. 50. In: *Canine and Feline Infectious Diseases.* Sykes, J.E. (ed.), Elsevier, St. Louis, MO, pp. 474–483.

Sykes, J.E., Hartmann, K., Lunn, K.F., *et al.* (2011) ACVIM small animal consensus statement on leptospirosis: diagnosis, epidemiology, treatment and prevention. *J Vet Intern Med.*, **25(1)**, 1–13.

Tully, C.C., Hinkle, M.K., McCall, S., *et al.* (2011) Efficacy of minocycline and tigecycline in a hamster model of leptospirosis. *Diag Microbiol Infect Dis.*, **71(4)**, 366–369.

Chapter 91: Lice

Description: Ecto parasite, Hexapoda insect, flat, gray
Zoonotic Potential: Species specific biting and sucking lice, not considered a zoonotic

Microbiology/epidemiology

Infestations are found worldwide but are very species specific. Dogs typically are infested with either biting lice (*Trichodectus canis, Heterodoxus spiniger*) that feed on skin and skin dander, or sucking lice (*Linognathus piliferus setosus*) that feed on canine blood. *T. canis* is found throughout the world and is a vector to the dog tapeworm (*D. caninum*). Sucking lice are most common in colder climates. Cats are only infected with *Felicols subrostratus*, which is a biting louse. Lice lay eggs (nits) that attach to the animal's hair shafts. The eggs are cemented to the hair shaft. Animals typically acquire the infection directly from another animal, but may also be transmitted by brushes, combs, or contaminated bedding. Very young, old, or debilitated animals are predisposed.

Clinical disease

T. canis typically causes little irritation unless there is very heavy infestation. Animals may present with damage from rubbing, scratching, and biting of the skin. Severe pruritus, restlessness, intense scratching, alopecia, and rough hair coats may be noted. Biting or chewing lice may be found on the head, tail, or neck of the animal, particularly around skin abrasions or body openings. Sucking lice are typically noted around the neck and shoulders or underneath a collar. Cats with biting or chewing lice are typically older or debilitated and infestations may go unnoticed.

Diagnosis

Diagnosis is based on demonstration of the eggs (nits) or adult lice on the animal.

Treatment

Animals can be easily treated with a variety of insecticide products. Bedding, leashes, kennels, and so on must be either discarded or washed with hot water and dried on a high heat cycle in the dryer. Follow-up treatment is usually required after a week to prevent reinfestation from hatching eggs or nymphs. Secondary bacterial infections should be treated with antibiotics that cover *Staphylococcus* species. Pruritus may continue to occur 2–4 weeks after the removal of lice. Hydroxyzine, diphenhydramine, or topical steroid sprays may be used for severe pruritus.

Drug therapy

- Fipronil
- Imidacloprid
- Selamectin

Drug therapy alternatives

Topical Permethrin (dogs only).

Further reading

Akucewich, L.H., Philman, K., Clark, A., *et al.* (2002) Prevalence of ectoparasites in a population of feral cats from north central Florida during the summer. *Vet Parasit.*, **109**, 129–139.

Arther, R.G. (2009) Mites and lice: Biology and control. *Vet Clin Small Anim.*, **39**, 1159–1171.

Endris, R.G., Reuter, V.E., Nelson, J., *et al.* (2001) Efficacy of a topical spot-on containing 65% permethrin against the dog louse, *Trichodectes canis* (*Mallophaga:Trichodectidae*). *Veterin Therap.*, **2**, 135–139.

Kuzner, J., Turk, S., Grace, S., *et al.* (2013) Conformation of the efficacy of a novel fipronil spot-on for the treatment and control of fleas, ticks and chewing lice on dogs. *Vet Parasit.*, **193(1–3)**, 245–251.

Shanks, D.J., Gautiers, P., McTier, T.L., *et al.* (2003) Efficacy of selamectin against lice on dogs and cats. *Vet Rec.*, **152(8)**, 234–237.

Stanneck, D., Kruedewagen, E.M., Fourie, J.J., *et al.* (2012) Efficacy of an imidacloprid/flumethrin collar against fleas, ticks, mites and lice on dogs. *Parasit Vectors.*, **5**, 102.

Chapter 92: *Malassezia*

Description: Lipophilic yeasts, skin flora
Zoonotic Potential: Environmental not considered a zoonotic

Microbiology/epidemiology

Malassezia is an indigenous flora of the skin. They are lipid dependent yeasts with at least 13 species. *M. pachydermatis* is one of the more common isolates from healthy animals. *Malassezia* primarily colonize the ear, lips, axillae, interdigital spaces, anal sacs, nose, and vagina. The yeast is noted in high concentrations in dogs with skin disease (allergic dermatitis, endocrinopathies, etc.). American cocker spaniels, West Highland terriers, Basset hounds, poodles, Australian silky terriers, and Sphynx and Devon Rex cats appear predisposed to *Malassezia* skin infections.

Clinical disease

Skin lesions may be local or generalized. Animals may present with erythema, pruritus, alopecia, scaling, and greasy exudate. Chronic infections may have hyperpigmentation, lichenification, or stenosis of the ear canals. A pungent, offensive odor may be present. Cats may present with a greasy dermatitis.

Diagnosis

Based on clinical signs, cytological exam and positive response to antifungals. Scotch tape tests with Diff-Quick stain will demonstrate wide-based budding yeasts that appear as footprints on microscopic exam.

Treatment

Treatment of underlying disease is mandatory along with antifungal therapy. Superficial, topical or systemic antifungals are useful. Multiple topical treatments with clotrimazole, miconazole, or posaconazole combined with steroids and an antibiotic are available for otic infections. Regular bathing with an antifungal shampoo (2% miconazole/2–3% chlorhexidine) is sufficient in many cases. For severe infections, systemic antifungals may be required for up to 3–4 weeks or even longer for nail bed infections.

Drug therapy

- Ketoconazole
- Fluconazole
- Itraconazole

Drug therapy alternatives

Terbinafine.

Further reading

Berger, D.J., Lewis, T.P., Schick, A.E., *et al.* (2012) Comparison of once-daily versus twice-weekly terbinafine administration for the treatment of canine *Malassezia* dermatitis: a pilot study. *Vet Dermatol.*, **23**, 418–429.

Perrins, N., Gaudiano, F., and Bond, R. (2007) Carriage of *Malassezia* spp. yeasts in cats with diabetes mellitus, hyperthyroidism and neoplasia. *Med Mycol.*, **45(6)**, 541–546.

Sykes, J.E., Nagle, T.M., and White, S.D. (2013) *Malassezia* infections. Ch. 59. In: *Canine and Feline Infectious Diseases*. Sykes, J.E. (ed.), Elsevier, St. Louis, MO, pp. 570–573.

Chapter 93: *Microsporidia*

Description: Intracellular fungi, single cell, obligate, spore forming
Zoonotic Potential: Can be transmitted from animals to immunosuppressed humans

Microbiology/epidemiology

Microsporidia are intracellular parasitic fungi that form spores that are released into the environment. In animals, the most common and important pathogen is *Encephalitozoon cuniculi*. This microorganism is distributed worldwide and is commonly found in domestic rabbits. Dogs are believed to acquire the disease by the oronasal route, when an animal licks/sniffs the spore-infected urine of another animal. Dogs may act as reservoirs of the disease with 20% seropositive animals in some areas. However, *E. cuniculi* clinical infections are relatively rare in dogs. It is also passed through the placenta and during nursing. Immunosuppressed animals may develop chronic disease and shed organisms into the environment.

Clinical disease

Most dogs are asymptomatic and will recover without treatment, but it may be fatal to puppies or immune suppressed animals. Puppies may be stillborn, show failure to thrive, or die shortly after birth. Puppies may also display stunted growth, small size, poor hair coat, anorexia, have neurologic complications (encephalitis) starting at 3 weeks of age, and begin to show signs of renal failure. Adults that acquire the infection may present with aggressive behavior, seizures, blindness, and progressive renal failure. In chronically infected dogs, a hyperimmune response may lead to progressive renal failure because of immunocomplex deposition.

Diagnosis

The oocysts are primarily identified in the stool, but may also be isolated from urine or histology samples of kidney, lung, nasal mucosa, skin, brain, cornea, jejunum, and duodenum. Demonstration of organisms in tissue sections, isolation in tissue culture, electron microscopy, serological tests, and molecular techniques such as PCR, are all ways to diagnose *Microsporidia*. On gross examination, lesions are characterized by lymphoplasmacytic or granulomatous interstitial cell infiltration in multiple sites, particularly in the kidney, liver, and brain, but also in the heart, brain, skeletal muscle, and placenta.

Treatment

Treatment has not been well established for this organism. Supportive therapy in combination with antifungal therapy is recommended. Human patients have been treated with albendazole and itraconazole with some success. Drug treatment must be prolonged (2–3 months). If severe brain or renal disease is present the prognosis is poor. Due to the zoonotic potential, dogs with the infection should be isolated to an area that can be sanitized. Animal contact with immunosuppressed individuals should be avoided.

Drug therapy

- Albendazole
- Itraconazole

Drug therapy alternatives

- Fenbendazole
- Ponazuril

Further reading

Cray, C. and Rivas, Y. (2013) Seroprevalence of *Encephalitozoon cuniculi* in dogs in the United States. *J Parasitol.*, **99(1)**, 153–154.

Jamshid, S.H., Tabrizi, A.S., Bahrami, M., *et al.* (2012) *Microsporidia* in household dogs and cats in Iran: A zoonotic concern. *Vet Parasit.*, **185(2–4)**, 121–123.

Lallo, M.A., daCosta, L.F., and de Castro, J.M. (2013) Effect of three drugs against *Encephalitozoon cuniculi* infection in immunosuppressed mice. *Antimicrob Agents Chemother.*, **57(7)**, 3067–3071.

McInnes, E.F. and Stewart, G.C. (1991) The pathology of subclinical infection of *Encephalitozoon cuniculi* in canine dams producing pups with overt encephalititozoonosis. *J S Af Vet Assoc.*, **62**, 51–54.

Rossi, P., Urbani, C., Donelli, G., *et al.* (1999) Resolution of microsporidial sinusitis and keratoconjunctivitis by itraconazole treatment. *Am J Ophthalmol.*, **127(2)**, 210–212.

Snowden, K.F., Lewis, B.C., Hoffman, J., *et al.* (2009) *Encephalitozoon cuniculi* infections in dogs: a case series. *J Am Anim Hosp Assoc.*, **45(5)**, 225–231.

Snowden, K., Logan, K., and Didier, E.S. (1999) *Encephalitozoon cuniculi* strain III is a cause of encephalitozoonosis in both humans and dogs. *J Infect Dis.*, **180(6)**, 2086–2088.

Chapter 94: *Mucor* Species

Description: Opportunistic zygomycetes fungus, sparsely septate mycelia, round sporangia
Zoonotic Potential: Not considered a zoonotic

Microbiology/epidemiology

Mucor species are opportunistic molds that are found worldwide. They grow in soil, dust, and spoiled fruit and bread. Mucormycosis is a fulminant, acute, invasive fungal infection that is often fatal. Animals typically acquire the infection by either direct inoculation through the skin or inhalation of fungal spores into the respiratory tract. Diabetic, immunosuppressed animals, or animals with malignancies may be at increased risk. Infections may also occur with disrupted skin barriers from trauma, maceration, or via intravenous catheters. Cats may be more prone to disease than dogs due to fighting.

Clinical disease

Infections may involve multiple anatomic sites including: rhinocerebral, pulmonary, cutaneous, gastrointestinal, and disseminated infections. Animals may present with a subcutaneous swelling of a non-healing scratch wound, sinusitis or periorbital cellulitis. This may be followed by fever, soft tissue swelling, loss of extraocular muscle function, cranial nerve involvement, and protosis. Infected tissues may appear normal at first and then progress through an erythematous phase, with or without edema. Tissues and pus may then become black. In uncontrolled diabetic patients, rhinocerebral mucormycosis appears the most common area affected. Animals may also present with pulmonary disease with fever, cough, and dyspnea. Both dogs and cats may present with gastrointestinal mucormycosis and show signs of nausea, vomiting, duodenal perforation, and abdominal fungal masses.

Diagnosis

Biopsied material may not always demonstrate growth. A definitive diagnosis is dependent on characteristic histopathology of infective material. CT and MRI are helpful to confirm the extent of spread but are frequently negative or only have subtle findings. MRI may be more sensitive than CT scans. Bony erosion of the sinuses may be noted. Surgical exploration with biopsy of the infected site may be most useful.

Treatment

Extensive surgical debridement of infected tissue may improve the prognosis. Correction of any underlying ketoacidosis or immune suppression is important to achieve therapeutic resolution. Empiric combination therapy should be instituted as soon as possible. Liposomal amphotericin B in combination with an echinocandin (caspofungin) or itraconazole or both may be the protocol of choice for severe mucormycosis if affordable. Small localized infections that can be debrided may be treatable with itraconazole or posaconazole. Prognosis is often poor for disseminated infections.

Drug therapy

- Liposomal Amphotericin B plus caspofungin +/− itraconazole
- Liposomal Amphotericin B plus itraconazole

Drug therapy alternatives

Posaconazole.

Further reading

Cunha, S.C., Aguero, C., and Damico, C.B. (2011) Duodenal perforation caused by *Rhizomucor* species in a cat. *J Feline Med Surg.*, **13(3)**, 205–207.

Denzoin-Vulcano, L., Fogel, F., Tapias, M.O., *et al.* (2005) Abdominal zygomycosis in a bitch due to *Absidia corymbifera*. *Rev Iberoam Micol.*, **22(2)**, 122–124.

English, M.P. and Lucke, V.M. (1970) Phycomycosis in a dog caused by unusual strains of *Absidia corymbifera*. *Sabouraudia.*, **8(2)**, 126–132.

Ossent, P. (1987) Systemic aspergillosis and mucormycosis in 23 cats. *Vet Rec.*, **120(14)**, 330–333.

Ravisse, P., Fromentin, H., Destombes, P., *et al.* (1978) Cerebral mucormycosis in the cat caused by *Mucor pusillus*. *Sabouraudia.*, **16(4)**, 291–298.

Loupal, G. (1982) Hemorrhagic lung infarct following mucormycosis in a cat suffering from diabetes mellitus. *Dtsch Tierarztl Wochenschr.*, **89(3)**, 104–107.

Wray, J.D., Sparkes, A.H., and Johnson, E.M. (2008) Infection of the subcutis of the nose in a cat caused by *Mucor* species: successful treatment using posaconazole. *J Feline Med Surg.*, **10(5)**, 523–527.

Chapter 95: *Mycobacterium* Species

Description: Acid fast aerobic bacteria, saprophytic, intracellular, non-spore forming
Zoonotic Potential: Significant zoonotic potential

Microbiology/epidemiology

Mycobacterium species are widely distributed in the environment. *Mycobacterium* species require selective media for growth. Canine and feline *Mycobacterium* are categorized into three broad groups based on their growth patterns:

1. Slow-growing obligate pathogens (*M. tuberculosis* and *M. bovis*) and non-tuberculin (*M. avium)* intracellular complex,
2. Rapid-growing (non-tuberculous) "atypical Mycobacteria", and
3. Difficult to grow (cause of leprosy/tuberculous syndromes).

In general, slow growing *Mycobacterium* cause more extensive disease. Most cases of mycobacteriosis in dogs and cats belong to the *M. avium-intracellulare* complex (MAC). Slow-growing *Mycobacterium* (*M. tuberculosis* and *M. bovis*) require reservoir mammalian hosts to survive (cattle, deer, badgers, etc.). Dogs and cats may be exposed to "atypical" *Mycobacterium* via direct contact or ingestion of organisms from soil, water, animal carcasses, or feces. Leprosy diseases of dogs and cats do not appear to be zoonotic and are believed to be transmitted by the bite of a rodent or insect. All species of non-tuberculous *Mycobacterium* are considered of low virulence, typically only causing disease in immunosuppressed individuals. Most cats are somewhat resistant to *M. avium* infections with the exception of Siamese cats.

Clinical disease

All mycobacterium cause granulomatous and pyogranulomatous disease. Localized infections may be asymptomatic leading to eventual dissemination. Gastrointestinal signs may include diarrhea, vomiting, and abdominal pain. Animals may develop fever, weight loss, anemia, elevated alkaline phosphatase, and organomegaly. Affected organs may have a yellowish appearance with granulomatous lesions observed. MAC may start following colonization of the gastrointestinal or respiratory tract. A localized infection may then develop leading to a chronic infection of the reticular endothelial system (RES) or organ systems. *M. avium* infection produces granulomatous lesions similar to tubercular lesions of *M. tuberculosis* and *M. bovis*. *Mycobacterium* produce a cell mediated, delayed type hypersensitivity response similar to granulomatous inflammation.

Diagnosis

Diagnosis can be made from cytology samples using Romanosky stains. Histology samples require acid fast staining and may require culture and/or PCR. Culture and/or PCR with gene sequencing are needed to make a definitive species identification.

Treatment

The potential for zoonotic transmission of *Mycobacteria* from animals to humans must be considered before initiating treatment. Evidence exists for the transmission of *M. bovis* and *M. tuberculosis* between dogs, cats, and humans. Risk is much higher for immunocompromised people. Leprosy *Mycobacteria* do not appear to be transmissible. The treatment of immunocompromised (cancer, FeLV, etc.) animals is not recommended due to poor prognosis. A good to poor prognosis in immunocompetent hosts is dependent on both the *Mycobacterium* species and disease distribution. Surgical excision of all lesions with appropriate reconstructive techniques should be performed prior to drug therapy. Long term treatment with multiple drugs is required for 6–8 weeks and up to 2 months after clinical resolution to prevent recurrence and resistance.

Drug therapy

Lepromatous/*M. avium*
- Clarithromycin with rifampin and/or clofazimine
- Azithromycin with rifampin and/or clofazimine

Atypical/*M. smegmatis, M. Fortuitum*, and *M. Chelonae*

Doxycycline in combination with enrofloxacin.

Further reading

Gunn-Moore, D.A. and Greene, C.E. (2006) Infections caused by slow-growing *Mycobacterium*. In: *Infectious Diseases of the Dog and Cat*. 3rd edn, Greene, C.E. (ed.). Saunders, Elsevier, St. Louis, MO, pp. 462–477.

Jang, S.S. and Hirsch, D.C. (2002) Members of the genus *Mycobacterium* affecting dogs and cats. *J Amer Anim Hosp Assoc.*, **38**, 217–220.

Malik, R., Wigney, D.I., Dawson, D., *et al.* (2000) Infection of the subcutis and skin of cats with rapidly growing *Mycobacteria*: A review of microbiological and clinical findings. *J Fel Med Surg.*, **2**, 35–48.

Chapter 96: *Mycoplasma* Species

Description: Cell wall-deficient bacteria, "fried egg" appearance on culture
Zoonotic Potential: Host specific not considered a zoonotic

Microbiology/epidemiology

Mycoplasma spp. are the smallest organisms known that are capable of free-living and self-replicating. They lack cell walls and have fastidious growth requirements. *Mycoplasma* spp. are commonly found on the mucous membranes (mouth, upper respiratory, and urogenital) of animals. *Mycoplasma* have been associated with significant disease in overcrowded, unhygienic kennels, and shelters. In dogs, *M. cynos* appears to be the pathogen associated with canine infectious respiratory disease (CIRD). Feline infectious anemia, which was due to the agent known as *H. felis*, has now been reassessed and was found to include three different species of *Mycoplasma* (*Mycoplasma haemofelis, Candidatus Mycoplasma turicensis*, and *Candidatus Mycoplasma haemominutum*). A cat becomes infected after being bite by infected fleas. The *Mycoplasma* organism attaches to the outside of red blood cells. The cat's immune system detects foreign proteins on the red blood cells and begins to attack them. Infected cats may be reservoirs of infection.

Clinical disease

In cats, *Mycoplasmas* are commonly associated with keratoconjunctivitis and upper respiratory tract disease. Cats may present with conjunctivitis, sneezing, and nasal discharge. Concurrent infections are common. In dogs and cats, pneumonia may occur with fever, cough, lethargy tachypnea, and decreased appetite. In dogs, epididymitis, prostatitis, and lower urinary tract infections may occur in patients with primary urinary tract diseases such as neoplasms, stones, and so on. Isolated cases of arthritis, bacteremia, pyothorax, and meningoencephalitis have also been reported. *M. haemofelis* is the most pathogenic species and causes hemolytic anemia in immunocompetent cats. Cats with *M. haemofelis* may present with pale mucus membranes, jaundice, weakness, fever, and anemia. Typically, cats with *Candidatus Mycoplasma turicensis* and *Candidatus Mycoplasma haemominutum* are not always associated with anemia, so other differential diagnosis should be made.

Diagnosis

Diagnosis of *Mycoplasma* is made on a clinical basis. Radiographs may demonstrate pleural effusion, interstitial to alveolar patterns or lung lobe consolidation. Joint radiographs may demonstrate soft tissue swelling and erosive changes to bone. For definitive diagnosis, either PCR assays or growth on special culture media are required. However, PCR results should be interpreted with clinical results due to common colonization without infection. PCR is the most effective tool in diagnosing *M. haemofelis*. The organism can be isolated from a transtracheal or bronchoalveolar lavage, synovial fluid, or CSF. Tissue swabs should be done vigorously and transported rapidly due to early fast deterioration. Molecular typing is required for speciation.

Treatment

Typically tetracyclines or fluoroquinolones are the drug of choice. Treatment should last for 2–3 weeks. Ulcerative keratitis can be treated with ofloxacin ophthalmic drops or oxytetracycline ointment.

Drug therapy

- Doxycycline
- Minocycline
- Fluoroquinolone

Further reading

Chalker, V.J., Owen, W.M., Paterson, C., *et al.* (2004) Mycoplasmas associated with canine infectious respiratory disease. *Microbiol.*, **150(10)**, 3491–3497.

Jang, S.S., Ling, G.V., Yamamoto, R., and Wolf, A.M. (1984) *Mycoplasma* as a cause of canine urinary tract infection. *J Am Vet Med Assoc.*, **185**, 45–47.

Kewish, K.E., Appleyard, G.D., Myers, S., *et al.* (2010) Feline hemotropic Mycoplasmas. *Vet Clin North Am Small Animal Pract.*, **40(6)**, 1157–1170.

Sykes, J.E. (2010) Feline hemotropic Mycoplasmas. *Vet Clin North Am Small Animal Pract.*, **40(6)**, 1157–1170.

Chapter 97: Myiasis (Maggots)

Description: Insect larva, maggots
Zoonotic Potential: Can infect humans in rural tropical regions where myiatic flies thrive

Microbiology/epidemiology

Myiasis involves the larvae (maggots) of two-winged (dipterous) flies. House flies (*Musca domestica*), blowflies or bottle flies (*Calliphora species, Phaenicia species, Lucilia species,* and *Phormia species*) and flesh flies (*Sarcophaga species*) all cause myiasis. Normally these flies lay their eggs on decaying meat or fecal matter. Typically, flies are attracted to open wounds and feces or urine soaked fur, some species (botfly, blowfly, and screwfly) can create an infestation on unbroken skin and can even use moist soil and non-myiatic flies as vectors for their parasitic larvae. Eggs hatch within 24 h and larva feed on decaying tissues for approximately 5–7 days. The larva drop off the animal, enter the soil, and emerge a few weeks later.

Clinical disease

Three types of cutaneous infestation exist. Cutaneous myiasis is skin infestation by the larvae of certain fly species. However, furuncular, wound and migratory myiasis may also occur. In some cases the nasopharynx, gastrointestinal and genital urinary tracts may also be involved. Furuncular myiasis is caused by *Dermatobia hominis*, which is more common in the tropics where larva burrow under the skin. *Dermatobia hominis* cause papules that later become a furuncular-like (boil-like) nodule with a central pore through which the organism breathes. Screwworms cause obligate myiasis that can infect dogs and other animals by laying eggs in a pre-existing wound in the skin or mucous membranes. The maggots bore their way into the tissues. Some species can bore into the skin causing a large subcutaneous lesion containing numerous maggots. Dogs with myiasis may present with a pungent odor and heavily infested dogs can even die of shock or infection.

Diagnosis

Diagnosis is based on visualization of fly larva (maggots) on the skin or within wounds.

Treatment

Hair should be shaved from the affected area and cleaned with soap (chlorhexidine/betadine solution) and water. Maggots should be mechanically or surgically removed. Animals with infected wounds should be treated with oral antibiotics. Drug therapy is often not required but can be given in cases with severe infection. Ivermectin (0.1–0.3 mg/kg) is typically the drug of choice. Nitenpyram (single dose orally or rectally) has been used anecdotally. Debilitated animals should remain indoors and frequently checked for further reinfestation. Pyrethrin shampoo may be of benefit in preventing reoccurrence in dogs.

Drug therapy

- Ivermectin
- Nitenpyram

Further reading

Anderson, G.S. and Huitson, N.R. (2004) Myiasis in pet animals in British Columbia: The potential of forensic entomology for determining duration of possible neglect. *Can Vet J.*, **45(12)**, 993–998.

McGraw, T.A. and Turiansky, G.W. (2008) Cutaneous Myiasis. *J Am Acad Dermatol.*, **58**, 907–926.

Urban, J.E. and Broce, A. (1998) Flies and their bacterial loads in greyhound dog kennels in Kansas. *Curr Microbiol.*, **36(3)**, 164–170.

Chapter 98: *Neospora Caninum*

Description: Coccidian protozoan parasite
Zoonotic Potential: Host specific, no clear evidence of transmission to humans

Microbiology/epidemiology

Neospora canium are obligate intracellular parasites found worldwide. Dogs are their definitive hosts and the only host where the entire life cycle is completed. *N. caninum* is the most common cause of infertility, abortion, and neonatal mortality in cattle. Herbivores acquire the infection via ingestion of oocyts shed in canine feces. Sheep, deer, and water buffalo are intermediate hosts. Dogs are infected via transplacental, transmammary, ingestion of raw infected tissues or infected bovine fetal membranes. Oocysts are infective 24–72 h after being shed. Sporozoites are released in the intestine and penetrate into intestinal epithelial cells that become bradyzoite cysts. Pregnancy can reactivate the infection and permit transplacental transmission. Rural or free roaming dogs, purebreds, and immunosuppressed animals have the highest risk of infection.

Clinical disease

Many dogs are asymptomatic. Puppies infected *in utero* may develop symptoms between 1–6 months of age. Involvement of the lumbosacral spinal nerve roots typically result in ascending paralysis, muscle atrophy, fibrous muscle and joint contracture, hyperextension of pelvic limbs, loss of patellar reflexes, exercise intolerance, ataxia, high-stepping or bunny-hopping gait, urinary incontinence, lethargy, tetraplegia, mandibular paralysis, dysphagia, vomiting, respiratory difficulty, and death. Adult dogs may present with polymyositis, neurologic symptoms, meningoencephalomyelitis, and infection of the heart, liver, pancreas, lungs, skin, and eyes.

Diagnosis

Diagnosis relies on serology, detection of protozoal organisms in body fluids, aspirates, or tissues using light microscopy or PCR. Fecal oocytes are typically not found. Serology (IFA and ELISA) of serum or CSF with a four-fold increase or >1:800 with clinical signs are suggestive of neosporosis.

Treatment

Treatment is challenging and often ineffective. The drug of choice is clindamycin. Other regimens that have been attempted have included TMS, pyrimethamine, and ponazuril. Treatment should continue for a minimum of 4 weeks. Early treatment may increase survival. Littermates of infected animals should be tested and early treatment should be initiated in seropositive puppies. Steroids have been suggested for meningoencephalomyelitis in combination with antiprotozoal therapy. Prevention involves containment of free roaming animals, muzzling to prevent predation on farms, and avoidance of raw meat or carcasses.

Drug therapy

- Clindamycin
- TMS
- Pyrimethamine
- Ponazuril

Further reading

Dubey, J.P. and Lappin, M.R. (2012) Toxoplasmosis and neosporosis. In: *Infectious Diseases of the Dog and Cat.* 4th edn. Greene, C.E., (ed.). Elsevier, Saunders, St. Louis, MO, pp. 754–775.

Dubey, J.P. and Schares, G. (2011) Neosporosis in animals-the last five years. *Vet Parasitol.*, **180**, 90–108.

Sykes, J.E. (2013) Neosporosis. Ch. 73. In: *Canine and Feline Infectious Diseases.* Sykes, J.E. (ed.), Elsevier, St. Louis, MO, pp. 704–712.

Chapter 99: *Neorickettsia Helminthoeca*

Description: Gram negative, obligate intracellular bacteria
Zoonotic Potential: Host specific, no clear evidence of transmission to humans

Microbiology/epidemiology

Neorickettsia helminthoeca is the organism underlying salmon poisoning disease (SPD) that affects animals in the Northwestern USA. The *Rickettsia* reside within trematode flukes (*Nanophyetus salmincola*) that commonly infect salmon in endemic areas. Dogs and other mammals acquire the infection by eating fish containing the vector trematode. The aquatic snail (*Oxytrema silicula*) is an intermediate host that limits the distribution of the organism. Dogs must ingest the encysted trematode metacercariae within uncooked or undercooked freshwater fish. Maturation of the metacercariae to the adult fluke in the intestine inoculates the *Rickettsia* into its host. Large breed, intact male dogs appear at highest risk potentially due to their popularity with fisherman.

Any breed ingesting raw or undercooked fish from endemic areas may acquire the infection.

Clinical disease

Dogs typically present with high fever (105°F/41°C), inappetence, lethargy, vomiting, diarrhea, hematochezia, weight loss, melena, polyuria, and polydipsia. Diarrhea may have melena, frank blood, or mucus. Neurologic signs have been reported. Lymphadenomegaly, dehydration, splenomegaly, tachypnea, tachycardia, sclera, or conjunctival injection, limb/cervical edema, mucosal pallor, cardiac arrhythmias, epistaxis, and hyphema may be present.

Diagnosis

Diagnosis is based on fecal sedimentation, cytology of lymph nodes or splenic aspirates, histopathology of biopsies, and PCR. Fecal sedimentation combined with zinc sulfate centrifugal fecal flotation of feces has specificity of 100% if performed by a parasitologist. Eggs are light brown, ovoid, with an operculum at one end.

Treatment

Treatment is with antibiotics and supportive care (antiemetics, fluids). Intravenous crystalloid fluid therapy, fresh frozen plasma, dextrans or hetastarch, whole blood, or packed RBCs may be required. Antibiotics should include intravenous doxycycline or oxytetracycline. Clinical improvement may occur within 1–4 days. The fluke infection should be treated with praziquantel (10–30 mg/kg PO q24 h × 1–2 days).

Drug therapy

- Doxycycline
- Oxytetracycline

Drug therapy alternatives

- Enrofloxacin
- Trimethoprim-sulfamethoxazole

Further reading

Mack, R.E., Bercovitch, M.G., Ling, G.V., *et al.* (1990) Salmon poisoning disease complex in dogs: A review of 45 cases. *Californ Vet.*, **44**, 42–45.

Sykes, J.E. (2013) Salmon poisoning disease. Ch. 31. In: *Canine and Feline Infectious Diseases.* Sykes, J.E. (ed.), Elsevier, St. Louis, MO, pp. 311–319.

Sykes, J.E., Marks, S.L., Mapes, S., *et al.* (2010) Salmon poisoning disease in dogs: 29 cases. *ZJ Vet Intern Med.*, **24(3)**, 504–513.

Chapter 100: *Nocardia* Species

Description: Aerobic acid fast bacteria, delicate, branching, beaded appearance
Zoonotic Potential: Environmental not considered a zoonotic

Microbiology/epidemiology

Nocardia are high-order, acid-fast bacteria that are only weakly gram positive. They are found worldwide in soil and decaying plant material. *Nocardia* are primarily isolated from respiratory tract infections but may also cause localized infections and disseminated disease mostly in immunocompromised animals. Animals with defective T-cell immunity, malignancy, or on immunosuppressive drugs (steroids, cyclosporine) may be at higher risk of infection. In humans, *Nocardia* infections are noted with neutrophil dysfunction, inflammatory bowel disease, vasculitis, sarcoidosis, and immunoglobulin deficiencies. In cats and dogs, *Nocardia nova* is a common isolate. *Nocardia* may be acquired via inhalation of organisms or inoculation through the skin. Infections typically result in local abscesses with an intact immune system.

Clinical disease

Dog and cat infections can be regional or disseminated. Local wound infections may extend to regional lymph nodes. Abscesses contain high numbers of polymorphonuclear leukocytes. Exudates are sanguinopurulent and may have soft granules consisting of bacteria, neutrophils, and debris.

Dogs and cats can develop debilitating, febrile illness. Pneumonia and suppurative pleuritis with empyema is common. In dogs, thoracic empyema with granulomatous serositis is reported. Dissemination occurs to the liver, bones, joints, and rarely, into the central nervous system, which often results in a poor prognosis.

Diagnosis

Nocardia can be isolated by bronchoscopy or aspirates from abscesses on aerobic culture. Increased carbon dioxide concentrations favor growth. Culture of "granules" typically offers the best chance of isolation.

Treatment

Abscesses, empyemas, and serosal effusions are treated by drainage and lavage. Antibiotic therapy with tri-methoprim-sulfamethoxazole appears to produce the best results. High doses are required if CNS infection is present. Alternative drugs include the tetracyclines. *Nocardia nova* may respond to tetracyclines and macrolides. Antibiotics should be given for 6–12 months due to the high recurrence rates of this organism.

Drug therapy

Trimethoprim-sulfamethoxazole.

Drug therapy alternatives

- Doxycycline/Minocycline
- Macrolides
- Amikacin plus Imipenem

Further reading

Ambrosioni, J., Lew, D., and Garbino, J. (2010) Nocardiosis: Updated clinical review and experience at a tertiary center. *Infection*, **38(2)**, 89–97.
Anagnostou, T., Arvanitis, M., Kourkoumpetis, T.K., *et al.* (2014) Nocardiosis of the central nervous system: experience from a general hospital and review of 84 cases from the literature. *Medicine*, **93(1)**, 19–32.
Hirsh, D.C. and Jang, S.S. (1999) Antimicrobial susceptibility of *Nocardia nova* isolated from five cats with nocardiosis. *J Am Vet Med Assoc.*, **215(6)**, 815–817.
Malik, R., Krockenberger, M.B., O'Brien, C.R., *et al.* (2006) *Nocardia* infections in cats: a retrospective multi-institutional study of 17 cases. *Aust Vet J.*, **84(7)**, 235–245.
Marino, D.J. and Jaggy, A. (1993) Nocardiosis. A literature review with selected case reports in two dogs. *J Vet Intern Med.*, **7(1)**, 4–11.
Riberiro, M.G., Salerno, T., Mattos-Guaraldi, A.L., *et al.* (2008) Nocardiosis: An overview and additional report of 28 cases in cattle and dogs. *Rev Inst Med Trop Sao Paulo.*, **50(3)**, 177–185.
Siak, M.K. and Burrows A.K. (2013) Cutaneous nocardiosis in two dogs receiving ciclosporin therapy for the management of canine atopic dermatitis. *Vet Derm.*, **24(4)**, 453–456.

Chapter 101: *Otodectes Cynotis* (Otodectic Mange)

Description: Psoroptidae insects, ectoparasitic mites
Zoonotic Potential: Does not infect humans

Microbiology/epidemiology

Otodectes cynotis mites are found worldwide and are a common cause of otitis externa in cats and dogs. Mites are highly contagious to both cats and dogs. Animals typically acquire the infection from direct contact with other infected animals. Mites typically infect the horizontal and vertical ear canal, but may also invade the body. Young cats and dogs are predisposed to infection.

Clinical Disease

Animals may present with head shaking, severe ear scratching, and suppurative otitis externa. The external ear flaps may be red, crusted, and excoriated, and scabs may be noted on the ear tips. The canals typically contain dark brown, crumbly, waxy discharge that is like coffee grounds in appearance. In severe cases, secondary bacterial infection may be present and the tympanic membrane may be ruptured.

Diagnosis

Mites are easily diagnosed by removing a small amount of wax from the ear canal using a cotton tip applicator and applying this to a microscope slide to look for adult mites. The mites can also be seen using a magnifying glass. They appear as white specks on a dark background that move.

Treatment

All animals should be treated at one time with appropriate therapy. The ears should be cleaned with a ceruminolytic agent prior to either topical or systemic therapy. Remaining wax may not allow for drugs to penetrate and may decrease efficacy of treatment. Local treatment inside the ear typically involves the use of a miticide. These must be applied according to the manufacturer and typically contain either pyrethrins or thiabendazole. Because the mites may also infect the body, the entire dog and all contacts may require treatment with a pyrethrin-based shampoo, or flea powder weekly for 4 weeks. For ears that appear infected with bacterial or fungal components, a product containing an antibiotic such as Tresaderm or Oridermyl (steroid/antibiotic/antifungal) may be of value. Systemic macrocyclic agents including selamectin (topically every 2 weeks × 3 treatments) and moxidectin/imidacloprid (topically every 2 weeks × 3 treatments) are effective spot-on treatments of ear mites. Ivermectin injectable has been used off-label (0.5 mL of 0.01% diluted solution AU × 1) for the treatment of *Otodectes* in kittens housed in shelters. This effectively killed mites within 72 h.

Drug therapy

- Topical mitacides (Acarexx, Cerumite, Mitox, Nolvamite, Oridermyl, Tresaderm)
- Selemectin
- Imidacloprid/moxidectin
- Ivermectin

Drug therapy alternatives

Pyrethrin shampoo/powder (dogs).

Further reading

Curtis, C.F. (2004) Current trends in the treatment of *Sarcoptes*, *Cheyletiella* and *Otodectes* mite infestations in dogs and cats. *Vet Dermatol.*, **15(2)**, 108–114.

Ghubash, R. (2006) Parasitic miticidal therapy. *Clin Tech Small Anim Pract.*, **21(3)**, 135–144.

Nunn-Brooks, L., Micahel, R., Ravitz, L.B., *et al.* (2011) Efficacy of a single dose of an otic ivermectin preparation or selamectin for the treatment of *Otodectes cynotis* infestation in naturally infected cats. *J Feline Med Surg.*, **13(8)**, 622–624.

Roy, J., Bedard, C., Moreau, M., *et al.* (2012) Comparative short-term efficacy of Oridermyl auricular ointment and Revolution selamectin spot-on against feline *Otodectes cynotis* and its associated secondary otitis externa. *Can Vet J.*, **53(7)**, 762–766.

Six, R.H., Clemence, R.G., Thomas, C.A., *et al.* (2000) Efficacy and safety of selamectin against *Sarcoptes scabiei* on dogs and *Otodectes cynotis* on dogs and cats presented as veterinary patients. *Vet Parasitol.*, **91(3–4)**, 291–309.

Chapter 102: Papilloma Virus

Description: Papillomavirus, non-enveloped, icosahedral shape
Zoonotic Potential: Host specific, not considered a zoonotic

Microbiology/epidemiology

Papilloma viruses are noted worldwide in many species, including cats and dogs. Exposure to the virus is widespread based on serology but congenital or acquired cell-mediated immune deficiencies may be required for the development of clinical disease. Clinical infection is rare in cats compared to dogs. *Canis familiaras* is associated with oral papillomas and cutaneous or invasive squamous cell carcinomas in dogs. In cats, papillomavirus infections are associated with plaque-like, dysplastic lesions, squamous cell carcinomas, Bowenoid *in situ* squamous cell carcinomas, and sarcoids.

Clinical disease

Oral papillomas may occur on the lips, mucus membranes, tongue, pharynx, eyelids, or skin. Lesions start as smooth and raised and enlarge into cauliflower-like lesions. Dogs may develop cutaneous exophytic papillomas that are wartlike on the lower limbs and feet. Endophytic or inverted papillomas have also been described.

Diagnosis

Based on history and gross appearance of lesions. Full thickness biopsy and histology are required to confirm the diagnosis. PCR, immunohistochemistry, *in-situ* hybridization, and electron microscopy can be used for analysis. PCR is often positive in healthy tissues so results must be interpreted along with clinical signs.

Treatment

Oral and cutaneous lesions may regress without treatment in young animals (4–8 weeks). Adult dogs should have lesions removed if there is physical obstruction, but reoccurrence is common. Underlying immune suppression should be evaluated in adults and any immunosuppressive therapy discontinued if possible. The current drug of choice has been azithromycin (10 mg/kg PO q24 h × 10 days) for oral and cutaneous papillomatosis. Antivirals (cidofovir) and immunomodulators (imiquimod cream applied topically 3× weekly) have been used in cats or dogs with localized lesions with some success. Imiquimod is an irritant to mucus membranes and care should be taken to prevent licking/grooming after application.

Drug therapy

Azithromycin

Drug therapy alternatives

- Cidofovir
- Imiquimod 5% cream

Further reading

Gill, V.L., Bergman, P.J., Baer, K.E., *et al.* (2008) Use of imiquimod 5% cream (Aldara) in cats with multicentric squamous cell carcinomas *in situ*: 12 cases (2002–2005). *Vet Comp Oncol.*, **6(1)**, 55–64.

Lange, C.E. and Favrot, C. (2011) Canine papillomaviruses. *Vet Clin North Am Smal Animal Pract.*, **41**, 1183–1195.

Sykes, J.E. and Luff, J.A. (2013) Viral papillomatosis. Ch. 26. In: *Canine and Feline Infectious Diseases*. Sykes, J.E. (ed.), Elsevier, St. Louis, MO, pp. 261–267.

Chapter 103: *Paragonimus* Species (Liver Flukes)

Description: Flatworms, or platyhelminths, oral suckers, parasitic flukes
Zoonotic Potential: Considered a zoonotic through increased environmental distribution of life cycle.

Microbiology/epidemiology

Paragonimus species are highly evolved parasites with a complex life cycle that involves at least three different hosts (snails, crustaceans, mammals). Nine species are known to cause paragonimiasis (liver flukes). P. westermani causes paragonimiasis in Asia. *P. kellicotti* is endemic in North America and is a well known pathogen of dogs, cats, and other domestic animals. It has been reported rarely in humans. Animals acquire the infection via ingestion of food that contains metacercariae (uncooked or raw crab meat, crayfish, or raw/uncooked meat from a paratenic host). These hatch and penetrate the intestinal wall and wonder into the peritoneal cavity, where they eventually pass into the lungs. Eggs are passed through the cyst wall, coughed up, swallowed, and passed in feces.

Clinical disease

Many infections may be asymptomatic. Clinical signs in symptomatic infections occur within 3 weeks after ingestion. Egg production takes approximately 8 weeks.

Abdominal pain, weakness, lethargy, intermittent cough, diarrhea, and fever may result from the animal's natural immune responses.

Diagnosis

Finding the characteristic eggs in sputum or feces is diagnostic. The eggs are golden brown, oval, and operculated (100×60 μm). Aberrant infections can be identified serologically.

Treatment

Animals should not be fed uncooked or raw meat (crab, crayfish, etc.). Bowls, utensils, and cutting boards should be cleaned thoroughly before using. The drugs of choice are praziquantel (25 mg/kg PO q8 h × 3 days), and fenbendazole (50 mg/kg PO 24 h × 10–14 days). Albendazole has also been effective.

Drug therapy

- Praziquantel
- Fenbendazole

Drug therapy alternatives

Albendazole

Further reading

Procop, G.W. (2009) North American paragonimiasis (caused by *Paragonimus kellicotti*) in the context of global paragonimiasis. *Clin Microb Rev.*, **22(3)**, 415–446.

Vélez, I., Velásquez, L.E., and Vélez, I.D. (2003) Morphological description and life cycle of *Paragonimus* sp. (Trematoda: Troglotrematidae): Causal agent of human paragonimiasis in Columbia. *J Parasitol.*, **89(4)**, 749–755.

Chapter 104: Parvovirus

Description: Parvovirus-2, small, non-enveloped, single-stranded DNA
Zoonotic Potential: Host specific, not a zoonotic threat to humans

Microbiology/epidemiology

Canine parvovirus (CPV-2) was responsible for a world-wide pandemic in dogs starting in the 1970s. It was believed to be derived from feline panleukopenia virus (FPV) and has undergone several mutations (CPV2a, CPV2b, CPV2c). The virus primarily affects canine species resulting in severe colitis but can also affect cats and foxes. CPV-2 can survive for up to a year in the environment and is typically transmitted by direct contact with virus in feces, vomit, or contact with fomites. Young dogs may develop more severe disease. Severity depends on the animal's immunity, viral strain, and environmental stresses.

Clinical disease

Incubation following exposure is typically 7–14 days. The virus replicates in oropharyngeal lymphoid tissues resulting in viremia. The virus then damages rapidly growing cells of the gastrointestinal tract, thymus, lymph nodes, and bone marrow. Clinically, animals have a fever (105°C), lethargy, weakness, dehydration, abdominal tenderness, vomiting, and diarrhea (sometimes bloody). Dogs may also present with intussusceptions, ulcerative glossitis, mucosal pallor, septic shock, occasional hypothermia, mentally obtunded, tremors, seizures, myocarditis, congestive heart failure, and rarely, erythema multiforme.

Diagnosis

In-house ELISA snap tests and hemagglutination assays from fecal swabs, histopathology, and PCR are diagnostic. ELISA tests have a high specificity (100%), but false positives can occur with live vaccines.

Treatment

Fluids, nutritional support, and electrolyte management are essential. Subcutaneous fluids and antibiotics can be prescribed for those animals where cost is an issue. For animals that can be hospitalized, intravenous routes are preferred. Supportive care (antiemetics, proton pump inhibitors, H2 blockers, blood transfusions, or plasma) and antibiotics for secondary bacterial infections are suggested. Single agent therapy with anaerobic coverage (metronidazole, ampicillin, amoxicillin/clavulanate) or enteric coverage (enrofloxacin) may be sufficient. For puppies with hemorrhagic diarrhea, combination therapy is advised with coverage for *C. perfringens* (metronidazole, beta-lactam, clindamycin). For severe infections, a carbapenem can also be used. Treatments with the anti-viral agents oseltamivir or recombinant feline interferon-omega (rfIFN-omega) have been suggested, but remain controversial.

Drug therapy

- Beta-lactam (Penicillin, Ampicillin, Amoxicillin/clavulanate)
- Metronidazole
- Enrofloxacin

Drug therapy alternatives

- Imipenem/meropenem
- Clindamycin

Further reading

Iris, K., Leonitides, L.S., Mylonakis, M.E., *et al.* (2010) Factors affecting the occurrence, duration of hospitalization and final outcome in canine parvovirus infection. *Res Vet Sci.*, **89**, 174–178.

Sykes, J.E. (2013) Canine parvovirus infections and other viral enteritides. Ch. 14. In: *Canine and Feline Infectious Diseases.* Sykes, J.E. (ed.), Elsevier, St. Louis, MO, pp. 141–151.

Unterer, S., Busch, K., Leipig, M., *et al.* (2014) Endoscopically visualized lesions, histologic findings, and bacterial invasion in the gastrointestinal mucosa of dogs with acute hemorrhagic diarrhea syndrome. *J Vet Intern Med.*, **28(1)**, 52–58.

Welborn, L.V., DeVries, J.G., Ford, R., *et al.* (2011) AAHA canine vaccination guidelines. *J Am Animal Hosp Assoc.*, **47**, 1–42.

Chapter 105: *Pasteurella* Species

Description: Gram negative coccobacillus, facultative anaerobes, endotoxins

Zoonotic Potential: Common zoonotic in animal handlers from bites, scratches

Microbiology/epidemiology

Pasteurella species are normal flora of the mouth in cats and dogs and are frequently found in infections caused by animal bites. There are more than six species of *Pasteurella* and many serotypes. *P. multocida* and *P. canis* are common isolates in dogs and cats.

Clinical disease

Animals may present with a bite or scratch wound. Soft tissue cellulitis and focal abscess formation may be apparent within 8–48 h after injury. Typically *Pasteurella* species are more progressive infections than those from other bacteria. Erythema, tenderness, swelling, and serosanguineous to purulent, malodorous, dark yellow discharge may occur. Lymphadenopathy and low grade fever may occur. Deeper infections and dissemination may cause septicemia, tenosynovitis, septic arthritis, osteomyelitis, meningitis, and smoldering abscesses. Upper and lower respiratory infections (bronchitis, pneumonia) may also be due to proliferation of *Pasteurella* species following viral infections or other impairment of bacterial clearance from the lungs.

Diagnosis

Both aerobic and anaerobic blood cultures and sensitivities are suggested.

Treatment

Penicillins are the drug of choice in animals with *Pasteurella* infections. Local infections may be treated with oral single agent beta-lactam therapy (amoxicillin, amoxicillin/clavulanate). Most isolates are also susceptible to fluoroquinolones and TMS. For deep infections or serious disseminated infections, parenteral penicillin, ampicillin/sulbactam, ticarcillin/clavulanate, piperacillin/tazobactam, cefoxitin, and carbapenems are effective. Macrolides, tetracyclines, aminoglycosides, and cephalosporins appear to have variable to poor coverage against *P. multocida*. Treatment should be given for 10–14 days. For tenosynovitis, septic arthritis, osteomyelitis, meningitis, and abscesses, 4–6 weeks of therapy starting with intravenous therapy is recommended.

Drug therapy

- Amoxicillin
- Amoxicillin/clavulanate

Drug therapy alternatives

- Penicillin parenteral
- Ampicillin/sulbactam
- Fluoroquinolones
- TMS
- Carbapenems

Further reading

Goldstein, E.J. and Citron, D.M. (1988) Comparative activities of cefuroxime, amoxicillin-clavulanic acid, ciprofloxacin, enoxacin, and ofloxacin against aerobic and anaerobic bacteria isolated from bite wounds. *Antimicrob Agents Chemother.*, **32(8)**, 1143–1148.

Goldstein, E.J., Citron, D.M., Merriam, C.V., *et al.* (1999) Activity of gatifloxacin compared to those of five other quinolones versus aerobic and anaerobic isolates from skin and soft tissue samples of human and animal bite wound infections. *Antimicrob Agents Chemother.*, **43(6)**, 1475–1479.

Griego, R.D., Rosen, T., Orengo, I.F., *et al.* (1995) Dog, cat, and human bites: A review. *J Am Acad Dermatol.*, **33(6)**, 1019–1029.

Kimura, R., Hayashi, Y., Takeuchi, T., *et al.* (2004) *Pasteurella multocida* septicemia caused by close contact with a domestic cat: Case report and literature review. *J Infect Chemother.*, **10(4)**, 250–252.

Kruth, S.A. (2006) Gram-negative bacterial infections. Ch. 37. In: *Infectious Diseases of the Dog and Cat.* 3rd Edn. Greene, C.E. (ed.), Saunders/Elsevier, St. Louis, MO, p. 325.

Stevens, D.L., Bisno, A.L., Chambers, H.F., *et al.* (2005) Practice guidelines for the diagnosis and management of skin and soft-tissue infections. *Clin Infect Dis.*, **41(10)**, 1373–1406.

Chapter 106: Poxvirus

Description: Large, enveloped, double stranded DNA virus
Zoonotic Potential: Zoonotic potential exists but not demonstrated

Microbiology/epidemiology

Poxvirus infections are uncommon in cats and dogs but can affect many other species, including cattle and humans. Cowpox, Raccoonpox, and Purapox virus infections have been identified in cats and dogs. Cowpox is the most commonly reported poxvirus in animals but is limited to Europe and Asia with reservoirs in wild rodents, voles, and mice. Both Raccoonpox and Purapox have been reported rarely in cats in North America. Poxvirus infections are typically acquired via inoculation through a break in the skin. Cats that are outdoor hunters appear to be at greatest risk.

Clinical disease

Cats may present with single or multiple popular or crusted skin lesions of the face or forelimb. They may also demonstrate lethargy, inappetence, or pneumonia.

Pneumonia can be fatal. A secondary rash (skin, mucosa) may occur with a second wave of viremia. The virus may spread to multiple organs including the spleen. Cats may also develop severe necrotizing facial dermatitis. Dogs rarely get poxvirus infections and typically have much less severe localized lesions.

Diagnosis

Diagnosis is often based on clinical signs and symptoms in endemic areas. Virus isolation, PCR, histopathology, and electron microscopy of skin biopsies may be used to confirm the diagnosis.

Treatment

Treatment has historically been supportive with fluids, nutrition and antibiotic therapy for skin lesions or pneumonia. Recent studies suggest a role for both antivirals (cidofovir) and immunostimulants (interferons), but these have only shown efficacy in laboratory animals to date. Most cats developing the infection will resolve completely if not immunosuppressed. Immunosuppressive therapy should be discontinued if possible in any animals acquiring poxvirus infections. If animals develop pneumonia, the prognosis is poor with high mortality rates.

Drug therapy

Supportive care

Drug therapy alternatives

* Cidofovir
* Interferon

Further reading

Bennett, M. (2013) Feline poxvirus infections. Ch. 24. In: *Canine and Feline Infectious Diseases*. Sykes, J.E. (ed.), Elsevier, St. Louis, MO, pp. 252–256.

Glatz, M., Richter, S., Ginter-Hanselmayer, G., *et al.* (2010) Human cowpox in a veterinary student. *Lancet Infect Dis.*, **10**, 288.

Smee, D.F. (2013) Orthopox virus inhibitors that are active in animal models: an update from 2008–2012. *Future Virol.*, **8(9)**, 891–901.

Yager, J.A., Hutchison, L., and Barrett, J.W. (2006) Raccoonpox in a Canadian cat. *Vet Dermatol.*, **17**, 443–448.

Chapter 107: *Proteus* Species

Description: Gram negative aerobic bacilli, facultative, enteric
Zoonotic Potential: Potential environmental/nosocomial source for humans

Microbiology/epidemiology

Proteus is a normal inhabitant of the gastrointestinal tract of animals. It can be recovered from water, soil, and fecal material. Clinically, *P. mirabilus* and *P. vulgaris* are important pathogens. *Proteus* species are capable of producing ureases that convert urea to ammonia hydroxide. This may result in the development of renal calculi and struvite stone precipitation in urinary tract infections due to *Proteus*. Nosocomial infections are common in human hospitals where the organisms readily contaminate equipment, catheters, and so on.

Clinical disease

Proteus may be isolated from the urinary tract, respiratory tract, ear infections, wounds, and the blood of veterinary patients. Catheter-related urinary tract infections and more life threatening systemic infections (pyelonephritis, pneumonia, septicemia) may also occur in debilitated patients. Cats may develop dermatologic infections including deep pyodermas, abscesses, and botryomycosis.

Diagnosis

Diagnosis of *Proteus* requires aerobic bacterial culture in association with cytologic evidence of inflammation and consistent clinical abnormalities. Susceptibility should also be requested due to the tendency of *Proteus* to be resistant to multiple antibiotics.

Treatment

Treatment should be based on culture and susceptibility results. *P. mirabilis* species are typically sensitive to extended spectrum penicillins, ceftriaxone, fluoroquinolones, and aminoglycosides. *P. vulgarisis* is more likely to be nosocomial and drug resistant. Resistance is emerging to both species so it is crucial to perform antimicrobial sensitivity testing. Animals presenting with renal or urinary stones should be further evaluated and treated accordingly to prevent reoccurrence. Urinary catheters and stones should be removed as they act as a nidus of infection.

Drug therapy

Cephalosporins

Drug therapy alternatives

- Fluoroquinolones
- Imipenem
- Meropenem
- Extended spectrum penicillins

Further reading

Gaastra, W., VanOosterom, R.A., Pieters, E.W., *et al.* (1996) Isolation and characterization of dogs uropathogenic *Proteus mirabilis* strains. *Vet Microbiol.*, **48(1–2)**, 57–71.

Grobbel, M., Lubke-Becker, A., Alesik, E., *et al.* (2007) Antimicrobial susceptibility of *Klebsiella* spp. and *Proteus* spp. from various organ systems of horses, dogs and cats as determined in the BfT-GermVet monitoring program 2004–2006. *Berl Munch Tierarztl Wochenschr.*, **120(9–10)**, 402–411.

Hordijk, J., Schoormans, A., Kwakernaak, M., *et al.* (2013) High prevalence of fecal carriage of extended spectrum B-lactamase/AmpC-producing Enterobacteriaceae in cats and dogs. *Front Microbiol.*, **16(4)**, 242.

Chapter 108: *Prototheca* Species

Description: Unicellular algae, fungal-like saprophytes
Zoonotic Potential: Not considered a zoonotic

Microbiology/epidemiology

Prototheca are ubiquitous in the environment and are recovered in soil, water, trees, and sewage. Protothecosis occurs in Europe, Asia, Africa, Oceania, and in North America. Infections in animals are uncommon and primarily reported in animals on immunosuppressive therapy. The pathogenesis in dogs and cats is not well understood but is believed acquired via ingestion, mucosal contact, or trauma. *P. zopfii* and *P. wickerhamii* are the most common isolates from cats and dogs. The organisms have an apparent tropism for the eye, central nervous system, bone, kidneys, and tissues with good blood supply. Young, medium to large breed, female dogs, and boxer breeds appear to be over represented. Only sporadic cases have been reported in cats.

Clinical disease

Animals may present with local skin or soft tissue infections. Lesions may develop post trauma and are non-healing. They may appear indurated, plaque-like, nodular, ulcerated, or vesicular. Following systemic dissemination, prognosis is poor with a median survival of 4 months in dogs. Dogs with systemic protothecosis may present with variable colitis (typically chronic diarrhea), ocular signs (exudative retinal separation, acute blindness), and/or neurologic signs. Bony lesions may be evident, as well as paraparesis and lumbar pain. In cats, dermal and nasal infections have been reported.

Diagnosis

Fungal culture of biopsy specimens may demonstrate *Prototheca*. Histopathology typically shows necrosis, giant cells, chronic inflammation, and/or microabscesses. Organisms stain readily with Gomori methenamine silver stain.

Treatment

Optimal treatment in veterinary species is unclear due to the lack of cases. Immunosuppressive therapies should be discontinued. Wide surgical excision and systemic drug therapy are recommended. Localized treatments with compounded topical amphotericin-B, iodine, peroxide, chlorhexidine, potassium permanganate, copper sulfate, ammonium compounds, and potassium iodide) in combination with oral therapy (itraconazole, doxycycline) have been attempted in humans with superficial infections with some success. Oral azole therapy alone (itraconazole, fluconazole, ketoconazole) has been used, but results are disappointing. Human studies suggest that fluconazole may be more effective than itraconazole, but that amphotericin B continues to be the most effective treatment. Amphotericin B in combination with doxycycline has also shown efficacy as well as itraconazole in combination with gamma interferon for 6 months. Prognosis of disseminated infections is often poor. Supportive care with fluid therapy, antiemetics, topical prednisolone ophthalmic drops, ocular enucleation to control pain, and metronidazole/sulfasalazine/dietary adjustments may help to treat colitis.

Drug therapy

Amphotericin B plus doxycycline

Drug therapy alternatives

- Itraconazole plus Gamma Interferon
- Fluconazole
- Ketoconazole

Further reading

Hollingsworth, S.R. (2000) Canine protothecosis. *Vet Clin North Am Small Animal Pract.*, **30(5)**, 1091–1101.

Lass-Florl, C. and Mayr, A. (2007) Human protothecosis. *Clin Microbiol Rev.*, **20**, 230–242.

Stenner, V.J., Mackay, B., King, T., *et al.* (2007) Protothecosis in 17 Australian dogs and a review of the canine literature. *Med Mycol.*, **45(3)**, 249–266.

Todd, J.R., King, J.W., Oberle, A., *et al.* (2012) Protothecosis: report of a case with 20-year follow-up, and review of previously published cases. *Med Mycol.*, **50(7)**, 673–689.

Torres, H.A., Bodey, G.P., Tarrand, J.J., *et al.* (2003) Protothecosis in patients with cancer: Case series and literature review. *Clin Microbiol Infect.*, **9**, 786–792.

Tortorano, A., Prigitano, A., Dho, G., *et al.* (2008) *In vitro* activity of conventional antifungal drugs and natural essences against the yeast-like alga *Prototheca*. *J Antimicrob Chemo.*, **61(6)**, 1312–1314.

Chapter 109: *Pseudomonas Aeruginosa*

Description: Nonfermenting, aerobic, gram negative bacillus
Zoonotic Potential: Multidrug resistant strains can colonize, be transmitted to humans

Microbiology/epidemiology

Pseudomonas aeruginosa is ubiquitous in the environment and lives on hospital equipment, sinks, cages, floors, and so on. Isolation of the organism itself may not be meaningful without clinical signs of infection. Debilitated animals, animals with tissue damage, burn patients, neutropenic, or immunosuppressed animals are at highest risk. Dogs commonly have Pseudomonas otitis, which may be highly multidrug resistant.

Clinical disease

P. aeruginosa is a common cause of otitis externa in dogs, but may also cause infections of the blood, lungs, heart, eye, urinary tract, gastrointestinal tract, and musculoskeletal system. *P. aeruginosa* is the most common organism isolated in chronic otitis externa in the dog. Clinically the ear is often ulcerated and filled with a purulent exudate. Hyperplasia of the canal, stenosis, and tympanic membrane ruptured are common.

Diagnosis

Culture and sensitivity in combination with relevant clinical signs are required for diagnosis. Dogs with Pseudomonas otitis will have a purulent exudate with numerous rod-shaped bacteria. These may be mixed with other cocci, rods, and/or Malassezia or may be present in pure culture. CT or radiographic examination of the bulla is recommended for chronic otitis under anesthesia.

Treatment

P. aeruginosa bacteria are typically multiple-drug resistant and antibiotic choice should be based on culture and sensitivities. Typically the most effective antibiotics include tobramycin, ticarcillin, polymyxin B, imipenem, amikacin, quinolones, and ceftazidime. For severe systemic infections, combination antibiotic therapy may be necessary. Ticarcillin, a fluoroquinolone or a carbapenum may be used in combination with aminoglycosides for severe infections. For urinary tract infections, fluoroquinolones alone may be effective. For more severe infections (pylonephritis) ceftazidime or extended spectrum penicillins may be administered systemically. For otitis externa, aminoglycosides may be ineffective in the presence of purulent discharge and enrofloxacin may develop rapid resistance. Steroids, either topical or systemic, may be necessary to open the ear canal and allow penetration of topical treatments. Ears should be flushed with saline prior to treatment under anesthesia with evaluation of the tympanic membrane. Empirically Tris-EDTA and enrofloxacin (22.7 mg/mL injectable instilled directly) twice daily may be effective. Tobramycin ophthalmic solution (1/2 mL into affected ear q12 h), or compounded Timentin solutions can be used. Silver sulfadiazine 1% (4.4 g) cream added to sterile water (29.3 mLs) and slightly heated until dissolved may also be effective.

Drug therapy

- Fluoroquinolones
- Tobramycin
- Ceftazidime plus aminoglycosides
- Ceftazidime plus extended spectrum penicillin

Drug therapy alternatives

- Fluoroquinolone plus aminoglycoside
- Carbapenum plus aminoglycoside
- Tris-EDTA (otitis)
- Compounded silver sulfadiazine or timentin solutions (otitis)

Further reading

Bennett, A.B., Martin, P.A., Gottlieb, S.A., *et al.* (2013) *In vitro* susceptibilities of feline and canine *Escherichia coli* and *Pseudomonas* spp. isolates to ticarcillin and ticarcillin/clavulanic acid. *Aust Vet J.*, **91(5)**, 171–178.

Buckley, L.M., McEwan, N.A., and Nuttall, T. (2013) Tris-EDTA significantly enhances antibiotic efficacy against multidrug-resistant *Pseudomonas aeruginosa in vitro*. *Vet Dermatol.*, **24(5)**, 519.

Hillier, A., Alcorn, J.R., Cole, L.K., *et al.* (2006) Pyoderma caused by *Pseudomonas aeruginosa* infection in dogs: 20 cases. *Vet Dermatol.*, **17(6)**, 432–439.

Papich, M.G. (2013) Antibiotic treatment of resistant infections in small animals. *Vet Clin North Am Small Anim Pract.*, **43(5)**, 1091–1107.

Chapter 110: Pseudorabies (Aujeszky's Disease)

Description: Suid Herpesvirus-1, alphaherpesvirus
Zoonotic Potential: Host specific, no zoonotic potential

Microbiology/epidemiology

Pseudorabies (SuHV-1) is a notifiable disease caused by a swine alpha-herpesvirus that can infect other species including cats and dogs. Its distribution is worldwide with the exception of Australia, but the disease is now considered rare due to vaccination of domestic pigs. Pockets of infection still persist in areas where feral pigs act as reservoirs (Southern USA, Europe). Clusters of canine infection have been noted in hunting dogs with wild swine contact. The disease is rare in dogs and has only occasionally been reported in cats. SuHV-1 infection is acquired by inhalation or ingestion of the virus following exposure to raw, uncooked offal, or carcasses. Feline predation may also increase the risk of infection from infected rodents.

Clinical disease

Following exposure, the virus replicates in the oropharynx and travels via retrograde axonal transport to the sensory nerve ganglia and into the CNS. This results in ganglioneuritis and encephalitis. It may also travel to the cardiac autonomic nerves resulting in myocardial degeneration or into the intestine. Incubation is typically 1–10 days. Animals typically present with hypersalivation, lethargy, fever, dysphagia, diarrhea, vomiting, respiratory distress, muscle stiffness, ataxia, head-pressing, and vestibular signs (circling, mydriasis, nystigmus), behavioral changes, seizures, coma, and cardiac arrhythmias. Death occurs in 48–96 h after symptom onset.

Diagnosis

Based on history of exposure to swine in areas known to harbor the infection, clinical signs, histopathology, PCR, or virus isolation. Most animals are diagnosed antemortem.

Treatment

There is no established treatment for SuHV-1 in dogs and cats. Vaccines are available for swine. Prevention of interactions between cats and dogs and feeding of raw or undercooked pork products may reduce the risk of infection.

Further reading

Cramer, S.D., Campbell, G.A., Njaa, B.L., *et al.* (2011) Pseudorabies virus infection in Oklahoma hunting dogs. *J Vet Diagn Invest.*, **23**, 915–923.

Muller, T., Hahn, E.C., Tottewitz, F., *et al.* (2011) Pseudorabies virus in wild swine: A global perspective. *Arch Virol.*, **156**, 1691–1705.

Sykes, J.E. and Cramer, S.D. (2013) Pseudorabies. Ch. 25. In: *Canine and Feline Infectious Diseases*. Sykes, J.E. (ed.), Elsevier, St. Louis, MO, pp. 257–260.

Chapter 111: Rabies Virus

Description: Single-stranded RNA virus, enveloped, bullet-shaped
Zoonotic Potential: Deadly zoonotic with dogs and bats being reservoirs

Microbiology/epidemiology

Rabies virus belongs to the family Rhabdovirdae. The virus is found throughout the world except in Taiwan, Australia, New Zealand, Iceland, the UK, Japan, Western Europe, Fiji, Hawaii, and Guam. It is a major zoonotic threat in many countries where animals are not vaccinated and stray animal populations are common. Wild canids, dogs, and bats are reservoirs of disease that can be transmitted to humans via bite wounds. Cats and other mammals contract the infection from wild animals (raccoons, skunks, etc.). Cats have a higher incidence most likely due to inadequate vaccination. Incubation is highly variable and can take between 4 days to 19 years. The virus survives 3–4 days in the environment and for up to a year under frozen conditions. The virus can be shed for up to 13 days prior to symptoms appearing in dogs. The virus is neurotropic and replicates in muscle with invasion into sensory and motor nerves.

Clinical disease

Most animals develop disease 1–2 months after exposure. Inoculation sites nearest the central nervous system have a shorter incubation period. Clinically, animals present with either excitatory (furious) or paralytic (dumb) symptoms. There may be evidence of a wound or history of one. A prodromal phase with lethargy, anorexia, apprehensive, restlessness, pain, papillary dilation, or licking at the bite site and variable fever may occur first (days 1–3). The excitable (furious phase) with bizarre behavior is demonstrated between 1–7 days. Symptoms of hyperesthesia, hypersalivation, vocalization, roaming, aggression, seizures, ataxia, and vestibular signs may be noted. Finally, the paralytic phase (dumb) follows with flaccid paralysis, laryngeal paralysis, hypersalivation, and dropped jaw. Death occurs rapidly (<10 days).

Diagnosis

Rabies may still occur in vaccinated animals. Any animal with sudden onset of bizarre behavior and flaccid paralysis in a rabies-endemic area should be suspect.

Reverse-transcriptase PCR, Direct fluorescent antibody testing, immunohistochemistry, and histopathology are used for confirmation. A national standardization protocol is published by the CDC and available via the Department of Public Health (www.cdc.gov/rabies/pdf/RabiesDFASPv2.pdf).

Treatment

There is no treatment for a rabid animal. If clinical signs are suggestive of rabies the animal should be euthanized and rabies testing performed. Otherwise, suspected exposures in vaccinated or unvaccinated animals should follow current *Rabies Compendium* CDC recommendations as mentioned.

Further reading

Lackay, S.N., Kuang, Y., and Fu, Z.F. (2008) Rabies in small animals. *Vet Clin North Am Small Animal Pract.*, **38**, 851–861.

McQuiston, J.H., Yager, P.A., Smith, J.S., *et al.* (2001) Epidemiology characteristics of rabies virus variants in dogs and cats in the United States, 1999. *J Am Vet Med Assoc.*, **218**, 1939–1942.

Sykes, J.E. and Chomel, B.B. (2013) Rabies. Ch. 13. In: *Canine and Feline Infectious Diseases*. Sykes, J.E. (ed.), Elsevier, St. Louis, MO, pp. 132–140.

Chapter 112: *Rhodococcus Equi*

Description: Gram positive, aerobic intracellular cocci or pleomorphic rods with branching
Zoonotic Potential: May act as reservoirs for immunocompromised humans

Microbiology/epidemiology

Rhodococcus equi is a soil borne saprophyte that typically causes pneumonia in foals and occasionally in immunosuppressed human hosts. It is frequently isolated from herbivore manure. It is acquired by inhalation of contaminated dust and only rarely causes infections in cats and dogs. Animals may also acquire the infection by inoculation following cutaneous trauma. *R. equi* has been isolated from lesions in dogs and abscesses in cats.

Clinical disease

Pyogranulomatous lesions of the extremities are the most common finding in cats. There may be localized peripheral abscesses, swelling, ulcerations, enlarged lymph nodes, fistulas, and purulent drainage. Fever, anorexia and pain are often absent. The infection may disseminate causing pylothorax, mediastinal lymphadenitis, anorexia, weight loss, and dyspnea. Abdominal distention, hepatomegaly, and mesenteric lymphadenopathy may also be noted. Disseminated infections in dogs are rare, but have included generalized hyperesthesia, necrotizing pyogranulomatous hepatitis, osteomyelitis, polymyositis, osteolytic/proliferative changes, and muscular swelling.

Diagnosis

Aerobic culture of percutaneous drainage or biopsy specimens is necessary for definitive diagnosis. Histopathology demonstrates inflammation and granuloma formation. Intracellular bacteria may be seen inside macrophages.

Treatment

Surgical excision and drainage of abscesses and lesions may be required, but often new lesions recur. Combination therapy is typically required to eradicate the infection. Due to the intracellular nature of *Rhodococcus* and its tendency to form granulomas, drug therapy must be selected that can penetrate intracellularly. Long term therapy (6–12 weeks) in equine patients has been successful with a combination of a macrolide (clarithromycin, azithromycin) along with rifampin. For macrolide resistant organisms, vancomycin, or a carbepenem may be effective. Long term therapy is generally required. Therapy should be continued for 14 days for localized lesions and potentially for 6–12 weeks for disseminated disease.

Drug therapy

- Azithromycin with rifampin
- Clarithromycin with rifampin

Drug therapy alternatives

- Imipenem
- Vancomycin

Further reading

Cantor, G., Byrne, B.A., Hines, S.A., *et al.* (1998) VapA-negative *Rhodococcus equi* in a dog with necrotizing pyogranulomatous hepatitis, osteomylitis and myositis. *J Vet Diagn Invest.*, **10(30)**, 297–300.

Farias, M.R., Takai, S., Ribeiro, M.G., *et al.* (2007) Cutaneous pyogranuloma in a cat caused by virulent *Rhodococcus equi* containing an 87 kb type 1 plasmid. *Aust Vet J.*, **85(1–2)**, 29–31.

Greene, C.E. (2006) Streptococcal and other gram-positive bacterial infections. Ch. 35. In: *Infectious Diseases of the Dog and Cat.* 3rd edn. Greene, C.E. (ed.) Saunders/Elsevier, St. Louis, MO, pp. 310–311.

Passamonti, F., Lepri, E., Coppola, G., *et al.* (2011) Pulmonary rhodococcosis in a cat. *J Feline Med Surg.*, **13(4)**, 283–285.

Chapter 113: *Rickettsia Rickettsii* (Rocky Mountain Spotted Fever)

Description: Gram negative coccobacillus, obligate intracellular bacteria
Zoonotic Potential: Tick-borne zoonotic transmission from animals to humans

Microbiology/epidemiology

R. rickettsii is the etiologic agent underlying Rocky Mountain Spotted Fever (RMSF). The geographic distribution follows the tick species *R. rickettsii* and is primarily noted in North Central and South America. Dogs are sentinels for rickettsioses in people. *R. rickettsii* and *R. conorii*, as well as other species, cause infections in dogs. Young animals and purebred dogs may be over represented. Antibodies to *Rickettsiae* are reported in cats in endemic areas, but clinical disease has not been well characterized. Dogs acquire the infection from *Ixodes* ticks (*Dermacetor*, *Rhipicephalus*, *Amblyomma*). Transmission occurs during feeding on mammalian hosts.

Clinical disease

Following infection, the parasite spreads through the lymphatics and goes into the bloodstream. Vasculitis and increased microvascular permeability occur due to endothelial cell damage. Animals may present with fever, myalgia, arthralgia, mucopurulent discharge, sclera and conjunctival injection, hemorrhage, conjunctivitis, uveitis, retinal hemorrhage, retinitis, lymphadenomegaly, splenomegaly, nasal discharge, epistasis, tachypnea, petechiae, ecchymosis, peripheral edema, hyperemia, necrosis, glomerulonephritis, gangrenous necrosis, orchitis, scrotal edema, arrhythmias, and CNS abnormalities (ataxia, vestibular signs, stupor, and seizures).

Diagnosis

A combination of diagnostic tests is necessary to confirm infection. PCR, immunohistochemistry, and serology along with clinical signs are diagnostic. Organisms can be identified in smears of infected tissues using the Gimenz method or immunofluorescence.

Treatment

Treatment should be initiated prior to diagnosis if richettsial disease is suspected. Most patients respond rapidly (24–48 h) to doxycycline treatment. Animals should be assessed for co-infections if not responding. Supportive care with colloid fluids is often required. Fluids should be given with caution to avoid exacerbation of interstitial edema. Glucocorticoids may be necessary in dogs with severe CNS manifestations or typically for treatment of ocular abnormalities. Doxycycline (7–14 days) is the treatment of choice. Typically seven days of treatment are sufficient for *Rickettsia*, but 14 days may be required for co-infections with *Ehrlichia* or other agents. Alternatively, chloramphenicol or a fluoroquinolone can be administered.

Drug therapy

Doxycycline

Drug therapy alternatives

• Chloramphenicol
• Enrofloxacin

Further reading

Gasser, A.M., Birkenheuer, A.J., and Breitschwerdt, E.B. (2001) Canine Rocky Mountain spotted fever: A retrospective study of 30 cases. *J Am Anim Hosp Assoc.*, **37(1)**, 41–48.
Kidd, L. and Breitschwerdt, E.B. (2013) Rocky Mountain spotted fever. Ch. 30. In: *Canine and Feline Infectious Diseases*. Sykes, J.E. (ed.), Elsevier, St. Louis, MO, pp. 300–310.

Nicholson, W.L., Allen, K.E., McQuuiston, J.H., *et al.* (2010) The increasing recognition of rickettsial pathogens in dogs and people. *Trends Parasitol.*, **26(4)**, 205–212.

Chapter 114: *Salmonella* Species

Description: Gram negative bacilli, Enterobacteriaceae, endotoxin producing
Zoonotic Potential: Animals may be a reservoir of infection for humans

Microbiology/epidemiology

Salmonella species are important causes of gastroenteritis and septicemia in humans and animals. *Salmonella* may colonize the gastrointestinal tract of animals but is not considered part of the normal flora in humans, cats or dogs. Dogs and cats may acquire the infection via ingestion of contaminated food (raw, dehydrated, improperly cooked meat, dog food, dog treats, eggs, and dairy) or water supplies. A very small inoculum (10^8) is required to cause disease. Cats appear to be more resistant then dogs to infection and dogs that roam or eat decaying food may have a much higher risk of infection. Young and old animals may have more severe disease.

Clinical disease

Animals may initially present with fever (104–106°F/40–41°C), lethargy, malaise, and anorexia. This may occur within hours of ingestion of contaminated food. This is followed by muscle tenderness, abdominal pain, hypersalivation (cats), nausea, vomiting, and watery to mucoid diarrhea. Symptoms are typically noted in 3–5 days after consumption. Symptoms may resolve without treatment after 2–7 days. Chronic diarrhea may last as long as 3–8 weeks. With more severe infections, animals may present with signs of systemic infection from bacteremia, endotoxemia, or localized infections (dehydration, shock, cardiovascular collapse, icterus, hypotension, end-organ damage, liver abscesses, osteomyelitis, septic arthritis, convulsions, hyperexcitability, blindness, incoordination, posterior paresis, and endocarditis). Pneumonia with coughing, dyspnea, and epistaxis have also been described. Abortion, stillbirth, and birth of weak, emaciated kittens or puppies may occur from *in utero* infections. Cats may present with chronic fever without other symptoms.

Following infection animals may remain colonized and shed bacteria for up to a year.

Diagnosis

Aerobic culture and sensitivity should be performed to confirm the diagnosis. Cultures can be done on blood, joint aspirates, and CSF. Stool and sputum cultures with multiple organisms require selective enrichment media. Serology may be diagnostic for systemic disease.

Treatment

Treatment should be based on susceptibility studies. Treatment of enterocolitis may not be required if self-limiting. Supportive care without antibiotics is advised in mild infections. In immunocompromised patients or severe systemic disease, antibiotics and intravenous fluids or plasma should be administered. *Salmonella* species are sensitive to many antibiotics (ampicillin, amoxicillin/clavulanate, fluoroquinolones, chloramphenicol, TMS, and third generation cephalosporins). In animals that are chronic carriers, antibiotics should be prescribed for up to 6 weeks. Avoid feeding raw meat to animals.

Drug therapy

- Ampicillin/Amoxicillin
- Chloramphenicol
- Cephalosporins, 3rd generation

Drug therapy alternatives

- TMS
- Amoxicillin/clavulanate
- Aminoglycosides
- Fluoroquinolones

Further reading

Ackers, M.L., Puhr, N.D., Tauxe, R.V., *et al.* (2000) Laboratory-based surveillance of *Salmonella* serotype Typhi infections in the United States: Antimicrobial resistance on the rise. *JAMA.*, **283**, 2668–2773.

Dow, S.W., Jones, R.L., Henik, R.A., *et al.* (1989) Clinical features of Salmonellosis in cats: six cases (1981–1986). *J Am Vet Med Assoc.*, **194(6)**, 1464–1466.

Greene, C.E. (2006) Salmonellosis. Ch. 39. In: *Infectious Diseases of the Dog and Cat.* 3rd edn. Greene, C.E. (ed.), Saunders/Elsevier, St. Louis, MO, pp. 355–360.

Manchanda, V., Bhalla, P., Sethi, M., *et al.* (2006) Treatment of enteric fever in children on the basis of current trends of antimicrobial susceptibility of *Salmonella enterica* serovar typhi and paratyphi A. *Indian J Med Microbiol.*, **24**, 101–106.

Chapter 115: *Sarcoptes Scabiei* (Sarcoptic Mange)

Description: Sarcoptic mite, ectoparasite, highly transmissible scabies
Zoonotic Potential: Can be transmitted to humans resulting in erythematous papules

Microbiology/epidemiology

Sarcoptic mange is a highly contagious ectoparasitic disease found worldwide on dogs. The *Sarcoptes scabiei var canis* mite is host specific but can temporarily affect humans and other animals, including cats. The mites have their entire life cycle (17–21 days) on the dog. Females burrow into the stratum corneum to lay eggs. Dogs acquire the infection by direct contact with other infected animals. Following exposure, the incubation period is between 10 days to 8 weeks.

Clinical disease

Dogs may present with lesions that appear as papular eruptions with thick crusts. Dogs typically have severe pruritus of sudden onset. Lesions typically start on the ventral abdomen, chest, ears, elbows, or hocks. Secondary bacterial or yeast infections may occur. If untreated, generalized disease may develop with seborrhea, severe thickening of the skin, fold formation, severe crusting, peripheral lymphadenopathy, emaciation, and even death. "Scabies incognito" is reported in dogs that are well groomed due to the removal of crusts and mites during bathing resulting in negative skin scrapings. Cats may acquire the infection rarely and present with crusty lesions on the bridge of the nose, pinnae, tail, or feet (pododermatitis).

Diagnosis

Diagnosis is based on clinical history. The onset of severe itching, possible exposure to infected dogs, and skin scrapings should be considered. Negative skin scrapings are common. Several scrapings of affected areas that are nonexcoriated may increase chances of finding mites, eggs, or feces. Fecal flotation may also be useful to reveal mites and eggs in heavy infestations.

Treatment

For dogs that present with typical clinical symptoms and history suggestive of mange, a treatment trial regardless of a negative skin scrapping is warranted. All dogs that have contact should be treated at the same time. Topical treatment with lime-sulfur dip (weekly × 2) may be effective and is safe for young animals. For more severe infections, dogs should be clipped and bathed with an antiseborrheic shampoo. Whole-body amitraz dips (0.025%) applied every 2 weeks along with a systemic avermectin is advised. Amitraz should not be used in Chihuahuas, pregnant or nursing bitches, or puppies <4 months of age. Selamectin can be given as a spot-on formulation to dogs 6 weeks of age or older (q2 weeks). Moxidectin/imidacloprid (topically q4 weeks × 1–2 doses) is also considered effective and safe. For refractory cases, ivermectin (0.2 mg/kg PO, SC q2 weeks × 2–4 doses) or milbemycin (2 mg/kg PO twice weekly for 3–4 weeks) is very effective. Avermectins are contraindicated in a number of breeds including collies and other herding breeds. Testing for MDR-1 gene mutations is advised (See Ivermectin). Treatment of cats is successful with moxidectin/imidacloprid (topically q2 weeks × 3 doses). Infected owners may be treated topically with pyrethrin containing creams on prescription.

Drug therapy

- Sulfer Dip
- Selemectin
- Ivermectin
- Moxidectin/imidacloprid
- Milbemycin

Drug therapy alternatives

Amitraz.

Further reading

Aydinqoz, I.E. and Mansur, A.T. (2011) Canine scabies in humans: A case report and review of the literature. *Dermatol.*, **223(2)**, 104–106.

Bandi, K.M. and Saikumar, C. (2013) Sarcoptic mange: A zoonotic ectoparasitic skin disease. *J Clin Diag Res.*, **7(1)**, 156–157.

Fourie, L.J., Heine, J., and Horak, I.G. (2006) The efficacy of an imidaclopride/moxidectin combination against naturally acquired *Sarcoptes scabiei* infestations on dogs. *Aust Vet J.*, **84(1–2)**, 17–21.

Huang, H.P. and Lien, Y.H. (2013) Feline sarcoptic mange in Taiwan: A case series of five cats. *Vet Derm.*, **24(4)**, 457–459.

Chapter 116: *Serratia* Species

Description: Gram negative aerobic bacilli, Enterobacteriaceae
Zoonotic Potential: Can be reservoir for multidrug resistant strains in humans

Microbiology/epidemiology

The bacterium lives in water, soil, plants, and the gastrointestinal tract of animals. *S. marcescens* and *S. liquefaciens* have been isolated from veterinary patients. *Serratia* are associated with endotoxins resulting in inflammatory responses (fever, leucopenia, hypotension, sepsis). *Serratia* can colonize the respiratory, urinary or gastrointestinal tract of animals. *Serratia* species are commonly reported nosocomial infections in humans. Immunocompromised patients are at highest risk. Transmission is often due to hand-to-hand contact, contaminated hospital equipment, and indwelling catheters. Immunocompromised animals are at highest risk. Contaminated benzalkonium chloride (0.025%) sponge pots have been identified as a source of infection in veterinary clinics.

Clinical disease

Serratia may result in lower respiratory tract infections of animals on ventilators. It may also cause urinary tract infections in animals with chronic bladder catheters. Bacteremia may also result from indwelling catheters, or post-instrumentation gastrointestinal or urinary procedures. Systemic infections such as endocarditis, necrotizing fasciitis, and nosocomial post-operative infections with lethargy, septicemia, and gastrointestinal upset may also occur.

Diagnosis

Aerobic culture and gram negative stain must be interpreted in combination with clinical signs due to the fact that isolation of organisms may only represent colonization rather than infection.

Treatment

Drug therapy can be challenging due to potential high level drug resistance. Drug therapy should therefore be based on culture and sensitivity results. Environmental hygiene (bleaching of water bowls, changing antiseptic solutions) may help reduce environmental contamination.

Drug therapy

- Extended spectrum penicillins
- Third generation cephalosporins

Drug therapy alternatives

- Imipenem
- Meropenem
- Fluoroquinolones

Further reading

Armstrong, P.J. (1984) Systematic *Serratia marcescens* infections in a dog and a cat. *J Am Vet Med Assoc.*, **184(9)**, 1154–1158.

Fox, J.G., Beaucage, C.M., Folta, C.A., *et al.* (1981) Nosocomial transmission of *Serratia marcescens* in a veterinary hospital due to contamination by benzalkonium chloride. *J Clin Microbiol.*, **14(2)**, 157–160.

Jenkins, C.M., Winkler, K., Rudloss, E., *et al.* (2001) Necrotizing fasciitis in a dog. *J Veter Emerg Crit Care.*, **11**, 229–305.

Lobetti, R.G., Joubert, K.E., Picard, J., *et al.* (2002) Bacterial colonization of intravenous catheters in young dogs suspected to have parvoviral enteritis. *J Amer Vet Med Assoc.*, **220**, 1321–1324.

Perez, C., *et al.* (2011) Fatal aortic endocarditis associated with community-acquired *Serratia marcescens* infection in a dog. *J Am Anim Hosp Assoc.*, **47(2)**, 133–137.

Chapter 117: *Shigella* Species

Description: Gram negative anaerobic rods, Shiga-toxin
Zoonotic Potential: Considered a zoonotic, animals may be a reservoir

Microbiology/epidemiology

Shigella species are found worldwide and are a common cause of gastrointestinal infections in people and animals. Multiple species exist with *S. sonnei* and *S. flexneri* being the most common isolates identified in the USA. *Shigella* species are capable of colonizing the intestinal epithelium by exploiting epithelial cell functions and circumventing the host's innate immune response. The most common mode of transmission is the fecal–oral route. Outbreaks of Shigellosis can occur in kennels, pet shops, and shelters via contaminated food or water bowls. Insects, particularly flies, can also play a role as mechanical vectors. Young animals are more susceptible. Immunosuppressed cats (FeLV, FIV) may be at increased risk. A low number of inoculum is required to produce disease. Incubation is between 16 h and 7 days.

Clinical disease

Shigella invades the intestinal cells of the gastrointestinal tract but rarely invades the mucosa. Clinical signs are rare in dogs, with intermittent or transient diarrhea. Mucosal ulcers may occur. Patients may present with fever, abdominal cramping, and large volume diarrhea due to enterotoxins. After 1–2 days, fever may resolve but frank bloody diarrhea with mucus may occur. Fecal urgency, tenesmus, diarrhea, and abdominal pain may remain. Animals may resolve the infection without treatment but may continue to act as reservoirs of infection by shedding of bacteria. In very young animals dissemination may occur resulting in seizures, septicemia, and hemolytic uremic syndrome.

Diagnosis

Shigella is diagnosed based on clinical and laboratory data. Patients with fever and diarrhea should be evaluated for *Shigella* in the stool. Stool fecal leukocytes are often found in sheets. Specific culture media may be required for the isolation of *Shigella* in the stool. Highest recovery of organisms is typically early in the disease process.

Treatment

Animals may resolve the infection without treatment but may remain reservoirs for other animal/human transmission. Antibiotics shorten the course and severity of infection. Treatment should be based on susceptibility data. Both TMS and fluoroquinolones are typically effective. The use of antimotility agents should be avoided due to increased risk of toxic megacolon.

Drug therapy

TMS.

Drug therapy alternatives

- Fluoroquinolones
- Ampicillin
- Third generation cephalosporins

Further reading

Floyd, T.M. (1955) Isolation of *Shigella* from dogs in Egypt. *J Bacteriol.*, **70(5)**, 621.

Priamukhira, N.S., Kilesso, V.A., and Tikhomirov, E.D. (1984) Animal carriers of *Shigella* and their possible epidemiological importance. *Zh Mikrobol Epidemol Immunobiol.*, **11(6)**, 20–24.

Sansonetti, P.J. (2001) Microbes and microbial toxins: Paradigms for microbial-mucosal interactions III. Shigellosis: from symptoms to molecular pathogenesis. *Am J Physiol Gastrointest Liver Physiol.*, **280**, 319–323.

Chapter 118: *Sporothrix* Species

Description: Saprophytic fungi, dimorphic
Zoonotic Potential: Environmental but can be transmitted via cat scratches, bites

Microbiology/epidemiology

The *Sporothrix* species lives in moist, humid soil and decaying vegetation (moss, wood, thorns, hay). It grows in tropical and temperate climates worldwide. At least six species exist with variable virulence and distribution. *S. schenckii*, *S. brasiliensis*, and *S. albicans* have been isolated from cats and *S. schenckii* and *S. luriei* have been isolated from dogs. Transmission between animals is thought to be from contaminated claw or bite wound infections. Inhalation of conidia may also occur as well as self-inoculation from grooming. Outdoor cats appear at highest risk due to cat fights. Sporothrichosis is relatively rare in dogs.

Clinical disease

Following inoculation, *Sporothrix* converts to a yeast form in tissues. Animals typically present with cutaneous lesions that are crust like, plaque-like, or nodular. These may ulcerate or drain serosanquineous fluid. Lesions may be single and localized, track along lymph nodes, or be multifocal. Lesions are typically found on the head, distal limbs, digits, or tail. Extracutaneous disease may disseminate to the respiratory tract (nasal cavity, lungs) of cats. Cats and dogs may also have sneezing, cough, tachypnea, increased respiratory effort, stertor, and/or nasal discharge. Cats may develop disseminated disease to the lungs, liver, spleen, kidneys, lymph nodes, and testicles. Often this is associated with fever, lymphadenopathy, anorexia, dehydration, vomiting, and weight loss. Dogs may have weight loss, vomiting, anorexia, and occasionally, lameness and synovial effusion from osteoarticular sporothrix.

Diagnosis

Diagnosis is based on clinical appearance of lesions and fungal isolation of organisms. Demonstration of *Sporothrix* in histopathologic samples is useful, but diagnosis is dependent on the isolation of *Sporothrix* in culture. Serology and PCR are available, but not used widely.

Treatment

Abscesses and local lesions may need to be excised and drained. Various alternative treatments have been attempted including cryotherapy and hyperthermia. The drug of choice is currently itraconazole. This may be used in combination with intralesional amphotericin-B for refractory cases. Other antifungal drugs have been used with variable success including fluconazole, ketoconazole, terbinafine, and potassium iodide.

Drug therapy

- Itraconazole
- Itraconazole plus intralesional amphotericin B

Drug therapy alternatives

- Fluconazole
- Ketoconazole
- Terbinafine
- Potassium iodide

Further reading

Crothers, S.L., White, S.D., Ihrke, P.J., *et al.* (2009) Sporothrichosis: A retrospective evaluation of 23 cases seen in northern California (1987–2007). *Vet Dermatol.*, **20(4)**, 249–259.

Madrid, I.M., Mattei, A.S., Fernandes, C.G., *et al.* (2012) Epidemiological findings and laboratory evaluation of sporo-thrichosis: A description of 103 cases in cats and dogs in Southern Brazil. *Mycopathol.*, **173(4)**, 265–273.

Schechtman, R.C. (2010) Sporotrichosis: Part I. *Skin Med.*, **8(4)**, 216–220.

Weingart, C., Lubke-Becker, A., Kohn, B. (2010) *Sporothrix schenckii* infection in a cat. *Berl Munch Tierarztl Wochenschr.*, **123(3–4)**, 125–129.

Welsh, R.D. (2003) Sporotrichosis. Vet Med Today: Zoonotic update. *JAVMA.*, **223(8)**, 1123–1126.

Chapter 119: *Staphylococcus* Species

Description: Gram positive aerobic cocci, non-spore forming, singles or pairs
Zoonotic Potential: Cats and dogs may act as reservoirs for human infection

Microbiology/epidemiology

Staphylococus species colonize the skin, perianal, vaginal, umbilical, ocular, nasal mucosa, and gastrointestinal tract of animals and humans. Hospitalized animals, those on immunosuppressants, and those with chronic disease (cancer, diabetes, etc.) have increased risk of colonization. Animals acquire the infection via skin trauma or inoculation. *Staphylococcus* species that infect cats and dogs primarily include *S. pseudintermedius*, *S. intermedius*, *S. aureus*. and coagulase negative *Staphylococcus* species. *S. pseudintermedius* is the most common species of bacteria found on dogs. A small percentage of dogs may develop skin infections caused by methicillin-resistant *S. pseudintermedius* (MRSP). All *Staphylococcus* species have the tendency to develop methacillin resistance, which is transmitted chromosomally. Nosocomial transmission of methacillin resistance is common in both human and veterinary medicine. *S. pseudintermedius* and *S. intermedius* are generally considered host specific for dogs and cats but can also be transmitted to immunosuppressed humans. Zoonotic transmission of methacillin resistant *S. pseudintermedius* between dogs and humans has been documented. *S. aureus*, which normally colonizes human and equine species is a common isolate in cats. Coagulase negative *Staphylococcus* (CNS) is innately resistance to many antibiotics. *S. epidermidis* species are common isolates of human skin and were considered a sampling contaminant until recently. It is now a recognized pathogen in humans and animals with prosthetic implants and innately resistant to many antibiotics.

Clinical disease

Animals typically present with localized skin infections (folliculitis, pyoderma, abscesses, etc.). Red papules, macules, vesicles, crusts, or bullous formations may be noted. Disseminated or deep tissue infections may involve mastitis, pneumonia, abscesses, toxic shock syndrome, osteomyelitis, septic arthritis, septicemia, or endocarditis. Gastrointestinal food poisoning due to *Staphylococcus* may also occur post ingestion of contaminated foods (2–6 h). Animals may present with salivation, nausea, vomiting, abdominal cramps, and watery, non-bloody diarrhea.

Diagnosis

Gram stain, aerobic culture, and sensitivity must be evaluated to confirm the diagnosis.

Treatment

Sensitive organisms can be treated with cephalosporins or clindamycin. *Staphylococcus* species are commonly positive for beta-lactamases so that antistaphylococcus antibiotics (dicloxacillin, oxacillin) are recommended. If sensitivity suggests the presence of methicillin resistant organisms, organisms are typically resistant to penicillins, antistaphylococcal penicillins, erythromycin, lincomycin, clindamycin, and intermediately resistant to aminoglycosides and chloramphenicol. Methicillin resistant *Staphylococcus* species are not responsive to cephalosporins even though *in vitro* results may suggest sensitivity. Doxycycline and TMS may be effective in mild infections if *in vitro* data suggests sensitivity. Vancomycin should be reserved for humans, but may be the only alternative for some highly resistant infections. If used, it should be combined with either aminoglycosides or rifampin and therapeutic plasma concentrations should be monitored. Linezolid has been successful in some cases. *S. epidermitis* (CNS) may be treated with penicillinase resistant penicillins, cephalosporins, clindamycin, or if resistant, chloramphenicol or vancomycin.

Drug therapy

- Penicillinase-resistant penicillins (dicloxacillin, oxacillin)
- Cephalosporins
- Clindamycin
- TMS

Drug therapy alternatives

- Vancomycin plus aminoglycoside (resistant cases only)
- Vancomycin plus rifampin (resistant cases only)
- Linezolid
- Chloramphenicol

Further reading

Mouney, M.C., Stiles, J., Townsend, W.M., *et al.* (2013) Prevalence of methacillin-resistant *Staphylococcus* spp. in the conjunctival sac of healthy dogs. *Vet Ophthal.*, **10**, 1111.

Van Hoovels, L., Vankeerberghen, A., Boel, A., *et al.* (2006) First case of *Staphylococcus pseudintermedius* infection in a human. *J Clin Microbiol.*, **44(12)**, 4609–4612.

Vengust, M., Anderson, M.E., Rousseau, J., *et al.* (2006) Methacillin-resistant staphylococcal colonization in clinically normal dogs and horse in the community. *Lett Appl Microbiol.*, **43(6)**, 602–606.

Vincenzo, S., Barbarini, D., Polakowska, K., *et al.* (2013) Methicillin-resistant *Staphylococcus pseudintermedius* infection in a bone marrow transplant recipient. *J Clin Microbiol.*, **51(5)**, 1636–1638.

Wang, N., Neilan, A.M., and Klompas, M. (2006) First Case of *Staphylococcus pseudintermedius* infection in a human. *J Clin Microbiol.*, **44(12)**, 4609–4612.

Chapter 120: *Streptococcus* Species

Description: Gram positive cocci, pairs and chains, facultative to strict anaerobes
Zoonotic Potential: Streptococcal species infecting dogs and cats may also be a reservoir for humans.

Microbiology/epidemiology

There are at least 40 species of *Streptococci* with high variation in host tropism and virulence. *S. canis* and *S. equi* subsp. *zooepidemus* are the most common isolates in dogs and cats. *S. bovis*, *S. dysgalactiae*, and *S. agalactiae* have been isolated, but are rare. *Streptococcus* infections are found worldwide and primarily cause infections in animals with atopic dermatitis, wounds, foreign bodies, or those with immune suppression (fetuses, neonates, immunosuppressive drugs, cancer).

Clinical disease

S. canis has been associated with a variety of clinical syndromes including pharyngitis, cervical lymphadenitis, endocarditis, urinary tract infections, postoperative infections, otitis externa, keratitis, bronchopneumonia, pyometra, metritis, meningoencephalitis, necrotizing fasciitis, toxic shock syndrome, neonatal bacteremia, rhinitis, sinusitis, pyrothorax, discospondylitis, arthritis, osteomyelitis, mastitis, cholangiohepatitis, and peritonitis. *S. equi* subsp. *zooepidemicus* has been associated with pneumonia, sinusitis and meningitis and is primarily isolated in group-housed animals.

Diagnosis

Diagnosis is based on isolation of organisms from blood, biopsies, body fluids, and lavage specimens. Antibiotic susceptibly testing for *Streptococci* is typically not performed due to innate penicillin susceptibility.

Treatment

Typically *Streptococci* infections are easily treated with a beta-lactam or a cephalosporin. Early diagnosis and treatment are essential to avoid toxic shock syndrome or necrotizing fasciitis. For animals that present with septic shock or severe pneumonia, a beta-lactam and an aminoglycoside should be used in combination for synergy.

Drug therapy

- Beta-Lactams (penicillin, ampicillin, amoxicillin)
- Cefazolin
- Cephalexin

Drug therapy alternatives

- Clindamycin with penicillin or ampicillin (necrotizing fasciitis or myositis)
- Aminoglycoside with penicillin or ampicillin (*S. equi*)
- Ceftriaxone (meningitis)
- Cefuroxime (meningitis)
- TMS (meningitis)

Further reading

Lappin, E. and Ferguson A.J. (2009) Gram positive toxic shock syndromes. *Lancet Infect Dis.*, **9**, 281–290.

Priestnall, S. and Erles K. (2011) *Streptococcus zooepidemicus*: An emerging canine pathogen. *Vet J.*, **188**, 142–148.

Sykes, J.E. (2013) Streptococcal and enterococcal infections. Ch. 34. In: *Canine and Feline Infectious Diseases*. Sykes, J.E. (ed.), Elsevier, St. Louis, MO, pp. 334–346.

Chapter 121: *Strongyloides* Species (Threadworms)

Description: Roundworm nematode, parasitic and free-living life cycles
Zoonotic Potential: Transmitted readily to humans in endemic areas

Microbiology/epidemiology

The *Strongyloides stercoralis* nematode can parasitize dogs, cats and humans. *S. canis* may also infect dogs and *S. felis* may infect cats. The adult parasitic stage lives in the mucosa of the small intestine. *Strongyloides* are found worldwide with higher prevalence in areas that have fecal contamination of soil or water and in tropical and subtropical climates. Outbreaks have been reported in kennels. A Strongyloid's life cycle is heterogenic in the environment but is homogenic in the animal. Animals acquire the infection via percutaneous, peroral, or transmammary transmission in addition to autoinfection (internal and external). Autoinfection may be induced by the use of corticosteroids or other factors that affect immunocompetence. Following penetration of the skin, larvae migrate to the blood where they go to pulmonary alveoli. Here, they are coughed up, swallowed, and invade intestinal mucosa (duodenum and jejunum). They molt twice and become adult female worms that produce eggs, which eventually produce rhabditiform larvae. The rhabditiform larvae are excreted in feces.

Clinical disease

S. stercoralis can cause both respiratory and gastrointestinal symptoms. Clinical disease can vary from mild tracheal irritation and dry cough to severe enteritis, pneumonia, and death. Animals may present with blood-streaked, mucoid diarrhea, emaciation, reduced growth rate in young animals, abdominal pain, nausea, vomiting, ileus, bowel edema, intestinal obstruction, mucosal ulceration, massive hemorrhage, and subsequent peritonitis or bacterial sepsis. In early infections, the appetite remains good and the animal is normally active. Without concurrent secondary infections, there is little or no fever. In advanced stages there may be shallow, rapid breathing, and fever, and the prognosis is often very poor. Respiratory symptoms may involve cough, wheezing, dyspnea, hoarseness, pneumonitis, hemoptysis, respiratory failure, and diffuse interstitial infiltrates. Other side effects may include; septic or gram negative meningitis, CSF larvae infection, peripheral edema, ascites, hypoalbuminemia, and bacteremia/sepsis.

Diagnosis

Larvae (rhabditiform or filariform) can be demonstrated in fresh stool samples using the Baermann technique. Other techniques used include culturing fecal samples on agar plates, serodiagnosis through ELISA, and duodenal fumigation. Still, diagnosis can be difficult because of the varying juvenile parasite load on a daily basis.

Treatment

Before antiparasitics are given, the environment should be cleaned of feces and all bedding should be washed and sterilized. Direct sunlight, increased temperatures, and desiccation assist in killing the larvae. Wooden and impervious surfaces should be washed, steamed or concentrated salt or lime solutions applied. This should be followed by rinsing with hot water. Dogs with diarrhea should be promptly isolated from dogs that appear healthy. Immunosuppressive therapy should be stopped or reduced if possible. All animals should be treated at the same time. Infections in dogs can be treated with ivermectin (0.2 mg/kg, SC or PO × 1 repeated in 4 weeks or 0.8 mg/kg PO once) or fenbendazole (50 mg/kg PO q24 h × 5 days, repeated 4 weeks later). In cats, fenbendazole (50 mg/kg PO q24 h for 3 days) can be used. Repeat fecals should be performed for at least 6 months after treatment to confirm efficacy.

Drug therapy

- Ivermectin
- Fenbendazole

Further reading

Johnston, F.H., Morris, P.S., Speare, R., *et al.* (2005) Strongyloidiasis: A review of the evidence for Australian practitioners. *The Austr J Rural Health.*, **13**(4), 247–54.

Marcos, L.A., Terashima, A., Dupont, H.L., *et al.* (2008) *Strongyloides* hyperinfection syndrome: An emerging global infectious disease. *Transact Royal Soc Trop Med Hygiene.*, **102(4)**, 314–318.

Safer, D., Brenes, M., and Dunipace, S. (2007) Urocanic acid is a major chemoattractant for the skin-penetrating parasitic nematode *Strongyloides stercoralis. Proceed Nat Acad Sci.*, **104(5)**, 1627.

Segarra-Newnham, M. (2007) Manifestations, diagnosis, and treatment of *Strongyloides stercoralis* infection. *Ann Pharmacother.*, **41(12)**, 1992–2001.

Chapter 122: *Toxocara Canis/Cati*

Type: Roundworms, helminthes, white to pale brown, up to 18 cm (7″) long
Description: Transmission to humans can result in significant zoonotic disease.

Microbiology/epidemiology

T. canis and *T. cati* are found worldwide in canine and feline hosts. The adult worms live in the hosts gut and disease is often asymptomatic. Massive infection in juveniles can be fatal. Incidental infections can occur in humans resulting in visceralis larva migrans and ocularis larva migrans. *Toxocara* species eggs are secreted in the feces of an infected host. Eggs may last in the feces for up to 3 weeks. A new host must ingest the embryonated eggs. After hatching, larvae migrate through body tissues into the lungs and are coughed up and swallowed. Larvae mature in the intestine to adult worms. Infection may also be transmitted either *in utero* or via transfer of L3 larvae in milk from bitches and queens to litters. Humans may contract infection via animal fur or feces.

Clinical disease

Many animals may be asymptomatic. Puppies may present with vomiting or defecating of roundworms. Typically there is a failure to gain weight, dull hair coat, anemia, loss of appetite, pot-bellied appearance, mucoid or bloody stool, diarrhea, and coughing. Rarely, animals may develop severe gastrointestinal obstruction.

Diagnosis

Fecal flotation of stool samples should demonstrate roundworm eggs. Notation of adult roundworms in feces or vomit is also diagnostic.

Treatment

Maintain good hygiene, remove waste regularly, prevent animals from eating prey (rodents), and children from exposure to animal feces. Fenbendazole, pyrantel pamoate, milbemycin oxime, moxidectin, ivermectin with either pyrantel pamoate or praziquantel, and febantel with pyrantel pamoate and praziquental are approved treatments. Selamectin is approved in cats. Residual larvae must be treated at 2 weekly intervals. Emodepside (0.4 mg) plus toltrazuril (9 mg/kg PO × 1) has been demonstrated to have greater than 94% efficacy against adults, immature adults, and L4 larvae of *T. canis*. All pups should be treated routinely with pyrantel pamoate at 2, 4, 6, and 8 weeks and then placed on monthly heartworm preventative. All kittens should be treated with pyrantel pamoate at 2 weeks (to cover hookworms and *T. cati*) and then on monthly heartworm treatment, which covers *Toxocara* sp. Nursing dams should be treated at the same time. Pregnant bitches may be treated with fenbendazole daily. Current recommendations can be found at capcvet.org.

Drug therapy

- Fenbendazole (pregnant animals)
- Pyrantel pamoate (pups/kittens)
- Milbemycin
- Moxidectin

Drug therapy alternatives

- Selemectin
- Pyrantel pamoate with ivermectin
- Praziquantel with ivermectin
- Fenbantal with pyrantel and praziquantel
- Emodepside with toltazuril

Further reading

Despommier, D. (2003) Toxocariasis: Clinical Aspects, epidemiology, medical ecology, and molecular aspects. *Clin Microbiol Rev.*, **16(2)**, 265–272.

Schimmel, A., Schroeder, I., Altreuther, G., *et al.* (2011) Efficacy of emodepside plus toltrazuril (Procox oral suspension for dogs) against *Toxocara canis, uncinaria stenocephala* and *Ancyclostoma canium* in dogs. *Parasitol Res.*, **109(Suppl 1)**, 1–8.

Wolken, S., Schaper, R., Mencke, N., *et al.* (2009) Treatment and prevention of vertical transmission of *Toxocara cati* in cats with an emodepside/praziquantel spot-on formulation. *Parasitol Res.*, **105**, 75–81.

Wolkin, S., Bohm, C., Schaper, R., *et al.* (2012) Treatment of third-stage larvae of *Toxocara cati* with Milbemycin oxime plus praziquantal tablets and emodepside plus praziquantel spot-on formulation in experimentally infected cats. *Parasitol Res.*, **111(5)**, 2123–2127.

Chapter 123: *Toxoplasma Gondii* (Toxoplasmosis)

Description: Coccidial protozoan
Zoonotic Potential: A significant zoonotic, teratogenic risk to human fetuses

Microbiology/epidemiology

Toxoplasmosis gondii is found worldwide in cat populations. Cats serve as the definition host where the protozoa complete their life cycle. Oocysts are only produced in cats, which are excreted into feces during the first 21 days. Oocysts are environmentally resistant and undergo sporulation 1–5 days after being shed in the environment. Sporozoites are released after ingestion that penetrate the intestine and undergo asexual replication in tissues where they become bradyzoites. These encyst in tissues (muscles, CNS, and visceral organs) resulting in chronic infections. Tissue cysts may be present for life in both cats, dogs, and other species. Cats may acquire the infection by ingestion of infected prey. Outdoor animals have the highest risk of infection.

Clinical disease

Clinical disease in rodent prey is associated with altered behavior increasing the likelihood of predator success and transmission to the definitive feline host. Following ingestion in cats, lethargy, anorexia, and respiratory distress may occur. Immunosuppressed animals and kittens are at risk of severe infection. Chronic infection may result in uveitis, chorioretinitis, cutaneous lesions, fever, muscle hyperesthesia, myocarditis, arrhythmias, weight loss, anorexia, seizures, ataxia, icterus, diarrhea, respiratory distress, and pancreatitis. Dogs typically have less severe disease, which may result in fever, vomiting, diarrhea, respiratory distress, ataxia, seizures, and icterus. Myositis, paralysis, weakness, stiff gait, muscle atrophy, polyradiculoneuritis, retinitis, uveitis, conjunctivitis, optic neuritis, and dermatitis (pustules, pruritus, subcutaneous nodules, and alopecia) can also occur.

Diagnosis

Fecal flotation and PCR may be useful but the oocyst shedding period is short so false negatives are high. PCR on blood and tissues in the presence of clinical symptoms is diagnostic. Serology on serum is useful but does not always correlate with active disease.

Treatment

Supportive care with antiemetics, fluids, and antiprotozoal therapy are required. Topical or systemic glucocorticoids may be required for *T. gondii* uveitis. Clindamycin or TMS are the drugs of choice. A positive response should be evident in the first week, if not another drug should be given. A full month of therapy is recommended due to high recurrence rates with shorter courses. Azithromycin or ponazuril has also been used but the duration of dosing remains to be determined for these. Disseminated disease in cats and dogs into the CNS, liver, or lungs carries a poor prognosis.

Drug therapy

- Clindamycin
- TMS

Drug therapy alternatives

- Azithromycin
- Ponazuril

Further reading

Dubey, J.P., Lindsay, D.S., and Lappin, M.R. (2009) *Toxoplasmosis and other intestinal coccidial infections in cats and dogs. Vet Clin North Amer Small Anim Pract.*, **39**, 1034.
Lappin, M.R. (2013) Toxoplasmosis. Ch. 72. In: *Canine and Feline Infectious Diseases.* Sykes, J.E. (ed.), Elsevier, St. Louis, MO, pp. 693–703.
Robert-Gangneux, F. and Dared, M.L. (2012) Epidemiology and diagnostic strategies for toxoplasmosis. *Clin Microb Rev.*, **25**, 264–296.

Chapter 124: *Trichomonas* Species

Description: Flagellate protozoan
Zoonotic Potential: Host specific, no known zoonotic transmission

Microbiology/epidemiology

Trichomonas foetus is an intestinal flagellate of cats and occasionally dogs. It is believed to infect animals worldwide. Animals acquire the infection via oral–fecal transmission. Cats in overcrowded conditions (e.g., shelters, breeders, and show cats), those that share litter boxes, and those that engage in mutual grooming are at highest risk. Organisms replicate by binary fission and are shed in feces. *T. foetus* can survive outside the host in cat food (0.5–2 h) and in hours to days in cat feces.

Clinical disease

T. foetus infects the ileum, cecum, and colon. Signs are often intermittent and can resolve following antibiotics, but may then recur. Cats may present with chronic intractable diarrhea or may be asymptomatic. Diarrhea, an increased frequency of defecation and passage of semiformed to liquid stool is typical. Feces may be foul smelling with fresh blood and mucus. The anus may be edematous and fecal incontinence may develop. Although diarrhea may be persistent, cats typically maintain an appetite and a good body score. Diarrhea may worsen if co-infection with *Cryptosporidium* species is present.

Diagnosis

Fecal culture (In-Pouch test) is considered the gold standard. PCR and cytologic examination may also be used but will have a higher level of false negatives.

Treatment

The treatment of choice is ronidazole. Tinidazole has been considered an alternative but is generally less effective (50%) than ronidazole at clearing infections.

Drug therapy

Ronidazole.

Drug therapy alternatives

Tinidazole.

Further reading

Gookin, J.L., Stauffer, S.H., Coccaro, M.R., *et al.* (2007) Efficacy of tinidazole for treatment of cats experimentally infected with *Tritrichomonas foetus*. *Am J Vet Res.*, **68**, 1085–1088.

Gookin, J.L., Copple, C.N., Papich, M.G., *et al.* (2006) Efficacy ofronidazole for treatment of feline *Tritrichomonas foetus* infection. *J Vet Intern Med.*, **20**, 536–543.

Kingsburg, D.D., Marks, S.L., Cave, N.J., *et al.* (2010) Identification of *Tritrichomonas foetus* and *Giardia* spp. infection in pedigree show cats in the New Zealand. *NZ Vet J.*, **58**, 6–10.

Scorza, V. and Lappin, M.R. (2010) Gastrointestinal protozoal infections. In: *Consultations in Feline Medicine*, 6th ed., August, J. (ed.), Elsevier, Philadelphia, p. 200.

Chapter 125: *Yersinia Pestis* (Plaque)

Description: Gram negative aerobic coccobacillus, non-motile, Enterobacteriaceae
Zoonotic Potential: Significant zoonotic potential via cat bites, scratches, or respiratory droplets inhalation or via carriage of infected fleas into the household

Microbiology/epidemiology

Yersinia pestis is the causative agent of plague. It causes disease in rabbits, rodents, cats, dogs, and humans, as well as other mammals. It has been eradicated in many countries, but is maintained in wild borrowing rodents in Asia, Africa, South America, and the South Western USA. Animals acquire the infection from infected fleas, which have fed on infected rodents. Ingestion of infected rodents or rabbits, or aerosolization of respiratory droplets by cats and/or dogs may also transmit disease. Human infections may occur following cat scratches, bites, or contact with aerosolized respiratory secretions. Incubation is typically 1–6 days after infection and death may occur in 2–3 days without therapy.

Clinical disease

Following infection, organisms are carried by lymphatics to regional lymph nodes. Cats typically have lethargy, dehydration, inappetence, variable fever (41°C/105°F) and enlarged, tender lymph nodes (Bubo). Lymph nodes may abscess and drain purulent material.

Mandibular or retropharyngeal lymph nodes may be involved. Localized development of Bubo is known as bubonic plaque, which is less fatal than the septicemic form that may lack Bubo. In some cases, dissemination may occur with bacteremia, endotoxemia, sepsis, and formation of hemorrhagic, neutrophilic, necrotizing, and lesions in many organs. Tachypnea, vomiting, tachycardia, bradycardia, and disseminated intravascular coagulation may occur. Pneumonic plaque occurs in 10% of infected cats and results in dyspnea and cough. Some cats (20%) may show no illness or a subacute infection with recovery. A transient febrile illness is commonly seen in dogs. Dogs typically present with fever, lethargy, mandibular, or cervical Bubo formation, oral ulceration, ptyalism, and cough.

Diagnosis

Diagnosis is based on clinical signs, history, and laboratory confirmation. A history of predation in endemic areas, physical signs consistent with *Y. pestis* and lymph node cytology (bipolar staining bacilli), supports the diagnosis. Culture of blood, lymph nodes, direct IFA, and serology are all required for confirmation but may take weeks.

Treatment

Animals suspected of plague should be isolated for at least 72 h after initiating antibiotics. Personnel protective gear (masks, goggles, gowns, gloves) should be worn by animal handlers and Public Health should be notified. Cats and dogs should be immediately treated for fleas (Capstar) and given supportive care along with antibiotics. Abscesses require lancing, draining, and flushing. All materials should be disposed of in biohazard waste with frequent disinfection. The drugs of choice include: Initial therapy with intravenous doxycycline (10 mg/kg IV q24 h for 10 days) or gentamycin for more serious infections is recommended. Oral therapy with doxycycline can be initiated after 72 h at the same dose. Both chloramphenicol and TMS are also active. The prognosis is good (90%) with antibiotic treatment.

Drug therapy

- Doxycycline
- Gentamycin

Drug therapy alternatives

- Chloramphenicol
- TMS

Further reading

Pennisi, M.G., Egberink, H., Hartmann K., *et al.* (2013) *Yersinia pestis* infection in cats: ABCD guidelines on prevention and management. *J Feline Med Surg.*, **15(7)**, 582–584.

Sykes, J.E. and Chomel, B.B. (2013) *Yersinia pestis* (Plaque) and other Yersinioses. Ch. 55. In: *Canine and Feline Infectious Diseases*. Sykes, J.E. (ed.), Elsevier, St. Louis, MO, pp. 531–545.

Watson, R.P., Blanchard T.W., Mense M.G., *et al.* (2001) Histopathology of experimental plague in cats. *Vet Pathol.*, **38(2)**, 165–172.

SECTION D

Antibiotics

Chapter 126: Amikacin

US Generic (Brand) Name: Amikacin (Amikin, Amiglyde-V, Amiject D, Amikacin C, Caniglide)
Availability: Human approved – Amikacin sulfate sterile injectable (50 mg/mL, 250 mg/mL × 2 mL, vials or 2 mL syringes). Veterinary approved – Amikacin sulfate sterile injectable (50 mg/mL × 50 mL bottles)
Resistance mechanisms: Aminoglycoside modifying enzymes, ribosome alteration, decreased permeability

Use

Serious gram negative infections due to *Pseudomonas, Proteus, Serratia,* or gram positive bacilli involving the respiratory tract, urinary tract, septicemia, endocarditis, or bone infections that are resistant to gentamycin and tobramycin. May be useful in severe bacterial endophthalmitis. Poor efficacy against intracellular bacilli, anaerobes, and mycoplasma. Only effective against some strains of *Mycobacteria* (*M. avium*), *Actinomyces, Nocardia* spp., *Corynebacterium,* and *Bacillus* spp.

Contraindications/warnings

Use with caution in animals with renal impairment, monitor the animal closely for signs of tubular necrosis (casts appear early in urine). Avoid use in animals with pre-existing vestibular impairment, electrolyte imbalances, and/or myasthenia gravis. Discontinue drug if signs of hypersensitivity, ototoxicity, or nephrotoxicity. Avoid use with other renal toxic drugs or prolonged therapy.

Dosage

Dosing should be individualized due to the low therapeutic index. Base the dose on ideal body weight in obese animals. Animals with endotoxemia may have increased risk of renal toxicity.

Canine

15–30 mg/kg IV, IM, SC q24 h. Dose reduce in greyhounds and sight hounds to 10–12 mg/kg IV, IM, SC q24 h. Use higher doses for sepsis (Papich 2002, Kukanich and Coetzee 2008).

Feline

10–14 mg/kg IV, IM, SC q24 h. SC dosing is preferred because of rapid absorption, good bioavailability and ease of administration (Jernigan *et al.,* 1988, Papich 2002).

Dose adjustments

Dose adjust in renal failure. Give a loading dose, then give 50% of the dose with moderate renal failure and 25% of the dose in severe renal failure. Monitor serum levels and adjust doses accordingly. No dose adjustment for hepatic insufficiency.

Administration

Hydrate animals prior to administration. SC or IV fluids are recommended to prevent renal toxicity. For IM or SC dosing, the dose should be drawn up from the 50 or 250 mg/mL vial and injected directly, either SC or in a large muscle. For IV administration the dose should be drawn up and diluted with 100–200 mL of a compatible solution (0.9% saline, 5% dextrose in water, lactated ringers, normosol, plasma-lyte 56 or 148, etc.). The infusion rate should be sufficient to provide the dose over 1–2 h in small animals or 0.5–1 h in larger animals.

Drug Therapy for Infectious Diseases of the Dog and Cat, First Edition. Valerie J. Wiebe.
© 2015 John Wiley & Sons, Inc. Published 2015 by John Wiley & Sons, Inc.

Electrolyte contents

Sodium concentration in one gram is 29.9 mg (1.3 mEq).

Storage/stability

May change to a light straw color, but not indicative of a loss in potency. Final concentrations between 0.25–5 mg/mL in most IV fluids are stable for 24 h at room temperature or 2 days under refrigeration when mixed with 5% dextrose in water, 0.9% saline, or lactated ringers. Dilute solutions (0.25 and 5 mg/mL) can be frozen at −15°C for 30 days if used within 24 h when brought to room temperature.

Adverse reactions

>10%
Renal toxicity is common at high doses (30 mg/kg/day) (gentamicin > amikacin > tobramycin). Nephrotoxicity is polyuric with increased fractional electrolyte excretion, glycosuria, and tubular casts, may progress to oliguria. Acute tubular necrosis manifested by increases in serum creatinine and BUN have been reported in dogs and cats. Renal damage is typically reversible if good urine output is maintained. Diarrhea, vomiting and injection site reactions (SC, IM doses) are reported commonly in dogs and cats.

1–10%
Ototoxicity may be irreversible. Neurotoxicity to the eighth cranial nerve (cochlear toxicity > vestibular toxicity with amikacin in dogs), vestibular injury and bilateral irreversible damage is related to the amount of drug given and duration of treatment. Cats may develop vestibular toxicity (ataxia, impaired righting, at high cumulative doses of 700 mg/kg) several days prior to renal toxicity. Vestibular toxicity following otic administration to animals with ruptured tympanic membranes has also been reported.

Other species
Hypotension, rash, eosinophilia, tremor, arthralgia, dyspnea, weakness, hypersensitivity reactions, drug fever, and anemia.

Drug interactions

Amikacin should not be admixed with other drugs. If a beta-lactam is being given it should be administered through a separate line or at a separate time following line flushing. Beta-lactams are synergistic with aminoglycosides against bacteria but inactivate aminoglycosides in serum samples if left sitting. Aminoglycoside assays must be assessed immediately after collection. Concurrent use with nephrotoxic drugs (amphotericin B, iron, calcium channel blockers, cisplatin, NSAIDs, vancomycin, and polymyxin) is reported to increase renal side effects in humans. Neuromuscular blocking drugs may prolong or increase risk of neuromuscular toxicities. Loop diuretics may increase nephrotoxicity and ototoxicity.

Monitoring

Establish baseline renal function, then monitor serum creatinine, urinalysis (casts). Draw blood for amikacin levels from alternative lumen or peripheral stick to avoid falsely high concentrations from central catheters. Both initial and periodic peak and trough levels should be obtained in patients with renal dysfunction or in serious infections. For serious infections, peak serum concentrations (30 min after a 30 minute IV infusion) should be in the range of 20–30 μg/mL and trough concentrations (30 min prior to the next dose) should be 4–8 μg/mL. Peak levels >35 μg/mL and troughs >10 μg/mL are considered toxic. Peak concentrations following IM or SC dosing should be drawn at 1 h after dosing.

Overdose

Maintain good urine output, polyionic electrolyte fluid therapy >3 weeks may be required to reverse renal damage. Oliguria is a poor prognostic sign. Edrophonium, neostigmine, calcium chloride, or calcium gluconate may be used to reverse muscle paralysis. Hemodialysis is typically not required, but can remove a significant amount of amikacin (50–100%).

Diagnostic test interference

Beta-lactams and cephalosporins may decrease measured serum concentrations in vitro.

Mechanism

Bactericidal. Aminoglycosides inhibit protein synthesis in susceptible bacteria by binding to the 30s and 50s ribosomal subunits. This results in a defective bacterial cell membrane.

Pharmacology/kinetics

Absorption

Poorly absorbed orally, rapid and complete absorption with IM injection. Bioavailability from extravascular injection sites (IM, SC) is >90%. The time to peak plasma concentrations following IM injection is 0.79 h and 0.89 h following SC dosing. Peak concentrations in healthy dogs after single IM and SC doses are 45 μg/mL and 31 μg/mL, respectively.

Distribution

Pleural and ascites fluid levels similar to serum levels. Amikacin achieves therapeutic concentrations in bone, heart, gallbladder, and lungs. The volume of distribution is smaller in greyhounds compared to other breeds and the clearance is significantly lower.

CNS penetration

Typically poor and variable penetration into CSF. Normal penetration is only 10–20% and maximum of 15–24% with inflammation.

Metabolism

Aminoglycosides are not metabolized and are almost entirely eliminated via renal elimination as intact drug. Within 6 h, >90% of amikacin is excreted in the urine of healthy dogs.

Half-life

The half-life is variable depending on renal function (0.5–2.0 h in cats and dogs). Following IM and SC dosing, the half-life is 1.4 and 1.8 h, respectively.

Pregnancy risk factor

Category C. Give only if benefit outweighs the risks. Renal toxicity in pregnant rats and their fetuses have been reported.

Lactation

Excreted into milk in low concentrations. Due to poor oral bioavailability, nursing animals would not be expected to absorb drug, but may develop diarrhea and altered gut flora.

References

Jernigan, A.D., Wilson, R.C., and Hatch, R.C. (1988) Pharmacokinetics of amikacin in cats. *Am J Vet Res.*, **49(3)**, 355–358.

Kukanich, B. and Coetzee, J.F. (2008) Comparative pharmacokinetics of amikacin in greyhound and beagle dogs. *J Vet Pharm and Therap.*, **31**, 102–107.

Papich, M.G. (2002) *Saunders Handbook of Veterinary Drugs*, 2nd edn. Winkel A. (ed.), W.B. Saunders Company, Philadelphia, pp. 17–19.

Further reading

Baggot, J.D., Ling, G.V., and Chatfield, R.C. (1985) Clinical pharmacokinetics of amikacin in dogs. *Am J Vet Res.*, **46(8)**, 1793–1796.

Christenson, E.F., Reiffenstein, J.C., and Madissoo, H. (1977) Comparative ototoxicity of amikacin and gentamycin in cats. *Antimicrob Agents Chemother.*, **12(2)**, 178–184.

Clark, C.H. (1977) Toxicity of aminoglycoside antibiotics. *Mod Vet Pract.*, **58(7)**, 594–598.

Zhenqing, D., Lin, Y., Yu, Y., *et al.* (2012) Pharmacokinetics of amikacin after intravenous, intramuscular and subcutaneous administration in German Shepherd dogs. *J Anim Veterin Advan.*, **11(8)**, 1145–1148.

Chapter 127: Amoxicillin

US Generic (Brand) Name: Amoxicillin (Amoxil, Amoxi-Tabs, Amoxi-Drops)
Availability: Human approved – Amoxicillin oral capsules (250, 500 mg), amoxicillin oral tablets (500, 875 mg), amoxicillin powder for oral suspension (200 mg/5 mL, 250 mg/5 mL, 400 mg/5 mL), chew tablets (125, 200, 250, 400 mg). Veterinary approved – Amoxicillin oral tablets (50, 100, 150, 200, 400 mg), amoxicillin powder for oral suspension (50 mg/mL × 15, 30 mL), amoxicillin sterile injection 250 mg/mL (IM/SC)
Resistance Mechanisms: Gene mutation (Amp C gene), altered TEM-1 B-lactamases

Use

In vitro activity is similar to ampicillin but absorption more reliable. Good activity against *Pasteurella multocida*, obligate anaerobes, non-penicillinase producing *Staphylococcus*, *Enterococcus faecalis*, *H. pylori*, and *C. perfringes*. Covers some *E. coli*, *Proteus*, and *Salmonella*. Used empirically for uncomplicated bladder infections. Also used for treatment of presumed gram positive infections of soft tissue, lung, sinus, and ear infections.

Contraindications/warnings

Avoid using in patients that are hypersensitive to penicillin or cephalosporins. In patients with renal failure, modify dose to the degree of renal impairment (see the following).

Dosage

Dogs/cats
Gram positive infections: 10 mg/kg PO, IM, SC q12 h for at least 2 days post symptoms subsiding.

Gram negative infections: 20 mg/kg IM, SC q8–12 h. In cases where endotoxic shock is present, there may be a decrease in elimination of amoxicillin as well as a substantial increase in the plasma concentrations potentially resulting in toxicity.

Dose adjustments

Reduce dose to every 12–18 h with moderate renal impairment and to every 24 h with severe renal impairment.

Administration

Amoxicillin is best absorbed on an empty stomach, if the animal does not tolerate it on an empty stomach, give with food.

Electrolyte contents

Not significant.

Storage/stability

Oral suspension is stable for 7 days at room temperature and for 14 days refrigerated after reconstitution. The tablets, chew tablets, capsules, and powder for oral suspension should be stored at room temperature in tight containers.

Adverse reactions

>10%
Salivation, anorexia reported in cats and dogs.

1–10%
Vomiting, diarrhea (less than ampicillin) reported in dogs and cats.

Other species
Seizures, hyperirritability, convulsions (at high doses or with renal impairment), fever, super-infection, hypersensitivity reactions (angioedema, rash, urticaria, anaphylaxis), anemia, hemolytic anemia, thrombocytopenia, eosinophilia, leucopenia, agranulocytosis, elevated liver enzymes, and cholestasis have been reported.

Drug interactions

Allopurinol increases amoxicillin concentrations in humans.

Monitoring

For prolonged therapy monitor renal, hepatic, and hematologic function.

Overdose

Acute toxicity may involve nausea, vomiting, seizures, muscle hyperirritability, and convulsions. Use supportive care and hemodialysis if available.

Diagnostic test interference

May interfere with urine glucose analysis if using the Clinitest. May inactivate aminoglycosides *in vitro* altering their concentrations.

Mechanism

Bactericidal aminopenicillin. Inhibits bacterial cell wall synthesis by binding to penicillin binding proteins resulting in inhibition of transpeptidation and bacterial cell wall autolysis.

Pharmacology/kinetics

Absorption
Oral absorption is >60%. Food may slow absorption but does not alter the amount absorbed.

Distribution

Widely distributed into most bodily fluids, urine, bile, lung, and bone. Does not penetrate into intracellular spaces or eye. Protein binding is only 13% in dogs.

CNS penetration

Has poor penetration into CNS (<1% serum concentrations). This increases to 8–90% with acute inflammation.

Metabolism

Amoxicillin undergoes hydrolysis to inactive penicilloic acids. Approximately 40–70% excreted unchanged in urine. Some biliary excretion also occurs.

Half-life

Half-life is 45–90 min in dogs and 1.2 h in cats. Increases with renal failure.

Pregnancy risk factor

Category B: doses up to 10-fold the human dose in rats and mice have shown no teratogenic effects in any species. Amoxicillin is considered safe to use in pregnancy.

Lactation

Amoxicillin is excreted into milk in low concentrations (0.68–1.3 µg/mL). Maximum concentrations are seen 4–5 h after an oral dose. Nursing animals may develop diarrhea and potential sensitization to penicillins.

Further reading

Aucoin, D. (2000) Antibiotic drug formulary. *Target: The Antibiotic Drug Guide to Effective Treatment*. North American Drug Compendiums Inc., Port Huron, MI, pp. 93–142.

Kung, K. and Wanner, M. (1994) Bioavailability of different forms of amoxicillin administered orally to dogs. *Vet Rec.*, **135(23)**, 552–554.

Marier, J.F., Beaudry, F., Ducharme, M.P., *et al.* (2001) A pharmacokinetic study of amoxicillin in febrile beagle dogs following repeated administrations of endotoxin. *J Vet Pharmacol Therap.*, **24(6)**, 379–383.

Sakamoto, H., Hirose, T., and Mine, Y. (1985) Pharmacokinetics of FK027 in rats and dogs. *J Antibiot (Tokyo)*, **38(4)**, 496–504.

Vree, T.B., Dammers, E., and VanDuuren, E. (2002) Variable absorption of clavulanic acid after an oral dose of 25 mg/kg of Clavubactin and Synulox in healthy cats. *Scientific World J.*, **2**, 1369–1378.

Vree, T.B., Dammers, E., and VanDuuren, E. (2003) Variable absorption of clavulanic acid after an oral dose of 25 mg/kg of Clavubactin and Synulox in healthy dogs. *J Vet Pharmacol Therp.*, **26(3)**, 165–171.

Chapter 128: Ampicillin

US Generic (Brand) Name: Ampicillin sodium or ampicillin trihydrate (Polycillin, Omnipen, Principen, Polyflex)

Availability: Human approved – Ampicillin oral capsules (ampicillin trihydrate or anhydrate-250, 500 mg), ampicillin trihydrate oral suspension 125 mg/5 mL, 250 mg/5 mL × 80, 100, 150, and 200 mL bottles), ampicillin sodium sterile powder for injection (125, 250, 500 mg and 1, 2, and 10 g vials). Veterinary approved – Ampicillin trihydrate sterile injectable 10 and 25 g vials

Resistance Mechanisms: Altered penicillin binding proteins and beta-lactamase (TEM-1) production

Use

Used for the treatment of infections due to most gram positive organisms (*Streptococcus* and *Staphylococcus*, with the exception of penicillinase-producing *Staphylococci*. Bacteriostatic against and some *Enterococcus* spp., but bactericidal in combination with aminoglycosides. Effective against some strains of gram negative aerobes including *E. coli*, *P. mirabilis*, and *Salmonella* spp. Used in the treatment of susceptible urinary tract infections, meningitis, and endocarditis. Systemic therapy should be instituted for severe infections due to the poor oral bioavailability of ampicillin.

Contraindications/warnings

Do not use in patients that are hypersensitive to penicillins. Avoid use of oral formulations in severely ill animals due to poor oral absorption.

Dosage

Canine

Ampicillin sodium: 10–20 mg/kg q6–8 h IV, IM, SC, or 20–40 mg/kg PO q8 h (doses as high as 100 mg/kg used in resistant *Enterococci* infections) or ampicillin trihydrate: 10–50 mg/kg IM, SC q12–24 h (Papich 2002).

Feline

Ampicillin sodium: 10–20 mg/kg q6–8 h IV, IM, SC or 20–40 mg/kg PO q8 h (doses as high as 100 mg/kg used in resistant enterococci infections) or ampicillin trihydrate: 10–20 mg/kg IM, SC q12–24 h (Papich 2002).

Dose adjustments

Decrease dosing frequency in renal failure or give 25–75% the normal dose. No changes in hepatic insufficiency.

Administration

Give ampicillin capsules or oral suspension on an empty stomach, either 1 h prior or 2 h after a meal. Following reconstitution with sterile water for injection, ampicillin sodium solutions for IM or IV should be administered within 1 h. Remaining solutions of ampicillin sodium 30 mg/mL in sterile water are stable refrigerated for 48 h. Intravenous administration should be used for moderate to severe infections due to the poor oral bioavailability of ampicillin in animals. Direct IV injections should be made slowly over 10–15 min to avoid seizures. For IV infusion, refer to the manufacturer's package insert for specifics on diluents, concentrations, and stabilities. In general, the rate of infusion should be adjusted so that the total dose of drug is administered before 10% or more of the drug is inactivated.

Electrolyte contents

Ampicillin 1 gram has 66.7 mg (3mEq) of sodium.

Storage/stability

Store capsules, powder for injection, powder for oral suspension at room temperature. Oral suspensions are stable after reconstitution at room temperature for 7 days or refrigerated for 14 days. Solutions for IM or direct IV use in general are good for 1 h. For IV infusion, stability is variable depending on the diluents, concentration and storage conditions (refer to manufacturer's package insert for specifics).

Adverse reactions

>10%
Diarrhea, nausea, and vomiting reported in cats and dogs.

1–10%
Injection site reactions, non-allergic rashes, allergic reactions (serum sickness, urticaria, angioedema, and bronchospasm) reported in cats and dogs.

Other species
Ataxia, neuromuscular hyperirritability, convulsions, penicillin encephalopathy, severe colitis, anemia, hemolytic anemia, elevated liver enzymes, eosinophilia, thrombocytopenia, granulocytopenia, and nephritis reported in other mammals, and with dogs at high doses.

Drug interactions

Synergistic with aminoglycosides and cephalosporins. May be less effective with bacteriostatic antibiotics (chloramphenicol, erythromycin, and tetracyclines). May decrease absorption of oral atenolol and estrogens in humans. Incompatible with heparin, cortisone, amphotericin B, aminoglycosides, metronidazole, and erythromycin in solution.

Monitoring

For chronic use, monitor renal, hepatic, and hematologic function.

Overdose

Symptoms of acute toxicity may include neurologic stimulation (agitation, encephalopathy, and seizures), neuromuscular hypersensitivity, or electrolyte imbalance (sodium, potassium). Hemodialysis decreases serum levels by 50%, supportive care is recommended.

Diagnostic test interference

May interfere with urinary glucose tests if using Clinitest. Can inactivate aminoglycosides and give falsely low concentrations if not assayed directly after blood draws.

Mechanism
A bactericidal aminopenicillin. Inhibits bacterial cell wall synthesis by binding to one or more penicillin binding proteins. This inhibits transpeptidation affecting peptidoglycan synthesis of bacterial cell walls.

Pharmacology/kinetics

Absorption
Ampicillin is poorly absorbed from the gastrointestinal tract of dogs (<32–42%), food decreases the rate and extent of absorption.

Distribution
It is widely distributed throughout body tissues. Attains therapeutic concentrations in the kidney, liver, heart,

skin, lungs, bile, bone, prostate, and pleural fluids. Concentrations in urine following a 55 mg/kg PO divided QID in dogs was 350 µg/mL. Protein binding is 15–20% in dogs.

CNS Penetration

Very poor penetration (<1%) into CSF, with inflammation this increases to <25% serum levels.

Metabolism

Ampicillin undergoes significant enterohepatic cycling. Only partially metabolized in the liver to penicilloic acids (10%). Excreted primarily via unchanged drug in urine (50%) with the remainder excreted into bile. Concentrations in bile can accumulate up to 40 times that in plasma.

Half-life

Half-life in dogs and cats is 45–80 min.

Pregnancy risk factor

Category B: Ampicillin has not been linked to any specific teratogenic effects in animals or humans and is considered safe in pregnancy.

Lactation

Excreted into milk in low concentrations. The milk to plasma ratio in humans is 0.2. Ampicillin may cause diarrhea and potential sensitization to penicillins in nursing animals.

Reference

Papich, M.G. (2002) *Saunders Handbook of Veterinary Drugs*, 2nd edn. Winkel, A. (ed.), W.B. Saunders Company, Philadelphia, pp. 33–34.

Further reading

Ling, G. and Gilmore, C. (1977) Penicillin G or ampicillin for oral treatment of canine urinary tract infections. *J Amer Vet Med Assoc.*, **171(4)**, 358–361.

Schulze, J.D., Peters, E.E., Vickers, A.W., *et al.* (2005) Excipient effects on gastrointestinal transit and drug absorption in beagle dogs. *Int J Pharm.*, **26(300)**, 67–75.

Voorde, G., Broeze, J., Hartman, E., *et al.* (1990) The influence of the injection site on the bioavailability of ampicillin and amoxicillin in beagles. *Vet Quart.*, **12(2)**, 73–79.

Chapter 129: Azithromycin

US Generic (Brand) Name: Azithromycin (Zithromax, Zmax)
Availability: Human approved – Azithromycin tablets (250, 500, and 600 mg), azithromycin oral packet (1 g), powder for oral suspension (100 mg/5 mL, 200 mg/5 mL), extend release oral suspension (2 g), sterile powder for injection (500 mg, 2.5 g)
Resistance Mechanisms: Ribosomal modification (erm gene), altered efflux (mefE gene)

Use

More active than erythromycin against *Spirochetes*, *Mycoplasma* and most gram negative organisms including *Enterobacteria*, *Moraxella*, *Pasteurella*, *Bordetella*, and *Brucella*. Somewhat ineffective against *E. coli*, *Salmonella*, *Shigella*, and *Yersinia* (MICs of 4–8 mg/mL). Somewhat less active than erythromycin against gram positive cocci. Active against *Toxoplasma*, *Chlamydia*, *Plasmodium* spp., and *Mycobacterium avium*. Used primarily for skin infections and upper respiratory infections (including *Bordetella* pneumonias) in dogs and cats. Has shown some efficacy in the treatment of papillomatosis as well as *Babesia* (combined with atovaquone) in dogs.

Contraindications/warnings

Hypersensitivity to macrolides. May cause liver failure in patients with pre-existing liver impairment. Avoid use or monitor closely any animals using other hepatotoxic drugs concurrently.

Dosage

Canine
Skin/soft tissue: 5–10 mg/kg PO qd × 3–5 days (Sykes and Papich 2013).

Papillomatosis: 10 mg/kg PO qd × 10 days (Yagci *et al.*, 2008).

Toxoplasmosis: 10 mg/kg PO qd × 4 weeks (Lappin 2013).

Babesia (B. conradae, B. gibsoni): 10–12.5 mg/kg PO q24 h with atovaquone 13.3 mg/kg PO q8 h for 10 days (DiCicco *et al.*, 2012).

Feline
Skin/soft tissue: 5–10 mg/kg PO qd × 3–5 days (Sykes and Papich 2013).

Feline Bartonellosis: 10 mg/kg PO qd × 21 days (Ketring 2009).

Toxoplasmosis: 10 mg/kg PO qd × 4 weeks (Lappin 2013).

Dose adjustments

No adjustment required in renal failure, the drug should be avoided in patients with significant hepatic impairment. No dose adjustments are suggested in humans with mild to moderate hepatic impairment, but liver panels should be closely monitored. Dosing needs further evaluation in cats and dogs. Due to high bioavailability and a long half-life, a loading dose of 10 mg/kg followed by a 2.5–5.0 mg/kg PO q24 h dose may be more appropriate, particularly in geriatric patients.

Administration

Suspension should be taken 1 h prior to meals or 2 h after eating. The tablets may be taken with food to decrease the gastrointestinal side effects. IV infusions should not be admixed with other drugs. The intravenous (500 mg) vial should be diluted with 4.8 mL of sterile water for injection to make 100 mg/mL. Reconstituted solutions should be further diluted to 2 or 1 mg/mL with 250 or 500 mL of a compatible IV solution (5% dextrose in water, lactated ringers, 0.45 or 0.9% sodium chloride, etc.). IV solutions containing 1 mg/mL should be infused over 3 h, solutions containing 2 mg/mL should be infused over 1 h.

Electrolyte contents

A 250 mg tablet contains 1.21 mg (0.05 mEq), a 500 mg tablet contains 2.42 mg (0.1 mEq) and an IV (500 mg) dose contains 114.1 mg (4.96 mEq) of sodium, respectively.

Storage/stability

Store tablets and undiluted oral and injectable powders at room temperature. Once diluted, store the oral powder for suspension in a closed container at room temperature. Unused suspension should be discarded after 10 days. Following dilution with sterile water for injection the injectable 100 mg/mL solution is good for 24 h at room temperature. Following further dilution in the manufacturer's recommended diluents, the dilute IV solution is good for 24 h at room temperature or 7 days refrigerated.

Adverse reactions

>10%
Diarrhea, nausea, vomiting, abdominal pain reported in dogs and cats.

1–10%
Allergic reactions, rashes, pruritus, anaphylaxis, angioedema, cholestatic jaundice, and elevated liver enzymes reported in dogs and cats.

<1%
Hepatic necrosis, fever, eosinophilia, thrombophlebitis, ventricular arrhythmias, nephritis, ototoxicity, and phospholipidosis reported in dogs.

Drug interactions

Azithromycin should not be taken with aluminum or magnesium containing antacids or vitamins due to reduced absorption of drug. Azithromycin may inhibit P450 liver enzyme activity causing increased levels of cyclosporine, digoxin, or midazolam. Ivermectin and albendazole may increase azithromycin concentrations. Concurrent use of hepatotoxic (rifampin), or cardiotoxic agents should be avoided or monitored closely.

Monitoring

Monitor liver enzymes and CBC with differential. Evaluate electrolytes (sodium) in patients where sodium loads may be a problem.

Overdose

Nausea, vomiting, diarrhea, and prostration are reported in human overdoses. Extreme overdoses may result in Torsade de pointes (Q-T interval prolongation), bradycardia, and complete heart block. Supportive care including epinephrine and atropine (if bradycardia) is recommended.

Diagnostic test interference

No test interactions reported.

Mechanism

A macrolide (azolide) antibiotic. Binds to bacterial 50s ribosomal subunit inhibiting protein synthesis. May be bacteriostatic at low concentrations or bactericidal at high concentrations, depending on the organism and growth phase. Typically more active in an alkaline pH.

Pharmacology/kinetics

Absorption
Rapidly absorbed from the gastrointestinal tract. Following a 5 mg/kg oral dose in cats, bioavailability was 58% with peak levels of 0.97 µg/mL at 0.85 h after the dose. In dogs, the bioavailability is 97%.

Distribution
Extensive distribution into tissues and intracellular penetration into macrophages. Distributes into skin, ocular spaces, muscle, fat, lungs, sputum, and milk. Protein binding is concentration dependent (7–50%). When compared to erythromycin, azithromycin has better tissue penetration, a longer half-life, better absorption, and fewer side effects (diarrhea) than erythromycin.

CNS penetration
Very poor penetration into the CSF.

Metabolism
Metabolism is primarily in the liver with three metabolites being identified in cats and dogs. Elimination (>50% of the dose) is via the bile as parent drug in cats and dogs. Less than 20% of the dose is excreted via the urine.

Half-life
The elimination half-life in tissue and in intracellular compartments does not reflect the serum half-life (35 h in cats). Tissue half-lives are highly variable (13 h in fat, 72 h in cardiac muscle).

Pregnancy risk factor

Category B: No teratogenic effects have been noted in humans, mice, or rats.

Lactation
Azithromycin accumulates in milk. Concentrations are reported to be as high as 2.8 µg/mL, 137 h after a 500 mg dose in humans. Nursing animals may be subject to altered gastrointestinal flora and potential sensitization to macrolides.

References

DiCicco, M.F., Downey, M.E., Beeler, E., *et al.* (2012) Re-emergence of *Babesia conradae* and effective treatment of infected dogs with atovoquone and azithromycin. *B Vet Parasitology.*, **187(1–2)**, 23–27.

Ketring, K. (2009) Feline Bartonellosis: The naysayers are wrong! It is the most under diagnosed feline ocular disease. *Proceedings WVC.*

Lappin, M.R. (2013) Toxoplasmosis. Ch. 72. In: *Canine and Feline Infectious Diseases*, Sykes, J.E. (ed.), Elsevier, St. Louis, MO, pp. 693–701.

Sykes, J.E. and Papich, M.G. (2013) Antibacterial drugs. Ch. 8. In: *Canine and Feline Infectious Diseases*, Sykes, J.E. (ed.), Elsevier, St. Louis, MO, pp. 66–86.

Yagci, B.B., Ural, K., Ocal, N., *et al.* (2008) Azithromycin therapy of papillomatosis in dogs: a prospective, randomized, double blinded, placebo-controlled clinical trial. *Vet Dermatol.*, **19(4)**, 194–198.

Further reading

Hunter, R.P., Lynch, M.J., Ericson, J.F., *et al.* (1995) Pharmacokinetics oral bioavailability and tissue distribution of azithromycin in cats. *J Vet Pharmacol Ther.*, **18(1)**, 38–46.

Chapter 130: Cefadroxil

US Generic (Brand) Name: Cefadroxil (Duricef, Ultracef, Cefa-drops, Cefatabs)
Availability: Human approved – Cefadroxil capsules (500 mg), cefadroxil tablets (1 g), powder for oral suspension (250 mg/5 mL, 500 mg/5 mL × 50, 100 mL). Veterinary approved – Variable availability: Cefatabs (50, 100, 200, and 1 g), Cefa-drops oral suspension (50 mg/mL × 15, 50 mL)
Resistance Mechanisms: Altered penicillin binding proteins, increased beta-lactamase production, altered permeability

Use

Activity is similar to other first generation cephalosporins (cephalexin). Its slightly longer half-life may provide some advantages clinically over cephalexin, although it has MICs 2–4 times higher for most gram positive cocci and gram negative bacilli. Cephalothin is used as a marker for cefadroxil sensitivity. Used in the treatment of gram positive cocci and bacilli (except *Enteroccus* spp.) skin and soft tissue infections, as well as UTIs in cats and dogs.

Contraindications/warnings

Hypersensitivity to cephalosporins or severe reactions to penicillins. Modify dose with renal impairment, prolonged use may cause superinfection.

Dosage

Canine

UTIs: 11–22 mg/kg PO q12 h × 7–30 days (Greene 2006).

Pyoderma: 22–35 mg/kg PO q12 h × 3–30 days (Greene 2006).

Systemic infections: 22 mg/kg PO q8–12 h × 30 days (Greene 2006).

Feline

UTIs: 22 mg/kg PO q24h < 21 days (Greene 2006).

Systemic infections: 22 mg/kg PO q12h (Greene 2006).

Dose adjustments

Adjust dose in renal impairment. For moderate renal impairment administer q24 h rather than q12 h; for severe impairment, administer q36 h.

Administration

Give with food to decrease gastrointestinal upset. Dilute oral suspension with water according to the manufacturer's directions. Shake well prior to dosing.

Electrolyte contents

Not significant.

Storage/stability

Store tabs, caps, or powder for suspension at room temperature. Refrigerate suspension after reconstitution. Expires 14 days after reconstitution.

Adverse reactions

>10%
Nausea, vomiting, and diarrhea commonly seen in dogs and cats.

1–10%
Lethargy, restlessness, and itching reported in dogs.

Other Species
Fever, jaundice, seizures, joint pain, eosinophilia, tachypnea, elevated liver enzymes, nephritis, and hives reported.

Drug interactions

Nephrotoxic drugs can contribute to an increase in potential plasma concentrations of cefadroxil as well as toxicities.

Monitoring

Monitor for allergic reactions. For patients with renal failure, on high doses, or with prolonged courses monitor CBC, hepatic, and renal function.

Overdose

Nausea, vomiting, and diarrhea are reported with moderate overdoses, significant overdoses may result in neurotoxicity (seizures). Most treatment would be supportive. Hemodialysis may be used in severe cases.

Diagnostic test interference

Positive direct Coomb's, false positive glucose with Clinitest, and false positive serum/urine creatinine with Jaffe reaction.

Mechanism

A bactericidal first generation cephalosporin. Inhibits bacterial cell wall synthesis by binding to penicillin binding proteins, resulting in the inhibition of the final transpeptidation step of peptidoglycan synthesis.

Pharmacology/kinetics

Absorption
Cefadroxil is rapidly and well absorbed from the gastrointestinal tract of cats and dogs. Peak absorption occurs in 2–2.5 h. Food does not appear to alter absorption.

Distribution
It is widely distributed throughout the body into most tissues and body fluids. Therapeutic concentrations are reached in synovial and pleural fluids, bile, gallbladder, skin, soft tissue, urine, and bone. The drug is approximately 20% protein bound in most species.

CNS penetration
Cefadroxil does not reach therapeutic concentrations in CSF even with inflammation.

Metabolism

Cefadroxil is primarily excreted unchanged by the kidneys. Approximately 50% of the dose is excreted in the urine of dogs within 24 h.

Half-life

The half-life is approximately 2 h in dogs and 2.5–3 h in cats. This may be prolonged in renal failure.

Pregnancy risk factor

Category B: Reproductive studies in mice and rats show no evidence of impaired fertility or fetal harm. No teratogenic effects reported in humans. Peak cord levels are high after oral doses (40% serum levels). Considered a drug of choice for susceptible organisms during pregnancy in canine patients.

Lactation

Only low concentrations are found in human milk (<0.019 milk/plasma ratios). It is considered safe while nursing.

Reference

Greene, C.K. (2006) Antimicrobial drug formulary. Appendix 8. In: *Infectious Diseases of the Dog and Cat*. Greene, C. (ed.) Elsevier, St. Louis, MO, pp. 1186–1383.

Further reading

Frank, L.A. and Kunkle, G.A. (1993) Comparison of the efficacy of cefadroxil and generic and proprietary cephalexin in the treatment of pyoderma in dogs. *J Am Vet Med Assoc.*, **203(4)**, 530–533.

Landsbergen, N., Pellicaan, C.H., and Schaefers-Okkens, A.C. (2001) The use of veterinary drugs during pregnancy of the dog. *Tijdschr Diergenees.*, **126(22)**, 716–722.

Westermeyer, R., Roy, A., Mitchell, M., *et al.* (2010) *In vitro* comparison of *Staphylococcus pseudintermedius* susceptibility to common cephalosporins used in dogs. *Vet Ther.*, **11(3)**, 1–9.

Chapter 131: Cefazolin

US Generic (Brand) Name: Cefazolin (Ancef, Kefzol, Zolicef)
Availability: Human approved – Sterile powder for injection (250, 500 mg and 1, 5, 10, and 20 g vials)
Resistance mechanisms: Altered penicillin binding proteins, increased beta-lactamase production, altered permeability

Use

Cefazolin is bactericidal for most gram-positive cocci (except *Enterococci*) and certain gram negative bacilli. *E. coli*, *Proteus*, and *Klebseilla* are generally susceptible. Cefazolin is frequently used for perioperative prophylaxis for various surgical procedures including procedures classified as contaminated or potentially contaminated (esophageal, gastroduodenal, obstetric, neurologic, orthopedic, and vascular surgeries) or where the risk of infection may be serious (cardiac, prosthetic material).

Contraindications/warnings

Hypersensitivity to cephalosporins or severe reactions to penicillins. Modify dose with renal impairment, prolonged use may cause superinfection.

Dosage

Canine

Susceptible organisms: 20–35 mg/kg IV, IM, SC q8 h or CRI: Loading dose: 1.3 mg/kg; then 1.2 mg/kg/h (Papich 2002).

Surgical prophylaxis: 22 mg/kg IV q2 h during surgery (Papich 2002).

Feline

Susceptible organisms: 20–35 mg/kg IV, IM, SC q8 h or CRI: Loading dose: 1.3 mg/kg; then 1.2 mg/kg/h (Papich 2002).

Surgical prophylaxis: 22 mg/kg IV q2h during surgery (Papich 2002).

Dose adjustments

Decrease dose frequency in moderate renal failure to q12 h dosing. For severe renal failure, administer dose q24 h.

Administration

Vials containing 500 mg or 1 gram of cefazolin should be diluted with 2 or 2.5 mL of sterile water for injection to provide a 225 or 330 mg/mL solution, respectively. These must be further diluted with 5 mL of sterile water. The calculated dose may be given IV over 3–5 min directly or deep IM or SC. IM or SC dosing may be painful. The dose may also be given by intermittent or continuous IV infusion (CRI) by placing the calculated dose into 50–100 mL of a compatible IV solution (dextrose 5% in water, lactated ringers, saline). The IV line should be flushed with saline or 5% dextrose in water before and after administration of the drug. Do not admix with aminoglycosides in the same bottle, syringe, or IV tubing.

Electrolyte contents

1 g of cefazolin sodium contains 47 mg (2 mEq) of sodium.

Storage/stability

Undiluted vials should be stored at room temperature. Reconstituted solutions are light yellow and should be protected from light. These are stable for 24 h at room temperature or 10 days under refrigeration. Once diluted (225 or 330 mg/mL) the drug may be frozen immediately after reconstitution at −20°C for up to 12 weeks. It should not be frozen or stored in plastic due to leaching of the plastic components into the solution. After thawing, the drug should be kept cool and not refrozen. Further dilution should be done according to the manufacturer's directions.

Adverse reactions

>10%
Pain at the injection site after IM/SC injections reported in dogs. Gastrointestinal upset, anorexia, and diarrhea are noted following rapid IV injection of large doses.

1–10%
Anaphylaxis, rashes, fever, eosinophilia, lymphadenopathy, and pruritus are reported in dogs and cats. In animals with renal failure both seizures and neuromuscular hyper-irritability can occur.

Other Species
Renal dysfunction, pseudomembranous colitis, thrombocytopenia, thrombocytosis, phlebitis, neutropenia, agranulocytosis, cholestasis, hemolytic anemia, prolonged prothrombin time, nephropathy, and superinfection are reported in mammals.

Drug interactions

Nephrotoxic drugs can decrease elimination of cefazolin and increase cefazolin plasma concentrations as well as toxicities. When mixed with certain drugs

(amikacin, cimetidine, calcium gluconate, erythromycin, lidocaine, pentobarbital, tetracycline, and vitamin B complex) incompatibility may occur. It is recommended that cefazolin is not to be mixed in an IV line with other medications, but rather to be given alone as a slow bolus.

Monitoring

Monitor renal function if used in combination with nephrotoxic drugs. Monitor hepatic function and CBC if used long term.

Overdose

High doses in renal failure may cause neuromuscular hypersensitivity and seizures. Hemodialysis removes 20–50% of a dose. Otherwise supportive care is targeted toward noted toxicities.

Diagnostic test interference

Positive direct Coomb's test, false positive serum or urine test with Jaffe reaction, and false-positive urinary glucose test with Clinitest.

Mechanism

Cefazolin is a semisynthetic first generation parenteral cephalosporin. It is bactericidal against sensitive organisms. Inhibits bacterial cell wall synthesis by binding to one or more penicillin binding proteins. This inhibits transpeptidation affecting peptidoglycan synthesis of bacterial cell walls.

Pharmacology/kinetics

Absorption
It is poorly absorbed via oral routes of administration and should be administered either by IV or IM injection. Following IM injection peak levels are noted within 30 min of injection.

Distribution
Cefazolin is widely distributed into most tissues including liver, gallbladder, kidneys, bone, sputum, bile, synovial, and pleural fluids. Protein binding is approximately 16–28% in dogs.

CNS penetration

The drug does not penetrate the CSF in adequate concentrations to treat meningitis.

Metabolism

Cefazolin is only minimally metabolized in the liver with the majority of drug (80–100%) being excreted unchanged in urine.

Half-life

The serum half-life in dogs is approximately 48 minutes and may be prolonged in renal failure.

Pregnancy risk factor

Category B: Cefazolin crosses the placenta into the cord serum and amniotic fluid. However, reproduction studies in mice, rats, and rabbits found no evidence of impaired fertility or fetal harm at doses up to 25 times the human dose.

Lactation

Cefazolin is excreted into milk in low concentrations but is considered safe in nursing animals.

Reference

Papich, M.G. (2002) *Saunders Handbook of Veterinary Drugs*. 2nd edn. Winkel A. (ed.), W.B. Saunders Company, Philadelphia, pp. 96–97.

Further reading

Arkaravichien, W., Tamungklang, J., and Arkaravichien, T. (2006) Cefazolin induced seizures in hemodialysis patients. *J Med Assoc Thai.*, **89(11)**, 1981–1983.

Bechtel, T.P., Slaughter, R.L., and Moore, T.D. (1980) Seizures associated with high cerebral fluid concentrations of cefazolin. *Am J Hosp Pharm.*, **37(2)**, 271–273.

Donnelly, R.F. (2011) Stability of cefazolin in polypropylene syringes and polyvinylchloride minibags. *Can J Hosp Pharm.*, **64(4)**, 241–245.

Donowitz, G.R. and Mandell, G.L. (1988) Beta-lactam antibiotics. *N Engl J Med.*, **318(7)**, 419–426.

Haslam, S., Yen, D., Dvirnik, N., *et al.* (2012) Cefazolin use in patients who report a non-IgE penicillin allergy: a retrospective look at adverse reactions in arthroplasty. *Iowa Orthop J.*, **32**, 100–103.

Marcellin-Little, D.J., Papich, M.G., Richardson, D.C., *et al.* (1996) Pharmacokinetic model for cefazolin distribution during total hip arthroplasty in dogs. *Am J Vet Res.*, **57(5)**, 720–723.

Chapter 132: Cefdinir

US Generic (Brand) Name: Cefdinir (Omnicef)
Availability: Human approved – Cefdinir oral capsules (300 mg), oral suspension 125 mg/5 mL, 250 mg/mL (60, 100 mL)
Resistance mechanisms: Altered penicillin binding proteins, increased beta-lactamase production, altered permeability

Use

An oral third generation cephalosporin used primarily in human medicine for pneumonia, bronchitis, otitis media, sinusitis, and uncomplicated skin and soft tissue infections. Not commonly used in veterinary medicine. Similar to cefpodoxime, it has expanded coverage against aerobic gram negative bacteria compared to first and second generation cephalosporins. It is more active than other oral third generation cephalosporins (cefpodoxime, ceftibuten) against most *Staphylococcus* and *Streptococcus*. It is reported to have efficacy against 96% of *E. coli* isolates in pediatric bladder infections and may be useful in canine bladder infections where cefdinir achieves very high concentrations. It is inactive against *Pseudomonas*, *Enterobacter*, *Enterococci*, and methacillin resistant *Staphylococcus*.

Contraindications/warnings

Hypersensitivity to cephalosporins or severe reactions to penicillins. Modify dose with renal impairment, prolonged use may cause superinfection.

Dosage

Doses have not been well established in veterinary medicine but laboratory studies indicate that dogs tolerate oral doses up to 800 mg/kg.

Canine

7 mg/kg PO q12 h (Papich 2002).

Feline

7 mg/kg PO q12 h (Papich 2002).

Dose adjustments

For severe renal impairment administer dose q24 h rather than q12 h.

Administration

Oral powder for suspension should be mixed with either 39 or 60 mL of water for the 65 or 120 mL bottle, respectively. Shake well before each dose. If taken concurrently with iron, aluminum, magnesium, or other antacids administer these either 2 h before or 1 h after cefdinir. The suspension is better absorbed than the capsules. Administration with a fatty meal may significantly decrease absorption by up to 40%.

Electrolyte contents

Not significant.

Storage/stability

Store oral powder for dilution and capsules at room temperature. After reconstitution, the oral suspension is stable at room temperature for 10 days.

Adverse reactions

>10%
Generally well tolerated in dogs, even at high doses (800 mg/kg). Diarrhea, nausea, vomiting, and salivation are the most common side effects reported in dogs.

1–10%
Frequent urination, change in stool color to a red/rust color from chelation of iron in the gastrointestinal tract of dogs. Can potentially decrease iron levels with long term use.

<1%
No information is available in cats. Side effects seen in other mammals include: anemia, thrombocytopenia, eosinophilia, neutropenia, nephritis, elevated BUN, serum creatinine, rash, urticaria, pruritus, elevated liver enzymes, cholestatic jaundice, arthralgia, and colitis.

Drug interactions

Co-administration with iron, magnesium, aluminum, or antacids reduces the rate and extent of absorption of cefdinir. Nephrotoxic drugs can contribute to an increase in potential plasma concentrations of cefdinir as well as toxicities.

Monitoring

Monitor renal function if used in combination with nephrotoxic drugs. Monitor hepatic function, CBC, and iron levels if used long term.

Overdose

High doses in renal failure may cause neuromuscular hypersensitivity and seizures. Hemodialysis removes 63% of a dose in 4 h. Otherwise supportive care is targeted toward noted toxicities.

Diagnostic test interference

Positive direct Coomb's test, false positive serum or urine test with Jaffe reaction, and false-positive urinary glucose test with Clinitest.

Mechanism

Cefdinir is a bactericidal third generation cephalosporin. It inhibits bacterial cell wall synthesis by binding to one or more penicillin binding proteins. This inhibits transpeptidation affecting peptidoglycan synthesis of bacterial cell walls.

Pharmacology/kinetics

Absorption
Oral doses of 20 mg/kg are well absorbed (60–70%) and produce peak concentrations of 43.1 µg/mL in dogs.

Distribution
Widely distributed in tissues and fluids including bronchial mucosa and epithelial lining, sinus tissue, middle ear, and blister fluid. High concentrations are noted in the gastrointestinal tract, kidney, and urinary bladder of dogs. Cefdinir is 90–93% bound to plasma proteins of dogs.

CNS penetration
Cefdinir has minimal penetration across the blood–brain barrier and would not be considered therapeutic for CNS infections.

Metabolism
Cefdinir is not appreciably metabolized and is primarily excreted unchanged in the urine as parent compound. Approximately 68% of a dose is excreted in the urine of dogs. Clearance is directly related to renal function.

Half-life

The half-life following an oral dose of 20 mg/kg is 3.4 h in dogs.

Pregnancy risk factor

Category B: Reproductive studies in rats and rabbits at 0.7–70 times the human dose have not shown any teratogenic effects. Cefdinir is considered safe in pregnancy.

Lactation

Cefdinir was not detected in milk following oral doses in humans. It is considered safe during nursing.

Reference

Papich, M.G. (2002) *Saunders Handbook of Veterinary Drugs*. 2nd edn. Winkel, A. (ed.), W.B. Saunders Company, Philadelphia, pp. 97–98.

Further reading

Bonsu, B.K., Shuler, L., Sawicki, L., *et al.* (2006) Susceptibility of recent bacterial isolates to cefdinir and selected antibiotics among children with urinary tract infections. *Acad Emergency Med.*, **13(1)**, 76–81.

Inamoto, Y., Chiba, T., Kamimura, T., *et al.* (1988) FK482, a new orally active cephalosporin synthesis and biological properties. *J Antibiot (Tokyo)*, **41(6)**, 28–830.

Sakamoto, H., Hirose, T., Nakamoto, S., *et al.* (1988) Pharmacokinetics of FK482, a new orally active cephalosporin in animals. *J Antibiot (Tokyo)*, **41(12)**, 1896–1905.

Chapter 133: Cefepime

US Generic (Brand) Name: Cefepime (Maxipime, Maxipime ADD-Vantage)

Availability: Human approved – Cefepime anhydrous sterile injectable powder for injection (500 mg, 1 g, 2 g) or cefepime HCL injectable solution in single dose frozen bags (20 mg/mL in dextrose) (1, 2 g)

Resistance mechanisms: Altered penicillin binding proteins, increased beta-lactamase production, altered permeability

Use

Cefepime is a fourth generation cephalosporin used in humans for uncomplicated and complicated UTIs and pyelonephritis. It is also used for skin and soft tissue infections, caused by *Streptococcus*. It covers most organisms causing pneumonia, including *Psuedomonas*, *Enterobacter*, and *Staphylococcus* (not methicillin resistant). Cefepime has greater activity against *Staphylococcus*, increased resistance to beta-lactamases and better penetration into gram negative organisms than the third generation cephalosporins. It should be reserved for use in severely ill patients that involve meningitis, intra-abdominal infections (combined with IV metronidazole) and penetrating head injuries where *Staphylococcus* spp., or aerobic gram negative bacteria (such as *Pseudomonas*) are suspected. May be used empirically in immune suppressed animals with severe infections.

Contraindications/warnings

Do not use in patients that are allergic to cephalosporins or if using the pre-mixed solution, allergies to corn products. Cefepime can accumulate in patients with renal failure.

Dosage

Canine

40 mg/kg q6 h IM or IV or CRI: 1.4 mg/kg Loading dose; followed by 1.1 mg/kg/h (Papich 2002).

Feline

No published dose.

Dose adjustments

Dose must be reduced in renal impairment. Reduce dose and dosing frequency according to severity of renal impairment. For moderate impairment give q12 h, for severe impairment give q24 h.

Administration

For intermittent IV infusion of vials containing 500 mg, 1 g, or 2 g of cefepime, add 5, 10, and 10 mL respectively of a compatible IV solution to make a concentration of 100, 100, and 160 mg/mL of drug. The appropriate dose should be withdrawn and added to a compatible IV solution. The dose must be given over 30 min. Alternatively the ADD-Vantage vials should only be administered via intermittent infusion and must be thawed and diluted according to the manufacturer's instructions. For IM injection the 500 mg or 1 g vial are reconstituted by adding either 1.3 or 2.4 mL of diluent (sterile water for injection, 0.9% saline, 5% dextrose, 0.5 or 1% lidocaine HCL, or bacteriostatic water) to provide a solution containing 280 mg/mL.

Electrolyte contents

Cefepime contains 750 mg L-arginine per 1 g of drug. High doses of arginine can alter glucose metabolism and elevate serum potassium transiently.

Storage/stability

Store powder for injection at room temperature. Store frozen bags in the freezer. Following dilution with NaCl (0.9%) or D5W the drug is stable for 24 h at room temperature or 7 days if refrigerated and protected from light. Yellowing of the solution may occur over time, but does not affect potency.

Adverse reactions

1–10%
Diarrhea, nausea, vomiting, and injection site reactions (swelling, pain, inflammation, phlebitis) have been reported in dogs.

Other species
Rashes, urticaria, pruritus, fever, neutropenia, thrombocytopenia, agranulocytosis, a positive Coomb's test, aplastic anemia, hemolytic anemia, anemia, pancytopenia, renal dysfunction, prolonged PT, decreased phosphorus, hypersensitivity, and neurotoxicity (fatal encephalopathy, myoclonus, seizures) are reported in other species.

Drug interactions

Other nephrotoxic drugs (aminoglycosides, amphotericin-B, furosemide) can decrease renal excretion of cefepime and increase toxicity. Many drugs are not compatible with cefepime when admixed. Check Manufacture's suggested guidelines before admixing.

Monitoring

Monitor for signs of anaphylaxis, CBC, and renal panel with prolonged dosing.

Overdose

Overdose symptoms may include nausea, vomiting, diarrhea, neuromuscular hyperirritability, seizures, and encephalopathy. Hemodialysis and supportive care (including anticonvulsant therapy) may be indicated.

Diagnostic test interference

Will cause a positive, direct Coomb's test, false positive urinary proteins and steroids, false positive serum or urinary creatinine with Jaffe, and false positive urinary glucose with Clinitest.

Mechanism

Bactericidal, fourth generation cephalosporin. Binds to bacterial penicillin binding proteins causing inhibition of transpeptidation step of peptidoglycan synthesis.

Pharmacology/kinetics

Absorption
Cefepime can only be given IV or IM. It is not absorbed orally. In humans, IM injections are painful but absorption is rapid and almost complete.

Distribution
Cefepime distributes into most tissues including the CNS, bronchial mucosa, inflammatory tissues, sputum, bile, urine, peritoneal fluid, gall bladder, and prostate. Protein binding is only 16–19% in humans.

CNS penetration
CSF penetration is variable (5–58%), but has demonstrated efficacy in a variety of human meningitis cases.

Metabolism
Metabolism is not well established in cats/dogs. In humans, cefepime has limited metabolism with the majority of drug being eliminated as parent compound in urine (85%). Partial metabolism results in a N-methylpyrrolidine (NMP) metabolite which is rapidly converted to N-oxide (NMP-N-oxide).

Half-life
In dogs the elimination half-life is 1.1 h, but may be significantly prolonged with renal impairment.

Pregnancy risk factor

Category B: No reports of causing teratogenic or embryotoxic effects in humans, rats, mice, or rabbits at high does (4× human dose). It is generally considered safe in pregnancy.

Lactation
Cefepime is excreted into milk in low concentrations (0.5 µg/mL). Nursing animals may have altered gastrointestinal flora resulting in diarrhea.

Reference

Papich, M.G. (2002) *Saunders Handbook of Veterinary Drugs*. 2nd edn. Winkel, A. (ed.), W.B. Saunders Company, Philadelphia, pp. 98–100.

Further reading

Barradell, L. and Bryson, H. (1994) Cefepime: A review of its antibacterial activity, pharmacokinetic properties and therapeutic use. *Drugs*, **47(3)**, 471–505.
Gardner, S. and Papich, M. (2001) Comparison of cefepime pharmacokinetics in neonatal foals and adult dogs. *J Vet Pharmacol Therap.*, **24**, 187–192.
Saez-Lloren, X. and O'Ryan, M. (2001) Cefepime in the empiric treatment of meningitis in children. *Pediatr Infect Dis J.*, **20(3)**, 356–361.
Stampley, A., Brown, M., Gronwell, R., *et al.* (1992) Serum concentrations of cefepime (BMY-28142) a broad spectrum cephalosporin in dogs. *Cornell Vet.*, **82**, 69–77.

Chapter 134: Cefotaxime

> **US Generic (Brand) Name:** Cefotaxime (Claforin)
> **Availability:** Human approved – Cefotaxime sterile powder for injection (500 mg, 1, 2, 10 g vials) or frozen pre-mix of sodium salt in D5W (1, 2 g bags)
> **Resistance mechanisms:** Altered penicillin binding proteins, increased beta-lactamase production, altered permeability

Use

Cefotaxime is active against most gram negative bacilli (not *Pseudomonas*) and gram positive cocci (not *Enterococcus*). It is active against *Enterobacteriaceae*, *Escherichia coli*, *Klebsiella* spp., *Pasteurella* spp., and *Streptococci*. It has variable coverage of most anaerobic bacteria and *Staphylococcus* spp. It is used to treat infections of the respiratory and urinary tract, skin, soft tissues, bone and joint, gynecologic, and septicemia. Due to its ability to penetrate into the CNS it can be used for meningitis cases due to susceptible bacteria.

Contraindications/warnings

Hypersensitivity to cephalosporins or severe reactions to penicillins. Modify dose with renal impairment, prolonged use may cause superinfection. Rapid bolus doses may cause arrhythmias. Minimize local tissue reactions by rotating injection sites.

Dosage

Dose according to the severity of the disease, IV is recommended for severe septicemia.

Canine
50 mg/kg IV, IM, or SC q12 h or CRI-3.2 mg/kg Loading dose; followed by 5mg/kg/h (Papich 2002).

Severe bacteremia: 20–80 mg/kg IV q6 h (Greene and Watson 1998).

Feline
20–80 mg/kg IV, IM q6 h (Papich 2002).

Dose adjustments

Reduce dose and/or dose frequency in moderate to severe renal impairment. For severe renal impairment, dose q24 h. Doses should also be reduced in patients with significant hepatic impairment.

Administration

Do not admix cefotaxime with aminoglycosides. Consult manufacturer's package insert for compatibility information. IV administration may result in inflammation, phlebitis, and thrombophlebitis. IM injections may result in pain and induration and SC injections may result in local tissue damage and abscess formation. Large doses of cefotaxime should be administered IV to avoid tissue irritation. To administer IM doses, add 2, 3, or 5 mL of sterile water for injection to the 500 mg, 1 g, or 2 g vial, respectively. This results in concentrations of 230, 300, or 330 mg/mL. Administer IM into a large, deep muscle mass. Doses >2 g should be split into divided doses. For IV injections, 10 mL of sterile water for injection should be added to the 500 mg, 1 g, or 2 g vial, respectively, resulting in a solution of 50, 95, or 180 mg. The appropriate dose can be injected into the vein over 3–5 min or via tubing with a free flowing compatible IV solution (NaCl, D5W). Do not administer faster due to risk of arrhythmias. For SC injections a solution of 1 g of cefotaxime per 14 mL of sterile water for injection is considered isotonic.

Electrolyte contents

Cefotaxime 1 g vials contain 50.6 mg (2.2 mEq) of sodium.

Storage/stability

Store unreconstituted powder at room temperature protected from light. Reconstituted solution is stable at room temperature for 24 h or 7 days if refrigerated. A change in color to an amber shade does not indicate instability. It can also be frozen for 13 weeks. If diluted in NS or D5W the solution is stable for 24 h at room temperature, 5 days in the refrigerator or 13 weeks frozen. Thawed solutions are stable for 24 h at room temperature or 10 days when refrigerated. Do not refreeze.

Adverse reactions

>10%
Diarrhea, vomiting, and nausea have been reported in dogs.

1–10%
Pain and inflammation at the injection site occurs in all species.

<1%
Seizures have not been reported in dogs, but may be seen in cats with high doses or with drug accumulation in renal impairment.

Other species
Anaphylaxis, rashes, pruritus, urticaria, colitis, superinfection, pancytopenia, neutropenia, thrombocytopenia, eosinophilia, fever, transaminase elevations, interstitial nephritis, elevated serum creatinine, BUN, hemolytic anemia, and hemorrhage are reported in other mammals.

Drug interactions

Other nephrotoxic drugs (aminoglycosides, amphotericin-B, furosemide) can decrease renal excretion of cefotaxime and increase toxicity.

Monitoring

Monitor renal panel, CBC, and for signs of anaphylaxis.

Overdose

Animal studies (rats, mice) suggest doses > 6 g/kg/day result in convulsions, dyspnea, hypothermia, and cyanosis. Due to CNS penetration seizures are likely with overdoses. Acute overdoses have also resulted in elevations of serum creatinine and BUN. Hemodialysis is moderately effective in removal of drug if available. Supportive care targeted at side effects is recommended.

Diagnostic test interference

Will cause a positive, direct Coomb's test, false positive serum or urinary creatinine with Jaffe, and false positive urinary glucose with Clinitest.

Mechanism

Third generation bactericidal cephalosporin. Inhibits cell wall synthesis by binding to one or more of the penicillin binding proteins. This in turn inhibits the final transpeptidation step of peptidoglycan synthesis in bacterial cell walls. Bacteria eventually lyse due to ongoing activity of cell wall autolytic enzymes while cell wall assembly is arrested.

Pharmacology/kinetics

Absorption
Not absorbed well orally. The bioavailability of cefotaxime following IM versus SC injection in dogs is 86.5 versus 100%, respectively. Bioavailability following IM injection in cats is approximately 94–98%.

Distribution
Widely distributed into most body tissues and fluids after IV, IM, or SC dosing. Penetrates into aqueous humor, prostatic fluids, and bones.

CNS penetration
May reach therapeutic levels in CSF for sensitive organisms when meninges are inflamed. Levels as high as 0.5–30 µg/mL have been reported in humans following IV injection.

Metabolism

Partially metabolized in the liver to an active metabolite (desacetyl-cefotaxime). After a dose of 20 mg/kg IV, both unchanged parent drug and 86% of the desacetyl metabolite is excreted into the urine of dogs. Urinary excretion is increased following IM injections in dogs. Approximately 50% protein binding in dogs.

Half-life

The half-life is dependent on the route of administration in dogs. After intravenous, intramuscular, and subcutaneous injections the mean biological half-lives were 0.74, 0.83, and 1.71 h, respectively. In cats, the half-life is reported to be 1 h after IV administration.

Pregnancy risk factor

Category B: There are no reports of embryotoxicity or teratogenicity in mice and rats receiving high doses of cefotaxime. Offspring did have a lower birth weight than controls.

Lactation

Cefotaxime is distributed into milk in significant concentrations. This may result in diarrhea and potential sensitization of nursing animals.

References

Greene, C. and Watson, A. (1998) Antimicrobial drug formulary. *Infectious Diseases of the Dog and Cat.* Greene, C. (ed.), W.B. Saunders, Philadelphia, pp. 790–919.

Papich, M.G. (2002) *Saunders Handbook of Veterinary Drugs.* 2nd edn. Winkel, A. (ed.), W.B. Saunders Company, Philadelphia, pp. 101–103.

Further reading

De Sarro, A., Ammendola, D., Zappala, M., *et al.* (1995) Relationship between structure and convulsant properties of some beta-lactam antibiotics following intracerebroventricular microinjection in rats. *Antimicrob. Agents Chemother.,* **39**, 232–237.

Guerrini, V.H., English, P.B., Filippich L.J., *et al.* (1986) Pharmacokinetics of cefotaxime in the dog. *Vet Rec.,* **119(4)**, 81–83.

Reid, K.H., Shields, C.B., Raff, M.J., *et al.* (1987) Effect of the topical application of some newer antibiotics on the cerebral cortex. *Neurosurgery,* **20(6)**, 868–870.

Sumano, H., Gutierrez, L., and Ocampo, L. (2004) Pharmacokinetics and clinical efficacy of cefotaxime for the treatment of septicaemia in dogs. *Acta Vet Hung.,* **52(1)**, 85–95.

Chapter 135: Cefovecin

US Generic (Brand) Name: Cefovecin (Convenia)
Availability: Veterinary approved – Convenia lyophilized sterile powder for injection (80 mg/mL × 10 mL)
Resistance mechanisms: Altered penicillin binding proteins, increased beta-lactamase production, altered permeability

Use

A long acting, third generation, single dose, injectable cephalosporin that is used in the treatment of small animals for soft tissue and bladder infections. It has gained popularity in the treatment of fractious cats and other animals where repetitive dosing may be difficult. It is active against *Pasturella multocida, S. intermedius, S. pseudintermedius,* and *S. canis.* It has also shown *in vitro* efficacy against anaerobes including *Prevotella* spp, *Porphyromonas* spp., *Peptostreptococcus* spp., *Fusobaterium* spp., *Bacteroides* spp., *Clostridium* spp., and *Corynebacterium* spp. Cefovecin is not active against systemic infections due to *E. coli, Pseudomonas* spp., or *Enterococci* due to its high protein binding. It is as effective as cephalexin against *E. coli* urinary tract infections in dogs where it may concentrate significantly. It is useful in the treatment of pyoderma, abscesses, and wound infections of dogs and cats.

Contraindications/warnings

Hypersensitivity to cephalosporins. Avoid use in severe renal impairment. Beware that adverse reactions may persist for up to 65 days due to the long half-life/clearance of the drug. Do not use in animals <8 weeks of age.

Dosage

Canine

Skin and soft tissue infections: 8 mg/kg SC once. May be repeated once in 7 days (for *S. pseudintermedius*) or 14 days (*S. canis*) if response is not complete (Pfizer Manufacturer's Label).

UTI: 8 mg/kg SC × 1 dose (Pfizer Manufacturer's Label).

Feline

Skin and soft tissue infections: 8 mg/kg SC once (Pfizer Manufacturer's Label), Drug accumulation occurs in cats with repeat dosing.

UTI: 8 mg/kg SC × 1 dose (Pfizer Manufacturer's Label).

Dose adjustments

Reduce dose in moderate renal impairment. Extend interval before second dose to 14 days instead of 7 days for *S. pseudintermedious*. Avoid use in severe renal impairment. Multiple doses in healthy cats show accumulation of drug. Only 50% of the dose is excreted in urine 14 days post-dose.

Administration

Reconstitute the lyophilized powder for injection with 10 mL of the sterile diluent supplied by the manufacturer. Shake well and allow the vial to sit until the antibiotic is completely dissolved. The resulting solution has 80 mg/mL of cefovecin and 12.3 mg/mL of benzyl alcohol.

Electrolyte contents

Cefovecin sodium (84 mg/mL) contains 80 mg/mL of cefovecin with the remainder being a monosodium salt. This amounts to 4 mg (0.173 mEq) of sodium per mL.

Storage/stability

Store the lyophilized powder in the refrigerator, protected from light. After dilution with the manufacturer's diluent, the reconstituted solution must be stored in the manufacturer's box in the refrigerator and protected from light. The multidose vial must be discarded 28 days after mixing. The solution color may vary from yellow to amber in color, but this does not affect potency if stored correctly.

Adverse reactions

>10%
Lethargy, depression, and decreased appetite, reported in dogs and cats.

1–10%
Vomiting, diarrhea, and elevated liver enzymes reported in dogs and cats.

<1%
Has caused anaphylactic reactions, tremors, ataxia, seizures, facial edema, pruritis, local reactions (alopecia, scabs, necrosis, erythema), and death in cats and dogs. Local reactions are dose and exposure related with irritation, edema occurring within 2 h of the injection.

Odd behavior, vocalization, inappropriate urination, hemolytic anemia, elevated BUN, and serum creatinine reported in cats.

Drug interactions

Other nephrotoxic drugs (aminoglycosides, amphotericin-B, furosemide) can decrease renal excretion of cefovecin and increase toxicity. Other highly protein bound drugs may be displaced by cefovecin with increased or decreased plasma concentrations.

Monitoring

Monitor renal function, CBC and for anaphylaxis particularly with repeat doses.

Overdose

Irritation, vocalization, injection site edema, swelling, and elevated liver enzymes have all been reported in cats and dogs at doses of 22.5 times the therapeutic dose. Cats receiving toxic doses also had reduced white blood cell counts and bilirubinuria. Supportive care should be given long term due to the long half-life of the drug. The drug is not expected to be dialyzable due to its high protein binding.

Diagnostic test interference

Although not reported for cefovecin, all cephalosporins can cause a positive, direct Coomb's test, false positive serum or urinary creatinine with Jaffe, and false positive urinary glucose with Clinitest.

Mechanism

Third generation bactericidal cephalosporin. Binds to penicillin binding proteins causing inhibition of transpeptidation step of peptidoglycan synthesis.

Pharmacology/kinetics

Absorption
Absorption is rapid (2–3 h) and complete in dogs and cats. Bioavailability after a subcutaneous injection is > 99%. In cats, peak serum concentrations of 141 μg/mL are measured at 2 h.

Distribution

Cefovecin is distributed throughout multiple tissues but its volume of distribution is low. Free concentrations of drug are higher in tissue exudates than in plasma. Protein binding in cats is >97% and in dogs is 96–98.7%.

CNS penetration

No data is reported on the CNS penetration of cefovecin. Due to the high protein binding, CSF concentrations are unlikely to be therapeutic.

Metabolism

Metabolism is not well understood in animals. Elimination occurs primarily via renal excretion of the parent compound. Urinary concentrations of >1 µg/mL are noted for up to 14 days in cats.

Half-life

The half-life in cats is 6.9 days (suggesting >65 days for 97% elimination of the drug). In dogs, the half-life is 5.5 days.

Pregnancy risk factor

Category has not been assigned, but no teratogenic effects have been noted in laboratory animals exposed to cefovecin. Due to its extensively long half-life and unknown effects on the fetus it is not recommended to give to pregnant animals.

Lactation

No studies have been performed in nursing animals. Due to its high protein binding and long half-life it would not be recommended in nursing animals.

Further reading

Passmore, C.A., Sherington, J., and Stegemann, M.R. (2007) Efficacy and safety of cefovecin (Convenia) for the treatment of urinary tract infections in dogs. *J Small Anim Pract.*, **48(3)**, 139–144.

Six, R., Chemi, J., Chesebrough, R., *et al.* (2008) Efficacy and safety of cefovecin in treating bacterial folliculitis, abscesses, or infected wounds in dogs. *J Am Vet Med Assoc.*, **233(3)**, 433–439.

Stegemann, M.R., Passmore, C.A., Sherington, J., *et al.* (2006) Antimicrobial activity and spectrum of cefovecin, a new extend-spectrum cephalosporin, against pathogens collected from dogs and cats in Europe and North America. *Antimicrob Agents Chemother.*, **50(7)**, 2285–2292.

Stegemann, M.R., Sherington., J., and Blanchfloue, S. (2006) Pharmacokinetics and pharmacodynamics of cefovecin in dogs. *J Vet Pharmacol Ther.*, **29(6)**, 501–511.

Chapter 136: Cefoxitin

US Generic (Brand) Name: Cefoxitin (Mefoxin)
Availability: Human approved – Infusion as a frozen pre-mix in D5W (1 g/50 mL, 2 g/50 mL), sterile powder for injection (1, 2, 10 g vials)
Resistance mechanisms: Altered penicillin binding proteins, increased beta-lactamase production, altered permeability

Use

Although a second generation cephalosporin, cefoxitin is active against many gram negative organisms including *E. coli*, *Klebsiella*, and *Proteus*. It is active against most *Staphylococcus* (including penicillin resistant strains) and *Streptococcus* spp. It is not effective against methicillin resistant *Staphylococcus* spp. or *Enterococcus* spp. It is also active against anaerobes including *Bacteriodes fragilis*, *Fusobacterium*, *Prevotella*, and some strains of *Clostridium*, *Propionibacterium*, and *Peptostreptococcus*. It is used in small animals for treatment of skin and soft tissue infections as well as intra-abdominal, bone/joint, urinary tract, gynecologic, septicemia, and other mixed infections.

Contraindications/warnings

Hypersensitivity to cephalosporins or severe reactions to penicillins. Modify dose with renal impairment, prolonged use may cause superinfection.

Dosage

Canine
30 mg/kg IV q6–8 h (Papich 2002).

Feline
30 mg/kg IV q6–8 h (Papich 2002).

Dose adjustments

Modify dose in renal impairment. Reduce the dosing frequency to q8–12 h in moderate renal impairment or to q12–48 h in severe impairment.

Administration

Cefoxitin should be administered intravenously. Reconstitute the 1 g and 2 g vials with 10 or 20 mL of sterile water for injection, respectively. This results in a 95 mg/mL solution. The appropriate dose can be injected over a 3–5 min period as an intermittent infusion. Larger doses should be given via a continuous rate infusion. The dose must be further diluted in 50–100 mL of 0.9% sodium chloride or D5W.

Electrolyte contents

1 g of cefoxitin has 53 mg (2.3 mEq) of sodium.

Storage/stability

Store vials at room temperature. After reconstitution, vials are stable for 24 h at room temperature or 48 h refrigerated. If made into an IV infusion with 0.9% NaCl or D5W the solution is stable for 24 h at room temperature, 7 days refrigerated, or 26 weeks if frozen. After thawing the solution is stable for 24 h at room temperature or 5 days refrigerated. Do not refreeze.

Adverse reactions

>10%
Thrombophlebitis, diarrhea reported in dogs and cats.

1–10%
Pruritus, rash reported in dogs.

Other species
Nausea, vomiting, angioedema, eosinophilia, hemolytic anemia, fever, hypotension, increased BUN/creatinine, nephrotoxicity, nephritis, increased transaminases, jaundice, leucopenia, prolonged PT, thrombocytopenia, colitis, pseudomembrane colitis, and toxic epidermal necrolysis have been reported.

Drug interactions

Other nephrotoxic drugs (aminoglycosides, amphotericin-B, furosemide) can decrease renal excretion of cefoxitin and increase toxicity.

Monitoring

Monitor for signs of anaphylaxis, CBC, and renal panel.

Overdose

High doses in renal failure may cause neuromuscular hypersensitivity and seizures. Hemodialysis may be required for extreme overdoses, otherwise supportive care is targeted toward noted toxicities.

Diagnostic test interference

Will cause a positive, direct Coomb's test, false positive serum or urinary creatinine with Jaffe, and false positive urinary glucose with Clinitest.

Mechanism

Bactericidal, second generation cephalosporin. Binds to penicillin binding proteins causing inhibition of transpeptidation step of peptidoglycan synthesis.

Pharmacology/kinetics

Absorption
Not absorbed orally, is absorbed after IM and SC injection, but is associated with significant injection site reactions.

Distribution
Cefoxitin is widely distributed throughout body tissues and fluids. It penetrates into bile, synovial, and pleural fluid. Cefoxitin is highly protein bound in most species.

CNS penetration
Less than 10% of the serum concentration is reported to cross into the CSF of dogs, so therapeutic concentrations may not be achieved in CNS infections.

Metabolism
Little is known about cefoxitin metabolism in cats and dogs. In humans, cefoxitin has very limited metabolism and is primarily secreted as parent drug via urinary excretion.

Half-life
The half-life in cats is reported to be 1.6 h and in dogs is 1.3 h after intravenous administration.

Pregnancy risk factor

Category B: No teratogenic effects have been noted in animals or humans. Transplacental passage has been documented for cefoxitin in humans, which amounts to

11–90% of the maternal serum concentrations. It is considered safe in pregnancy.

Lactation

Cefoxitin is excreted in milk but in very low concentrations. Due to poor oral absorption it is considered safe in lactating animals.

Reference

Papich, M.G. (2002) *Saunders Handbook of Veterinary Drugs*. 2nd edn. Winkel, A. (ed.), W.B. Saunders Company, Philadelphia, pp. 104–105.

Further reading

Greene, C., Hartmann, K., *et al.* (2006) Antimicrobial drug formulary. Appendix 8. In: *Infectious Disease of the Dog and Cat*. Greene, C. (ed.), Elsevier, St. Louis, MO, pp. 1186–1333.

Hardie, E. (2000) Therapeutic management of sepsis. In: *Kirk's Current Veterinary Therapy XIII, Small Animal Practice*. Bonagura, J. (ed.), W.B. Saunders Company, Philadelphia, pp. 272–275.

Massip, P., Kitzis, M.D., Tran, V.T., *et al.* (1979) Penetration of cefoxitin into cerebral fluid of dogs with and without experimental meningitis. *Rev Infect Dis.*, **1(1)**, 132–133.

Chapter 137: Cefpodoxime

US Generic (Brand) Name: Cefpodoxime (Vantin, Simplicef)
Availability: Human approved – Cefpodoxime proxetil oral tablets (100, 200 mg) and oral granules for suspension (50 mg/5 mL, 100 mg/5 mL) (50, 75, 100 mL). Veterinary Labeled – Simplicef tablets (100, 200 mg)
Resistance mechanisms: Altered penicillin binding proteins, increased beta-lactamase production, altered permeability

Use

Labeled for use in dogs for the treatment of skin infections (wounds and abscesses) caused by susceptible strains of *S. intermedius*, *S. aureus*, *Streptococcus canis*, *E. coli*, *Pasteurella multocida*, and *Proteus mirabilis*. Used for uncomplicated infections of the sinus, otitis media, pharyngitis, bronchitis due to *Streptococcus* spp., and *M. catarrhalis*. Also covers uncomplicated skin infections due to *S. intermedius*, *S. aureus*, *S. pseudintermedius*, and *S. pyogenes*. May also be effective in simple, uncomplicated urinary tract infections due to *E. coli*, *Klebsiella*, and *Proteus*.

Contraindications/warnings

Hypersensitivity to cephalosporins or severe reactions to penicillins. Modify dose with renal impairment, prolonged use may cause superinfection.

Dosage

Canine
Susceptible infections: 10 mg/kg PO q24 h for 5–7 days or 2–3 days past resolution of clinical signs. (Max 28 days) (Zoetis Manufacturer's Label).

Feline
Susceptible infections: 5 mg/kg PO BID (Greene and Watson 1998).

Dose adjustments

Doses and or dosing frequency should be adjusted in severe renal impairment. Twice daily dosing should be decreased to once daily and once daily dosing should be reduced according to the severity of impairment (q48–72 h).

Administration

Tablets and suspension should be given with food. Low gastric pH and food increases oral absorption. Refrigeration improves flavor of the lemon flavored suspension. Do not freeze.

Electrolyte contents

Not significant.

Storage/stability

Store film coated tablets and granules for suspension at room temperature. After reconstitution of granules, store in the refrigerator and discard after 14 days.

Adverse reactions

>10%
Diarrhea, inappetence reported in dogs.

1–10%
Lethargy, vomiting reported in dogs.

<1%
Pemphigus-like skin reaction noted in one dog.

Other species
Rash, itching, anaphylaxis, anxiety, epistaxis, fever, fatigue, flushing, cough, hypotension, nephritis, colitis, weakness, tinnitus, agranulocytosis, aplastic anemia, eosinophilia, leukocytosis, leucopenia, neutropenia, lymphocytopenia, hyperglycemia, hyperkalemia, hyponatremia, increased BUN, serum creatinine, elevated AST, ALT, alkaline phosphatase, bilirubin, and fungal skin infections.

Drug interactions

Other nephrotoxic drugs (aminoglycosides, amphotericin-B, furosemide) can decrease renal excretion of cefpodoxime and increase toxicity. Antacids and H-2 antagonists reduce absorption and serum concentrations of cefpodoxime.

Monitoring

Monitor for allergic reactions. For patients with renal failure, on high doses, or with prolonged courses monitor CBC, hepatic, and renal function.

Overdose

Overdose symptoms may include nausea, vomiting, diarrhea, neuromuscular hyperirritability, seizures, and encephalopathy. Institute gastrointestinal decontamination. Hemodialysis and supportive care (including anticonvulsant therapy) may be indicated.

Diagnostic test interference

Will cause a positive, direct Coomb's test, false positive serum or urinary creatinine with Jaffe, and false positive urinary glucose with Clinitest.

Mechanism

A bactericidal third generation cephalosporin. Binds to penicillin binding proteins causing inhibition of transpeptidation step of peptidoglycan synthesis.

Pharmacology/kinetics

Absorption
Oral absorption is rapid in dogs (0.5 h). Bioavailability of the tablets and oral suspension in dogs is 35–36%. Food may decrease the rate but not the extent of absorption. Following oral doses of 5 and 10 mg/kg, peak concentrations are 14 and 27–33 μg/mL, respectively.

Distribution
Cefpodoxime is readily distributed into the skin and soft tissues of dogs. Following doses of 10 mg/kg therapeutic skin concentrations for most bacteria are achieved. Protein binding in dog plasma is high (82.6%).

CNS penetration
CSF concentrations are reported to be very low in other species (5% of plasma concentrations in pigs), suggesting insufficient concentrations to be therapeutic.

Metabolism
Cefpodoxime proxetil is a prodrug that is hydrolyzed by intestinal esterases to cefpodoxime. The major route of elimination is via urine as unchanged drug.

Half-life
The half-life in dogs following oral doses of 5 and 10 mg/kg is 3–5.7 h.

Pregnancy risk factor

Category B: No teratogenic effects have been noted in mice, rabbits or humans. Generally considered safe during pregnancy.

Lactation
Low concentrations are reported in human milk (<16% of serum concentrations). Altered bowel flora and sensitization of nursing animals may occur.

Reference

Greene, C. and Watson, A. (1998) Antimicrobial drug formulary. *Infectious Diseases of the Dog and Cat*. Greene, C. (ed.), W.B. Saunders Company, Philadelphia, pp. 790–919.

Further reading

Bryan, J., Frank, L.A., Rohrbach, B.W., *et al.* (2012) Treatment outcome of dogs with methicillin-resistant and methicillin-susceptible *Staphylococcus pseudintermedius* pyoderma. *Vet Dermatol.*, **23(4)**, 361–368.

Papich, M., Davis, J.L., and Floerchinger, A.M. (2010) Pharmacokinetics, protein binding and tissue distribution of orally administered cefpodoxime proxetil and cephalexin in dogs. *Am J Vet Res.*, **71(12)**, 1484–1491.

Chapter 138: Ceftazidime

US Generic (Brand) Name: Ceftazidime (Fortaz, Ceptaz, Tazicef,Tazidime)
Availability: Human approved – Sterile powder for injection (500 mg, 1, 2, 6 g) and frozen pre-mixed infusion (1, 2 g/ 50 mL)
Resistance Mechanisms: Altered penicillin binding proteins, increased beta-lactamase production

Use

Active against *Burkholderia* spp., *Pseudomonas* spp., and *Stenotrophomonas*. Used in veterinary medicine primarily for severe infections caused by *Pseudomonas* spp. and other gram negative aerobic organisms. Can be used for severe sepsis, pneumonia, endophthalmitis, severe otitis externa, and sinusitis. Due to excellent penetration across the blood brain barrier it can be used in cases of meningitis.

Contraindications/warnings

Hypersensitivity to cephalosporins or severe reactions to penicillins. Modify dose with renal impairment, prolonged use may cause superinfection.

Dosage

Canine
Susceptible infections: 30 mg/kg IV, IM q6 h or 30 mg/kg SC q4–6 h or CRI: Loading dose 12 mg/kg followed by 1.56 mg/kg/h (Papich 2002).

Feline
Susceptible infections: 30 mg/kg IV, IM q6 h (Papich 2002).

Dose adjustments

Decrease dose frequency in moderate renal failure proportional to the degree of renal failure. In severe renal failure administer dose q12–24 h.

Administration

The IV injectable powder must be diluted with sterile water for injection according to the manufacturer's directions. The drug may be administered either by intravenous push over 3–5 min or intermittent infusion over 15–30 min. Final concentrations should not exceed 100 mg/mL. For IM injections, ceftazidime should be diluted with sterile water for injection, bacteriostatic water for injection, or 0.5–1% lidocaine hydrochloride injection (1.5 mL to a 500 mg vial) to concentrations of 280 mg/mL. Local pain at the injection site occurs for 2–3 min after the injection.

Electrolyte contents

One gram of ceftazidime has 54 mg of sodium (2.3 mEq). The product also contains benzyl alcohol as a preservative.

Storage/stability

Vials need to be stored at room temperature and protected from light. The frozen ceftazidime pre-mix must be stored at (−20°C). Following reconstitution the IV solution is stable for 12 h at room temperature or 3 days refrigerated. When ceftazidime solutions are diluted to 100–170 mg/mL with 0.9% sodium chloride they can be frozen immediately and are stable for 3 months. These can be thawed at room temperature and used within 12 h or refrigerated for 3 days. A change in color from yellow to amber may occur with time that does not affect the potency.

Adverse reactions

>10%
Diarrhea is reported in dogs.

1–10%
Nausea, vomiting, and pain at injection site in dogs.

Other species
Anaphylaxis, angioedema, fever, erythema, rash, asterixis, elevated liver enzymes, hemolytic anemia, elevated BUN/serum creatinine, leucopenia, thrombocytosis, neuromuscular excitability, paresthesia, phlebitis, pruritus, and colitis.

Drug interactions

Other nephrotoxic drugs (aminoglycosides, amphotericin-B, furosemide) can decrease renal excretion of cephalosporins and increase toxicity.

Monitoring

Monitor for signs of anaphylaxis, CBC, and renal panel. For long term therapy, monitor hepatic and hematologic function periodically.

Overdose

Overdose symptoms may include nausea, vomiting, diarrhea, neuromuscular hyperirritability, seizures, and encephalopathy. Supportive care (including anticonvulsant therapy) may be indicated. Hemodialysis removes 50–100% of the drug.

Diagnostic test interference

Will cause a positive, direct Coomb's test, false positive serum or urinary creatinine with Jaffe, and false positive urinary glucose with Clinitest.

Mechanism

A bactericidal third generation cephalosporin. Binds to penicillin binding proteins causing inhibition of transpeptidation step of peptidoglycan synthesis.

Pharmacology/kinetics

Absorption
Ceftazidime is poorly absorbed orally and must be given by IV, IM, or SC administration. Following SC administration of 30 mg/kg to dogs, plasma concentrations remain above the MIC of *Pseudomonas* for at least 4 h. In cats, IM injections are absorbed well with a maximum concentration of 89 μg/mL at 0.48 h after injection. Bioavailability after IM injection is 82% in cats.

Distribution
Widely distributed throughout tissues and fluids including the bone, bile, skin, heart, endometrium, lymphatic fluids, and CSF.

CNS penetration
Ceftazidime readily penetrates the blood brain barrier and can be used for meningitis. Levels in humans reach 10–30 μg/mL at 2–4 h after a dose. Inflammation can increase penetration.

Metabolism
Ceftazidime is not highly metabolized and is excreted primarily as unchanged drug into urine. In dogs, 86% of the drug is excreted unchanged in urine within 24 h.

Half-life
The half-life in dogs following SC administration is reported to be 0.8 h.

Pregnancy risk factor

Category B: Ceftazidime has not been associated with any teratogenic effects in animal or human studies. It achieves high concentrations in amniotic fluid and fetal tissues.

Lactation
Ceftazidime is excreted into milk in low concentrations, which could result in diarrhea and sensitization of nursing animals. However, it is considered safe for use during nursing.

Reference

Papich, M.G. (2002) *Saunders Handbook of Veterinary Drugs*. 2nd edn. Winkel, A. (ed.), W.B. Saunders Company, Philadelphia, pp. 107–109.

Further reading

Albarellos, G., Ambros, L., and Landoni, M. (2008) Pharmacokinetics of ceftazidime after intravenous and intramuscular administration to domestic cats. *Vet J.*, **178(2)**, 238–243.
Matsui, H., Komiya, M., Ikeda, C., *et al.* (1984) Comparative pharmacokinetics of YM-13115, ceftriaxone, and cetazidime in rats, dogs, and Rhesus monkeys. *Antimicrob Agents Chemother.*, **26(2)**, 204–207.
Moore, K. and Trepanier, L. (2000) Pharmacokinetics of ceftazidime in dogs following subcutaneous administration and constant infusion and association with *in vitro* susceptibility of *Pseudomonas aeruginosa*. *Am J Vet Res.*, **61(10)**, 1204–1208.

Chapter 139: Ceftiofur

US Generic (Brand) Name: Ceftiofur sodium (Naxcel)
Availability: Veterinary approved – Ceftiofur sterile powder for injection (1, 4 g vials)
Resistance mechanisms: Altered penicillin binding proteins, increased beta-lactamase production, altered permeability

Use

Ceftiofur sodium is used only rarely in small animals. It is labeled for daily subcutaneous administration for the treatment of urinary tract infections in dogs. Ceftiofur has activity against gram negative bacilli including *E. coli*, *Klebsiella* spp., and *Salmonella*. Due to the fact that it causes bone marrow toxicity with prolonged dosing, it is not a common drug of choice in small animals.

Contraindications/warnings

Hypersensitivity to cephalosporins or severe reactions to penicillins. Modify dose with renal impairment, prolonged use may cause superinfection. High doses (>6.6 mg/kg) in dogs may cause bone marrow suppression (thrombocytopenia, anemia).

Dosage

Canine
UTI: 2.2–4.4 mg/kg SC q24 h (Papich 2002) or 1 mg/lb SC q24 h for 5–14 days (Pfizer Manufacturer's Label).

Feline
Not recommended.

Dose adjustments

Hypersensitivity to cephalosporins or severe reactions to penicillins. Modify dose with renal impairment, prolonged use may cause superinfection.

Administration

Mix the 1 g or 4 g vial with 20 mL or 80 mL of sterile water for injection respectively, to make a 50 mg/mL suspension. Shake well and refrigerate.

Electrolyte contents

Cetiofur has 50 mg (2.2 mEq) of sodium per mL.

Storage/stability

Store undiluted vials at room temperature. Once reconstituted, the solution is stable at room temperature for up to 12 h or refrigerated for up to 7 days. It should be protected from light. A one-time salvage procedure can be performed by freezing the remaining product before it expires for up to 8 weeks. To thaw, the vial can be held under warm water. The color of the solution may change to a slight yellowish color, which does not affect potency.

Adverse reactions

>10%
Thrombocytopenia has been reported in dogs after 15 days and anemia after 36 days of therapy. Bone marrow dysplasia, extramedullary hematopoiesis, and thymic atrophy were seen microscopically at all dose levels in dogs following prolonged treatment.

1–10%
Noted to cause irreversible thrombocytopenia/ bone marrow suppression in dogs at doses >25 times the recommended dose. Vomiting and soft stools have also been reported in dogs.

Other species
In other mammals there are reports of allergic reactions including rashes, fever, eosinophilia, lymphadenopathy, and anaphylaxis.

Drug interactions

Other nephrotoxic drugs (aminoglycosides, amphotericin-B, furosemide) can decrease renal excretion of cephalosporins and increase toxicity.

Monitoring

Monitor for signs of anaphylaxis, CBC, and renal panel.

Overdose

High doses in renal failure may cause neuromuscular hypersensitivity and seizures. Hemodialysis may be required for extreme overdoses, otherwise supportive care is targeted toward noted toxicities.

Diagnostic test interference

No data reported for ceftiofur. In general, cephalosporins cause a positive, direct Coomb's test, false positive serum or urinary creatinine with Jaffe, and false positive urinary glucose with Clinitest.

Mechanism

A bactericidal, third generation cephalosporin. Binds to penicillin binding proteins causing inhibition of transpeptidation step of peptidoglycan synthesis.

Pharmacology/kinetics

Absorption
Ceftiofur is poorly absorbed after oral administration. It is rapidly absorbed after intramuscular and subcutaneous administration.

Distribution
Ceftiofur is widely distributed throughout fluid compartments and is found in high concentrations in tissues.

CNS penetration
CSF penetration in foals is <3% of plasma concentrations, suggesting that therapeutic concentrations are unlikely to be achieved in other species.

Metabolism
Ceftiofur is metabolized in the liver to an active metabolite, desfuroylceftiofur, which is less active than the parent compound. The majority of the metabolite is excreted in urine of dogs with a small amount excreted in feces.

Half-life
The half-life reported in dogs is 4.1 h.

Pregnancy risk factor

Ceftiofur does penetrate in high concentrations across the placental membranes. However, no teratogenic effects were noted in mice and rats even at high doses.

Lactation
Ceftiofur is excreted into milk in significant concentrations as demonstrated in cattle. Due to the limited oral absorption of the drug, systemic concentrations in nursing animals would be negligible. Altered bowel flora and sensitization of nursing animals may occur.

Reference

Papich, M.G. (2002) *Saunders Handbook of Veterinary Drugs*. 2nd edn. Winkel, A. (ed.), W.B. Saunders Company, Philadelphia, pp. 112–114.

Further reading

Craigmill, A.L., Brown, S.A., Wetzlich, S.E., *et al.* (1997) Pharmacokientics of ceftiofur and metabolites after single intravenous and intramuscular administration and multiple intramuscular administrations of ceftiofur sodium to sheep. *J Vet Pharmacol Therap.*, **20**, 139–144.

Greene, C., Hartmann, K., *et al.* (2006) Antimicrobial drug formulary. Appendix 8. In: *Infectious Disease of the Dog and Cat.* Greene, C. (ed.), Elsevier, St. Louis, MO, pp. 1186–1333.

Pharmacia and Upjohn Company. (2001) Naxcel Sterile Powder. NADA 140–338. *Freedom of Information Summary 2001*; May.

Chapter 140: Cefuroxime

US Generic (Brand) Name: Cefuroxime axetil and Cefuroxime sodium (Ceftin, Kefurox, Zinacef)
Availability: Human approved – Cefuroxime axetil oral tablets (125, 250, 500 mg), and powder for oral suspension 125 mg/5 mL (50, 100, 200 mL). Cefuroxime sodium sterile powder for injection (750 mg, 1.5 g, and 7.5 g) or frozen premix (750 mg/50 mL, 1.5 g/50 mL).
Resistance mechanisms: Altered penicillin binding proteins, increased beta-lactamase production, altered permeability

Use

Active against *Staphylococcus*, Group B *Streptococcus*, *E. coli*, *Enterobacter*, *Salmonella*, and *Klebsiella*. Used in respiratory tract and sinus infections, uncomplicated skin and soft tissue infections, bone and joint, urinary tract, and sepsis. Due to excellent penetration into the CNS, cefuroxime has been used in human cases of meningitis.

Contraindications/warnings

Hypersensitivity to cephalosporins or severe reactions to penicillins. Modify dose with renal impairment, prolonged use may cause superinfection.

Dosage

Canine
Susceptible infections: 5–10 mg/kg IV or deep IM injection q8 h (Greene 2006) or 20–30 mg/kg PO q12 h.

Meningitis: 30 mg/kg IV q8 h (Greene *et al.*, 2006).

Feline

Susceptible infections: 5–10 mg/kg IV or deep IM injection q8 h (Greene *et al.*, 2006).

Dose adjustments

Decrease dose frequency in moderate renal failure to twice daily dosing. In severe renal failure, administer dose every 24 h.

Administration

Cefuroxime oral powder for suspension should be mixed with the amount of water specified to make a 125 or 250 mg/mL suspension. It should be mixed well and refrigerated. Doses should be given with food. For direct intermittent IV injection, 8 or 16 mL of sterile water for injection is added to the 750 mg or 1.5 g vial to make a 90 mg/mL solution of cefuroxime sodium. The appropriate dose should be injected IV over 3–5 min or injected into a free flowing compatible IV solution. Do not admix with other drugs, especially aminoglycosides. For intermittent or continuous IV infusions the drug must be further diluted with 100 mL of sterile water for injection, D5W, or 0.9% sodium chloride to make a concentration of 7.5 or 1.5 mg/mL, respectively. The dose should be administered over 15–60 min. For IM injections add 3 mL of sterile water for injection to a 750 mg vial to make a suspension of 220 mg/mL. The appropriate dose can be given by deep IM injection into a large muscle.

Electrolyte contents

Sodium content is 54.2 mg (2.4 mEq) per 1 g of cefuroxime sodium.

Storage/stability

Store tablets, injectables, and un-reconstituted oral powder at room temperature. The oral suspension must be refrigerated after reconstitution and should be discarded after 10 days. After reconstitution the sterile injectable solution is good for 24 h at room temperature and 48 h when refrigerated. The IV infusion in normal saline or D5W is stable for 24 h at room temperature, 7 days refrigerated, and 26 weeks frozen. After thawing, the solution is good for 24 h at room temperature or 21 days when refrigerated.

Adverse reactions

>10%

Weight loss and localized site reactions following IM injections have been reported in dogs and cats.

1–10%

At high doses a decrease in hematocrit, erythrocytes, and prolonged clotting times has been reported in dogs. There has also been a reduction in plasma protein, albumin, and cholesterol.

<1%

Heinz body hemolytic anemia has been reported in dogs on high dose cefuroxime.

Other species

Vomiting, diarrhea, gastrointestinal bleeding, colitis, eosinophilia, leucopenia, neutropenia, increased transaminases, increased alkaline phosphatase, anaphylaxis, fever, erythema, nephritis, increased BUN, and serum creatinine are reported.

Drug interactions

Other nephrotoxic drugs (aminoglycosides, amphotericin-B, furosemide) can decrease renal excretion of cephalosporins and increase toxicity.

Monitoring

Monitor for signs of anaphylaxis, CBC, and renal panel. For long term therapy monitor hepatic and hematologic function periodically.

Overdose

Overdose symptoms may include nausea, vomiting, diarrhea, neuromuscular hyperirritability, seizures, and encephalopathy. Gastrointestinal lavage, hemodialysis and supportive care (including anticonvulsant therapy) may be indicated. Approximately 25% of a dose is dialyzable.

Diagnostic test interference

Will cause a positive, direct Coomb's test, false positive serum or urinary creatinine with Jaffe, false positive urinary glucose with Clinitest.

Mechanism

A bactericidal, second generation cephalosporin. Binds to penicillin binding proteins causing inhibition of transpeptidation step of peptidoglycan synthesis.

Pharmacology/kinetics

Absorption
Oral absorption after a 20 mg/kg dose in dogs results in peak concentrations of 10.09 µg/mL at 60 min. Well absorbed after IM injection in humans. Maximum absorption occurs in 1–2 h.

Distribution
Widely distributed throughout tissues including the lungs, bone, bile, gallbladder, and CSF. Protein binding in dogs is 19.6%.

CNS penetration
Cefuroxime penetrates into the CSF in high concentrations (0.15–2.03 µg/mL) and has been used in human cases of meningitis.

Metabolism
Cefuroxime is excreted primarily as parent drug both in urine and in feces. In dogs, 29.4% of drug is excreted in urine within 24 h.

Half-life
The half-life in dogs is reported to be short (70 min).

Pregnancy risk factor

Category B. Cefuroxime has not been associated with any teratogenic effects in animal or human studies. It achieves high concentrations in amniotic fluid and fetal tissues. It is generally considered safe in pregnancy.

Lactation
Cefuroxime is excreted into milk in low concentrations which could result in diarrhea and sensitization of nursing animals.

Reference

Greene, C., Hartmann, K., *et al.* (2006) Antimicrobial drug formulary. Appendix 8. In: *Infectious Disease of the Dog and Cat*. Greene, C. (ed.), Elsevier, St. Louis, MO, pp. 1186–1333.

Further reading

Spurling, N.W., Harcourt, R.A., and Hyde, J.J. (1986) An evaluation of the safety of cefuroxime axetil during six months of oral administration to beagle dogs. *J Toxicol Sci.*, **11(4)**, 237–277.

Zhao, L., Li, Q., Li, X., *et al.* (2012) Bioequivalence and population pharmacokinetic modeling of two forms of antibiotic, cefuroxime lysine and cefuroxime sodium after intravenous infusion in Beagle dogs. *J Biomed Biotechnol.*, doi 507294: July 15.

Chapter 141: Cephalexin

US Generic (Brand) Name: Cephalexin (Keflex, Rilexine)
Availability: Human approved – Cephalexin oral capsules (250, 500 mg), oral tablets (1 g) and powder for oral suspension (125 mg/5 mL, 250 mg/5 mL in 100 and 200 mL bottles). Veterinary approved – Rilexine (75, 150, 300, and 600 mg chew tabs)
Resistance Mechanisms: Altered penicillin binding proteins, increased beta-lactamase production,

Use

Labeled for use in the treatment of canine secondary superficial bacterial pyoderma caused by *Staphylococcus pseudintermedius*. In addition, it covers group A beta-hemolytic *Streptococcus, Staphylococcus, Klebsiella, E. coli, Proteus, Shigella,* and *Pasteurella*. Not effective against methicillin resistant *Staphylococcus, Pseudomonas,* or many other gram negative bacilli. Used in lower respiratory, urinary, skin, and soft tissue infections. Also used for prophylaxis and treatment of bone and joint infections.

Contraindications/warnings

Hypersensitivity to cephalosporins and severe reactions to penicillins. Use with caution in animals with renal failure or those on prolonged use.

Dosage

Canine
Susceptible infections: 10–30 mg/kg PO q6–12 h (Papich 2002).

Pyoderma: 22–35 mg/kg PO q12 h (Papich 2002) or 30–60 mg/kg PO q24 h (Toma *et al.,* 2008) or 22 mg/kg PO q12 h × 28 days (Rilexine package insert-Virbac).

Feline

Susceptible infections: 15–20 mg/kg PO q12 h (Papich 2002).

Dose adjustment

Decrease dose and adjust dosing frequency in severe renal impairment, give q24 h with severe impairment.

Administration

Give on an empty stomach (1 h before or 2 h after a meal) to increase absorption. If not tolerated give with food.

Electrolyte contents

Not significant.

Storage/stability

Store oral capsules, chew tablets and powder for suspension at room temperature. Once reconstituted, the oral suspension should be refrigerated according to the manufacturer and must be discarded after 14 days. Further studies suggest that cephalexin monohydrate oral suspension reconstituted from powder as a suspension and repackaged in clear polypropylene oral syringes is stable for 90 days when stored under ambient, refrigerated, and frozen conditions.

Adverse reactions

>10%
Anorexia, nausea, vomiting, diarrhea, and salivation reported in dogs and cats.

1–10%
Rashes, tachypnea, lethargy, pruritus, and erythema have been reported in dogs and fever has been reported in cats.

Other species
Anaphylaxis, seizures, neuromuscular hypersensitivity, colitis, thrombocytopenia, phlebitis, eosinophilia, neutropenia, toxic neutropenia, transient increases in serum aminotransferases, agranulocytosis, cholestasis, hemolytic anemia, hypoprothrombinemia, prolonged prothrombin time, platelet dysfunction, nephritis, epidermal necrolysis (cats), and superinfection (prolonged use).

Drug interactions

Other nephrotoxic drugs (aminoglycosides, amphotericin-B, and furosemide) can decrease renal excretion of cephalexin and increase toxicity.

Monitoring

Monitor for allergic reactions. For patients with renal failure, on high doses or with prolonged courses, monitor CBC, hepatic, and renal function.

Overdose

With an acute overdose, the animal may have nausea, salivation, lethargy, vomiting, and diarrhea. Increased ALT, decreased total protein and/or globulin, neuromuscular hypersensitivity, and seizures are also possible, particularly with high doses in renal insufficiency. Hemodialysis may be helpful but generally not required. Supportive care and gastrointestinal decontamination are generally indicted rather than hemodialysis.

Diagnostic test interference

Will cause a positive, direct Coomb's test, false positive serum or urinary creatinine with Jaffe, and false positive urinary glucose with Clinitest.

Mechanism

Bactericidal, first generation cephalosporin. Inhibits bacterial cell wall synthesis by binding to penicillin binding proteins, resulting in the inhibition of the final transpeptidation step of peptidoglycan synthesis.

Pharmacology/kinetics

Absorption
Cephalexin is well absorbed orally. Oral absorption is 75–90% in dogs and 56% in cats. Maximum concentrations (17–22 µg/mL) occur at 1.2–1.4 h. Food may delay/lower peak concentrations but not the total amount absorbed. As is in humans, severe illness (shock, septicemia, etc.) and age (neonates, youth) may decrease overall absorption.

Distribution
Distributes into most body fluids and tissues. Therapeutic concentrations are noted in the gallbladder, liver, bile, kidneys, bone, pleural, and synovial fluids. Protein binding is low (9–30%) in dogs.

CNS penetration

CSF penetration is low, even with inflammation.

Metabolism

The majority of drug (80–100%) is excreted as parent drug in urine.

Half-life

The terminal half-life is 4.7–9 h in dogs. In cats, it is 1–2 h.

Pregnancy risk factor

Category B: Animal studies have not demonstrated any teratogenic or adverse effects in first trimester or later stages of pregnancy. Cephalexin is considered to be a drug of choice in pregnant canine patients for bacterial infections that are susceptible.

Lactation

Cephalexin is readily excreted into milk in humans and achieves a maximum concentration of 4 µg/mL at 4 h after an oral dose. Altered bowel flora and sensitization of nursing animals may occur.

References

Papich, M.G. (2002) *Saunders Handbook of Veterinary Drugs.* 2nd edn. Winkel, A. (ed.), W.B. Saunders Company, Philadelphia, pp. 114–115.

Toma, S., Colombo, S., Cornegliania, L., *et al.* (2008) Efficacy and tolerability of once-daily cephelexin in canine superficial pyoderma: an open controlled study. *J Small Anim Pract.*, **49(8)**, 384–391.

Further reading

Crosse, R. and Burt, D.G. (1984) Antibiotic concentration in the serum of dogs and cats following a single oral dose of cephalexin. *Vet Rec.*, **115(5)**, 106–107.

Papich, M., Davis, J.L., and Floerchinger, A.M. (2010) Pharmacokinetics, protein binding and tissue distribution of orally administered cefpodoxime proxetil and cephalexin in dogs. *Am J Vet Res.*, **71(12)**, 1484–1491.

Silley, P., Rudd, A.P., Symington, W.M., *et al.* (1988) Pharmacokinetics of cephalexin in dogs and cats after oral, subcutaneous and intramuscular administration. *Vet Rec.*, **122(1)**, 15–17.

Sylvestri, M.F., Makoid, M.C., and Cox, B.E. (1988) Stability of cephalexin monohydrate suspension in polypropylene oral syringes. *Am J Hosp Pharm.*, **45(6)**, 1353–1356.

Chapter 142: Chloramphenicol

US Generic (Brand) Name: Chloramphenicol (Chloromyceton, Chloramphenicol sodium succinate, Chloroptic, AK-Chlor)
Availability: Human approved – Chloramphenicol succinate sterile powder for injection (1 g) (Availability is currently questionable). Veterinary approved – Chloramphenicol base oral tablets (50, 100, 250, 500 mg, and 1 g)
Resistance Mechanisms: Reduced membrane permeability, mutation of 50s ribosomes

Use

Only use for severe infections due to organisms resistant to less toxic drugs or infections located in hard to penetrate spaces (CNS). Wide spectrum of activity against gram positive and gram negative organisms. Active against *Salmonella*, *Brucella*, *Yersinia*, vancomycin resistant *Enterococci*, methicillin resistant *Staphylococcus* spp., *Shigella*, and *Francisella*. Also has activity against anaerobes, *Bacteriodes*, *Clostridium*, and *Fusobacterium*. Covers some atypical organisms including *Nocardia*, *Chlamydia*, *Mycoplasma*, and *Richettsia*.

Contraindications/warnings

Hypersensitivity to chloramphenicol, avoid use in severe hepatic impairment and in neonatal animals. Dose related side effects (bone marrow suppression) may be more common in renal/hepatic impairment. Warn clients of risks of human exposure (rare idiosyncratic aplastic anemia in 1/10,000). Consult on wearing gloves, eye/skin protection when handling drug, feces, and urine. Avoid contact if pregnant or lactating.

Dosage

Canine

Susceptible infections: 40–50 mg/kg PO q8 h or 40–50 mg/kg IV, IM q6–8 h (Papich 2002).

Meningitis: 35 mg/kg IV q8 h × 5 days; followed by oral therapy for 3 weeks (Greene 2013).

Feline

Susceptible infections: 12.5–20 mg/kg PO q12 h or 12.5–20 mg per cat IV, IM q12 h (Papich 2002).

Dose adjustments

Do not use in severe hepatic impairment. Increase dosing interval (q12–24 h) in severe renal impairment.

Administration

Tablets or capsules should be administered whole to prevent human exposure. If tablets require cutting, this should be done either in a chemical hood or wearing gloves using a tablet splitter within a plastic enclosure (Zip-Lock bag). Gloves and eye wear should be used when administering the drug or handling excreta. Wash off immediately if skin or mucus membranes are exposed. To prepare a 10% (100 mg/mL) IV, SC, IM solution, add 10 mL of sterile water or 5% dextrose into each 1 g vial. Administer the IV injection over 1 min. The IV succinate ester salt is a prodrug that must be hydrolyzed to chloramphenicol base. Hydrolysis is incomplete so that 30% of the dose is lost in urine. Therefore, serum concentrations of chloramphenicol following IV administration are only 70% of those following oral administration. Oral therapy is preferred therapeutically if tolerated.

Electrolyte contents

One gram of chloramphenicol succinate contains 51.8 mg (2.25 mEq) of sodium.

Storage/stability

Store tablets, capsules, and IV injectable at room temperature.

Adverse reactions

>10%
Gastrointestinal side effects are common. Nausea and vomiting in both cats and dogs has been reported.

1–10%
Weight loss, inappetence, dehydration, and CNS depression reported in dogs and cats.

<1%
Bone marrow suppression is reported in cats receiving 60 mg/kg/day after 1–2 weeks of treatment. Cats appear more sensitive than dogs.

Other species
In humans, rare but fatal, idiosyncratic aplastic anemia developing weeks to months after oral (1/10,000) or topical exposure (1/224,716) are reported. A dose related reversible bone marrow suppression (anemia, neutropenia) is also noted at plasma concentrations > 25 μg/mL. Gray syndrome (circulatory collapse, cyanosis, acidosis, neurotoxic reactions, optic neuritis, peripheral neuritis, abdominal distention, myocardial depression, coma, and death) is reported in neonates and adults with severe liver impairment where high plasma concentrations (40–200 μg/mL) may occur.

Drug interactions

Erythromycin and chloramphenicol compete for the same binding site on the ribosome and are antagonistic. Phenobarbital and rifampin can decrease chloramphenicol concentrations. Chloramphenicol increases concentrations of digoxin and pentobarbital. Chloramphenicol decreases the intestinal absorption of riboflavin, pyridoxine, and vitamin B12.

Monitoring

Monitor CBC, liver, and renal function. Monitor chloramphenicol concentrations if available. Peak concentrations should be 15–20 μg/mL and troughs 5–10 μg/mL. Toxicity occurs at >40 μg/mL.

Overdose

Nausea, vomiting weight loss, dehydration, metabolic acidosis, hypotension, hypothermia, CNS depression, and bone marrow suppression may all occur. Gastrointestinal decontamination and supportive care should be instituted. Hemodialysis removes 5–20% of the dose.

Diagnostic test interference

None noted.

Mechanism

Reversibly binds to 50s ribosome in susceptible bacteria causing inhibition of bacterial protein synthesis.

Pharmacology/kinetics

Absorption
The palmitate salt given orally is well absorbed in dogs, but poorly in cats. The injectable succinate salt is well absorbed after SC and IM injection in animals but must

be hydrolyzed to become active. Plasma levels after IV administration are only 70% of those following oral therapy.

Distribution
Distributes throughout body tissues and fluids, including CNS, aqueous, and vitreous humor. High concentrations are found in the liver and kidneys of dogs.

CNS penetration
Excellent CNS penetration (>50%) and improves with inflammation.

Metabolism
The oral palmitate salt must be hydrolyzed in the intestine to the active base. The injectable succinate salt must be hydrolyzed by estrases to the active base. Metabolism occurs in the liver to inactive glucuronidated metabolites. Elimination is primarily renal, 55% of a dose is recovered in the urine of dogs. Inactive metabolites account for the majority of drug recovered (80%).

Half-life
The half-life in dogs is 1.2 h and 5 h in cats. The longer half-life may be due to the limited glucuronidation capacity of cats.

Pregnancy risk factor

Category C: Chloramphenicol crosses into the placenta in high concentrations and should not be given to pregnant animals due to its inherent toxicity in neonates/fetuses

Lactation
Chloramphenicol readily distributes into milk and should be avoided in nursing animals due to the risk of toxicity (Gray Syndrome) in neonatal animals.

References

Greene, C.E. (2013) Bacterial meningitis. Ch. 90. In: *Canine and Feline Infectious Diseases*, Sykes, J.E. (ed.), Elsevier, St. Louis, MO, pp. 886–892.

Papich, M.G. (2002) *Saunders Handbook of Veterinary Drugs*. 2nd edn. Winkel, A. (ed.), W.B. Saunders Company, Philadelphia, pp. 123–125.

Further reading

Kauffman, R.E., Thirumoorthi, M.C., Buckley, J.A., *et al.* (1981) Relative bioavailability of intravenous chloramphenicol succinate and oral chloramphenicol palmitate in infants and children. *J Pediatr.*, **99(6)**, 963–967.

Watson, A.D. (1977) Chloramphenicol toxicity. *Res Vet Sci.*, **23(1)**, 66–69.

Watson, A.D. and Middleton, D.J. (1978) Chloramphenicol toxicosis in cats. *Am J Vet Res.*, **39(7)**, 1199–1203.

Chapter 143: Ciprofloxacin

US Generic (Brand) Name: Ciprofloxacin (Cipro, Cipro IV, Ciloxan, ProQuin XR)
Availability: Human approved – Ciprofloxacin oral tablets (100, 250, 500, 750 mg), oral extend release tablets (500 mg, 1 g), oral suspension 250 mg/5 mL (20 mL), 500 mg/5 mL (100 mL), IV injectable concentrate 10 mg/mL (20, 40 mL), pre-mix IV solution (2 mg/mL in 5% dextrose), otic suspension 0.2% with hydrocortisone, ophthalmic oint. 3.33 mg/g (3.5 g)
Resistance Mechanisms: Bacterial topoisomerase mutations, altered membrane permeability and efflux pumps

Use

Treatment of infections of the lower respiratory tract, sinuses, skin, otitis, endometritis, bone/joints, UTI, prostatitis, bacteremia, and systemic infections. Indicated for gram negative organisms including *Pseudomonas, E. coli, Klebsiella, Enterobacter, Citrobacter, Salmonella, Moraxella, Campylobacter, Brucella,* and *Pasteurella.* It is typically more effective against *Pseudomonas* than other veterinary fluoroquinolones. Gram positive organisms including *Staphylococcus* and some strains of *Streptococcus* are susceptible. Covers some intracellular organisms and other atypical organisms including; *Mycoplasma, Leptospira, Borrelia, Chlamydia, Mycobacterium tuberculosis* (not *M. avium*). Does not cover obligate anaerobes, *Enterococcus, Actinomyces,* or *Nocardia.*

Contraindications/warnings

Hypersensitivity to fluoroquinolones. Avoid or reduce dose in patients with renal failure. Avoid in pregnant, lactating, or young animals due to arthropathy. Large, rapidly growing dogs 4–28 weeks of age are most susceptible. Use with caution in patients with known or suspected CNS disorders, since CNS stimulation can occur. May prolong Q-T interval, use with caution in patients with pre-existing cardiac disease.

Dosage

Canine

Susceptible Infections: 10–20 mg/kg PO q24 h or 5–10 mg/kg IV q12 h (Papich 2002). Use lower doses for less severe infections (UTIs) and higher doses for more severe infections.

Feline

Susceptible Infections: 20 mg/kg PO q24 h or 10 mg/kg IV q24 h (Papich 2002).

Dose adjustments

Dose adjust in patients with moderate to severe renal impairment. Extent dosing interval to q18–24 h for IV dosing in dogs or q48 h in place of q24 h in cats.

Administration

Best absorbed on an empty stomach, but may be administered with food to decrease gastrointestinal upset. The extend release tablets are best with food but may not be well absorbed in animal patients. Maintain hydration and urinary output. The oral suspension should not be administered via a stomach tube and when given orally it should be followed with water to avoid animal from chewing the microcapsules. The intravenous solution concentrate should be further diluted to no greater than 2 mg/mL in an appropriate diluent and infused IV over 60 min. Animals should avoid long term exposure to UV light while on ciprofloxacin due to photosensitivity reactions.

Electrolyte contents

Not significant.

Storage/stability

Ciprofloxacin tablets, suspension and IV products should be stored at room temperature and protected from light. The reconstituted oral suspension should be stored at room temperature or refrigerated, protected from freezing and is stable for 14 days. The reconstituted IV injectable solution in LRS, D5W, 0.9% NaCl (0.5–2 mg/mL) is stable for 14 days at room temperature or refrigerated.

Adverse reactions

>10%
Nausea and salivation reported in cats and dogs. Cats appear to have more inappetence and malaise.

1–10%
Vomiting and diarrhea reported in dogs and cats.

<1%
CNS side effects: tremors, seizures, and restlessness have been reported with high doses in dogs and cats. Mydriasis, retinal degeneration, and blindness are reported in cats on high doses of enrofloxacin and may also occur with other fluoroquinolones including ciprofloxacin.

Other species
Elevated liver enzymes, hypertension, rash, photosensitivity skin reactions, elevated serum creatinine, arthralgia, cartilage damage, lameness, cataracts, tendon rupture, allergic reactions, agranulocytosis, prolongation of the Q-T interval, angina, palpitations, myocardial infarction, toxic epidermal necrolysis, pseudomembranous colitis, visual disturbances, acute renal failure, anemia, and agranulocytosis.

Drug interactions

Bioavailability is decreased by enteral feedings containing cations. Aluminum or magnesium products (antacids), sucralfate, calcium, iron, zinc, and multiple vitamins with minerals may all decrease absorption by >90%. Give these agents at least 2–4 h from dosing, consider switching to an H_2 antagonist or omeprazole. Theophylline and NSAIDs may increase the CNS stimulation of ciprofloxacin. H_2 antagonists and loop diuretics may inhibit renal elimination of quinolones, antineoplastics may decrease absorption of ciprofloxacin, ciprofloxacin may increase cyclosporine concentrations. Avoid use with agents that can cause prolongation of the Q-T interval (cisapride, macrolides, etc.).

Monitoring

Monitor for hypersensitivity reactions and CNS stimulation. Monitor for mydriasis and retinal degeneration with long term use in cats.

Overdose

Acute renal failure and seizures may result. Gastrointestinal decontamination and supportive care are recommended. Charcoal hemoprofusion has markedly reduced plasma concentrations of enrofloxacin and may be effective in severe overdoses of ciprofloxacin.

Diagnostic test interference

None noted.

Mechanism

A bactericidal fluoroquinolone. Promotes breakage of double stranded bacterial DNA. Inhibits DNA-gyrase in susceptible organisms and stops relaxation of supercoiled DNA.

Pharmacology/kinetics

Absorption
Inconsistent oral absorption in dogs. Because of the wide range in oral absorption of tablets, the dose needed to reach the target concentration to inhibit bacteria ranges from 12 to 52 mg/kg with a mean dose of 25 mg/kg q24 h for bacteria with a minimum inhibitory concentration ≤0.25 μg/mL.

Distribution
Distributes widely into tissues. Concentrations exceed serum concentrations in kidneys, gallbladder, liver, lungs, prostate, and urogenital tissues. Present in high concentrations in most fluids (saliva, nasal, and bronchial secretions, sputum, lymph, peritoneal fluid, and bile). Lowest concentrations are reported from bone, muscle, fat, and skin.

CNS penetration
CSF concentrations are less than 10% unless inflammation is present, which increases penetration.

Metabolism
Ciprofloxacin is partially metabolized in the liver with <37% of the drug excreted into the urine as unchanged drug.

Half-life
The plasma elimination half-life in dogs is 2–3 h which is similar to other species.

Pregnancy risk factor

Category C: No evidence of teratogenic effects in laboratory animals or human exposures to ciprofloxacin. However, due to potential fetal cartilage effects the drug is not recommended in pregnant patients.

Lactation
Ciprofloxacin is excreted into milk in significant concentrations and may have adverse effects (cartilage damage) on nursing animals.

Reference

Papich, M.G. (2002) *Saunders Handbook of Veterinary Drugs*. 2nd edn. Winkel, A. (ed.), W.B. Saunders Company, Philadelphia, pp. 132–134.

Further reading

Papich, M.G. (2012) Ciprofloxacin pharmacokinetics and oral absorption of generic ciprofloxacin tablets in dogs. *Am J Vet Res.*, **73(7)**, 1085–1091.

Chapter 144: Clarithromycin

US Generic (Brand) Name: Clarithromycin (Biaxin)
Availability: Human approved – Film coated oral tablets (250, 500 mg), extend release tablets (500 mg), granules for oral suspension 125 mg/5 mL (50, 100 mL), 250 mg/5 mL (50, 100 mL)
Resistance Mechanisms: Ribosomal modification (erm gene), altered efflux (mefE gene)

Use

Active against *Streptococcus* spp., *M. catarrhalis*, *Mycoplasma*, *S. aureus*, *S. pseudintermedias*, *Bordetella*, *Chlamydia*, *Ureaplasma*, *M. avium*, and *M. intracellular*. Also active against *R. equi*. Frequently used in small animals for disseminated mycobacterial infections often in combination with rifampin, clofazimine or a fluoroquinolone. Can also be used for sinusitis, otitis media, and uncomplicated skin and soft tissue infections.

Contraindications/warnings

Avoid use in patients that are hypersensitive to macrolides or patients with uncorrected hypokalemia or hypomagnesemia. Use with caution in geriatric patients with impaired renal/hepatic function. Reduce dose with severe renal impairment. Monitor closely for colitis. Clarithromycin has been associated with Q-T prolongation (torsade de pointes) and ventricular arrhythmias. Use with caution in patients with pre-existing arrhythmias.

Dosage

Canine
Susceptible Infections: 7.5 mg/kg PO q12 h (Papich 2002).

Leproid granuloma: 7.5–15 mg/kg PO q12 h plus rifampin or clofazimine (Malik *et al.*, 2013).

Feline

Susceptible Infections: 7.5 mg/kg PO q12 h (Papich 2002).

Cutaneous/Pulmonary Mycobacterium Complex: 7.5 mg/kg PO q12 h combined with marbofloxacin 2.75–5.5 mg/kg/day PO and rifampin 5–10 mg/kg PO q12 h × 2 months followed by clarithromycin and marbofloxacin continuous treatment for 6 months (Sykes and Papich, 2013). Cats may need treatment for months to life to prevent recurrence.

Dose adjustments

Reduce dose in renal impairment. Give a normal loading dose; followed by a decreased dose or prolonged dosing interval (i.e., 50% dose or once daily dosing for severe impairment).

Administration

Give with food. Do not crush oral-extend release tablets.

Electrolyte contents

Not significant.

Storage/stability

Store the tablets and granules for suspension at room temperature. Once diluted, store the suspension at room temperature, do not refrigerate or this will cause the micro-encapsulated granules to form a gel.

Adverse reactions

>10%
Loose stool, nausea, and diarrhea have been reported in dogs/cats.

1–10%
Vomiting, inappetence, jaundice, elevated AST, alkaline phosphatase, bilirubin, pinnal, and generalized erythema in cats/dogs. Conjunctival injection and lacrimation reported in dogs.

Other species
Altered taste, colitis, ventricular tachycardia, prolonged Q-T interval, decreased white blood count, elevated prothrombin time, thrombocytopenia, elevated BUN and serum creatinine, tremor, anxiety, and hypoglycemia.

Drug interactions

Clarithromycin increases concentrations of benzodiazepams, cyclosporine, theophylline, digoxin, tacrolimus, omeprazole, cisapride, itraconazole, and sildenafil. Fluconazole increases concentrations of clarithromycin. Clarithromycin prolongs the Q-T interval and should be used with caution with other drugs that prolong the Q-T interval (cisapride, amiodarone, fluoroquinolones, etc.).

Monitoring

Monitor CBC, liver, and cardiac function in patients on long term therapy and particularly in geriatric patients. Monitor liver enzyme activity frequently if combined with rifampin, and Q-T interval prolongation if combined with a fluoroquinolone.

Overdose

Symptoms of acute toxicity in dogs have included nausea, vomiting, diarrhea, pancreatitis, and liver toxicity. Ataxia, hearing loss, and behavioral changes are noted in humans. Gastrointestinal decontamination and supportive care is indicated for acute overdoses. Dialysis does not reduce plasma concentrations of clarithromycin.

Diagnostic test interference

None reported.

Mechanism

Binds to bacterial 50s ribosomal subunit causing inhibition of bacterial protein synthesis.

Pharmacology/kinetics

Absorption
Oral absorption is greater than 70% in dogs. This is increased with the oral suspension or in the fasted state.

Distribution
Distributes widely into most tissues, particularly lung tissue and gastric mucosa. Extensive intracellular penetration. Highly protein bound.

CNS penetration

Minimal penetration into the CNS.

Metabolism

Clarithromycin is metabolized in the liver to an active metabolite (14-OH clarithromycin). *In vitro* this metabolite is twice as active as the parent drug. Clarithromycin is primarily secreted via feces (70–80%) with the remaining eliminated renally (20–30%).

Half-life

The half-life is non-linear due to saturation of hepatic metabolism and ranges from 2–6 h in dogs.

Pregnancy risk factor

Category C: Animal studies have shown an increase in spontaneous abortions, cleft palates, and cardiac malformations. It is contraindicated in pregnant patients.

Lactation

Clarithromycin and its active metabolite are secreted in milk. Nursing animals may develop diarrhea and become sensitized.

References

Malik, R., Smits, B., Reppas, G., *et al.* (2013) Ulcerated and nonulcerated nontuberculous cutaneous mycobacterial granulomas in cats and dogs. *Vet Dermatol.*, **24(1)**, 146–153.

Papich, M.G. (2002) *Saunders Handbook of Veterinary Drugs*. 2nd edn. Winkel, A. (ed.), W.B. Saunders Company, Philadelphia, pp. 137–138.

Sykes, J.E. and Papich, M.G. (2013) Antibacterial drugs. Ch. 8. In: *Canine and Feline Infectious Diseases*, Sykes, J.E. (ed.), Elsevier, St. Louis, MO, pp. 886–892.

Further reading

Katayama, M., Nishijima, N., Okamura, Y., *et al.* (2012) Interaction of clarithromycin with cyclosporin in cats: pharmacokinetic study and case report. *J Feline Med Surg.*, **14(4)**, 257–261.

Vilmanyi, E., Kung, K., Riond, J.L., *et al.* (1996) Clarithromycin pharmacokinetics after oral absorption with or without fasting in cross breed beagles. *J Small Anim Pract.*, **37(11)**, 535–539.

Zhang, X.R., Zhang, Y.F., Wang, J., *et al.* (2008) Pharmacokinetics of clarithromycin citrate salt after oral administration to beagle dogs and food effects on its absorption. *PDA J Pharm Sci Technol.*, **62(6)**, 445.

Chapter 145: Clavamox

US Generic (Brand) Name: Amoxicillin/clavulanic acid (Clavamox, Augmentin)
Availability: Human approved – Amoxicillin/clavulanic acid film coated tablets (250/125, 500/125, 875/125 mg/mg), chew tablets (125/31.25, 200/28.5, 250/62.5, 400/51 mg/mg), powder for oral suspension (125/31.25, 200/28.5, 250/62.5, 400/57, 600/42.9 mg per 5 mL). Veterinary approved – Clavamox tablets (50/12.5, 100/25, 200/50, 300/75 mg/mg), Clavamox powder for oral suspension (50 mg/12.5 mg/mL)
Resistance Mechanisms: Increased beta-lactamases, decreased membrane permeability, increased OXA-type enzymes

Use

The combination of amoxicillin with clavulanic acid expands the activity of amoxicillin to cover gram positive organisms including beta-lactamase producing *S. aureus* and *S. pseudintermedius*. It also covers gram negative organisms such as *E. coli*, *Klebsiella*, and *Proteus*, but not *Pseudomonas* or *Enterobacter*. The clavulanic acid also improves amoxicillin's anaerobic coverage including some *Bacteriodes* spp. isolates. It is commonly used in veterinary medicine to treat a variety of infections including: skin and soft tissue, urinary tract infections, bronchitis, and sinusitis.

Contraindications/warnings

Hypersensitivity to penicillins, aminopenicillins, cephalosporins, or clavulanic acid. In patients with renal failure, the dose should be modified. Caution in patients with pre-existing hyperkalemia.

Dosage

Dosing is based on the combination of amoxicillin plus clavulanic potassium. Continue treatment for at least 2 days beyond resolution of clinical signs. Do not exceed 30 days of treatment.

Canine
Gram positive infections: 10 mg/kg PO q12 h (Aucoin 2000).

Gram negative infections: 20 mg/kg PO q8 h (Aucoin 2000).

UTIs: 12.5 mg/kg PO q8 h (Greene *et al.*, 2006).

Pyoderma: 22 mg/kg PO q12 h or 13.75 mg/kg PO q8 h (Summers *et al.*, 2012).

Feline
Gram positive infections: 10 mg/kg PO q12 h (Aucoin 2000).

Gram negative infections: 20 mg/kg PO q8 h (Aucoin 2000).

UTIs: 62.5 mg/cat PO q12 h (Greene *et al.*, 2006).

Dose adjustments

In moderate renal impairment the dosing frequency should be expanded to q12 h instead of q8 h or the dose slightly reduced. In severe renal failure, doses should be given q24 h rather than q12 h.

Administration

Administer oral tablets and suspensions with food. Be aware that the amoxicillin to clavulanic ratio varies between brands and formulations so human and veterinary products may not be entirely interchangeable. Mix Clavamox or Augmentin powder for oral suspension with the specified amount of water, shake well, and refrigerate.

Electrolyte contents

Potassium content = 0.16 mEq per 31.25 mg of clavulanic potassium.

Storage/stability

Store products at room temperature. Keep tablets in the manufacturer's foil. If splitting tablets, the remaining portion should be tightly re-wrapped in foil. Products are sensitive to humidity and moisture. Once reconstituted the oral suspensions can be refrigerated for up to 10 days. The suspension may be left out of the refrigerator at room temperature for up to 48 h.

Adverse reactions

>10%
Dose related diarrhea, nausea, vomiting, and flatulence (increased incidence due to clavulanic acid) in cats/dogs.

1–5%
Rashes, urticaria, gastritis, hypersensitivity reactions (angioedema, rash, urticaria, anaphylaxis), and anemia reported in dogs and cats.

Other species
Ataxia, fever, elevated liver enzymes, hepatic dysfunction, anaphylaxis, neurotoxicity at high doses (particularly with renal failure), seizures, hyperirritability, convulsions, super-infection, hemolytic anemia, thrombocytopenia, eosinophilia, leucopenia, agranulocytosis, and cholestasis have been reported.

Drug interactions

Allopurinol can increase amoxicillin concentrations.

Monitoring

Monitor for hypersensitivity reactions. With prolonged use, monitor CBC, liver, and renal function. Electrolytes should be monitored carefully particularly in renal failure due to high potassium content.

Overdose

Acute toxicity may involve nausea, vomiting, muscle hyperirritability, seizures, and convulsions. Electrolyte imbalance particularly in renal failure. Use supportive care and hemodialysis if available. Both amoxicillin and clavulanic acid are removed with hemodialysis and clavulanic acid is removed by peritoneal dialysis.

Diagnostic test interference

May interfere with urine glucose analysis if using the Clinitest. May inactivate aminoglycosides *in vitro* altering their concentrations.

Mechanism

A bactericidal aminopenicillin with a beta-lactamase inhibitor. Similar to amoxicillin, but the clavulanic acid inactivates beta-lactamases preventing their inactivation of amoxicillin. This improves the spectrum to cover beta-lactamase producing anaerobes and gram negative organisms.

Pharmacology/kinetics

Absorption
Amoxicillin is well absorbed orally. Clavulanic acid has highly variable absorption (5-fold) in animals. Extend release forms have not been studied in animals and are not well absorbed in fasted humans or following a high fat meal.

Distribution
Following administration, both amoxicillin and clavulanic acid are widely distributed into tissues and fluids (lungs, pleural fluids, peritoneal fluids, soft tissue, prostate, liver, muscle, gallbladder, and urine). Protein binding in dogs is approximately 13% for amoxicillin. Protein binding in humans for clavulanic acid is 22–30%.

CNS penetration
Amoxicillin has poor penetration into CNS (<1% serum concentrations). This increases to 8–90% with inflammation. CNS penetration of amoxicillin/clavulanate is not reported.

Metabolism
Amoxicillin is mainly excreted unmetabolized into urine, with only 10–25% excreted as penicilloic acid. In dogs, clavulanic acid is metabolized to L-amino-4-hydroxybutan-2-one, which is found in the urine. Approximately 34–52% is excreted via urine, 25–27% via feces and 16–33% via respired air.

Half-life
The half-life of Clavamox in dogs is 1.5 h for amoxicillin and 0.76 h for clavulanic acid.

Pregnancy risk factor

Category B: Both drugs penetrate into the placenta but are not associated with any teratogenic effects to date. It is generally considered safe in pregnancy.

Lactation
Amoxicillin is excreted into milk in low concentrations (0.68–1.3 µg/mL). The maximum concentration is seen 4–5 h after an oral dose. No data is available on clavulanic acid but due to its low molecular weight it would be expected to be excreted into milk. Consequences may be diarrhea and potential hypersensitization of nursing animals.

References

Aucoin, D. (2000) Antibiotic drug formulary. Target. *The Antibiotic Drug Guide to Effective Treatment*. North American Drug Compendiums Inc., Port Huron, MI, pp. 93–142.

Greene, C., Hartmann, K., *et al.* (2006) Antimicrobial drug formulary. Appendix 8. In: *Infectious Disease of the Dog and Cat*. Greene, C. (ed.), Elsevier, St. Louis, MO, pp. 1186–1333.
Summers, J.F., Bradbelt, D.C., Forsythe, P.J., *et al.* (2012) The effectiveness of systemic antimicrobial treatment in canine superficial and deep pyoderma; a systemic review. *Vet Dermatol.*, **23(4)**, 305–329.

Further reading

Kung, K. and Wanner, M. (1994) Bioavailability of different forms of amoxicillin administered orally to dogs. *Vet Rec.*, **135(23)**, 552–554.
Marier, J.F., Beaudry, F., Ducharme, M.P., *et al.* (2001) A pharmacokinetic study of amoxicillin in febrile beagle dogs following repeated administrations of endotoxin. *J Vet Pharmacol Therap.*, **24(6)**, 379–383.
Sakamoto, H., Hirose, T., Mine, Y. (1985) Pharmacokinetics of FK027 in rats and dogs. *J Antibiot (Tokyo)*, **38(4)**, 496–504.
Vree, T.B., Dammers, E., and VanDuuren, E. (2002) Variable absorption of clavulanic acid after an oral dose of 25 mg/kg of Clavubactin and Synulox in healthy cats. *Scientific World J.*, **2**, 1369–1378.
Vree, T.B., Dammers, E., and VanDuuren, E. (2003) Variable absortion of clavulanic acid after an oral dose of 25 mg/kg of Clavubactin and Synulox in healthy dogs. *J Vet Pharmacol Therp.*, **26(3)**, 165–171.

Chapter 146: Clindamycin

US Generic (Brand) Name: Clindamycin (Cleocin, Cleocin phosphate, Cleocin T, Clinda-Derm Topical Solution, Aquadrops, Clinsol, Clintabs, Antirobe)
Availability: Human approved – Clindamycin oral capsules (75, 150, 300 mg), oral solution (75 mg/5 mL × 100mL), sterile injectable (150 mg/mL × 2, 4, 5, 50, 60 mL), lotion 1% (60 mL), topical gel 1% (7.5, 30 g). Veterinary approved – Oral tablets and capsules 25, 75, 150, and 300 mg, oral solution 25 mg/mL (30 mL)
Resistance Mechanisms: Bacterial ribosomal target modification

Use

Active against anaerobes (including *Bacteriodes* spp.), aerobic and anaerobic *Streptococcus* spp., *Staphylococcus* spp., and *Actinomyces*. Also active against *Mycoplasma hominis*, *Babesia microti*, and *Toxoplasma gondi*. Useful in the treatment of brain and lung abscesses, endometritis, osteomyelitis, sinusitis, pneumonia, and other skin and soft tissue infections. Often used for periodontal infections involving anaerobic bacteria.

Contraindications/warnings

Hypersensitivity to clindamycin. Use with caution in atopic patients, hepatic impairment, and prior pseudomembranous colitis.

Dosage

Canine
Anaerobic/Periodontal: 11–33 mg/kg PO q12 h or 10 mg/kg IV, IM q12 h (Papich 2002).

Gram positive Prostatitis: 11–33 mg/kg PO q12 h for 6 weeks (Sykes and Westropp 2013).

Toxoplasmosis: 10–12 mg/kg PO q12 h × 4 weeks (Lappin 2013).

Hepatozoon: 10 mg/kg PO q8h with pyrimethamine 0.25 mg/kg PO q24 h and trimethoprim/sulfamethoxazole 15 mg/kg PO q12 h for 2–4 weeks. Follow with decoquinate (MacIntire *et al.*, 2006).

Babesia (alternative therapy): 25 mg/kg PO q12 h for 1–2 weeks (Wulansari *et al.*, 2003).

Feline
Anaerobic Infections/Sepsis: 5–11 mg/kg IV, SC, PO q8–12 h for 3–5 days (Greene 2006).

Toxoplasmosis: 12.5–25 mg/kg PO q12 h for 4 weeks or 10 mg/kg IV, IM q12 h (Papich 2002).

Dose adjustments

Reduce dose in severe hepatic impairment. No adjustments in renal impairment.

Administration

Follow oral medications with water to prevent esophageal strictures. Clindamycin phosphate must be diluted prior to IV administration. The concentration of clindamycin in diluent for IV infusion should not exceed 18 mg/mL. Infusion rates should not exceed 30 mg per minute. A dose of 300 mg in 50 mL may be given over 10 min, 600 mg/50 mL over 20 min or > 900 mg/100 mL over 30 min. Single intramuscular injections of greater than 600 mg are not recommended.

Electrolyte contents

Not significant.

Storage/stability

Store capsules, oral suspension, topical, and injectable solutions at room temperature. After reconstitution of the oral solution, do not refrigerate. Store at room temperature for up to 2 weeks. The IV infusion solution in normal saline or dextrose 5% in water is stable for 16 days at room temperature.

Adverse reactions

>10%
Loose stool, diarrhea, and esophagitis reported in cats and dogs.

1–10%
Nausea, vomiting, rashes, and injection site reactions reported in dogs and cats.

<1%
Colitis and esophageal strictures reported in dogs and cats.

Other species
Elevated liver enzymes, eosinophilia, granulocytopenia, neutropenia, thrombocytopenia, polyarthritis, thrombophlebitis, urticaria, severe profuse diarrhea, *C. difficile* overgrowth, and decreased renal function.

Drug interactions

Clindamycin can increase concentrations of pancuronium and other neuromuscular blocking agents. Antagonism has been demonstrated *in vitro* with erythromycin. Clindamycin may decrease levels of cyclosporine.

Monitoring

Monitor CBC, liver, and renal function for prolonged therapy. Observe closely for signs and symptoms of colitis, *C. difficile* overgrowth.

Overdose

Typically results in nausea, vomiting, and diarrhea. Gastrointestinal decontamination and supportive care are indicated. Hemodialysis is not effective.

Diagnostic test interference

None noted.

Mechanism

A bacteriostatic or bactericidal lincosamide. Binds to bacterial 50s ribosomal subunit resulting in inhibition of bacterial protein synthesis.

Pharmacology/kinetics

Absorption
Clindamycin is well absorbed following oral administration (72%). Peak concentrations following oral dosing occur at 1.25 h in dogs and 1 h in cats. Following IM injection in dogs the bioavailability is 87%.

Distribution
Widely distributed in fluids, tissues, bone, and urine.

CNS penetration
Diffuses poorly into the CSF.

Metabolism
Is metabolized in the liver to an active metabolite (N-dimethylclindamycin). In dogs, 1/3 of the dose is excreted into urine and the remaining is secreted into feces.

Half-life
The half-life in dogs is 4–5 h and 7.5 h in cats.

Pregnancy risk factor

Category B: Studies in rats and mice have not shown any teratogenic effects.

Lactation
Penetrates into milk and may cause sensitization or diarrhea in nursing animals.

References

Greene, C. (2006) Gastrointestinal and intra-abdominal infections. In: *Infectious Disease of the Dog and Cat.* Greene, C. (ed.), Elsevier, St. Louis, MO, pp. 883–912.

Lappin, M.R. (2013) Toxoplasmosis. Ch. 72. In: *Canine and Feline Infectious Diseases*, Sykes, J.E. (ed.), Elsevier, St. Louis, MO, pp. 693–701.

MacIntire, D., Vincent-Johnson, N., *et al.* (2006) *Hepatazooan americanum* infection. In: *Infectious Disease of the Dog and Cat.* Greene, C. (ed.), Elsevier, St. Louis, MO, pp. 705–711.

Papich, M.G. (2002) *Saunders Handbook of Veterinary Drugs.* 2nd edn. Winkel, A. (ed.), W.B. Saunders Company, Philadelphia, pp. 140–142.

Sykes, J.E. and Westropp J.L. (2013) Bacterial infections of the genitourinary tract. Ch. 89. In: *Canine and Feline Infectious Diseases*, Sykes, J.E. (ed.), Elsevier, St. Louis, MO, pp. 871–885.

Wulansari, R., Wijaya, A., Ano, H., *et al.* (2003) Clindamycin in the treatment of Babesia gibsoni infections in dogs. *J Am Anim Hosp Assoc.,* **39(6)**, 558–562

Further reading

Batzias, G.C., Delis, G.A., and Athanasiou, L.V. (2005) Clindamycin bioavailability and pharmacokinetics following oral administration of clindamycin capsules in dogs. *The Vet J.,* **170(3)**, 339–345.

Budsberg, S.C., Kemp, D.T., and Wolski, N. (1992) Pharmacokinetics of clindamycin phosphate in dogs after single intravenous and intramuscular administration. *Am J Vet Res.,* **53(12)**, 2333–2336.

Sun, F.F. and His, R.S. (1973) Metabolism of clindamycin. I. Absorption and excretion of clindamycin in the rat and dog. *J Pharm Sci.,* **62(8)**, 1265–1269.

Chapter 147: Dicloxacillin

US Generic (Brand) Name: Dicloxacillin (Dycill, Dynapen, Pathocil)
Availability: Human approved – Oral capsules as dicloxacillin sodium (125, 250, 500 mg).
Resistance Mechanisms: Altered penicillin binding proteins, increased beta-lactamase production, altered permeability

Use

Used for skin and soft tissue infections, otitis externa, mastitis, septic arthritis, pneumonia, and osteomyelitis caused by penicillinase producing *Staphylococcus* spp. Not for use in severe, life-threatening infections.

Contraindications/warnings

Contraindicated in penicillin and cephalosporin allergic patients.

Dosage

Canine
Susceptible Infections: 11–55 mg/kg PO q8 h (Papich 2002).

Feline
Susceptible Infections: 11–55 mg/kg PO q8 h (Papich 2002).

Dose adjustments

No dose adjustments are necessary in renal impairment.

Administration

Administer capsules 1 h prior or 2 h after a meal. Food decreases absorption rate and amount.

Electrolyte contents

One 250 mg capsule contains 13 mg (0.6 mEq) of sodium.

Storage/stability

Capsules should be stored at room temperature in tight containers.

Adverse reactions

>10
Nausea and anorexia reported in dogs.

1–10%
Vomiting and diarrhea reported in dogs.

<1%
At high doses, ataxia, tachypnea, edema, and tachycardia are reported in dogs.

Other species
Elevated liver enzyme activity, BUN and creatinine, agranulocytosis, eosinophilia, anemia, leucopenia, neutropenia, serum sickness, seizures, colitis, fever, rashes, and hematuria are reported.

Drug interactions

Dicloxacillin decreases the effects of cyclosporine. Allopurinol and renal toxic drugs can increase dicloxacillin plasma concentrations and toxicity.

Monitoring

For prolonged therapy, get baseline CBC and renal and liver panels.

Overdose

Similar to other penicillins, neuromuscular hypersensitivity, encephalopathy, seizures, and electrolyte imbalances (potassium, sodium), especially in renal failure. Gastrointestinal decontamination and supportive care may be required. Hemodialysis only removes 0–5% of the dose.

Diagnostic test interference

False-positive urine/serum proteins, uric acid, and urinary steroids. Alters urine glucose with Clinitest.

Mechanism

A bactericidal antistaphylococcal penicillin. Inhibits bacterial cell wall synthesis by binding to penicillin binding proteins, resulting in the inhibition of the final transpeptidation step of peptidoglycan synthesis.

Pharmacology/kinetics

Absorption
Oral absorption is variable and minimal in dogs (23%). Food decreases the rate and extent of absorption. Intramuscular administration shows no advantage over oral dosing in dogs.

Distribution
Widely distributed throughout body fluids and tissues including synovial fluid, bone, liver, kidney, and bile. Protein binding in dogs is 90%.

CNS penetration
Penetration into the CNS in all species studied is minimal and not therapeutic.

Metabolism
Dicloxacillin is hydrolyzed to inactive penicilloic acids and hydroxylated to active metabolites. Elimination of the parent drug is primarily renal with a small amount excreted via biliary elimination. Approximately 62% of the parent drug and 10–20% of the active metabolite is excreted in canine urine.

Half-life

The half-life is variable in dogs and reported to be between 20 min and 2.6 h.

Pregnancy risk factor

Category B: Dicloxacillin crosses the placenta but has not been associated with any teratogenic effects in laboratory animals or humans.

Lactation

Dicloxacillin crosses into milk, which may result in diarrhea and hypersensitization of nursing animals.

Reference

Papich, M.G. (2002) *Saunders Handbook of Veterinary Drugs*. 2nd edn. Winkel, A. (ed.), W.B. Saunders Company, Philadelphia, pp. 137–138.

Further reading

Dimitrova, D.J., Pashov, D.A., and Dimitrov, D.S. (1988) Dicloxacillin pharmacokinetics in dogs after intravenous, intramuscular and oral administration. *J Vet Pharmacol Therap.*, **21**, 414–417.

Vasilev, V.K. (1977) Study of the pharmacokinetics of dicloxacillin used parenterally in an experiment. *Antibiotiki.*, **22(5)**, 414–417.

Chapter 148: Doxycycline

US Generic (Brand) Name: Doxycycline hyclate, doxycycline monohydrate (Atridox, Doxy, Bio-tab, Periostat, Vibramycin, Vibra-Tabs)
Availability: Human approved: Doxycycline hyclate tablets and capsules (20, 50, 100 mg), Doxycycline monohydrate tablets and capsules (50, 75, 100, 150 mg), Vibramycin powder for oral suspension (monohydrate) 5 mg/mL (60 mL), oral syrup (calcium) 10 mg/mL (473 mLs), sterile injectable powder (hyclate) (100, 200 mg vials), Compounded oral suspension.
Resistance mechanisms: Increased efflux, ribosomal protection, tetracycline modification.

Use

Primarily used to treat atypical infections caused by *Rickettsia*, *Chlamydia*, and *Mycoplasma*. It also covers some gram negative/positive organisms, including some vancomycin-resistant *Enterococci*. Has activity against *Actinomyces* spp., *Bartonella* spp., *Borrelia burgdorferi*, *Brucella* spp., *Campylobacter jejuni*, *Chlamydia* spp., *Coxiella* spp., *Erlichia* spp, *Enterococcus* spp., *Leptospira interrogans*, *Mycoplasma* spp., *Neisseria* spp., *Rickettsia* spp., *Staphylococcus aureus* (methacillin-resistant), *Stenotrophomonas* spp., *Treponema* spp., *Ureaplasma*, *Vibrio cholera*, and *Yersinia pestis*. Commonly used for *Wolbachia* in heartworm positive animals.

Contraindications/warnings

Hypersensitivity to tetracyclines. Contraindicated in pregnant, lactating, or young/growing animals as well as in severe liver impairment or esophageal inflammation/strictures. Follow oral doses with water. Do not use expired drug or unstable compounded drug suspensions (see stability).

Dosage

Canine

Ehrlichiosis: 10 mg/kg PO, IV q12–24 h for 30 days (Greene *et al.*, 2006).

Wolbachia: 10 mg/kg PO once daily for 30 days with ivermectin/pyrantel pamoate 6–14 µg/kg PO once every 15 days for 6 months (Grandi and Quintavalla 2010).

Salmon poisoning (neosrickettsia helmintheca): 5 mg/kg PO, IV q12 h × 14 days with praziquantel 10–30 mg/kg PO q24 h × 1–2 days to cover flukes (Sykes and Papich 2013).

Feline

Systemic infections: 5–11 mg/kg PO, IV q12 h (Greene *et al.*, 2006).

Ehrlichiosis/Anaplasmosis: 5–10 mg/kg PO q12 h × 21 days (Greene *et al.*, 2006).

Dose adjustments

Do not give to patients with severe liver impairment; reduce dose frequency with moderate to severe renal impairment.

Administration

The tablets should be administered with food to decrease gastrointestinal upset. Oral doses should be followed with food and water to assure that the dose does not dissolve in the esophagus causing irritation and esophageal strictures. The sterile intravenous powder is reconstituted with either 10 or 20 mL of sterile water for injection and then diluted further with normal saline or dextrose 5% in water. Each 100 mg should be diluted with 100 mL to 1 L of solution (0.1–1 mg/mL). Concentrated solutions may be very irritating to the tissues if given IM or SC. Intravenous doses should be administered over 1–4 h. Avoid extravasation. Keep animal out of direct sunlight to avoid photosensitivity reactions.

Electrolyte contents

Not significant.

Storage/stability

Store tablets, capsules, oral powder, oral powder, injectable powder at room temperature, in a tight container, protected from light. Following reconstitution the oral suspension should be refrigerated and discarded after 14 days. Following reconstitution of the injectable powder the vial is good for 12 h at room temperature or 72 h refrigerated. Compounded products are not recommended due to their instability in many solutions. The commercially available doxycycline hyclate tablets can be mixed with ora-plus/ora-sweet (1:1), which is stable for only 7 days at room temperature or refrigerated at concentrations of 33.3 and 166.7 mg/mL. Do not use compounded suspensions beyond 7 days unless stability information can be confirmed. All tetracyclines degrade into toxic metabolites when exposed to light, heat, humidity, or air. Avoid using expired drug or compounded drugs that may not be efficacious and may contain significant amounts of renal toxic degradation products (anhydro-4-epitetracycline).

Adverse reactions

>10%
Vomiting, nausea, loss of appetite, and elevated ALT reported in cats and dogs. For oral administration, the monohydrate salt is preferred, which is shown to have less gastrointestinal upset than the hyclate salt.

1–10%
Anorexia, diarrhea, and fever have been reported in cats and dogs. Severe esophagitis, esophageal adhesions and strictures are reported in dogs and cats if oral doses of doxycycline are not followed with food or water.

Other species
Hepatotoxicity (hyperbilirubinemia, hepatic cholestasis, hepatitis), tooth discoloration, and altered bone growth rates, eosinophilia, phlebitis, photosensitivity, urticarial, neutropenia, rash, hemolytic anemia, thrombocytopenia, dose-related increase in BUN, and intracranial hypertension have been reported.

Drug interactions

Concurrent administration with divalent or trivalent cations (aluminum, calcium, magnesium, iron) in antacids, bismuth subsalicylate or vitamins (VAL syrup) may decrease doxycycline oral bioavailability if taken concurrently. Barbiturates (phenobarbital), bile acid sequestrants, sulcrafate, nafcillin, and rifamycins can decrease the half-life of doxycycline. Doxycycline can increase the effects/toxicity of benzodiazepams (midazolam), calcium channel blockers, cyclosporine, mirtazepine, quinidine, sildenafil, tacrolimus, and cisapride.

Monitoring

Monitor liver function, efficacy, and gastrointestinal side effects.

Overdose

May result in nausea, vomiting, diarrhea, elevated liver enzymes, and hypotension. Gastrointestinal decontamination and supportive care should be instituted. Dialysis only removes 5% of the drug.

Diagnostic test interference

False negative urine glucose using Clinistix Test-Tape.

Mechanism

A bacteriostatic tetracycline. Binds to 30s and 50s bacterial ribosomes resulting in protein synthesis inhibition.

Pharmacology/kinetics

Absorption
Excellent oral absorption in cats and dogs (>75%). Drug interactions can significantly reduce oral absorption.

Distribution

Distributes widely into fluids and tissues including aqueous humor, prostate, seminal fluid, pleural space, and synovial fluid. Urinary concentrations in cats and dogs following a 5 mg/kg PO q12 h dose were reported to be sufficient to inhibit the growth of a significant number of urinary tract pathogens at 4 h after the dose.

CNS penetration

Poor penetration into the CNS.

Metabolism

Not metabolized in the liver, primarily gets inactivated in the gastrointestinal tract by chelate formation. Elimination is via both feces and urine.

Half-life

Following intravenous administration the half-life in dogs is 7 h and in cats is 5 h.

Pregnancy risk factor

Category D: Readily crosses the placenta. Use in pregnancy causes permanent yellow-gray-brown discoloration of teeth. Also forms complex in bone-forming tissues leading to decreased fibula growth rates.

Lactation

Readily crosses into milk and is not recommended due to side effects in growing animals.

References

Grandi, G. and Quintavalla, C. (2010) A combination of doxycycline and ivermectin is adulticidal in dogs with naturally acquired heartworm disease (*Dirofilaria immitis*). *Vet Parasit.*, **169**, 347–351.

Greene, C.K., Hartmann, K., *et al.* (2006) Antimicrobial drug formulary. In: *Infectious Disease of the Dog and Cat*. Greene, C. (ed.). Elsevier, St. Louise, MO, pp. 1186–1333.

Sykes, J.E. and Papich, M.G. (2013) Antibacterial drugs. Ch. 8. In: *Canine and Feline Infectious Diseases*, Sykes, J.E. (ed.), Elsevier, St. Louis, MO. pp. 66–86.

Further reading

Papich, M.G., Davidson, G.S., Fortier, L.A., *et al.* (2013) Doxycycline concentration over time after storage in a compounded veterinary preparation. *J Amer Vet Med Assoc.*, **242(12)**, 1674–1678.

Riond, J.L., Vaden S.L., and Riviere, J.E. (1990) Comparative pharmacokinetics of doxycycline in cats and dogs. *J Vet Pharmacol Ther.*, **13(4)**, 415–424.

Schulz, B.S., Hupfauer, S., Ammer, H., *et al.* (2011) Suspected side effects of doxycycline use in dogs: a retrospective study of 386 cases. *Vet Record.*, **169**, 229–233.

Schulz, B.S., Zauscher, S., Ammer, H., *et al.* (2013) Side effects suspected to be related to doxycycline use in cats. *Vet Record.*, **172**, 184–185.

Wilson, B.J., Norris, J.M., Malik, R., *et al.* (2006) Susceptibility of bacteria from feline and canine urinary tract infections to doxycycline and tetracycline concentrations attained in urine four hours after oral dosage. *Aust Vet J.*, **84(1–2)**, 8–11.

Wilson, R.C., Kemp, D.T., Kitzman, J.V., *et al.* (1988) Pharmacokinetics of doxycycline in dogs. *Can J Vet Res.*, **52(1)**, 12–14.

Chapter 149: Enrofloxacin

US Generic (Brand) Name: Enrofloxacin (Baytril)
Availability: Veterinary approved – Enrofloxacin film coated and flavored tablets (22.7, 68, 136 mg), sterile injectable for small animals (22.7 mg/mL × 20 mL) and cattle (100 mg/mL × 100 mL), compounded oral suspension (22.95 mg/mL)
Resistance mechanisms: Altered DNA gyrase and topoisomerase, altered drug accumulation

Use

Treatment of infections of the lower respiratory tract, sinuses, skin, otitis, endometritis, bone/joints, UTI, prostatitis, bacteremia, and systemic infections. Indicated for gram negative organisms including *Pseudomonas*, *E. coli*, *Klebsiella*, *Enterobacter*, *Proteus*, *Citrobacter*, *Salmonella*, *Moraxella*, *Campylobacter*, *Brucella*, and *Pasteurella*. Also covers *Serratia*, *Shigella*, *Yersinia*, and *Vibrio* spp. It is typically less effective than ciprofloxacin against *Pseudomonas*. Gram positive organisms including *Staphylococcus* spp. and some strains of *Streptococcus* spp. are susceptible. Covers some intracellular organisms and other atypical organisms including; *Mycoplasma*, *Leptospira*, *Borrelia*, *Isospora*, *Chlamydia*, *Mycobacterium tuberculosis* (not *M. avium*). Does not cover obligate anaerobes, *Enterococcus*, *Actinomyces*, or *Nocardia*.

Contraindications/warnings

Avoid in pregnant or lactating animals. Use with caution in patients with pre-existing cardiac disease due to prolongation of the Q-T interval. Use only with extreme caution in young animals due to arthropathy. Large, rapidly growing dogs 4–28 weeks of age are most susceptible. Use with caution in patients with known or suspected CNS disorders due to CNS stimulation. Reduce dose, use divided doses, and avoid intravenous bolus dosing in geriatric cats with renal impairment to avoid retinal degeneration. Avoid physically stressing, over exercising animals during therapy due to increased predisposition to tendon inflammation, rupture. Use of cattle injectable is alkaline (pH = 10.5) and contains benzyl alcohol and L-arginine, which is contraindicated in small animals due to injection site irritation, abscess formation, and thrombophlebitis if given intravenously. Avoid long term exposure to UV light due to photosensitivity reactions.

Dosage

May give in divided doses if high single doses are not tolerated, or in geriatric cats.

Canine

Susceptible infections: 5–20 mg/kg q24 h IM, IV, or PO (Papich 2002), use higher doses for *Pseudomonas* infections.

Gram negative chronic prostatitis: 20 mg/kg q24 h PO × 6 weeks (Sykes and Westropp 2013).

Uncomplicated bladder infections: 20 mg/kg PO q24 h × 3 days (Daniels *et al.*, 2014).

Feline

Susceptible infections: 5 mg/kg q24 h PO, IM (avoid IV use in cats) (Papich 2002).

Dose adjustments

Reduce dose frequency in severe renal impairment (48 h instead of q24 h).

Administration

Oral doses best absorbed on an empty stomach, but may be administer with food to decrease gastrointestinal upset. Maintain hydration and urinary output. The injectable solution is labeled for IM injection and not approved for IV dosing, but has been administered safely to dogs if infused slowly. Do not administer IV to cats. Enrofloxacin (22.7 mg/mL) can be diluted with 0.9% saline > 1:1 dilution and administered IV slowly over 15–30 min. Subcutaneous dosing has also been safely performed in dogs.

Electrolyte contents

Not significant.

Storage/stability

Store tablets and injectable solution at room temperature in tight containers protected from light. Do not freeze. A compounded oral suspension can be made with Baytril film tablets in cherry syrup to make a 22.95 mg/mL suspension. This is stable for 56 days at room temperature or refrigerated.

Adverse reactions

>10%

Nausea, diarrhea, and anorexia reported in dogs and cats.

1–10%

Vomiting and elevated liver enzyme activity in dogs and cats.

<1%

Concentration dependent reversible CNS toxicity (ataxia, depression, lethargy, nervousness, seizures, and vocalization) reported in cats and dogs. Mydriasis, retinal degeneration, and blindness in cats following high doses (>20 mg/kg, accumulation in renal failure, bolus IV injections).

Other species

Fluoroquinolone use in other species has resulted in elevated liver enzyme activity, crystaluria, hypertension, angina pectoris, myocardial infarction, cardiopulmonary arrest, dyspnea, photosensitivity, rash, elevated serum creatinine, arthralgia, cartilage damage, lameness, cataracts, spermatogenesis, tendon rupture, allergic reactions, agranulocytosis, prolongation of the Q-T interval, erythema multiforme, toxic epidermal necrolysis, and pseudomembranous colitis.

Drug interactions

Bioavailability is decreased by enteral feedings containing cations. Aluminum or magnesium products, sucralfate, calcium, iron, zinc, and multiple vitamins with minerals may all decrease absorption by >90%. Give these agents at least 2–4 h from the dose and consider switching to an H_2 antagonist or omeprazole. Theophylline and NSAIDs may increase the CNS stimulation of enrofloxacin. H_2 antagonists and loop diuretics may inhibit renal elimination of quinolones, antineoplastics may decrease absorption of enrofloxacin, enrofloxacin may increase cyclosporine concentrations. Use with caution with other agents that can cause prolongation of the Q-T interval (cisapride, macrolides, etc.).

Monitoring

Monitor for hypersensitivity reactions and CNS stimulation. Monitor cats for mydriasis and discontinue if it develops.

Overdose

Acute renal failure and seizures may result. Gastrointestinal decontamination and supportive care are recommended. Charcoal hemoprofusion has been reported to markedly reduce plasma concentrations of enrofloxacin in a cat with a severe (10×) overdose.

Diagnostic test interference

Enrofloxacin may cause a false positive result on urine glucose tests with Clintest.

Mechanism

A bactericidal fluoroquinolone. Inhibits bacterial DNA gyrase resulting in inhibition of relaxation of supercoiled DNA and double stranded DNA breaks.

Pharmacology/kinetics

Absorption
Following oral doses, bioavailability is 80% in dogs. Plasma concentrations in dogs are proportional to the oral dose. It is unknown in cats. Rapid and almost complete absorption occurs within 30 min following IM doses in dogs.

Distribution
Distributes widely into tissues. High concentrations in kidneys, gallbladder, liver, lungs, prostate, and urogenital tissues. Present in very high concentrations in dog urine and most other fluids (saliva, nasal and bronchial secretions, sputum, lymph, peritoneal fluid, and bile). Lowest concentrations are reported from bone, muscle, fat, and skin. Protein binding in dogs is only 27%.

CNS penetration
Enrofloxacin has limited penetration into the CSF (<10%).

Metabolism
Enrofloxacin is metabolized in the liver of cats and dogs to ciprofloxacin, an active desmethyl metabolite accounting for approximately 10–20% of the plasma concentration. Enrofloxacin and ciprofloxacin are eliminated via renal and non-renal routes. Approximately 30–50% is excreted in urine.

Half-life
The half-life in dogs is 4–5 h and 6 h in cats.

Pregnancy risk factor

Category C: No evidence of teratogenic effects in laboratory animals. However, due to potential fetal cartilage effects, the drug is not recommended in pregnant patients.

Lactation
Enrofloxacin is excreted into milk in significant concentrations and may cause damage to the cartilage of nursing animals.

References

Daniels, J.B., Tracy, G., Irom, S.J., *et al.* (2014) Fluoroquinolone levels in healthy dog urine following a 20-mg/kg oral dose of enrofloxacin exceed mutant prevention concentration targets against *Escericha coli* isolated from canine urinary tract infections. *J Vet Pharmacol Ther.*, **37(2)**, 201–204.

Papich, M.G. (2002) *Saunders Handbook of Veterinary Drugs.* 2nd edn. Winkel, A. (ed.), W.B. Saunders Company, Philadelphia, pp. 236–237.

Sykes, J.E. and Westropp, J.L. (2013) Bacterial infections of the genitourinary tract. Ch. 89. In: *Canine and Feline Infectious Diseases*, Sykes, J.E. (ed.), Elsevier, St. Louis, MO. pp. 871–885.

Further reading

Petritz, O.A., Guzman, D.S., Wiebe, V., and Papich, M. (2013) Stability of three commonly compounded extemporaneous enrofloxacin suspensions for oral administration to exotic animals. *J Am Med Assoc.*, **243(1)**, 85–90.

Walker, R.D., Stein, G.E., Hauptmam, J.G., *et al.* (1992) Pharmacokinetic evaluation of enrofloxacin administration orally to healthy dogs. *Am J Vet Res.*, **53(12)**, 2315–2319.

Wiebe, V. and Hamilton, P. (2002) Fluoroquinolone-induced retinal degeneration in cats. *J Am Vet Med Assoc.*, **221(11)**, 1568–1571.

Chapter 150: Erythromycin

US Generic (Brand) Name: Erythromycin (Ery-tabs, Erythromycin Filmtabs, EYRC, PCE Dispertab, EES Granules, EES tabs, EryPed 400, Eryped drops, Eythrocin, Eryzole, Pediazole, Gallimycin)
Availability: Human approved – Erthromycin base oral delayed release caps (250 mg), delayed release tabs (250, 333, 500 mg), film coated tabs (250, 500 mg), erythromycin estolate oral capsules (250 mg) and suspension (125 mg/5 mL, 250 mg/5 mL), eryth-romycin ethylsuccinate oral film tabs (400 mg), chew tabs (200 mg), suspension (100 mg/2.5 mL, 200 mg/5 mL, 400 mg/5 mL), erthromycin lactobi-onate sterile intravenous injection (500 mg, 1 g), and erthromycin stearate oral film tablets (250, 500 mg). Veterinary approved – Erthromycin IM injection (100 mg/mL × 100 mL)
Resistance mechanisms: Ribosomal modification (erm gene), altered efflux (mefE gene)

Use

Used primarily for skin infections and upper respiratory infections (including *Bordetella* pneumonias) in dogs and cats. Limited spectrum of activity, primarily active against gram positive aerobic bacteria (*S. aureus*, *S. pseudintermedius*, *Streptococcus* spp.) and some atypical organisms (*Rhodococcus, Chlamydia, Corynebacterium*). Has more limited spectrum and greater toxicity than clar-ithromycin and azithromycin so is less commonly used. Has been used in small animals for gastroparesis.

Contraindications/warnings

Hypersensitivity to macrolides, hepatic impairment, concomitant use with cisapride or other drugs with Q-T prolongation. Do not use IM injectable intravenously. Do not use the lactobionate injectable in animals due to high benzyl alcohol content. Avoid use in combination with other hepatotoxic drugs.

Dosage

Canine
Susceptible infections: 10–20 mg/kg PO q8–12 h (Papich 2002).

Prokinetic effects: 0.5–1 mg/kg PO q8–12 h (Hall and Washabau 2000).

Feline
Susceptible infections: 10–20 mg/kg PO q8–12 h (Papich 2002).

Prokinetic effects: 0.5–1 mg/kg PO q 8–12 h (Hall and Washabau 2000).

Dose adjustments

Do not use with significant hepatic impairment. No dose adjustment needed in renal impairment.

Administration

Store tablets, capsules, and suspensions according to the manufacturer's directions. Shake suspensions well prior to administering. The stearate salt and non-delayed release base formulations should be administered on an empty stomach while the others may be given with food to decrease gastrointestinal upset. Erythromycin lactobi-onate sterile vials containing 500 mg or 1 g should be diluted with 10 or 20 mL of sterile water (without preservative), respectively. This results in a solution con-taining 50 mg/mL. This must be further diluted with 0.9% NaCl, LRS, or other manufacturer-recommended solutions to a concentration of 1 mg/mL. A continuous IV infusion is required due to local irritating effects of bolus administration.

Electrolyte contents

Filmtablets (250 mg) have 70 mg (3mEq) sodium and oral suspension (ethylsuccinate) 200 mg/5 mL has 29 mg (1.3 mEq) sodium. The injectable solution also contains benzyl alcohol, which may be toxic to animals.

Storage/stability

Store tablets and capsules at room temperature in tight containers. Erythromycin estolate suspension should be refrigerated. The ethylsuccinate suspension should be refrigerated until dispensed to preserve taste, but is stable for 14 days at room temperature. The ethylsucci-nate granules for oral suspension are stored at room temperature and stable refrigerated for 10 days. EryPed (ethylsuccinate suspension) is stored at room tempera-ture prior to reconstitution and is stable for 35 days if kept at <25°C. Following reconstitution, the injectable solution (50 mg/mL) is stable for 24 h at room temper-ature or 2 weeks refrigerated.

>10%

Nausea, vomiting, and diarrhea reported in dogs and cats.

1–10%

Elevated liver enzyme activity and hypersensitivity reactions reported in dogs and cats.

<1%

Neurologic toxicity reported in dogs.

Other species

In other mammals, cholestatic jaundice (primarily with estolate), phlebitis, eosinophilia, fever, hypertrophic pyloric stenosis, rash, pseudomembranous colitis, thrombocytopenia, ventricular arrhythmias, and torsade de pointes (Q-T prolongation) have been reported.

Drug interactions

Erythromycin decreases clearance and increases toxicity of cyclosporine, digoxin, bromocriptine, methylprednisolone, alfentanil, sildenafil, theophylline, warfarin, vinblastine and midazolam, alprazolam, and triazolam. Antifungal agents (itraconazole, ketoconazole, etc.), diltiazem, verapamil, and omeprazole may increase erythromycin plasma concentrations and increase toxicity. *In vitro* antagonism is seen with chloramphenicol, clindamycin, and lincomycin. Concomitant use with cisapride, quinidine, and disopyramide may increase risk of Q-T prolongation. Sucralfate may decrease absorption and should be administered 2 h apart from erythromycin.

Monitoring

Monitor liver enzyme activity and electrolytes (sodium) in patients where sodium loads may be a problem.

Overdose

Symptoms of nausea, vomiting, and diarrhea may result. Supportive care is recommended. Extreme overdoses may result in Torsade de pointes (Q-T interval prolongation), bradycardia, and complete heart block. Supportive care including epinephrine, atropine (if bradycardia) is recommended. Hemodialysis removes 5–20% of the drug.

Diagnostic test interference

False positive urinary catecholamines.

Mechanism

Bacteriostatic macrolide. Binds to bacterial 50s ribosomal subunit inhibiting protein synthesis. May be bacteriostatic at low concentrations or bactericidal at high concentrations, depending on the organism and growth phase.

Pharmacology/kinetics

Absorption

Absorption of erythromycin is variable and dependent on the formulation used. Salt forms are better absorbed than the base. Ethylsuccinate is better absorbed with food, but neither the tabs or suspensions are absorbed in cats and only the suspension (EryPed, EES) is absorbed well in dogs. The estolate salt (capsules, suspension) appears to have the best oral absorption in dogs.

Distribution

Widely distributed throughout body tissues and fluids including lungs, prostate, liver, and bile. Protein binding is dependent on the salt form and is between 70–96%.

CNS penetration

Penetration into the CSF is low (2–13%).

Metabolism

Erthromycin is metabolized in the liver. The parent drug and the inactive N-desmethyl metabolite are excreted primarily via biliary excretion into feces. Only small amounts are excreted into urine (2–15%).

Half-life

The half-life after oral absorption is variable in dogs and cats and is dependent on the formulation used. In dogs and cats it is reported to be around 1.5–2.9 h.

Pregnancy risk factor

Category B: Erthromycin penetrates across the placenta, fetal levels are approximately 5–20% of maternal levels. Studies in rats and mice have not shown any teratogenic effects.

Lactation

Erthromycin is excreted into milk and may result in diarrhea in nursing animals.

References

Hall, J. and Washabau, R. (2000) Gastric prokinetic agents. *Kirk's Current Veterinary Therapy: XIII. Small Animal Practice.* Bonagura, J. (ed.), W.B. Saunders Company, Philadelphia, pp. 609–617.

Papich, M.G. (2002) *Saunders Handbook of Veterinary Drugs.* 2nd edn. Winkel, A. (ed.), W.B. Saunders Company, Philadelphia, pp. 246–247.

Further reading

Albarello, G.A., Kreil, V.E., Ambros, L.A., *et al.* (2008) Pharmacokinetics of erythromycin after administration of intravenous and various oral dosage forms to dogs. *J Vet Pharmacol Ther.*, **31(6)**, 496–500.

Albarellos, G.A., Montoya, L., and Landoni, M.F. (2011) Pharmacokinetics of erythromycin after intravenous, intramuscular and oral administration to cats. *Vet J.*, **187(1)**, 129–132.

Kunkle, G.A., Sundloft, S., and Keisling, K. (1995) Adverse side effects of oral antibacterial therapy in dogs and cats: an epidemiologic study of pet owner's observations. *J Am Animal Hospital Assoc.*, **31(1)**, 46–55.

Chapter 151: Florfenicol

US Generic (Brand) Name: Florfenicol (Nuflor, Aquaflor)
Availability: Veterinary approved – Florfenicol sterile injectable solution (300 mg/mL) for cattle or 23 mg/mL oral solution to be added to drinking water for pigs
Resistance Mechanisms: Reduced membrane permeability, mutation of 50s ribosomes, increased chloramphenicol acetyltransferases

Use

Florfenicol has not been studied in depth in small animals. It is a derivative of chloramphenicol and has a similar spectrum of activity. It is more active than chloramphenicol and like chloramphenicol it is lipophilic and can cross the blood brain barrier as well as penetrate intracellularly. It has been substituted in small animals when chloramphenicol has not been available. It should only be used for severe infections due to organisms resistant to less toxic drugs or infections located in hard to penetrate spaces (CNS). It has a wide spectrum of activity against gram positive and negative organisms. Active against *Pasteurella multocida*, *Streptococococcus* spp., *Salmonella*, *Brucella*, *Richettsia*, vancomycin resistant *Enterococci*, methicillin resistant *Staphylococcus* spp., *Shigella*, and *Haemophilus*. Also has activity against anaerobes, *Bacteriodes*, *Clostridium*, and *Fusobacterium*.

Contraindications/warnings

Hypersensitivity to chloramphenicol or florfenicol, avoid use in severe hepatic impairment and neonatal animals, dose related side effects (bone marrow suppression) may be more common in renal/hepatic impairment. Avoid contact if pregnant or lactating.

Dosage

Only use when other antibiotics cannot be employed.

Canine
Severe infections: 20 mg/kg IM q8 h for 3–5 days (Greene *et al.*, 2006).

Feline
Severe infections: 22 mg/kg IM, PO q12 h for 3–5 days (Greene *et al.*, 2006).

Dose adjustments

Do not use in severe hepatic impairment. Increase dosing interval in severe renal impairment (q12 h versus q8 h).

Administration

There is little data on administration of florfenicol to small animals and few studies on long term use. Florfenicol injectable (Nuflor) 300 mg/mL is made for IM injection into cattle and can cause tissue irritation via this route. References using oral dosing in small animals have used bulk chemical rather than the commercial product (Nuflor). If oral dosing is used, a Pharmacy Compounding specialist should be consulted to either dilute the commercial product or obtain the chemical powder formulation.

Electrolyte contents

Not significant.

Storage/stability

Store florfenicol (Nuflor) injectable at room temperature and protect from freezing. Do not store in metal containers. Once opened the multidose vial should be discarded after 28 days.

Adverse reactions

>10%

Gastrointestinal side effects (nausea, vomiting) in both cats and dogs has been reported.

1–10%

Weight loss, dehydration, and CNS depression reported in dogs and cats.

<1%

Although dose related bone marrow suppression is reported at high doses (100 mg/kg) in dogs, florfenicol lacks a nitro group that has been associated with chloramphenicol induced, non-dose related irreversible aplastic anemia in people. A reversible dose-related bone marrow suppression (anemia, neutropenia) may still be seen.

Drug interactions

Erythromycin, clindamycin, lincomycin, and florfenicol compete for the same binding site on the ribosome and are antagonistic. Phenobarbital and rifampin may decrease florfenicol concentrations. Florfenicol may increase concentrations of digoxin, phenytoin and pentobarbital.

Monitoring

CBC, liver, and renal panel with prolonged dosing.

Overdose

Large doses administered to dogs have resulted in hepatotoxicity (elevated liver enzyme activity), CNS effects (vocalization), hematopoietic changes, renal tubule dilation, and testicular atrophy. Gastrointestinal decontamination and supportive care should be instituted. Hemodialysis is not expected to remove significant amounts of drug.

Diagnostic test interference

None noted.

Mechanism

A bacteriostatic thiamphenicol derivative. Reversibly binds to 50s ribosome in susceptible bacteria causing inhibition of protein synthesis.

Pharmacology/kinetics

Absorption

Good oral absorption in dogs (95%), but poor concentrations following subcutaneous injections. Oral and IM absorption in cats is around 100%. Cats maintain levels above the MIC of organisms following both oral and intramuscular injections.

Distribution

Distributes throughout the body including the CSF. High concentrations are found in lung, heart, pancreas, muscle, spleen, synovial, bile, kidney, urine, and aqueous humor. Protein binding in most species studied is between 12–19%.

CNS penetration

Readily penetrates across the blood brain barrier (25–50% plasma concentration) so therapeutic levels are achieved in the CSF.

Metabolism

Florfenicol is metabolized in the liver to florfenicol amine. Elimination is primarily renal with some biliary excretion.

Half-life

The half-life is short in dogs (only 1 h with IV injections), following oral administration, the concentrations remain above the MIC for 4 h. In cats, the half-life is much longer (IM: 5.6 h and PO: 7.8 h).

Pregnancy risk factor

Not studied (potentially Category C). Is expected to pass into the placenta in high concentration and may have significant toxicities in growing fetuses and neonatal animals.

Lactation

Readily distributes into milk. Due to potential toxicities in neonates, it is not recommended in nursing animals.

Reference

Greene, C., Hartmann, K., *et al.* (2006) Antimicrobial drug formulary. Appendix 8. In: *Infectious Disease of the Dog and Cat.* Greene, C. (ed.), Elsevier, St. Louis, MO, pp. 1186–1333.

Further reading

Cannon, M., Harford, S., and Davies, J. (1990) A comparative study on the inhibitory actions of chloramphenicol, thiamphicol and some fluorinated derivatives. *J Antimicrob Chemother.*, **26**, 307–317.

Freedom of Information Summary (n.d.) *Nuflor Injectable solution for the treatment of bovine interdigital phlegmon.* NADA 141–063. Schering-Plough Animal Health.

Papich, M.G. (2002) *Saunders Handbook of Veterinary Drugs.* 2nd edn. Winkel, A. (ed.), W.B. Saunders Company, Philadelphia, pp. 266–267.

Park, B.K., Lim, J.H., and Kim, M.S. (2008) Pharmacokinetics of florfenicol and its metabolite florfenicol amine in dogs. *Res Vet Sci.*, **84(1)**, 85–90.

Chapter 152: Gentamicin

US Generic (Brand) Name: Gentamicin (Garamycin, Gentamax, Gentafuse, Gentaved, Gentozen)
Availability: Human approved – Gentamicin sulfate injectable (IM, IV) 10 mg/mL and 40 mg/mL. Gentamicin sulfate in NaCl IV infusion (0.4 mg/mL, 0.6 mg/mL, 0.8 mg/mL, 1 mg/mL, 1.2 mg/mL, 1.6 mg/mL, 2 mg/mL, 2.4 mg/mL). Veterinary approved – Gentamicin sulfate 100 mg/mL (100, 250 mL)
Resistance Mechanisms: Aminoglycoside modifying enzymes, ribosome alteration, decreased permeability

Use

Used in serious gram negative infections due to *Pseudomonas, Proteus, Serratia* or gram positive infections involving the respiratory tract, soft tissue, urinary tract, septicemia, endocarditis, or bone infections. May be effective in severe bacterial endophthalmitis. Active against *Staphylococcus* spp. (including methicillin resistant strains), *Brucella, Enterococcus* spp., *Francisella tularensis, Streptococcus viridians,* and *Yersinia pestis.* Poor efficacy against intracellular *Bacilli,* anaerobes, and *Mycoplasma* spp. Only effective against some strains of *Mycobacteria* (*M. avium*), *Actinomyces, Nocardia* spp., *Corynebacterium,* and *Bacillus* spp. Amikacin is typically more effective against multidrug resistant strains and tobramycin is more effective against *Psuedomonas* spp.

Contraindications/warnings

Avoid use in animals with pre-existing renal impairment, vestibular impairment, electrolyte imbalances, and myasthenia gravis. Discontinue the drug if there are signs of hypersensitivity, ototoxicity, or nephrotoxicity. Provide subcutaneous fluid hydration in animals receiving subcutaneous amikacin. Avoid use of other renal toxic drugs in combination or prolonged therapy.

Dosage

Use ideal body weight in obese animals rather than total body weight, otherwise overdosing may occur. Once daily dosing is associated with less renal toxicity.

Canine

Susceptible infections: 2–4 mg/kg SC, IM, IV q8 h or 9–14 mg/kg SC, IM, IV q24 h (Papich 2002).

Feline

Susceptible infections: 3 mg/kg SC, IM, IV q8 h or 5–8 mg/kg SC, IM, IV q24 h (Papich 2002).

Dose adjustments

Dosing must be adjusted in renal failure. The dose can be reduced and the interval frequency extended in the presence of mild renal impairment. Give a loading dose to achieve adequate therapeutic concentrations, then give <50% of the total daily dose with moderate renal failure and <25% dose in severe renal failure. No dose adjustment for hepatic insufficiency.

Administration

Hydrate animals and evaluate renal parameters prior to administration. For IM, SC injection, draw up appropriate dose in a concentration of 10 or 40 mg/mL and give undiluted. For IV administration, the appropriate dose of 10 or 40 mg/mL solution should be withdrawn and diluted with 0.9% sodium chloride or 5% dextrose injection (50–200 mL) in an amount sufficient to allow infusion over 30 min to 2 h. Gentamicin should not be admixed with other drugs.

Electrolyte contents

Not significant.

Storage/stability

Store IV injectable solutions at room temperature in a tight, sealed container, protected from light. Do not refrigerate. Dilute solutions are stable in normal saline or D5W for 24 h at room temperature or in the refrigerator. Multidose vials should be discarded 28 days after opening.

Adverse reactions

>10%
Diarrhea, vomiting and injection site reactions (SC, IM doses) reported in dogs and cats. Renal toxicity is common at high doses (30 mg/kg q24 h) (Gentamicin > Amikacin > Tobramycin). Nephrotoxicity is polyuric, with increased fractional electrolyte excretion, glycosuria, and tubular casts, this may progress to oligouria. Typically reversible if a good urine output is maintained.

1–10%
Ototoxicity, high frequency hearing loss after prolonged therapy, may be irreversible. Neurotoxicity to the eighth cranial nerve (cochlear toxicity > vestibular toxicity), vestibular injury and bilateral irreversible damage is related to the amount of drug given and duration of treatment. Cats may have vestibular toxicity (ataxia, impaired righting) several days prior to renal toxicity. Gentamicin doses >40 mg/kg cause acute renal necrosis, neuromuscular blockade, and respiratory paralysis in cats.

Other species
Hypotension, rash, eosinophilia, tremor, arthralgia, dyspnea, weakness, hypersensitivity reactions, drug fever, and anemia.

Drug interactions

Concurrent use with nephrotoxic drugs (amphotericin-B, iron, calcium channel blockers, cisplatin, NSAIDs, vancomycin, and polymyxin) may increase renal side effects. Neuromuscular blocking drugs may prolong or increase risk of neuromuscular toxicities. Loop diuretics may increase nephrotoxicity and ototoxicity. Beta-lactam antibiotics are synergistic against some types of bacteria. Beta-lactams inactivate aminoglycosides *in vitro* in serum samples obtained from patients receiving concomitant therapy which may result in falsely decreased aminoglycoside concentrations. Aminoglycoside assays must be assessed immediately after collection.

Monitoring

Establish baseline renal function then monitor serum creatinine, urinalysis. Monitor animal closely for signs of tubular necrosis (casts appear early in urine). If possible, monitor peak and trough gentamicin concentrations. Trough concentrations should be <1 µg/mL for serious infections and <2 µg/mL for life threatening infections.

Overdose

Symptoms may include nausea, vomiting, diarrhea, acute renal failure, neurotoxicity, and neuromuscular paralysis. Maintain good urine output, polyionic electrolyte fluid therapy >3 weeks may be required to reverse renal damage. Oliguria is a poor prognostic sign. Edrophonium, neostigmine, calcium chloride, or calcium gluconate may be used to reverse muscle paralysis. Hemodialysis is typically not required, but can remove 30% of a dose.

Diagnostic test interference

Beta-lactams and cephalosporins may decrease aminoglycoside serum concentrations *in vitro*.

Mechanism

A bactericidal aminoglycoside. Inhibits protein synthesis in susceptible bacteria by binding to the 30s and 50s ribosomal subunits. This results in a defective bacterial cell membrane.

Pharmacology/kinetics

Absorption
Poor oral absorption, but has excellent absorption from IM and SC sites in cats and dogs. In dogs, bioavailability following IM and SC administration is 93–96% and in cats is 68–76%.

Distribution
Widely distributed throughout body fluids and tissues. Pleural and ascites fluid levels similar to serum levels. Gentamicin achieves therapeutic concentrations in bone, heart, gallbladder, and lungs. The volume of distribution is increased with edema, ascites, and fluid overload and is decreased with dehydration. Protein binding is <10% in dogs.

CNS penetration
The drug has minimal penetration across the blood brain barrier, even with inflammation (<30%).

Metabolism
Gentamicin is not metabolized to any significant degree and is primarily excreted in dogs and cats by glomerular filtration. Approximately 95% of the gentamicin dose is excreted in the urine of dogs.

Half-life

The half-life of gentamicin in dogs is between 54–68 min following IV administration.

Pregnancy risk factor

Category C. Gentamicin readily crosses the placenta and is shown to produce significant hypertension and renal toxicity in fetal animals. Although it does not appear to be teratogenic, due to it embryotoxic effects it is not recommended in pregnant animals.

Lactation

Gentamicin is excreted into milk (milk:plasma ratio = 0.1–0.4). Although aminoglycosides are not absorbed significantly from the gastrointestinal tract, nursing animals may still develop diarrhea.

Reference

Papich, M.G. (2002) *Saunders Handbook of Veterinary Drugs*. 2nd edn. Winkel, A. (ed.), W.B. Saunders Company, Philadelphia, pp. 287–289.

Further reading

Albarellos, G., Montoya, C., Ambros, L., *et al.* (2004) Multiple once daily dose pharmacokinetics and renal safety of gentamycin in dogs. *J Vet Pharmacol Ther.,* **27(1)**, 21–25.

Isoherranen, N., Lavy, E., and Soback, S. (2000) Pharmacokinetics of gentamycin C1, C1a and C2 in beagles after a single intravenous dose. *Antimicrob Agents Chemother.,* **44(6)**, 1443–1447.

Jernigan, A.D., Wilson, R.C., Hatch, R.C., *et al.* (1988) Pharmacokinetics of gentamicin after intravenous, intramuscular and subcutaneous administration in cats. *Am J Vet Res.,* **49(1)**, 32–35.

Wilson, R.C., Duran, S., Horton, C.R., *et al.* (1989) Bioavailability of gentamycin in dogs after intramuscular or subcutaneous injections. *Am J Vet Res.,* **50(10)**, 1748–1750.

Chapter 153: Imipenem and Cilastatin

US Generic (Brand) Name: Imipenem and cilastatin (Primaxin)
Availability: Human approved – Imipenem and cilastatin injectable for IM administration (500 mg imipenem/500 mg cilastatin, 750 mg imipenem/750 mg cilastatin), imipenem for IV administration (250 mg imipenem/250 mg cilastatin, 500 mg imipenem/500 mg cilastatin)
Resistance Mechanisms: Altered outer membrane protein (OprD) and increase in extended spectrum cephalosporinases (ESACs)

Use

Reserved for serious infections that include resistant gram negative bacilli, gram positive bacteria (methacillin sensitive), and anaerobes. Active against *Acinetobacter* spp., *Bacteriodes* spp., *Campylobacter* spp., *Bacillus* spp., *Prevotella* spp., *Bordetella* spp., *Citrobacter* spp., *E. coli, Erysipelthrix, Klebsiella* spp., *Proteus* spp., *Providencia* spp., *Pseudomonas* spp., *Rhodococcus* spp., *Serratia* spp., and *Nocardia* spp. Used for sepsis, liver abscess, osteomyelitis, pancreatitis, and peritonitis. Slightly less effective than meropenem against most organisms, imipenem is not active against methicillin-resistant *Staphylococcus* spp. or resistant strains of *Enterococcus faecium*.

Contraindications/warnings

Hypersensitivity to imipenem, penicillins or amide local anesthetics (if giving IM with lidocaine). Use with caution in renal impairment. Use with caution in patients with a history of seizures. Do not use the IM injectable intravenously.

Dosage

Canine
Susceptible infections: 3–10 mg/kg IV, IM q6–8 h, Typically 5 mg/kg IV, IM, SC q6–8 h (Papich 2002).

Feline
Susceptible infections: 3–10 mg/kg IV, IM q6–8 h, Typically 5 mg/kg IV, IM, SC q6–8 h (Papich 2002).

Dose adjustments

For moderate to severe renal failure, reduce dose and administer at the same interval or give normal dose with prolonged interval (q12–24 h).

Administration

Deep IM injections should be administered using a 21 gauge, 2 inch needle. IM injections may be painful so lidocaine is advised. The IM vial should be diluted with

2 or 3 ml of 1% lidocaine HCL (without epinephrine) into the 500 or 750 mg vials, respectively. The dose is withdrawn and injected deep IM into a large muscle. Large doses should be split. SC injections may be given by preparing the IV product with saline to 11 mg/mL and injection of the dose in the interscapular region. For intravenous infusion, the vial contents must be diluted with 10 mL of a compatible solution (0.9% NaCl, 5 or 10% dextrose, 5% dextrose with 0.9% NaCl, or 5 or 10% mannitol, etc.) and transferred to a minimum of 100 mL of infusion solution (<5 mg/mL). Infuse slowly to prevent seizures (500 mg/30 min or 1 g/60 min). Slow infusion if nausea and/or vomiting develop. Do not admix with other antibiotics, drugs.

Electrolyte contents

The sodium content for 1 g of IM injectable is 64.4 mg (2.8 mEq) and for the IV injectable is 73.6 mg (3.2 mEq).

Storage/stability

Store vials at room temperature. After reconstitution the solution is stable for 10 h at room temperature and 48 h refrigerated if diluted with normal saline. If diluted with 5 or 10% dextrose injection, 5% dextrose and 0.9% sodium chloride, it is stable for 4 h at room temperature and 24 h when refrigerated.

Adverse reactions

>10%
Nausea, salivation, and vomiting reported in cats and dogs.

1–10%
Diarrhea, injection site pain (vocalization), and irritation reported in dogs and cats.

<1%
Transient elevations in liver enzyme activity (ALT), eosinophilia, urine casts, and WBCs have been reported in dogs. Nephrotoxicity and seizures (imipenem > meropenem) have been reported with high doses in dogs.

Other species
Elevated BUN, Scr, elevated liver enzyme activity, anemia, eosinophilia, hypotension, neutropenia, palpitations, thrombocytopenia, rash, *C. difficile* colitis, and positive Coomb's tests have been reported.

Drug interactions

Nephrotoxic drugs (aminoglycosides, amphotericin, etc.) can contribute to an increase in potential plasma concentrations of imipenem as well as toxicities. Antagonism may occur with other penicillins and chloramphenicol. Imipenem is synergistic with aminoglycosides.

Monitoring

Monitor for allergic reactions. Monitor CBC and renal, hepatic panels with prolonged courses.

Overdose

Overdose symptoms may include nausea, vomiting, diarrhea, neuromuscular hyperirritability, seizures, and encephalopathy. Gastrointestinal lavage, hemodialysis, and supportive care (including anticonvulsant therapy) may be indicated. Approximately 20–50% of a dose is dialyzable.

Diagnostic test interference

Alters urinary glucose determination with Clinitest.

Mechanism

Bactericidal carbapenem. Binds bacterial penicillin-binding proteins (PBP-I) that result in more rapid weakening and interference of the cell wall then other beta-lactams. Cilastatin is not active against bacteria, it inhibits renal dipeptidases that block renal tubular metabolism of imipenem.

Pharmacology/kinetics

Absorption
Imipenem and cilastatin are poorly absorbed via oral administration. Following IM injection bioavailability is 60–75% in dogs and 93.25% in cats. Following SC injection, absorption in dogs and cats is complete (100–107.9%). Following a 5 mg/kg dose IV, IM, and SC, concentrations remained above the MIC of organisms for at least 9 h.

Distribution
Imipenem is widely distributed in fluids and tissues including the saliva, sputum, aqueous humor, bone, bile, reproductive tissues, heart valves, intestine,

peritoneal, interstitial, blister, and wound fluids. Imipenem is minimally bound to plasma proteins (<20%).

CNS penetration

Minimal penetration into the CSF (1–10%). Concentrations achieved after a 25 mg/kg IV dose q6 h to pediatric patients ranged from 0.27–3.5 µg/mL at 1.5–3.6 h after the dose.

Metabolism

Imipenem is partially metabolized by hydrolysis in the kidneys by dehydropeptidase to an inactive metabolite. The addition of cilastatin allows up to 70% of imipenem to be excreted into urine unchanged.

Half-life

The half-life in cats and dogs following IV, IM, and SC administration is between 0.8–1.5 h. The time above the MIC appears best for SC administration in both species.

Pregnancy risk factor

Category C: Imipenem crosses the placenta to the fetus. The drug does not appear to cause teratogenic effects but has increased embryonic loss and has shown increased maternal toxicity in pregnant monkeys.

Lactation

Only small amounts of drug pass into milk which would not be considered a significant risk to nursing animals. Diarrhea and altered gastrointestinal flora would be expected.

Reference

Papich, M.G. (2002) *Saunders Handbook of Veterinary Drugs*. 2nd edn. Winkel, A. (ed.), W.B. Saunders Company, Philadelphia, pp. 323–324.

Further reading

Albarellos, G.A., Denamiel, G.A., Montoya, L., *et al.* (2013) Pharmacokinetics of imipenem after intravenous, intramuscular and subcutaneous administration to cats. *J Feline Med Surg.*, **15(6)**, 483–487.

Barker, C.W., Zhang, W, Sanchez, S., *et al.* (2003) Pharmacokinetics of imipenem in dogs. *Am J Vet Res.*, **64(6)**, 694–699.

Chapter 154: Linezolid

US Generic (Brand) Name: Linezolid (Zyvox)
Availability: Human approved – Linezolid oral film coated tablets (400, 600 mg), oral suspension 20 mg/mL (150 mL), sterile injectable solution 2 mg/mL (100, 200, 300 mL)
Resistance Mechanisms: Altered ribosomal binding sites (23s rRNA)

Use

Limited use in veterinary medicine. Reserved for humans with vancomycin resistant *Enterococcus* spp. infections or methicillin resistant *Staphylococcal* spp. infections where no other alternative antibiotics can be used. Not indicated for gram negative infections. Its use in human medicine has been limited due to bone marrow suppression with long-term use. Has activity against *E. faecalis* (vancomycin resistant), *E. faecium* (vancomycin susceptible), *Staphylococcus epidermidis* (methacillin resistant), *S. haemolyticus*, Viridians group *Streptococci* spp., and *Pasteurella multocida*. Used in skin and soft tissue infections as well as osteomyelitis.

Contraindications/warnings

Hypersensitivity to linezolid. Use with extreme caution in patients with uncontrolled hypertension, pheochromocytoma, carcinoid syndrome, or untreated hyperthyroidism. Avoid use in patients with pre-existing blood dyscrasias or myelosuppressive disorders. Limit prolonged use (>14 days) due to potential for bone marrow suppression. Check for drug interactions prior to use.

Dosage

Canine

10 mg/kg PO or IV q8–12 h (Papich 2002).

Feline

10 mg/kg PO or IV q8–12 h (Papich 2002).

Dose adjustments

No dose adjusting mild to moderate renal or hepatic impairment. Accumulation of inactive metabolites may occur in severe renal impairment.

Administration

Give tablets with or without food. Limit quantity of tyramine-containing foods (smoked meats, cheese, etc). Reconstitute the oral powder with 123 mL of distilled water (2 portions), gently invert. Do not shake. Administer the IV pre-mix solution slowly over 30–120 min without further dilution. Do not mix with or administer with other medications.

Electrolyte contents

Not significant.

Storage/stability

Store tablets, oral suspension, and IV pre-mix solution at room temperature, protected from light. Following reconstitution the orange flavored suspension should be stored at room temperature and discarded after 21 days. The single-use pre-mix IV solution should remain in the manufacturer's overwrap and protected from freezing. It may slightly yellow, which does not affect its potency.

Adverse reactions

>10%
Loose stools and diarrhea have been reported in dogs and cats.

1–10%
Nausea and vomiting reported in dogs.

<1%
Pure red blood cell aplasia reported in one cat.

Other species
Hypertension, insomnia, pancreatitis, fever, rash, lactic acidosis, thrombocytopenia, leucopenia, neutropenia, elevated liver/renal enzymes, fungal infections, peripheral and optic neuropathy, blurred vision, and convulsions.

Drug interactions

Linezolid is an MAO inhibitor. Serotonin syndrome may occur if combined with the following agents: TCAs, SSRIs, meperidine, and dextromethorphan. Agents with adrenergic activity (phenylpropanolamine, sympathomimetic agents, vasopressors, and dopamine) may cause significant hypertension when combined with linezolid.

Rifampin can significantly decrease the peak concentrations and AUC of linezolid. Avoid use of concomitant drugs with myelosuppressive effects.

Monitoring

Monitor blood pressure, CBC, and platelet counts. CBC with differential should be monitored weekly. Bone marrow suppression is frequently seen in humans with prolonged use (>2 weeks).

Overdose

Side effects may include hypertension, agitation, and fever. For acute oral doses induce vomiting and institute GI decontamination. Supportive care including antihypertensives is indicated. Dialysis removes approximately 30% of a dose if available.

Diagnostic test interference

None noted.

Mechanism

A bacteriostatic oxazolidinone. It binds to the 23S ribosomal RNA of the 50S bacterial subunit causing inhibition of protein synthesis.

Pharmacology/kinetics

Absorption
Very well absorbed orally in dogs (>95%). High fat foods may slow the absorption but not the total amount absorbed.

Distribution
Distributes throughout fluid and tissue compartments that are well profused. Limited cortical bone exposure in dogs due to low water content. Protein binding is <35% in dogs.

CNS penetration
Measurable, but not therapeutic concentrations are reported in the brains of dogs.

Metabolism
Linezolid is metabolized in the liver to two inactive metabolites (aminoethoxy acetic acid and hydroxyethyl glycine). Renal excretion of the parent drug was noted

to be equivalent to fecal elimination in dogs, suggesting enterohepatic recirculation.

Half-life

In dogs, the half-life following oral administration was 3.6 h and after IV infusion was 3.9 h.

Pregnancy risk factor

Category C: No teratogenic effects noted in mice, rats, or rabbits, but embryo and fetal toxicities (total litter loss, decreased weights, and increased incidence of costal cartilage fusion) were noted.

Lactation

Linezolid and its metabolites are excreted in the milk of rats. Concentrations are similar to plasma concentrations. Diarrhea may occur in nursing animals.

Reference

Papich, M.G. (2002) *Saunders Handbook of Veterinary Drugs*. 2nd edn. Winkel, A. (ed.), W.B. Saunders Company, Philadelphia, pp. 370–371.

Further reading

Slatter, J.G., Adams, L.A., Bush, E.C., *et al.* (2002) Pharmacokinetics, toxicokinetics, distribution, metabolism and excretion of linezolid in mouse, rat and dog. *Xenobiotica.*, **32(10)**, 907–924.
Sykes, J.E. and Papich, M.G. (2013) Antibacterial drugs. Ch. 8. In: *Canine and Feline Infectious Diseases*, Sykes, J.E. (ed.), Elsevier, St. Louis, MO. pp. 66–86.

Chapter 155: Marbofloxacin

US Generic (Brand) Name: Marbofloxacin (Zeniquin)
Availability: Veterinary approved – Marbofloxacin oral tablets (25, 50, 100, 200 mg)
Resistance Mechanisms: Altered DNA gyrase and topoisomerase, altered drug accumulation

Use

Treatment of infections of the lower respiratory tract, sinuses, skin, otitis, endometritis, bone, joints, UTI, prostatitis, bacteremia, and systemic infections.

Marbofloxacin has a similar spectrum of activity compared to other veterinary fluoroquinolones. Indicated for gram negative organisms including *Pseudomonas, E. coli, Klebsiella, Enterobacter, Citrobacter, Salmonella, Moraxella, Campylobacter, Brucella,* and *Pasteurella.* May be less effective against *Pseudomonas* than ciprofloxacin. Gram positive organisms including *Staphylococcus* and some strains of *Streptococcus* are susceptible. Covers some intracellular organisms and other atypical organisms including; *Mycoplasma, Leptospira, Borrelia, Chlamydia, Mycobacterium tuberculosis* (not *M. avium*). Does not cover obligate anaerobes, *Enterococcus, Actinomyces,* or *Nocardia.*

Contraindications/warnings

Avoid or reduce dose in patients with renal failure. Avoid in pregnant or lactating animals or those with pre-existing cardiac disease involving Q-T prolongation. Use only with extreme caution in young animals due to arthropathy. Large, rapidly growing dogs 4–28 weeks of age are most susceptible. Use with caution in patients with known or suspected CNS disorders, since CNS stimulation can occur. Avoid long term UV exposure due to potential photosensitivity reactions.

Dosage

Canine
Susceptible infections: 2.75–5.5 mg/kg PO q24 h for 2 days beyond cessation of clinical signs or 10 days for UTI. Maximum of 30 days (Pfizer Manufacturer's Insert).

Feline
Susceptible infections: 2.75–5.5 mg/kg PO q24 h for 2 days beyond cessation of clinical signs or 10 days for UTI. Maximum of 30 days (Pfizer Manufacturer's Insert).

Dose adjustments

Marbofloxacin and its metabolite do not accumulate significantly in mild renal impairment in dogs, but doses may need adjusting in severe renal impairment. Extend dosing interval to q 48 h in severe renal failure.

Administration

Best absorbed on an empty stomach, but may be administered with food to decrease gastrointestinal upset. Avoid antacid use or concurrent administration with divalent or trivalent cations (iron, calcium, and aluminum). Maintain hydration and urinary output.

Electrolyte contents

Not significant.

Storage/stability

Store tablets at room temperature in tight containers protected from light. Do not freeze.

Adverse reactions

>10%
Nausea, anorexia, and soft stools reported in cats and dogs.

1–10%
Vomiting and diarrhea reported in cats and dogs.

<1%
Salivation, pytyalism, redness of the ear pinnae (eosinophilic dermatitis), and decreased absolute neutrophil counts have been reported in cats at high doses, no retinal degeneration was reported in healthy young cats at 10× the dose by the manufacturer, but post-market reports to FDA suggest 14 reports associated with blindness in cats. Lameness and articular cartilage lesions reported in 3–4 month-old large breed dogs with 11 mg/kg q24 h dosing.

Other species
Fluoroquinolone use in other species has resulted in elevated liver enzymes, crystalluria, hypertension, angina pectoris, myocardial infarction, cardiopulmonary arrest, dyspnea, photosensitivity, rash, elevated serum creatinine, arthralgia, cartilage damage, lameness, cataracts, tendon rupture, allergic reactions, agranulocytosis, prolongation of the Q-T interval, erythema multiforme, toxic epidermal necrolysis, and pseudomembranous colitis.

Drug interactions

Bioavailability is decreased by enteral feedings containing cations. Aluminum or magnesium products, sucralfate, calcium, iron, zinc, and multiple vitamins with minerals may all decrease absorption by >90%. Give these agents at least 2–4 h from the dose, consider switching to an H_2 antagonist or omeprazole. Theophylline and NSAIDs may increase the CNS stimulation of marbofloxacin. H_2 antagonists and loop diuretics may inhibit renal elimination of quinolones, antineoplastics may decrease absorption of marbofloxacin, and marbofloxacin may increase cyclosporine concentrations. Avoid use with agents that can cause prolongation of the Q-T interval (cisapride, macrolides, etc.).

Monitoring

Monitor for hypersensitivity reactions and CNS stimulation. Monitor cats for mydriasis and discontinue if develops.

Overdose

High doses of 55 mg/kg q24 h in dogs have resulted in anorexia, vomiting, dehydration, lethargy, tremors, red skin, and facial edema. Acute renal failure and seizures may result. Gastrointestinal decontamination and supportive care are recommended. Charcoal hemoprofusion has been reported to markedly reduce plasma concentrations of enrofloxacin and may be successful in severe cases of marbofloxacin overdoses.

Diagnostic test interference

None noted.

Mechanism

A bactericidal fluoroquinolone. Promotes breakage of bacterial double stranded DNA. Inhibits DNA-gyrase in susceptible organisms, stops relaxation of supercoiled DNA.

Pharmacology/kinetics

Absorption
Oral doses are well absorbed in dogs with a bioavailability of 94%.

Distribution
Marbofloxacin is widely distributed throughout tissues and fluids. The highest concentrations in dogs are found in kidney, lymph nodes, and prostate. Protein binding is 9.1% in dogs and 7.3% in cats.

CNS penetration
Marbofloxacin has minimal penetration across the blood brain barrier. Therapeutic CSF concentrations would not be expected for most organisms.

Metabolism

About 10–15% of marbofloxacin is metabolized in the liver to N-oxide-marbofloxacin. Both the parent drug and metabolite are eliminated via renal and biliary excretion. Approximately 40% of parent drug is eliminated via urine in dogs and up to 70% in cats.

Half-life

In dogs, the half-life is approximately 10 h and in cats is 12 h.

Pregnancy risk factor

Not studied (potentially Category C): Most fluoroquinolones do not show evidence of teratogenic effects in laboratory animals but due to potential fetal cartilage effects, this category of drugs is not recommended in pregnant patients.

Lactation

Studies have not been performed, but most fluoroquinolones are excreted into milk in significant concentrations and may cause damage to the cartilage of nursing animals.

Further reading

Lefebvre, H.P., Schneider, M., Dupouy, V., *et al.* (1998) Effect of experimental renal impairment on disposition of marbofloxacin and its metabolites in the dog. *J Vet Pharmacol Therap.*, **21(6)**, 453–461.

Marbofloxacin Freedom of Information Summary. Supplemental approval for use in cats. Pfizer Inc. NADA #141–151.

Schneider, M., Thomas, V., Boisrame, B., *et al.* (1996) Pharmacokinetics of marbofloxacin in dogs after oral and parenteral administration. *J Vet Pharmacol Therap.*, **19(1)**, 56–61.

Chapter 156: Meropenem

US Generic (Brand) Name: Meropenem (Merrem)
Availability: Human approved – Meropenem powder for injection (500 mg and 1 g)
Resistance Mechanisms: Altered outer membrane protein (OprD) and increase in extended spectrum cephalosporinases (ESACs)

Use

Should be restricted for use to organisms that are resistant to all other alternative antibiotics. Reserved for serious infections that include resistant gram negative bacilli, gram positive bacteria (methacillin sensitive), and anaerobes. Active against *Acinetobacter* spp., *Bacteriodes* spp., *Prevotella* spp., *Bordetella* spp., *Citrobacter* spp., *E. coli*, *Erysipelthrix*, *Klebsiella* spp., *Proteus* spp., *Providencia* spp., *Pseudomonas* spp., *Rhodococcus* spp., and *Serratia* spp. Use for sepsis, liver abscess, intra-abdominal infections, osteomyelitis, pancreatitis, and peritonitis. Slightly more effective than imipenem against most organisms. The main advantage of meropenem over imipenem is that it is more soluble and can be administered in less fluid volume and more rapidly. It may also have less potential for inducing seizures.

Contraindications/warnings

Hypersensitivity to meropenem or penicillins. Reduce dose in renal impairment. Use with caution in patients with a history of seizures.

Dosage

Canine
UTI: 8 mg/kg SC q12 h (Papich 2002).

Severe Systemic infections: 8.5 mg/kg SC q12 h or 24 mg/kg IV q12 h (Papich 2002).

Pseudomonas/Other resistant infections: 12 mg/kg SC q8 h or 25 mg/kg IV q8 h (Papich 2002).

Feline
UTI: 8 mg/kg SC q12 h (Papich 2002).

Severe Systemic infections: 8.5 mg/kg SC q12 h or 24 mg/kg IV q12 h (Papich 2002).

Pseudomonas/Other resistant infections: 12 mg/kg SC q8 h or 25 mg/kg IV q8 h (Papich 2002).

Dose adjustments

For moderate to severe renal failure, reduce dose and administer at the same interval or give normal dose with prolonged interval.

Administration

For direct intermittent intravenous injection, add 10 or 20 mL of sterile water for injection to the 500 mg or 1 g vial, respectively. This makes a final concentration of

50 mg/mL. Shake until dissolved and let clear. Administer dose over 3–5 min. For IV infusion, vials may be diluted as mentioned or can be diluted with another compatible solution 0.45 or 0.9% sodium chloride injection, or 5% dextrose injection (500 mg in 100 mL or 1 g in 100 mL). The dose is then administered over 15–30 min. For SC administration, meropenem may be diluted with 0.9 % NaCl to concentrations <20 mg/mL and the appropriate dose administered SC.

Electrolyte contents

Not significant.

Storage/stability

According to the Manufacturer, if reconstituted with sterile water for injection the vial is stable at room temperature for up to 2 h or for 12 h under refrigeration. If reconstituted for an IV infusion with 0.9% sodium chloride, it is stable for 2 h at room temperature or up to 18 h under refrigeration. If reconstituted with 5% dextrose it is stable for 1 h at room temperature or up to 8 h under refrigeration. Meropenem 4 mg/mL in 0.9% NaCl was stable for at least 7 days in PVC bags and elastomeric infusion containers when stored at 5°C. Meropenem 10 and 20 mg/mL in 0.9% NaCl was stable for at least 5 days in both containers at 5°C. The Manufacturer states that the drug should not be frozen. However, meropenem has been diluted in concentrations of 1–22 mg/mL in D5W or 0.9% NaCl and frozen for up to 14 days with <10% loss (Plumb 2011).

Adverse reactions

>10%
Nausea, salivation, and vomiting reported in cats and dogs.

1–10%
Diarrhea, skin irritation, and hair loss at SC injection site reported in dogs and cats.

<1%
Transient elevations in liver enzyme activity (ALT), eosinophilia and urine casts, WBCs have been reported in dogs. Nephrotoxicity, seizures (imipenem > meropenem) is reported with high doses in dogs.

Other species
Elevated BUN, Scr, elevated liver enzyme activity, anemia, eosinophilia, hypotension, neutropenia, palpitations, thrombocytopenia, colitis, rash, and Coomb's tests is reported.

Drug interactions

Nephrotoxic drugs (aminoglycosides, amphotericin, etc.) can contribute to an increase in potential plasma concentrations of imipenem as well as toxicities. Antagonism may occur with other penicillins and chloramphenicol.

Monitoring

Monitor for allergic reactions. Monitor renal, hepatic, and CBC.

Overdose

Overdose symptoms may include nausea, vomiting, diarrhea, neuromuscular hyperirritability, seizures, and encephalopathy. Gastrointestinal lavage, hemodialysis, and supportive care (including anticonvulsant therapy) may be indicated. Approximately 20–50% of a dose is dialyzable.

Diagnostic test interference

Alters urinary glucose determination with Clinitest.

Mechanism

A bactericidal carbapenem. Binds penicillin-binding proteins (PBP-I) that results in more rapid weakening and interference of the cell wall then other beta-lactams.

Pharmacology/kinetics

Absorption
Bioavailability orally is very poor. Following SC administration in dogs, the bioavailability is 84%.

Distribution
Meropenem is widely distributed into tissues and body fluids. Protein binding in dogs is 11.87%.

CNS penetration
Meropenem does cross the blood/brain barrier, but not readily (CSF/plasma ratio = 0.02–0.1). It has been used to treat meningitis in pediatric patients but only at very high doses.

Metabolism

Meropenem is primarily excreted renally in dogs with 90–100% of the dose excreted in urine within 24 h. This consists of 36–43% of the parent compound and 34–51% of an opened-ring metabolite.

Half-life

The half-life in dogs after IV and SC administration in tissues is 0.98–1 h.

Pregnancy risk factor

Category B: There is no evidence of embryotoxicity or teratogenicity in laboratory animals receiving four times the human dose of meropenem. It is expected to cross the placenta into fetal tissues which may result in toxicity to fetuses but evidence to date considers it safe.

Lactation

Meropenem has been measured in milk with a calculated exposure to the drug of 0.18% of the maternal dose. This potentially could cause diarrhea or altered flora of a nursing animal but at this time it is considered safe during nursing.

References

Papich, M.G. (2002) *Saunders Handbook of Veterinary Drugs*. 2nd edn. Winkel, A. (ed.), W.B. Saunders Company, Philadelphia, pp. 408–409.

Plumb, D.C. (2011) *Plumb's Veterinary Drug Handbook*. 7th edn. Plumb, D.C. (ed.), Wiley-Blackwell, Ames, Iowa, p. 652.

Further reading

Bidgood, T. and Papich, M. (2002) Plasma pharmacokinetics and tissue fluid concentrations of meropenem after intravenous and subcutaneous administration in dogs. *Am J Vet Res.*, **63(12)**, 1622–1628.

Harrison, M.P., Moss, S.R., Featherstone, A., *et al.* (1989) The disposition of meropenem in laboratory animals and man. *J Antimicrob Chemother.*, **24(Suppl A)**, 265–277.

Jaruratanasirikul, S. and Sriwiryajan, S. (2003) Stability of meropenem in normal saline solution after storage at room temperature. *Southeast Asian J Trop Med Public Health.*, **34(3)**, 627–629.

Smith, D.L., Bauer, S., and Nicolau, D.P. (2004) Stability of meropenem in polyvinyl chloride bags and an elastomeric infusion device. *Am J Health-System Pharm.*, **61(16)**, 412–421.

Walker, S.E., Varrin, S., Yannicelli, D., *et al.* (1998) Stability of meropenem in saline and dextrose solutions and compatibility with potassium chloride. *Can J Hosp Pharm.*, **5**, 156–168.

Chapter 157: Metronidazole

US Generic (Brand) Name: Metronidazole (Flagyl, Metrogel-Topical, Metrogel-Vaginal, Metro-IV injection, Noritate cream, Protostat oral)

Availability: Human approved – Metronidazole oral film tablets (250, 500 mg), oral extend release tablets (750 mg), oral capsules (75 mg), powder for injection (500 mg), premix-RTU 5 mg/mL (100 mL), topical gel 0.75% (30 g), vaginal gel 0.75% (70 g), compounded oral suspension 50 mg/mL

Resistance Mechanisms: Decreased uptake, increased efflux, increased oxygen scavenging

Use

Treatment of anaerobic infections and protozoal infections. Active against *Bacteriodes* spp., *Blastocystis hominis*, *Clostridium* spp., *Entamoeba histolytica*, *Giardia lamblia*, *H. pylori*, *Microsporidia*, and *Trichomonas*. Used for soft tissue infections, intra-abdominal infections, CNS infections, bone infections, periodontal disease, systemic infections due to anaerobes, inflammatory bowel disease, and empiric treatment of diarrhea. Inactive against most aerobic bacteria, use appropriate antibiotics in conjunction with metronidazole for mixed infections (cefepime, ciprofloxacin, etc.).

Contraindications/warnings

Hypersensitivity to metronidazole, pregnant animals. Reduce dose frequency with severe liver, renal, and CNS disease. Use with caution in patients with a history of blood dyscrasias, seizures, those receiving corticosteroids, congestive heart failure, or sodium retention due to the high sodium content of the intravenous solution. Discontinue drug if neurotoxicity develops.

Dosage

All doses are based on 1 mg of metronidazole base rather than the benzoate salt. If using the benzoate salt multiply the dose by 1.6. The benzoate salt is not available commercially in the US but is more palatable to cats and available via Compounding Pharmacies: Double check dosing.

Canine

Anaerobic Infections: 15 mg/kg IV q12 h (Hall 2000) or 15 mg/kg PO q12 h (Sykes and Papich 2013).

Entamoeba histolytica: 25 mg/kg PO q12 h for 8 days (Lappin 2000).

Giardia: 15 mg/kg PO q12 h for 8 days (Sykes and Papich 2013). Can combined with fenbendazole 50 mg/kg PO once daily for 3–5 days for resistant cases (Payne and Artzer 2009).

Feline
Anaerobic Infections: 15 mg/kg IV q12 h (Hall 2000) or 10–15 mg/kg PO q24 h (Sykes and Papich 2013).

Entamoeba histolytica: 25 mg/kg PO q 12 h for 8 days (Lappin 2000).

Giardia: 15 mg/kg PO q12 h for 8 days (Sykes and Papich 2013). Can add fenbendazole 50 mg/kg PO once daily for 3–5 days for resistant cases (Payne and Artzer 2009).

Dose adjustments

Not required in mild liver disease. Reduce dose in severe liver disease. For severe liver failure, increase dose interval to twice daily versus three times daily. Reduced doses may be necessary in geriatric patients.

Administration

Oral film tablets are best absorbed with food in dogs. The intravenous preparations should not be mixed with other drugs and due to the low pH may interact with aluminum causing a red/brown discoloration of the solution. Aluminum hub needles should not be used. Intravenous RTU solutions are ready to use and should be administered by intermittent or continuous infusion. The 500 mg powder vial for injection must be reconstituted with 4.4 mL of sterile water or bacteriostatic water, 0.9% saline, or bacteriostatic saline to produce a 100 mg/mL solution. This must be diluted further with 0.9% saline injection, 5% dextrose, or LRS to <8 mg/mL. This must be neutralized with 5 mEq of sodium bicarbonate injection for each 500 mgs of metronidazole. Remove any resulting gas before administration. A compounded oral suspension (50 mg/mL) can be made with commercial metronidazole tablets in Ora-Plus, Karo syrup, and DI water that is stable for 60 days refrigerated.

Electrolyte contents

500 mg of IV solution contains 322 mg (14 mEq) of sodium.

Storage/stability

Store injectables, tablets, and topicals at room temperature. Avoid exposure to direct light. Prolonged exposure to light will cause a darkening of the solution. Exposure to room light short term does not affect stability. The pre-mix is stable until the manufacturer's expiration date unless removed from its overwrap. Stability is only 30 days without the overwrap.

Adverse reactions

>10%
Nausea, salivation, and appetite loss reported in cats and dogs.

1–10%
Ataxia, depression, and hepatotoxicity in cats and lethargy, vomiting, diarrhea, and neutropenia reported in dogs.

<1%
Most toxicities are dose related. Neurotoxicity at large doses including seizures, more common in cats (50 mg/kg/day), recumbency, opisthotonus, positional nystagmus, and muscle spasms.

Other species
Sensory polyneuropathy, syncope, nervousness, transient leukopenia, thrombocytopenia, bone marrow aplasia, polyuria, red/brown urine, photosensitivity, furry tongue, and metallic taste.

Drug interactions

Metronidazole increases the effects of oral anticoagulants, phenobarbital decreases the serum half-life of metronidazole, and cimetidine increases metronidazole concentrations and toxicity.

Monitoring

CBC, get baseline total and differential leukocyte count, monitor liver enzyme activity.

Overdose

Symptoms may include nausea, vomiting, ataxia, seizures, and neuropathy. Mydriasis, nystagmus, and bradycardia in dogs >60 mg/kg/day or with chronic dosing at 30 mg/kg/day. Gastrointestinal decontamination and diazepam (0.43 mg/kg) IV or PO q8 h × 3 days are effective. Hemodialysis removes 50–100% of a dose.

Diagnostic test interference

Can alter ALT, AST, triglycerides, glucose, and LDH testing.

Mechanism

Bactericidal nitroimidazole: Metronidazole is reduced to a compound that interacts with DNA resulting in bacterial, protozoal DNA damage, and inhibition of protein synthesis.

Pharmacology/kinetics

Absorption
Metronidazole is well absorbed in dogs after oral administration (50–100%). Food increases the absorption in dogs. In cats, 65% of a dose is absorbed orally. Rectal administration has not been evaluated in small animals, but is approximately 50% absorbed in horses.

Distribution
Distributed widely to most body tissues and fluids, including bone, abscesses, CNS, and seminal fluid. Protein binding is 20%.

CNS penetration
CNS concentrations are 43% of plasma concentrations and can be up to 100% with inflamed meninges.

Metabolism
Extensively metabolized in the liver by hydroxylation, oxidation, and glucuronide conjugation. The primary metabolite (2-hydroxy-metronidazole) is active. Elimination is via renal and biliary routes with the majority excreted renally.

Half-life
The half-life in dogs is 3–13 h and is 5 h in cats.

Pregnancy risk factor

Category B: Metronidazole crosses the placenta and should not be used in the first trimester of pregnancy where the drug has been shown to be teratogenic (cleft palate).

Lactation
Metronidazole readily penetrates into milk and has been noted to be tumorigenic. The risks most likely outweigh the benefits in nursing animals.

References

Hall, J. (2000) Diseases of the stomach. *Textbook of Veterinary Internal Medicine: Diseases of the Dog and Cat, Vol. 2.* 2nd edn, Ettinger, S. and Feldman, E. (eds), Elsevier, St. Louis, MO, pp. 1154–1182.

Lappin, M. (2000) Protozoal and miscellaneous infections. *Textbook of Veterinary Internal Medicine: Diseases of the Dog and Cat, Vol. 1.* Ettinger, S. and Feldman, E. (eds), Elsevier, St. Louis, MO, pp. 408–417.

Payne, P.A. and Artzer, M. (2009) The biology and control of *Giardia* spp. and *Tritrichomonas foetus. Vet Clin North Amer Sm Anim Pract.,* **39(6)**, 939–940.

Sykes, J.E. and Papich, M.G. (2013) Antibacterial drugs. Ch. 8. In: *Canine and Feline Infectious Diseases.* Sykes, J.E. (ed.), Elsevier, St. Louis, MO. pp. 66–86.

Further reading

Fitch, R., Moore, M., Roen, D., *et al.* (1991) A warning to clinicians: metronidazole neurotoxicity in a dog. *Prog Vet Neurol.,* **2**, 307–309.

Olson, E.J., Morales, S.C., McVey, A.S., *et al.* (2005) Putative metronidazole neurotoxicosis in a cat. *Vet Path.,* **42**, 665–669.

Sekis, I., Ramstead, K., Rishniw, M., *et al.* (2009) Single dose pharmacokinetics and genotoxicity of metronidazole in cats. *J Fel Med Surg.,* **11(2)**, 60–68.

Chapter 158: Minocycline

US Generic (Brand) Name: Minocycline (Minocin, Dynacin, Vectrin)
Availability: Human approved – Minocycline oral tablet and capsules (50, 75, 100 mg), minocycline HCL sterile injectable (100 mg) (availability may be limited)
Resistance Mechanisms: Tetracycline resistance genes (tet-M and tet-O) ribosomal protection, tetracycline modification

Use

Active against some gram negative and gram positive organisms as well as atypical infections. Active against; *Bacillus anthrax, Burkholderia cepacia, Streptococcus* spp.,

Staphylococcus spp., *Bartonella* spp., *Brucella* sp., *Campylobacter fetus*, *Francisella tularensis*, *Haemophilus* spp., *Vibrio cholera*, *Yersina pestis*, *Acinetobacter*, *Enterobacter* spp., *E. coli*, *Klebsiella*, *Neisseria* spp., *Shigella* spp., *Stenotrophomonas*, *Borrelia*, *Chlamydia* spp., *Clostridia* spp., *Entamoeba*, *Mycobacterium marinum*, *Mycoplasma*, *Nocardia*, and *Richettsia*. In penicillin allergic patients, minocycline can be used against *Fusobacterium* and *Actinomyces*. Has enhanced activity against Lyme disease due to its increased CNS penetration compared to other tetracyclines. *In vitro*, minocycline is more active against *Wolbachia* spp. then doxycycline. Minocycline shows immunomodulatory activity similar to doxycycline.

Contraindications/warnings

Hypersensitivity to tetracyclines, contraindicated in pregnant, lactating, or young/growing animals as well as severe liver/renal impairment, or esophageal inflammation/strictures. Contraindicated in patients with known autoimmune hepatitis and lupus. Do not use expired or unstable compounded drug. The degradation product (anhydro-4-epitetracycline) is renal toxic.

Dosage

Canine
Soft tissue infections/ehrlichiosis: 5–12 mg/kg PO, IV q12 h for 7–14 days or for ehrlichiosis × 28 days (Greene *et al.*, 2006).

Brucellosis: 25 mg/kg PO q day × 4 weeks with gentamicin 5 mg/kg SC q day × 7 days, off 7 days, repeat 7 days (Hartmannn and Greene *et al.*, 2006).

Feline
Susceptible infections: 5–12.5 mg/kg PO, IV q12 h (Papich 2002).

Dose adjustments

Decrease dose and/or frequency in renal impairment. Antianabolic effects can cause an increase in BUN, azotemia, hyperphosphatemia, and acidosis.

Administration

Give capsules and tablets on an empty stomach 1 h before or 2 h after a meal. If not tolerated, give with food to reduce gastrointestinal side effects. Try to prevent chewing of tablet/capsule, follow with water to prevent esophagitis. Do not administer with antacids, iron containing products, vitamins, or dairy products. The intravenous injectable should be reconstituted with 5 mL of sterile water to make a 20 mg/mL solution. Each 100 mg must be further diluted with 500 mL–1 L of compatible solution (0.9% saline, D5W, 5% dextrose, and NaCl, or LRS). Infuse over 6 h.

Electrolyte contents

Not significant.

Storage/stability

Store capsules in tight, light resistant container at controlled room temperature. Protect from moisture, heat, and freezing. The reconstituted IV solution (20 mg/mL) is stable for 24 h at room temperature.

Adverse reactions

>10%
Nausea and vomiting, diarrhea in dogs and cats. Erythema, papules with high doses in dogs.

1–10%
Esophagitis if not followed with water in dogs and cats.

<1%
Hepatotoxicity (hyperbilirubinemia, hepatic cholestasis, and hepatitis), lethargy, ataxia, tooth discoloration, and altered bone growth rate in growing dogs and cats. Urticaria, cardiovascular depression, and hypotension reported in dogs with rapid IV infusion. Thyroid hyperplasia occurs if used long term in dogs. Intravascular hemolysis, hypercoagulation, decreased packed cell volume, and hemoglobin.

Other species
Photosensitivity, fever, skin discoloration, auto-immune hepatitis, lupus, vestibular disturbances, intracranial hypertension, renal toxicity, agranulocytosis, and hemolytic anemia.

Drug interactions

Concurrent administration with sucralfate or divalent or trivalent cations (aluminum, calcium, magnesium, and iron) in antacids or bismuth subsalicylate may decrease oral bioavailability if taken concurrently (separate doses by 2 h). Avoid use in combination with bactericidal drugs (penicillin, cephalosporins, etc.). Concurrent methoxyflurane anesthesia reported to cause fatal nephrotoxicity. Barbiturates, bile acid sequestrants, nafcillin, and rifamycins can decrease minocycline effects.

Monitoring

Monitor renal, hepatic, and CBC with long term therapy. Monitor for signs of thyroid cancer and autoimmune reactions.

Overdose

Results in nausea, vomiting, anorexia, and diabetes insipidus. Following gastrointestinal decontamination, administer supportive care with fluid therapy. Dialysis only removes 0–5% of a dose.

Diagnostic test interference

May cause false elevations of urinary catecholamine levels due to interference with fluorescence test.

Mechanism

A bacteriostatic tetracycline. Binds to 30s and 50s bacterial ribosomes resulting in protein synthesis inhibition.

Pharmacology/kinetics

Absorption
Oral absorption in canine patients is 50%. Food delays absorption and can decrease absorption by 20–27%. Drug interactions may significantly affect absorption.

Distribution
More lipophilic than other tetracyclines, so there is greater penetration into the prostate and CNS. Less concentrated in urine than other tetracyclines, so not the preferred drug for urinary infections. Protein binding is between 60–72%.

CNS penetration
CNS penetration is good, 30% of plasma concentration. Three fold CNS concentrations in dogs compared to doxycyline.

Metabolism
Minocycline is deactivated in the intestine by chelate formation to inactive metabolites and is primarily excreted in feces with a small amount (20–30%) excreted via urine.

Half-life
The half-life in dogs following oral administration of 5 mg/kg PO BID is 4.1 h in plasma and 7.4 h in intrastitial fluid.

Pregnancy risk factor

Category D: Readily crosses the placenta and causes embryotoxic effects. Causes retardation of skeletal development in laboratory animals.

Lactation
Readily crosses into milk. Not recommended in nursing animals, due to toxicities.

References

Greene, C., Hartmann, K., *et al.* (2006) Antimicrobial drug formulary. Appendix 8. In: *Infectious Disease of the Dog and Cat*. Greene, C. (ed.), Elsevier, St. Louis, MO, pp. 1186–1333.

Hartmannn, K. and Greene, C. (2006) Diseases caused by systemic bacterial infections. *Textbook of Veterinary Internal Medicine: Diseases of the Dog and Cat, Vol. 2*. 6th edn., Ettinger, S. and Feldman, E. (eds), Elsevier, St. Louis, MO, pp. 1186–1333.

Papich, M.G. (2002) *Saunders Handbook of Veterinary Drugs*. 2nd edn. Winkel, A. (ed.), W.B. Saunders Company, Philadelphia, pp. 441–443.

Further reading

Barza, M., Brown, R.B., Shanks, C., *et al.* (1975) Relationship between lipophilicity and pharmacological behavior of minocycline, doxycycline, tetracycline, and oxytetracycline in dogs. *Antimicrob Agents Chemother.*, **8(6)**, 713–720.

Katzman, J.V., Kemp, D.T., *et al.* (1985) Compartmental and non-compartmental pharmacokinetics of minocycline HCL in the dog. *AJVR.*, **46(6)**, 1316–1318.

Maaland, M.G., Guardabassi, L., and Papich, M. (2014) Minocycline pharmacokinetics and pharmacodynamics in dogs: Dosage recommendations for treatment of methicillin-resistant *Staphylococcus pseudintermedius* infections. *Vet Derm.*, **25**, 182–190.

Chapter 159: Nitrofurantoin

US Generic (Brand) Name: Nitofurantoin (Furadantin, Furalan, Furan, Macrobid, Macrodantin)
Availability: Human approved – Nitrofurantoin oral capsules (50, 100 mg), nitrofurantoin macrocrystal oral capsules (25, 50, 100 mg), nitrofurantoin macrocrystal/monohydrate-(Macrobid or Macrodantin 100 mg), nitrofurantoin oral suspension 25 mg/5 mL (470 mL)
Resistance Mechanisms: Upregulation of nsfA and nfsB genes that encode oxygen-insensitive nitroreductases

Use

To prevent or treat urinary tract infections due to susceptible gram negative and some gram positive organisms. Nitrofurantoin is typically not used as first line therapy for UTIs but has shown efficacy in multidrug resistant *E. coli, Enterococcus faecalis,* and multidrug resistant *S. pseudintermedius* UTI infections and may help prevent the overuse of carbepenems. Resistant mutants are rare. It is also active against *E. coli, Enterococci, Enterobacter, Klebsiella, Citrobacter, Salmonella, Shigella, Corynebacterium,* and *Staphylococcus* spp. It is not active against *Pseudomonas* spp. or *Proteus* spp. The drug concentrates in urine where it is converted to reactive intermediates with antibacterial properties, so therapeutic concentrations are not reached elsewhere, only in urine.

Contraindications/warnings

Hypersensitivity to nitrofurantoin leads to renal impairment. Urine concentrations of drug may be sub therapeutic. Use with caution in very young or geriatric patients where enzymes (glutathione) may be immature or impaired (increased risk of hemolytic anemia). Do not use in pregnant or lactating animals. Caution with patients that have anemia, vitamin B deficiency, diabetes, and electrolyte abnormalities. Avoid prolonged therapy.

Dosage

Canine/feline
UTI: Nitrofurantoin 10 mg/kg q24 h PO divided into four daily treatments for 4–10 days. Then 1 mg/kg q24 h (give at bedtime after urination); or Macrocrystalline formulations (Macrobid, Macrodantin): 2–3 mg/kg PO q8 h. Then 1–2 mg/kg q24 h (at bedtime) (Papich 2002).

Recurrent UTI: Nitrofurantoin 4 mg/kg PO q8 h for 4–10 days; Prophylactic dose 3–4 mg/kg PO q24 h (after micturition immediately before bedtime) (Polzin and Osborne 1985).

Dose adjustments

Do not use in renal impairment, decrease dose in geriatric patients with liver impairment.

Administration

Give capsules with food to decrease gastrointestinal upset. Food slows the rate of absorption. The microcrystalline capsules are rapidly absorbed versus the macrocrystalline capsules, which are slowly absorbed and cause less gastrointestinal upset. The suspension can be mixed with food or flavored broths to improve palatability. Give prophylactic doses after micturition just prior to bedtime.

Electrolyte contents

Not significant.

Storage/stability

Store capsules and suspension at room temperature in tightly sealed containers away from light.

Adverse reactions

>10%
Discoloration of urine to dark yellow or brownish, nausea reported in dogs and cats.

1–10%
Vomiting and anorexia reported in dogs and cats.

<1%
Myasthenic-like effects reported in dogs. Yellow discoloration of the teeth reported in very young animals.

Other species
Hepatopathy has been noted in laboratory animals. Cholestatic jaundice, hepatic necrosis, hepatitis, acute pulmonary interstitial pneumonitis, pulmonary fibrosis, eosinophilia, fever, hypersensitivity reactions, dyspnea and pleural effusion, rashes, erythema multiforme, angioedema, peripheral neuropathy, polyneuropathy,

nystagmus, hemolytic anemia, agranulocytosis, methemoglobinemia, renal impairment, anemia, diabetes, electrolyte imbalances, and vitamin B deficiency.

Drug interactions

Antacids containing magnesium salts decrease absorption of nitrofurantoin. Food and anticholinergic drugs may increase the absorption of nitrofurantoin. Nitrofurantoin antagonizes the effects of fluoroquinolones.

Monitoring

Get baseline CBC, liver, and renal panel prior to prolonged therapy. Monitor for signs of toxicity (hepatic, hemolytic anemia, interstitial pneumonitis, eosinophilia, and peripheral neuropathy).

Overdose

Overdoses may result in vomiting and CNS involvement (excitation, tremors, convulsions, and peripheral neuritis). Gastrointestinal decontamination and supportive care may be required.

Diagnostic test interference

Causes false positive urine glucose with Clinitest.

Mechanism

Bacteriostatic urinary antiseptic. Inhibits bacterial enzymes (acetyl coenzyme A) involved in bacterial metabolism and cell wall synthesis.

Pharmacology/kinetics

Absorption
Oral absorption is rapid and variable (38–120%) depending on the formulation. Food and anticholinergics may slow gastrointestinal transit time and increase absorption.

Distribution
Nitrofurantoin has poor tissue penetration. It only reaches therapeutic concentrations in urine and should not be used for pyelonephritis, renal abscesses, or prostatitis. It concentrates in acidic urine. The drug is metabolized in the liver and excreted (16–22%) primarily via renal elimination at low doses (<6 mg/kg), but has increased biliary excretion at higher doses where it undergoes enterohepatic circulation. Protein binding is 20–60% in dogs.

CNS penetration
Nitrofurantoin does not penetrate into the CNS in therapeutic concentrations.

Metabolism
Nitrofurantoin is partially metabolized in the liver, the majority of drug (40–50%) is excreted unchanged into the urine where it is converted to its active metabolites by bacterial flavoproteins.

Half-life
The half-life is 19–87 min in dogs.

Pregnancy risk factor

Category B: No teratogenic effects have been noted in rats and rabbits. Nitrofurantoin does cross the placenta but systemic concentrations are very low. Nitrofurantoin can induce hemolytic anemia in glucose-6-phosphate dehydrogenase (G-6-PD)-deficient human patients and in patients with red blood cells deficient in reduced glutathione. This is noted in newborn humans and animals, so it is not advised near delivery.

Lactation
Nitrofurantoin is actively transported into milk resulting in 6% of the maternal plasma concentration. Although exposure is low it is not recommended in nursing animals.

References

Papich, M.G. (2002) *Saunders Handbook of Veterinary Drugs.* 2nd edn. Winkel, A. (ed.), W.B. Saunders Company, Philadelphia, pp. 468–469.

Polzin, D.J. and Osborne, C.A. (1985) Diseases of the urinary tract. In: *Handbook of Small Animal Therapeutics.* Davis, L.E. (ed.), Churchill Livingstone, New York, pp. 333–395.

Further reading

Conkling, J.D. and Wagner, D.L. (1977) Excretion of nitrofurantoin in dog hepatic bile. *Br J Pharmacol.,* **43(1)**, 140–150.

Maaland, M. and Guardabassi, L. (2011) *In vitro* antimicrobial activity of nitrofurantoin against *Escherichia coli* and *Staphylococcus pseudintermedius* isolated from dogs and cats. *Vet Microbiol.,* **151(3–4)**, 396–399.

Niazi, S., Vishrupad, K.S., and Veng-Pederson, P. (1983) Absorption and distribution characteristics of nitrofurantoin in dogs. *Biopharm Drug disposition*, **4(3)**, 213–223.

Pomba, C., Couto, N., and Moodley, A. (2010) Treatment of a lower urinary tract infection in a cat caused by a multidrug methacillin resistant *Staphylococcus pseudintermedius* and *Enterococcus faecalis*. *J Feline Med Surg.*, **12(10)**, 802–806.

Chapter 160: Orbifloxacin

US Generic (Brand) Name: Orbifloxacin (Orbax)
Availability: Veterinary approved – Orbax oral suspension (30 mg/mL × 20 mL), Orbax tablets (5.7, 22.7, 68 mg)
Resistance Mechanisms: Bacterial topoisomerase mutations, altered membrane permeability

Use

Orbifloxacin is used in the treatment of skin and soft tissue infections (wounds and abscesses) in cats and dogs. It covers most strains of *Pasteurella multocida*, *Escherichia coli*, and *Staphylococcus* spp. It is also used in the treatment of canine urinary tract infections (cystitis) caused by susceptible strains of *Pasteurella multocida*, *Proteus mirabilis*, *Pseudomonas* spp., *Staphylococcus* spp., *E. coli*, *Klebsiella* spp., *Enterobacter* spp., *Citrobacter* spp., *Streptococcus* spp., *and Enterococcus faecalis*.

Contraindications/warning

Hypersensitivity to fluoroquinolones. Avoid or reduce dose in patients with renal/hepatic impairment. Contraindicated in young, pregnant, or lactating animals due to arthropathy. Do not use in young small to medium breed dogs (<8 months) or large breeds (<18 months) or those with pre-existing articular cartilage lesions. Use with caution in patients with known or suspected CNS disorders, since CNS stimulation can occur. May prolong Q-T interval, use with caution in patients with pre-existing cardiac disease or in those on other drugs that prolong the Q-T interval.

Dosage

The oral suspension is not bioequivalent to the tablets on a mg/kg basis in cats. Tablets provide higher less variable plasma concentrations.

Dogs
UTI, Wound/soft tissue infections: 2.5–7.5 mg/kg PO q24 h (Minimum of 10 days for suspension) or for 2–3 days beyond cessation of clinical signs (Max 30 days) (Intervet Manufacturer's Package Insert).

Feline
Wound/soft tissue infections: Suspension 7.5 mg/kg q24 h (Maximum dose: Do not exceed due to variability in absorption) or tablets (5–7.5 mg/kg q24 h) (Intervet Manufacturer's Package Insert).

Dose adjustments

Dose reductions in renal failure have not been established for this drug. Due to primarily renal excretion it would be expected to accumulate in severe renal failure. A reduction in the dose frequency in severe renal impairment (q48 h) instead of q24 h may be indicated.

Administration

Before initial use of the suspension, shake well, remove the cap, and insert the syringe adaptor by pressing firmly into top of bottle. Insert the syringe tip into the adaptor opening and invert the bottle. Withdraw the required dose with the calibrated syringe. After use, replace cap, leaving adaptor in the bottle, and rinse the syringe with water. The tablets are enteric coated to hide the bitter taste, do not crush or split tablets.

Electrolyte contents

Not significant.

Storage/stability

Store at room temperature. After opening, store in the tightly closed bottle provided at room temperature.

Adverse reactions

>10%
Salivation, vomiting, and white to yellow discoloration of feces reported in dogs. Vomiting reported in cats.

1–10%
Anorexia, diarrhea, and depression/lethargy reported in dogs and cats.

<1%

Convulsions reported in dogs. At high doses glucosuria, low urine pH, hepatic necrosis, bile duct hyperplasia, elevated bilirubin, and hepatic enzymes are reported in dogs. Blindness (potentially reversible), mydriasis, ataxia, convulsions, ophthalmic changes, lacrimation, and retinal degeneration reported in cats.

Drug interactions

Bioavailability is decreased by dairy products and enteral feedings containing cations. Aluminum or magnesium products, sucralfate, calcium, iron, zinc, and multiple vitamins with minerals may all decrease absorption. Give these agents at least 2–4 h from the dose, consider switching to an H_2 antagonist or omeprazole. Theophylline and NSAIDs may increase CNS stimulation of orbifloxacin, H_2 antagonists, and loop diuretics may inhibit renal elimination of quinolones, antineoplastics may decrease absorption of quinolones, and orbifloxacin may increase cyclosporine and digoxin concentrations. Avoid use with agents that can cause prolongation of the Q-T interval (cisapride, etc.).

Monitoring

Monitor for hypersensitivity reactions, CNS stimulation, and mydriasis in cats.

Overdose

Acute renal failure and seizures may result. Gastrointestinal decontamination and supportive care are recommended. Although hemodialysis is not recommended in fluoroquinolone overdose, charcoal hemoprofusion, and dialysis have been reported to markedly reduce plasma concentrations of enrofloxacin and may work for orbifloxacin.

Diagnostic test interference

None noted.

Mechanism

A bacteriocidal fluoroquinolone. Promotes breakage of double stranded DNA. Inhibits DNA-gyrase in susceptible organisms and stops relaxation of supercoiled DNA.

Pharmacology/kinetics

Absorption

Orbifloxacin is well absorbed orally on an empty stomach (100%) in dogs. The effects of food on absorption in dogs is unknown. In cats, food increases total absorption (32%) but delays the time to peak concentrations.

Distribution

Orbifloxacin is widely distributed into tissues and body fluids following oral dosing. It is reported to concentrate in prostate, kidneys, liver, bile, lungs, lymph nodes, small intestine, cartilage, muscle, salivary glands, and testes. Protein binding in cats is low (18%).

CNS penetration

No information is reported to date on penetration into the CNS. In general, fluoroquinolones have limited penetration into the CNS.

Metabolism

Orbifloxacin is metabolized in the liver. In dogs, 40% of the drug is excreted unchanged in urine within 24 h.

Half-life

The half-life in dogs is 5–6 h in the fasted state and 7.5 h in cats.

Pregnancy risk factor

Category C: Orbifloxacin has not been studied in pregnant animals but most fluoroquinolones penetrate the placenta and have the potential to cause teratogenic effects and fetal cartilage effects so it is considered contraindicated in pregnant animals.

Lactation

Orbifloxacin excretion into milk is unknown. However, other fluoroquinolones are excreted into milk and can cause arthropathy in nursing animals.

Further reading

Freedom of Information Summary (2009) *Original New Animal Drug Application* (NADA 141–305). *Orbax*, Oral Suspension. Roseland, NJ: Intervet Inc. July 1.

Ganiere, J.P., Medaille, C., and Etoré F. (2004) *In vitro* antimicrobial activity of orbifloxacin against *Staphylococcus intermedius* isolates from canine skin and ear infections. *Res Veterin Sci.*, **77**, 67–77.

Chapter 161: Oxytetracycline

US Generic (Brand) Name: Oxytetracycline (Liquamycin, Terramycin, Biomycin, Oxytet, Oxyject, Biocyl)
Availability: Veterinary approved – Oxytetracycline HCL injectable (50, 100 mg/mL), oxytetracycline base injectable (200 mg/mL–LA 200), tablets (250, 500 mg)
Resistance Mechanisms: Increased efflux, ribosomal protection, tetracycline modification

Use

Treatment of aerobic and anaerobic gram negative and gram positive organisms that are susceptible. Not effective against *Pseudomonas, Proteus, Serratia, Klebsiella, Arcanobacterium* spp., or pathogenic *E. coli*. Less effective against *Staphylococcus* spp. than doxycycline or minocycline. Effective on some atypical intracellular organisms. Used in small animals for severe infections due to *Rickettsia, Mycoplasma, Chlamydia,* and *Spirochetes*. Some efficacy against protozoa (*Amebae*).

Contraindications/warnings

Do not administer to animals with a hypersensitivity to tetracyclines, those that are pregnant, lactating, or still growing. Contraindicated for animals with significant hepatic/renal impairment. Avoid using with other nephrotoxic or hepatotoxic drugs.

Dosage

Canine
Susceptible infections: 7.5–10 mg/kg IV q12 h or 20 mg/kg PO q12 h (Papich 2002).

Salmon poisoning (Neorickettsia helminthoeca): Give 10 mg/kg IV loading dose; followed by 7 mg/kg IV q8 h × 3–5 days. Doxycycline may be more effective, start doxycycline orally as soon as animal can tolerate oral therapy. Give praziquantel 10–30 mg/kg q24 h × 1–2 doses PO or SC to eradicate the associated liver fluke (*Nanophyetus salmincola*).

Feline
Susceptible infections: 7.5–10 mg/kg IV q12 h or 20 mg/kg PO q12 h (Papich 2002).

Dose adjustments

Doses should be decreased in patients with severe liver or renal impairment. Decrease dosing to every 12–24 h with severe renal disease.

Administration

Dehydrated animals should be rehydrated prior to administering. For oral medication give 1 h prior or 2 h after meals or other drugs that may interact (antacids, vitamins, etc.). The presence of food, dairy products, antacids, vitamins, or other products containing calcium, iron, aluminum, magnesium, and so on can decrease absorption of oxytetracycline by up to 50%. Follow dosage with sufficient water to avoid esophagitis. For injectable oxytetracycline administration, follow the manufacturer's directions. The veterinary labeled products remaining on the market in the United States are labeled for large animals. IM injections may cause tissue necrosis and pain at the injection site. Products labeled for IV injection may contain significant amounts of propylene glycol that may cause intravascular hemolysis and cardiac depressant effects if administered without dilution. Others may contain high concentrations of povidine, which is also toxic to small animals. Bolus injections have also resulted in renal toxicity. Dilution in LRS or NaCl (0.9%) (>250 mL) and administration over 1 h has demonstrated a reduction in renal toxicity in healthy dogs.

Electrolyte contents

Not significant.

Storage/stability

Store oxytetracycline at room temperature in air tight, light resistant vials. Avoid freezing. Oxytetracycline is not compatible with most diluents and should only be diluted just prior to use with products recommended by the manufacturer (only use D5W, 0.9% NaCl, or LRS as diluents). All tetracycline products are unstable in aqueous solutions and are inactivated by heat, light, oxygen, altered pH, and cations. Inactivated products are renal toxic.

Adverse reactions

>10%
Nausea, vomiting, diarrhea, tooth discoloration, enamel hypoplasia, and esophagitis (if given orally) reported in dogs and cats.

1–10%

Photosensitivity, thrombophlebitis, acute renal failure (rapid IV infusion), and injection site reactions reported in dogs and cats. Fever, depression, and hair loss reported in cats.

<1%

Hepatotoxicity, colitis, anaphylaxis, dermatitis, superinfections, hair loss in cats, and uroliths in dogs. The long acting formulation (LA-200) can cause significant tissue irritation, necrosis, and abscess formation in small animals.

Drug interactions

Do not administer any cation containing products (antacids, vitamins, etc.) with orally administered oxytetracycline. Barbiturates decrease oxytetracycline's half-life. Theoretically, bacteriostatic drugs should not be given prior to bactericidal drugs.

Monitoring

Monitor hydration, and renal and hepatic function.

Overdose

Symptoms may include nausea, vomiting, anorexia, and diarrhea. Oral doses up to 400 mg/kg/day did not cause significant toxicity in dogs. Supportive care is recommended, including gastrointestinal decontamination, fluid therapy, and electrolyte replacement.

Diagnostic test interference

Elevated levels of urine catecholamines if using fluorometric assays and false positive urinary glucose if using Clinistix.

Mechanism

Bacteriostatic tetracycline. Inhibits protein synthesis by binding to the bacterial 30s ribosomal subunit.

Pharmacology/kinetics

Absorption

Oxytetracycline is readily absorbed following oral administration (60–80%). Following IM injection of the non-long acting formulations, peak concentrations occur in 30–120 min. The long acting formulation (LA-200) has a much slower absorption.

Distribution

Oxytetracycline is widely distributed into most tissues including, heart, kidney, muscle, pleural, bronchial, sputum, urine, synovial fluid, aqueous humor/vitreous humor, and prostate. Protein binding is 10–40% in dogs.

CNS penetration

CNS penetration remains poor due to low lipophilicity. Therapeutic concentrations cannot be achieved.

Metabolism

Primarily metabolized in the liver and excreted via bile. Some elimination occurs via urine with concentrations above the MIC for some organisms.

Half-life

The elimination half-life is 4–6 h in dogs and is highly dependent on the product used and the animals liver function.

Pregnancy risk factor

Category D: Retards fetal skeletal development and discolors tooth enamel in growing fetuses.

Lactation

Oxytetracycline is excreted into milk and absorption over time may cause harm to suckling animals (bone/teeth).

Reference

Papich, M.G. (2002) *Saunders Handbook of Veterinary Drugs*. 2nd edn. Winkel, A. (ed.), W.B. Saunders Company, Philadelphia, pp. 492–494.

Further reading

Booth, A.J., Stogdale, L., Griger, J.A., *et al.* (1984) Salmon poisoning disease in dogs on Southern Vancouver Island. *Canadian Vet J.*, **25(1)**, 2–6.

Headley, S.A., Scorpio, D.C., Vidotto, O., *et al.* (2011) *Neorickettsia helminthoeca* and salmon poisoning disease: A review. *The Vet Jour.*, **187**, 165–173.

Chapter 162: Penicillin

US Generic (Brand) Name: Penicillin G potassium (Pfizerpen), penicillin G sodium, penicillin G procaine (Wycillin, Bicillin CR), penicillin G benzathine (Bicillin LA, Bicillin CR, Permapen), penicillin V potassium (PenVK).
Availability: Human approved – Penicillin G benzathine sterile suspension (300,000 µ/mL × 10 mL) and (600,000 µ/mL × 1, 2, or 4 mL), penicillin benzathine with penicillin G procaine (PB: 150,000 µ/mL and PP: 150,000 µ/mL × 10 mL, PB: 300,000 µ/mL and PP: 300,000 µ/mL × 1, 2, or 4 mL, PB: 450,000 µ/mL and PP: 150,000 µ/mL × 2 mL), penicillin G potassium Inj. (5 MU, 20 MU) or frozen in dextrose (1, 2, or 3 MU), penicillin G sodium (5 MU), penicillin G procaine sterile suspension (600,000 µ/mL × 1, 2 mL), penicillin V potassium oral powder for suspension (125 mg/ mL and 250 mg/mL), penicillin V potassium oral tablets (250, 500 mgs), and penicillin V-film coated tablets (250, 500 mg). Veterinary Labeled – Penicillin G procaine sterile suspension 300,000 µ/mL (100, 250 mL) and penicillin G benzathine (150,000 µ/mL with penicillin G procaine 150,000 µ/mL × 100, 200 mL)
Resistance Mechanisms: Beta-lactamase inactivation, altered penicillin binding proteins (PBP), decreased penetration to target PBP site

Use

Use in small animal medicine has declined due to resistance. Natural penicillins are still useful for a variety of infections caused from gram positive and negative aerobic cocci, gram positive aerobic bacilli, gram-positive anaerobic bacteria, and spirochetes. Penicillins are typically active against *Streptococcus* spp., *Fusobacterium, Actinomyces* spp., *Bacillus anthrax*, *Borrelia burgdorferi*, *Clostridium* spp. (not *C. difficile*), *Corynebacterium* spp., *Enterococcus* spp. *(with aminoglycosides)*, *Erysipelothrix*, *Leptospira*, and *Pasteurella multocida*.

Contraindications/warnings

Hypersensitivity to penicillins, cephalosporins or procaine (if using PPG). Caution in patients with renal/ hepatic impairment, pre-existing seizure disorders, pre-existing electrolyte imbalances or congestive heart failure. Avoid IV, intravascular, or intra-arterial administration of penicillin G procaine since this may cause irreversible neurovascular damage.

Dosage

Penicillin G (1 MU = 625 mg) and Penicillin V (250 mg = 400,000 units).

Canine
Bacteremia, systemic infections: Penicillin G potassium 20,000–40,000 µ/kg IV q4–6 h (Greene *et al.*, 2006).

Soft tissue infections: Penicillin G procaine 20,000–40,000 µ/kg IM, SC q12–24 h or penicillin G benzathine 40,000 µ/kg IM q120 h (5 days) or penicillin V 10 mg/kg PO q8 h for 7 days (Greene *et al.*, 2006).

Leptospiremia: Penicillin G potassium 25,000–40,000 µ/kg IV q12h for 14 days followed by doxycycline 5–10 mg/ kg PO q12 h for 14 days (Ross and Rentko 2000).

Feline
Soft tissue/systemic infections: Penicillin G procaine 20,000 µ/kg IM, SC q12 h or Penicillin V 10 mg/kg PO q8 h for 7 days (Greene *et al.*, 2006).

Actimomyces: Penicillin G procaine 50,000–100,000 µ/kg IM, SC q12 h (Greene *et al.*, 2006).

Dose adjustments

In patients with severe renal and hepatic impairment, doses and/or frequency of administration should be modified in response to the degree of impairment, severity of the infection, and susceptibility of the organism. Give one half of the dose or double the interval between dosing.

Administration

Give oral medications on an empty stomach (1 h prior to meals or 2 h after meals). For intramuscular injections, shake suspensions well prior to pulling up the dose and inject dose carefully into a deep muscle, avoiding nerves and vessels. Penicillin G sodium or potassium should be diluted according to the manufacturer's directions and the route to be administered. Generally, powders for injection should be diluted with sterile water for injection, dextrose 5% injection or 0.9% sodium chloride. For intravenous infusions of penicillin G sodium or penicillin G potassium, infusions should be done over 0.5–2 h.

Electrolyte contents

Penicillin V has 0.7 mEq of potassium per 250 mg of penicillin. Penicillin G potassium has 1.7 mEq potassium and 0.3 mEq of sodium per 1 MU of penicillin. Penicillin G sodium has 2 mEq sodium per 1 MU of penicillin.

Storage/stability

Store the suspension of penicillin G benzathine refrigerated. Penicillin G potassium powder is stable stored at room temperature. The reconstituted solution is stable for 7 days refrigerated. If admixed with normal saline or dextrose 5% it is stable for 24 h. Penicillin V potassium powder for oral suspension and tablets are stored at room temperature. After reconstitution of oral powder, the suspension is stable refrigerated for 14 days.

Adverse reactions

>10%
Pain at injection site and mild diarrhea reported in dogs and cats.

1–10%
Sterile abscesses at injection site, drowsiness, anorexia, and vomiting.

<1%
CNS stimulation, ataxia, and hypersensitivity reactions reported in dogs.

Other species
Interstitial nephritis, seizures, electrolyte imbalances, fever, thrombophlebitis, neutropenia, serum sickness, hemolytic anemia, positive Coomb's reaction, elevated liver enzymes, tachypnea, dyspnea, edema, tachycardia, and rashes.

Drug interactions

Synergistic with aminoglycosides, antagonism with tetracyclines, chloramphenicol, and macrolides *in vitro*. Penicillin can increase bleeding risks with heparin and increase NSAID concentrations/toxicity. Combination with potassium sparing diuretics may increase the risk of hyperkalemia.

Monitoring

Monitor for signs of allergies. For prolonged therapy, monitor renal function, CBC, and electrolytes (sodium/potassium).

Overdose

Neuromuscular hypersensitivity, seizures, and electrolyte imbalances (sodium/potassium) may occur. Inadvertent administration of the penicillin procaine/benzathine intravenously has resulted in muscle tremor, seizures, blindness, vocalization, agitation, loss of vision, hypothermia, pruritus, hypotension in dogs, and cardiac arrest in cats. Supportive care should be instituted. Hemodialysis removes 20–50% of the dose.

Diagnostic test interference

False positive or negative glucose determination using Clinitest, positive direct Coomb's test, false-positive urinary and/or serum proteins, and false positive serum uric acid with copper-chelate methods. Falsely low aminoglycoside concentrations if samples are allowed to sit prior to analysis.

Mechanism

Bactericidal beta-lactam. Inhibits bacterial cell wall synthesis by binding to penicillin binding proteins, resulting in the inhibition of the final transpeptidation step of peptidoglycan synthesis.

Pharmacology/kinetics

Absorption
Oral absorption is highly variable and dependent on the formulation, acidity, presence of food in the stomach. Penicillin V is the most acid stable and is the formulation used for oral administration. Absorption is >60% in dogs. Following IM administration, penicillin G (sodium/potassium) absorption is rapid (0.5–1 h) and complete due to its high degree of solubility. Absorption of organic esters in microsuspensions (penicillin G procaine or benzathine) are gradually absorbed over 1–3 days and act as depot drugs.

Distribution
Penicillins are widely distributed in body fluids and tissues, including liver, bile, intestines, muscle, and lungs. Penicillin does not penetrate intracellularly and has poor penetration into some tissues such as the CNS, cornea, bronchial secretions, prostate, cartilage, and bone. Protein binding is 50%.

CNS penetration
Penicillins have very poor penetration into the CSF (<1%), but increase with inflammation (3–6%). High doses with inflammation may provide temporary therapeutic concentrations.

Metabolism
Both procaine and benzathine penicillins are hydrolyzed to the parent compound after IM injection. Penicillin G is primarily excreted unchanged in urine.

Most of a dose (60–90%) is excreted into urine by tubular secretion with approximately 20% being excreted by glomerular filtration. Anuria may significantly increase the half-life.

Half-life

The half-life of penicillin in dogs is only 30 min. Procaine and benzathine penicillin have much longer half-lives but may not reach peak concentrations sufficient to be effective against some bacteria.

Pregnancy risk factor

Category B: No reports of embryotoxic or teratogenic effects in laboratory animals or humans. Penicillins are considered safe in pregnancy.

Lactation

Penicillin is excreted into milk in very low concentrations with milk to plasma rations of 0.2. It is considered safe for nursing animals.

References

Greene, C., Hartmann, K., *et al.* (2006) Antimicrobial drug formulary. Appendix 8. In: *Infectious Disease of the Dog and Cat*. Greene, C. (ed.), Elsevier, St. Louis, MO, pp. 1186–1333.

Ross, L. and Rentko, V. (2000) *Leptosirosis. Kirk's Current Veterinary Therapy: XIII Small Animal Practice*. Bonaggura, J. (ed.), W.B. Saunders, Philadelphia, pp. 298–300.

Further reading

Kaplan, M.I., Lee, J.A., Hovda, L.R., *et al.* (2011) Adverse effects associated with inadvertent intravenous penicillin procaine-penicillin G benzathine administration in two dogs and a cat. *JAVMA*, **238(4)**, 507–510.

Chapter 163: Pradofloxacin

US Generic (Brand) Name: Pradofloxacin (Veraflox)
Availability: Veterinary approved – Pradofloxacin oral suspension 25 mg/mL (15, 30 mL)
Resistance Mechanisms: Bacterial topoisomerase mutations, altered membrane permeability and efflux pumps

Use

Labeled for use in cats only for the treatment of skin infections caused by *Pasteurella multocida, Streptococcus canis, Staphylococcus aureus, S. pseudintermedius,* and *S. felis*. Active against some gram negative (*E. coli, Proteus*), gram positive, and anaerobic bacteria (*Fusobacterium, Porphyromonas gingivivalis*). Also active against *B. henselae, Mycoplasma* spp., *Rickettsia* spp., and *Mycobacterium* spp. Not active against *Nocardia spp.* Used clinically for wound infections, abscesses, upper respiratory infections, conjunctivitis, feline infectious anemia, and lower urinary tract infections in cats. Pradofloxacin has been used in Europe in dogs for deep pyoderma, UTIs, and as adjuvant therapy for periodontal infections.

Contraindications/warnings

Hypersensitivity to fluoroquinolones. Caution in dogs due to bone marrow toxicity. Avoid or reduce dose in patients with renal failure. Contraindicated in young, pregnant, or lactating animals due to arthropathy. Do not use in cats <6 weeks of age or those with pre-existing articular cartilage lesions. Use with caution in patients with known or suspected CNS disorders, since CNS stimulation can occur. May prolong Q-T interval, use with caution in patients with pre-existing cardiac disease or in those on other drugs that prolong the Q-T interval. Do not use more than 7 days in cats due to increased risk of bone marrow toxicity. Feline leukemia positive cats at higher risk of leucopenia and neutropenia.

Dosage

A trend toward decreased neutrophil counts is a function of dosage and the number of days dosed.

Feline

Wound/soft tissue infections: 7.5 mg/kg PO q24 h for 7 days (Bayer Manufacturer's Package Insert).

Upper Respiratory/Acute Infections: 7.5 mg/kg PO q 24 h for 5 days (Bayer Manufacturer's Package Insert).

Dose adjustments

Dose reductions in renal failure have not been established for this drug. Due to primarily renal excretion it would be expected to accumulate in severe renal failure. A reduction in the dose frequency in severe renal impairment (q48 h) instead of q24 h may be indicated.

Administration

Shake well. Use dosing syringe provided to ensure accuracy to the nearest 0.1 mL. Rinse syringe between administrations. Best absorbed on an empty stomach, but may be administered with food to decrease gastrointestinal upset. Avoid antacid use or concurrent administration with divalent or trivalent cations (iron, calcium, aluminum). If given orally, separate doses by 2–4 h. Maintain hydration and urinary output. A vanilla flavoring is added to the suspension, which is reported to be palatable to cats. Animal should avoid long term exposure to UV light while taking due to potential photosensitivity reactions.

Electrolyte contents

Not significant. Pradofloxacin suspension vehicle contains an undisclosed quantity of propylene glycol.

Storage/stability

Store at room temperature. After opening, store in the tightly closed bottle provided at room temperature. The bottle is stable for 60 days after opening.

Adverse reactions

>10%
Salivation reported in cats.

1–10%
Diarrhea and loose stools reported in cats.

<1%
Dose dependent side effects in cats have included vomiting, hypersalivation, leukocytosis, neutrophilia, photoreceptor degeneration via electron microscopy (differing from enrofloxacin) reported in one cat, decreased left ventricular performance, vocalization, and ataxia. Bone marrow toxicity has been reported in dogs.

Other species
Fluoroquinolones may also cause elevated liver enzymes, crystaluria, hypertension, angina pectoris, myocardial infarction, cardiopulmonary arrest, dyspnea, photosensitivity, rash, elevated serum creatinine, arthralgia, cartilage damage, lameness, cataracts, tendon rupture, allergic reactions, agranulocytosis, prolongation of the Q-T interval, erythema multiforme, toxic epidermal necrolysis, and colitis.

Drug interactions

Bioavailability is decreased by dairy products and enteral feedings containing cations. Aluminum or magnesium products, sucralfate, calcium, iron, zinc, and multiple vitamins with minerals may all decrease absorption. Give these agents at least 2–4 h from the dose, consider switching to an H_2 antagonist or omeprazole. Theophylline and NSAIDs may increase CNS stimulation of pradofloxacin, H_2 antagonists and loop diuretics may inhibit renal elimination of quinolones, antineoplastics may decrease absorption of quinolones, pradofloxacin may increase cyclosporine and digoxin concentrations. Avoid use with agents that can cause prolongation of the Q-T interval (cisapride, etc.).

Monitoring

Monitor for hypersensitivity reactions and CNS stimulation. Get baseline CBC with differential and monitor closely for unexplained drop in leukocyte, neutrophil, or lymphocyte counts.

Overdose

Acute renal failure and seizures may result. Gastrointestinal decontamination and supportive care are recommended. Although hemodialysis is not recommended in fluoroquinolone overdose, charcoal hemoprofusion and dialysis have been reported to markedly reduce plasma concentrations of enrofloxacin and may work for pradofloxacin.

Diagnostic test interference

None noted.

Mechanism

Bactericidal third generation fluoroquinolone. Promotes breakage of double stranded bacterial DNA. Inhibits DNA-gyrase in susceptible organisms, stops relaxation of supercoiled DNA.

Pharmacology/kinetics

Absorption
Pradofloxacin is well absorbed orally on an empty stomach (70%) in cats. Food markedly decreases absorption (53% decrease in the peak concentration and 26% decrease in the AUC).

Distribution

Pradofloxacin is widely distributed into tissues and is reported to concentrate in the skin of dogs by up to 7 times the plasma concentration. Protein binding is 30% in cats.

CNS penetration

No information is reported to date on penetration into the CNS. In general, fluoroquinolones have limited penetration into the CNS.

Metabolism

Pradofloxacin is metabolized in the liver. Elimination is via glucuronidation in cats and primarily renal excretion. In dogs, 40% of the drug is excreted unchanged in urine.

Half-life

The half-life in cats is 7.3 h in the fasted state and 6.4 h after feeding.

Pregnancy risk factor

Category C: Penetrates the placenta and was shown to cause teratogenic effects (eye malformations) in fetal rats. It also has potential fetal cartilage effects so it is considered contraindicated in pregnant animals.

Lactation

Pradofloxacin is excreted into milk and was demonstrated to cause arthropathy in nursing puppies following maternal exposure.

Further reading

Biswas, S., Maggi, R., Papich, M., *et al.* (2010) Comparative activity of pradofloxacin, enrofloxacin and azithromycin against *Bartonella henselae* isolates collected from cats and a human. *J Clin Microbiol.*, **48(2)**, 617–618.

Less, P. (2013) Pharmacokinetics, pharmacodynamics and therapeutics of pradofloxacin in the dog and cat. *J Vet Pharmacol Ther.*, **36(3)**, 209–221.

Liu, X., Boothe, D., Jin., Y., *et al.* (2013) *In vitro* potency and efficacy favor later generation fluoroquinolones for the treatment of canine and feline *Escherichia coli* uropathogens in the United States. *World J Microbiol Biotech.*, **29(2)**, 347–354.

Messias, A., Gekeler, F., Wegener, A., *et al.* (2008) Retinal safety of a new fluoroquinolone, pradofloxacin in cats: Assessment with electroretinography. *Documenta Ophthal.*, **116(3)**, 777–191.

Schink, A.K., Kadlec, K., Hauschild, T., *et al.* (2013) Susceptibility of canine and feline bacterial pathogens to pradofloxacin and comparison with other fluoroquinolones approved for companion animals. *Vet Microbiol.*, **162**, 116–126.

Chapter 164: Rifampin

US Generic (Brand) Name: Rifampin (Rifadin, Rimactane)
Availability: Human approved – Rifampin oral capsules (150, 300 mg), rifampin powder for injection (600 mg), compounded oral suspension (10 mg/mL)
Resistance Mechanisms: Altered RNA polymerase

Use

Used in combination with other antibiotics for synergistic effects. Should not be used alone due to rapid onset of resistance. Active against a variety of organisms including gram positive and facultative anaerobic organisms. Most gram negative bacteria should be considered resistant. Rifampin is considered especially active in the treatment of Staphylococcal infections and in the eradication of pathogens located inside phagocytic cells. It is effective in the treatment of *Staphylococcus* spp. infections (including methicillin resistant) and *Streptococcus* spp. infections (including drug resistant) when combined with other agents. It is very active in combination with other agents against biofilm infections involving prosthetic joints. It is active against a variety of intracellular organisms including *Corynebacterium*, *Ehrlichia*, and *Rhodococcus*. It may also be used in combination with dapsone, fluoroquinolones, clofazimine, or a macrolide in the treatment of *Mycobacterium* infections. Rifampin has been used in the treatment of Brucellosis in combination with doxycycline and an aminoglycoside.

Contraindications/warnings

Hypersensitivity to rifampin. Caution in patients with liver impairment or on other hepatotoxic drugs.

Dosage

Rifampin should never be used as monotherapy, doses presented here are in combination with various other drugs (macrolides, fluoroquinolones, vancomycin, etc.) that are synergistic to improve efficacy.

Canine

Susceptible infections: 5 mg/kg PO q12–24 h (Papich 2002).

Feline

Susceptible infections: 5 mg/kg PO q12–24 h (Papich 2002).

Dose adjustments

Doses should be reduced in patients with moderate to severe hepatic impairment.

Administration

Administer on an empty stomach if tolerated. Food decreases the extent of rifampin's absorption. Administer 1 h prior or 2 h after a meal or antacids. Follow oral administration with water. Give with food if nausea or vomiting occurs. For IV infusion, add 10 mL of sterile water for injection into the 600 mg vial to make a 60 mg/mL solution. Swirl gently, draw up the appropriate dose, and add to 100 mL of 5% dextrose injection. Infuse at a rate that allows complete infusion over 30 min. IV infusion solutions in dextrose must be used within 4 h of reconstitution due to precipitation. Do not administer IM or SC due to tissue irritation.

Electrolyte contents

Not significant.

Storage/stability

Store capsules and injectable vials at room temperature. Avoid exposure to light and heat. After the sterile vial is reconstituted it is stable for 24 h at room temperature. For small oral doses, a liquid suspension (10 mg/mL) can be compounded with one of the following syrups (Syrup NF, simple syrup, raspberry syrup, or Syrpalta). Empty the contents of four (300 mg) capsules into a 4 oz plastic oral dispensing vial. Add sufficient amount of syrup up to the 120 mL mark and shake well until dissolved. This is stable for 4 weeks refrigerated or at room temperature.

Adverse reactions

>10%

Elevated liver enzymes have been reported in a small number of cats and up to 20% of dogs receiving 5–10 mg/kg/day. This may be related to the high serum concentrations achieved in dogs compared to other species and the fact that canine patients have limited acetylation capacity. Nausea, vomiting, and orange colored urine/feces are reported in dogs and cats.

1–10%

Lethargy, anorexia, bilirubinemia, and bilirubinuria reported in dogs.

Other species

Rashes, pruritus, urticaria, edema, eosinophilia, leucopenia, hemolytic anemia, hemolysis, thrombocytopenia, pancreatitis, colitis, elevated BUN and serum uric acid concentration, nephritis, acute renal failure, behavioral changes, ataxia, myalgia, weakness, osteomalacia, visual changes, and pemphigoid reactions.

Drug interactions

In humans, rifampin decreases plasma concentrations of calcium channel blockers (verapamil, diltiazem, nifedipine), digoxin, cyclosporine, corticosteroids, anticoagulants, theophylline, barbiturates, chloramphenicol, azole antifungals, benzodiazepams, beta-blockers, enalapril, sulfa-drugs, dapsone, anti-arrhythmics, fluoroquinolones, tetracyclines, and levothyroid. TMS increases rifampin concentrations. Antacids decrease rifampin concentrations. Hepatotoxic drugs (macrolides, antifungals) may increase hepatotoxicity. In humans, ciprofloxacin and clarithromycin have produced a lupus like reaction if used concomitantly with rifampin.

Monitoring

Establish baseline CBC, liver, and renal function. Monitor AST and bilirubin at 2, 4, 6, and 8 weeks of therapy and then monthly for prolonged therapy. Owners should monitor for vomiting, dark urine, yellow discoloration of eyes, pale stools, or unusual bleeding or bruising.

Overdose

Symptoms of overdose may include nausea, vomiting, erythema, and hepatotoxicity. Supportive care and gastrointestinal decontamination with activated charcoal may be required. Active diuresis may promote excretion of the drug. If severe hepatic impairment lasts more than 24–48 h, charcoal hemoprofusion can be considered. Hemodialysis does not effectively remove the drug.

Diagnostic test interference

Rifampin can alter vitamin B12 and folate assays. It may also cause a positive Coomb's reaction, transient increases in liver function tests, and decreased excretion of contrast media.

Mechanism

Bacteriostatic rifamycin. Binds to the B-subunit of bacterial DNA-dependent RNA polymerase causing inhibition of RNA transcription.

Pharmacology/kinetics

Absorption
Rifampin is well absorbed orally. Absorption occurs within 2 h of an oral dose in dogs. Absorption is decreased with food.

Distribution
Rifampin has excellent penetration into most tissues and fluids. It penetrates into cells and is found in high concentrations in all tissues including milk, bone, CSF, exudates, ascetic fluid, and soft tissues. Protein binding is >70% in humans.

CNS penetration
Rifampin has good penetration into the CSF with CSF:plasma ratios of 0.52–1.17 in rabbits.

Metabolism
Rifampin metabolism is not well understood in dogs and cats. In humans, it is metabolized in the liver to an active metabolite (Desacetylrifampin), which is primarily excreted via bile. The parent compound undergoes significant enterohepatic recycling. Autoinduction of liver enzymes causes an increase in its own metabolism over time.

Half-life
The half-life in dogs is 8 h following a 10 mg/kg oral dose.

Pregnancy risk factor

Category C: Rifampin has demonstrated teratogenic effects in laboratory animals at high doses and should be avoided in pregnant animals.

Lactation
Rifampin is excreted into milk, with milk to serum concentrations of 0.9–1.28. This may cause adverse reactions (elevated liver enzymes, diarrhea, etc.) in nursing animals.

Reference

Papich, M.G. (2002) *Saunders Handbook of Veterinary Drugs*. 2nd edn. Winkel, A. (ed.), W.B. Saunders Company, Philadelphia, pp. 586–587.

Further reading

Ackerman, L. (1987) Cutaneous bacterial granuloma (botryomycosis) in five dogs: Treatment with rifampin. *Mod Vet Pract.*, **68(7/8)**, 404–409.

Beck, D.M. (1987) Can rifampin help manage CNS infections and internal abscesses in cats? *Vet Med.*, **82(12)**, 1239–1240.

Finel, J.M., Pittillo, R.F., and Mellett, L.B. (1971) Flourometric and microbiological assays for rifampin and the determination of serum levels in the dog. *Chemother.*, **16**, 380–388.

Gunn-Moore, D.A., Jenkins, P.A., and Lucke, V.M. (1996) Feline tuberculosis: a literature review and discussion of 19 cases caused by an unusual mycobacterial variant. *Vet Rec.*, **138(3)**, 53–58.

Senturk, S., Ozel, E., and Sen, A. (2005) Clinical efficacy of rifampin for treatment of canine pyoderma. *Acta Vet Brno.*, **74**, 117–122.

Chapter 165: Potentiated Sulfas

US Generic (Brand) Name: Sulfamethoxazole/trimethoprim (TMS), Co-trimazole (Bactrim, Bactrim DS, Cotrim, Cotrim DS, Septra, Septra DS, Uroplus SS, Uroplus DS, and Sulfamethoxazole/ormetoprim (Primor)

Availability: Human approved – Sulfamethoxazole/trimethoprim (single strength: 400/80 mg tablets, double strength: 800/160 mg), oral suspension (sulfamethoxazole 40 mg/mL/trimethoprim 8 mg/mL), sterile injectable solution (sulfamethoxazole 80 mg/trimethoprim 16 mg per mL). Veterinary approved – Sulfadimethoxine and ormetoprim oral tablets (100 mg/20 mg, 200 mg/40 mg, 500 mg/100 mg, 1000 mg/200 mg)

Resistance Mechanisms: Altered bacterial binding sites (dihydropteroate synthase: DHPS)

Use

Active against *Streptococcus* spp., *Staphylococcus* spp., *E. coli*, *Klebsiella*, *Enterobacter* spp., *Proteus*, *Aeromonas*, *Bordetella* spp., *Burkheria*, *Cyclospora*, *Isospora*, *Moraxella*, *Shigella*, *Stenotrophomonas*, and anaerobes. Commonly used to treat urinary tract infections, sinusitis, and prostatitis. Can be used intravenously to treat disseminated *Nocardia*, *Salmonella*, and *Brucella* spp. Also active against *Toxoplasma* and *Coccidia*.

Contraindications/warnings

Hypersensitivity to sulfas or trimethaprim/ormetoprim. Avoid in severe liver and renal impairment, anemia, dehydration, malnutrition, thyroid dysfunction, animals with blood dyscrasias, or very young animals. Do not use in pregnant or lactating animals. Doberman pinchers more susceptible to idiosyncratic sulfonamide toxicosis compared to other breeds. Slow acetylators (canines) are at increased risk of toxicities. Avoid in animals with pre-existing urinary obstruction or urolithiasis.

Dosage

Doses are based on combined sulfa/trimethoprin unless specified otherwise.

Canine
Skin and soft tissue: 15 mg/kg PO q12 h × 14 days or Primor – 55 mg/kg PO loading dose (based on combined sulfa/ormetoprim); then 27.5 mg/kg PO q24 h for at least 2 days after resolution (max. of 21 days) (Primor Manufacture's Package insert).

Meningitis: Septra – 25 mg/kg sulfamethoxazole and 5 mg/kg trimethoprim IV q12 h (Greene 2013).

Systemic infections, Bacteremia: Septra – 30–45 mg/kg PO q12 h for 3–5 days (Greene *et al.*, 2006).

Toxoplasmosis: Septra – 15 mg/kg PO q12 h for 4 weeks (Lappin 2013).

Neospora: Septra – 15 mg/kg PO q12 h for 4 weeks. Use with Clindamycin (10–12 mg/kg PO q8 h × 4 weeks) or pyrimethamine (1 mg/kg PO q24 h for 4 weeks) (Sykes 2013).

Hepatazoon cani: Septra – 15 mg/kg PO q12 h for 2–4 weeks. Use with Clindamycin (10 mg/kg PO q8 h) and pyrimethamine (0.25 mg/kg PO q24 h) (Lappin 2013).

Feline
Soft tissue/UTI: Septra – 15 mg/kg PO q12 h for 7–14 days (Greene *et al.*, 2006).

Toxoplasmosis: Septra – 15 mg/kg PO q12 h for 4 weeks (Lappin 2013).

Nocardia: Septra – 30–60 mg/kg PO q12 h (Ford and Aronson, 1985). High doses and prolonged therapy (12 weeks) are used in humans for this innately resistant organism, particularly with abscesses and CNS infections. Monitor closely for bone marrow toxicity and hepatotoxicity.

Dose adjustments

Doses should be reduced in impaired renal function. The dose and/or frequency should be modified in response to the degree of renal impairment. Doses should be reduced by approximately 50% in patients with significant renal impairment.

Administration

If oral therapy is not feasible, IV therapy may be given. Do not administer IM. For IV administration dilute 5 mL of the concentrated solution containing 80 mgs/mL of sulfamethoxizole and 16 mg/mL trimethoprim with 125 mL of 5% dextrose. If fluid restriction is required, dilute with 75 mL. Infuse intravenously over 60–90 min. The injectable concentrate contains sodium metabisulfate that may cause anaphylaxis in some animals. Do not admix with other drugs or solutions. Shake the oral solution well before administering. Maintain hydration at all times during therapy.

Electrolyte contents

Septra single strength tablets have 1.8 mEq (0.08 mEq) and the double strength tablets have 3.6 mg (0.16 mEq) of sodium. Injectable vial contains benzyl alcohol and sodium metabisulfate.

Storage/stability

Store tablets, oral solution, and injectable solutions at room temperature, protected from light. Do not refrigerate the injectable or use normal saline as a diluent. Stability of admixtures in D5W are concentration dependent (5 mL/125 mL: 6 h, 5 mL/100 mL: 4 h, 5 mL/75 mL: 2 h). The injectable vial is stable for 48 h after first entry.

Adverse reactions

>10%
Keratoconjunctivitis sicca (up to 15% in small dogs <12 kg), nausea, vomiting, and anorexia reported in dogs. Anorexia reported in cats.

1–10%
Diarrhea, depression, fever, pruritus, and facial swelling reported in dogs. Leukopenia and anemia reported in cats.

<1%

Idiosyncratic toxicosis reported in dogs at 8–20 days after starting treatment (blood dyscrasias including anemia, leucopenia, and thrombocytopenia), fever, focal retinitis, lymphadenopathy, non-septic polyarthritis, polymyositis, and skin rash (greater in Doberman pinschers and with prior sulfa exposure). Samoyeds and miniature Schnauzers may also have an increased risk of toxicities. Typically reversible 2–5 days after sulfa is discontinued. Non-regenerative anemia with high dose, long term (60–120 mg/kg/day) therapy. Iatrogenic hypothyroidism in dogs with high doses (25 mg/kg q12 h × 6 weeks), hemolytic/aplastic anemia, cutaneous drug eruptions, erythema multiforme, perforating folliculitis, fever, severe hepatitis, aggression, ataxia, thrombocytopenia, seizures, hyperexcitability, and polyuria/polydipsia.

Other species

Side effects in humans and other mammals: crystallization of acetylated sulfa metabolite in urine with acidura, dehydration, nephritis, hyperkalemia, hyper/hypoglycemia, pancreatitis, fatal hepatitis and dermatologic reactions, and kernicterus in neonates.

Drug interactions

Potentiated sulfas may increase arrhythmias and hypotensive effects of detomidine. Potentiated sulfas may increase the plasma concentrations/toxicity of bone marrow suppressants, dapsone, amantidine, sulfonylureas, digoxin, oral anticoagulants, and procainamide. Sulfas may decrease the efficacy of tricyclic antidepressants, and cyclosporine. Hepatotoxic drugs may increase the risk of hepatotoxicity from sulfas. Thiazide diuretics may increase sulfa-induced thrombocytopenia and pyrimethamine may increase the risk of sulfa induced megaloblastic anemia. Sulfas may increase the risk of hyperkalemia from ACE inhibitors and may decrease the efficacy of live vaccines.

Monitoring

Monitor CBC, platelets and Schirmer's tear test closely if on long term therapy. Monitor for signs/symptoms of allergic/autoimmune disease. Monitor serum potassium if on concurrent ACE inhibitors.

Overdose

At five-fold the labeled dose of Primor, convulsions and hypoglycemia were reported in dogs. Nausea, vomiting and colitis may also be seen. Delayed toxicity may include bone marrow suppression and hepatotoxicosis. Gastrointestinal decontamination/lavage, fluid therapy, and diazepam for seizures are advised. Acidification of urine will increase renal elimination of the trimethoprim. Anemia may be reversible with folinic acid (Leucovorin) supplementation. Hemodialysis only removes a small portion of the drug.

Diagnostic test interference

False positive urine glucose (Benedict's), elevated (10%) creatinine with Jaffe reaction, false positive urine protein, and false positive urine urobilinogen test, Thyroid tests (T4 and thyrotropin stimulation) may be significantly reduced (no alteration in T3).

Mechanism

Bacteriostatic sulfonamide. Inhibits bacterial utilization of para-aminobenzoic acid (PABA) for folic acid synthesis. It inhibits dihydrofolic acid formation. Trimethoprim and ormetroprim inhibits dihydrofolic acid reduction to tetrahydrofolate resulting in dual inhibition of enzyme in the folic acid pathway.

Pharmacology/kinetics

Absorption

Sulfamethozaxole, sulfadimethoxazole, trimethoprim, and ormetoprim are rapidly and almost completely absorbed following oral doses in cats and dogs (>90%).

Distribution

Potentiated sulfas are widely distributed throughout most tissues and fluids, including the middle ear, prostate, bile, aqueous humor, CSF, peritoneal fluid, synovial fluid, and urine. Trimethoprim appears to have much better penetration than sulfamethoxazole in some tissues. In dogs, concentrations of trimethoprim in prostatic fluid reach as high as three-fold serum concentrations while sulfamethoxizole may reach only 10% of concurrent serum concentrations. Protein binding in cats and dogs is >75%.

CNS penetration

Penetration of trimethoprim into the CSF is approximately 50% of serum concentrations compared to only 2.7% of sulfadimethoxine at the same time after single doses. However, sulfas accumulate in the CSF over time with repeat dosing, which may lead to therapeutic concentrations.

Metabolism

Trimethoprim is metabolized in the liver to oxide and hydroxylated metabolites, which have between 2.5–39.5% the activity of the parent drug. Trimethoprim, its metabolites and sulfas are primarily excreted via glomerular filtration and tubular secretion. Only small amounts of trimethoprim are excreted into feces via biliary excretion. Sulfas are metabolized in the liver/tissues in most species (cats, humans) to N-acetyl metabolites. These metabolites are then glucuronidated and excreted into urine where their poor solubility may be the cause of crystalluria. In dogs, acetylation is limited, so sulfas are primarily excreted as the active parent compound, with two-thirds of a dose being excreted within 24 h via renal excretion. The parent drug is more soluble in urine and less likely to precipitate out to cause crystalluria.

Half-life

The half-life of trimethoprim in dogs is short (2.5 h) compared to sulfamethoxazole (13.1 h). In cats, the half-life of sulfamethoxizole is 10.2 h.

Pregnancy risk factor

Category C–D: Sulfonamides and trimethoprim cross the placenta and are reported to cause significant teratogenic effects in mice and rats (malformations and cleft palates). Fetal toxic effects are also reported in late term pregnancy in humans.

Lactation

Sulfonamides and trimethoprim are distributed into milk in small quantities. Approximately 0.5–2% of maternal plasma concentrations of sulfonamides and 1–3.5 % of trimethoprim are excreted into milk.

References

Ford, R.B. and Aronson, A.L. (1985) Antimicrobial drugs and infectious disease. In: *Handbook of Small Animal Therapeutics*. Davis, L.E. (ed.), Churchill Livingstone, New York, pp. 45–88.

Greene, C.E. (2013) Bacterial meningitis. Ch. 90. In: *Canine and Feline Infectious Diseases*, Sykes, J.E. (ed.), Elsevier, St. Louis, MO. pp. 886–892.

Greene, C., Hartmann, K., *et al.* (2006) Antimicrobial drug formulary. Appendix 8. In: *Infectious Disease of the Dog and Cat*. Greene, C. (ed.), Elsevier, St. Louis, MO, pp. 1186–1333.

Lappin, M.R. (2013) Toxoplasmosis. Ch. 72. In: *Canine and Feline Infectious Diseases*, Sykes, J.E. (ed.), Elsevier, St. Louis, MO. pp. 693–701.

Sykes, J.E. (2013) Neosporosis. Ch. 73. In: *Canine and Feline Infectious Diseases*, Sykes, J.E. (ed.), Elsevier, St. Louis, MO. pp. 704–711.

Further reading

Baggot, J.D. (1977) Pharmacokinetics of sulfadimethoxine in cats. *Aust J Exp Biol Med Sci.*, **55(6)**, 663–670.

Baggott, J.D., Ludden, T.M., and Powers, T.E. (1976) The bioavailability, disposition kinetics and dosage of sulphadimethoxine in dogs. *Can J Comp Med.*, **40**, 310–317.

Morgan, R.V. and Bachrach, A. (1982) Keratoconjunctivitis sicca associated with sulfonamide therapy in dogs. *J Am Vet Med Assoc.*, **180**, 432–434.

Rowland, P.H., Center, S.A., and Dougherty, S.A. (1992) Presumptive trimethoprim-sulfaciazine-related hepatotoxicosis in a dog. *J Am Vet Med Assoc.*, **200(3)**, 348–350.

Weiss, D.J. and Klausner, J.S. (1990) Drug-associated aplastic anemia in dogs: eight cases (1984–1988). *J AmVet Med Assoc.*, **196(3)**, 472–475.

Chapter 166: Timentin

US Generic (Brand) Name: Ticarcillin disodium/clavulanate potassium (Timentin)
Availability: Human approved – Timentin sterile powder for injection (ticarcillin/clavulanate 3 g/0.1 g). Frozen pre-mix 3.1 g (ticarcillin/clavulanate 3 g/0.1 g × 100 mL) (availability varies)
Resistance Mechanisms: Increased beta-lactamases, decreased membrane permeability, increased OXA-type enzymes

Use

Used for the treatment of severe infections due to gram negative, gram positive, and anaerobic bacteria. Commonly used for *Pseudomonas, Bacteriodes, E. coli, Pasturella, Klebsiella, Proteus,* and *Staphylococcus* spp. (including beta-lactamase producing) infections. Can be used to treat respiratory, bone, joint, septicemia, skin and soft tissue, urinary tract, cholangitis, pancreatitis, peritonitis, and liver abscesses. Not effective for the treatment of methicillin or oxacillin resistant strains of *Staphylococcus* spp.

Contraindications/warnings

Hypersensitivity to ticarcillin, clavulanate, penicillins, or cephalosporins. Use with caution and adjust dose in renal failure. Caution in chronic heart failure or those with pre-existing electrolyte imbalances due to high sodium concentration.

Dosage

Dosed on ticarcillin fraction, IM injections should only be for uncomplicated UTIs.

Canine
Susceptible infections: 33–50 mg/kg IV, IM q4–6 h (Papich 2002).

Feline
Susceptible infections: 33–50 mg/kg IV, IM q4–6 h (Papich 2002).

Dose adjustments

Adjust dose in renal impairment. Decrease frequency of dosing proportional to the degree of renal impairment (q12 h in moderate renal failure/q24 h in severe renal failure). For patients with renal and hepatic impairment, dosing frequency and dose should be adjusted.

Administration

For IV infusions, reconstitute the vial with 13 mL of sterile water for injection or sodium chloride to provide a 200 mg of ticarcillin per mL and 6.7 mg of clavulanic acid per mL. The dose should then be further diluted to a concentration of 10–50 mg/mL in a compatible IV solution (D5W, normal saline, or LRS). Intermittent IV infusions should be infused over 30 min. If giving aminoglycosides, give at least 1 h apart from ticarcillin. For IM injections 1% lidocaine may be used for dilution to decrease pain. Reconstitute each gram of ticarcillin with 2 mL of sterile water, sodium chloride or 1% lidocaine to make a solution of 385 mg/mL. The IM dose should not exceed 2 g/dose or 1 g/site (2.6 mL). Deep IM injections should be done into large muscles.

Electrolyte contents

1 g of Timentin has 109.3 mg (4.75 mEq) of sodium and 0.15 mEq of potassium.

Storage/stability

Store the powder at room temperature, not to exceed 24°C or this will cause degradation of clavulanate. Initial reconstituted solution is stable for 6 h at room temperature or 72 h refrigerated. After further dilution with LRS or normal saline 0.9% to concentrations of 10–100 mg/mL, Timentin is stable for 24 h at room temperature, 7 days refrigerated, or 30 days frozen. If using D5W, solutions are stable for 24 h at room temperature, 3 days refrigerated, and up to 7 days frozen. Frozen solutions once thawed should not be refrozen and are stable for 8 h. Darkened solutions indicate a loss in potency of clavulanate and should not be used.

Adverse reactions

>10%
Pain at IM injection site, thrombophlebitis, and electrolyte imbalances reported in dogs

1–10%
Lethargy, diarrhea, and colitis reported in dogs

Other species
Rash, pruritus, erythema, fever, dermal necrolysis, eosinophilia, thrombocytopenia, positive Coomb's, vomiting, colitis, hyperkalemia, hypokalemia, hypernatremia, elevated serum creatinine, BUN, elevated liver enzymes, neuromuscular hyperirritability, seizures, abnormal platelet aggregation, and prolonged prothrombin time.

Drug interactions

Other nephrotoxic drugs (aminoglycosides, amphotericin-B, and furosemide) can decrease renal excretion of ticarcillin and increase toxicity. Many drugs are not compatible with ticarcillin when admixed. Check the manufacturer's suggested guidelines before admixing. Do not admix with bicarbonate or aminoglycosides.

Monitoring

Monitor sodium and potassium concentrations. For prolonged therapy, monitor CBC, liver, and renal function.

Overdose

Neuromuscular hypersensitivity and seizures may occur. Provide supportive care and diazepam for seizures. Hemodialysis removes 20–50% of a dose.

Diagnostic test interference

Alters urinary glucose tests if using Clinitest. False positive urinary and serum proteins. Inactivates aminoglycosides *in vitro*, so alters tests for aminoglycoside therapeutic testing, false positive Coomb's test.

Mechanism

Extended spectrum penicillin with beta-lactamase inhibitor. Bactericidal. Inhibits bacterial cell wall synthesis by binding to one or more penicillin binding proteins. This inhibits transpeptidation affecting peptidoglycan synthesis of bacterial cell walls. Clavulanate binds to beta-lactamases and inactivate them. This extends the spectrum of ticarcillin to cover beta-lactamase producing strains.

Pharmacology/Kinetics

Absorption

Clavulanate is well absorbed orally, but ticarcillin is poorly absorbed so must be given parenterally. IM administration has variable absorption in dogs and should be limited to treatment of uncomplicated UTIs.

Distribution

Both drugs are widely distributed throughout tissues and fluids including peritoneal fluids and bone. Protein binding is only 13% for ticarcillin in dog plasma.

CNS penetration

CSF penetration is poor (6%). Although this may increase with inflamed meninges it is not considered therapeutic.

Metabolism

In dogs, clavulanate is metabolized to 1-amino-4-hydroxybutan-2-one which is excreted in urine. Overall, 34–52%, 25–27%, and 16–33% of a dose is excreted in urine, feces, and respired air, respectively. Ticarcillin is excreted primarily as unchanged drug in urine accounting for about 60% of a dose.

Half-life

The half-life in dogs and cats is between 45–80 min.

Pregnancy risk factor

Category B: Not demonstrated to be teratogenic in laboratory animals (mice, rats) or humans. Ticarcillin crosses the placenta and has a fetal: maternal ratio of 0.91. Timentin is considered safe in pregnancy.

Lactation

Ticarcillin is excreted into milk in low concentrations and is not considered a risk to nursing animals due to its limited oral absorption.

Reference

Papich, M.G. (2002) *Saunders Handbook of Veterinary Drugs*. 2nd edn. Winkel, A. (ed.), W.B. Saunders Company, Philadelphia, pp. 648–649.

Further reading

Bennett, A.B., Martin, P.A., Gottieb, S.A., *et al.* (2013) *In vitro* susceptibilities of feline and canine *Escherichia coli* and *Pseudomonas* spp. isolates to ticarcillin and ticarcillin–clavulanic acid. *Aust. J. Vet Med.*, **29(5)**, 171–178.

Garg, R.C., Keefe, T.J., and Vig, M.M. (1987) Serum levels and pharmacokinetics of ticarcillin and clavulanic acid in dogs following parenteral administration of Timentin. *J Vet Pharmacol Ther.*, **10(4)**, 324–330.

Greene, C., Hartmann, K., *et al.* (2006) Antimicrobial drug formulary. Appendix 8. In: *Infectious Disease of the Dog and Cat*. Greene, C. (ed.), Elsevier, St. Louis, MO, pp. 1186–1333.

Mealey, K.L. (2001) Penicillin and B-lactamase inhibitor combinations. *JAVMA*, **218**, 1893–1896.

Chapter 167: Tobramycin

US Generic (Brand) Name: Tobramycin sulfate (Nebcin, Tobrex, TOBI, AKTob)
Availability: Human approved –Tobramycin sulfate injectable (10, 40 mg/mL), powder for injection (1.2 g vial), inhalation solution (60 mg/mL × 5 mL), ophthalmic solution 0.3% (5 mL), ophthalmic oint. 0.3% (3.5 g)
Resistance Mechanisms: Aminoglycoside modifying enzymes, ribosome alteration, decreased permeability

Use

Treatment of severe gram negative bacilli infections. More active against *Pseudomonas aeruginosa* than gentamicin or amikacin. Also active against *Citrobacter* spp., *Klebsiella* spp., *Proteus* spp., *Serratia* spp., *Enterobacter* spp., *Morganella morganii*, *Proteus* spp., *E. Coli.*, and *Providencia* spp. Used for pneumonia, sepsis, and endophthalmitis.

Contraindications/warnings

Use with caution in animals with renal impairment, monitor animal closely for signs of tubular necrosis (casts appear early in urine). Avoid use in animals with pre-existing vestibular impairment, electrolyte imbalances, or myasthenia gravis. Discontinue the drug if signs of hypersensitivity, ototoxicity, or nephrotoxicity. Provide subcutaneous fluid hydration in animals receiving subcutaneous tobramycin. Avoid use of other renal toxic drugs in combination or prolonged therapy.

Dosage

Canine
Susceptible infections: 2 mg/kg IV, IM, SC q8 h or 4–6 mg/kg IV, IM, SC q24 h for 5 days or less (Greene *et al.*, 2006).

Feline
Susceptible infections: 2 mg/kg IV, IM, SC q8 h or 4–6 mg/kg IV, IM, SC q24 h for 5 days or less (Greene *et al.*, 2006).

Dose adjustments

No dose adjustment should be given for hepatic impairment. Avoid in severe renal impairment. The dose and interval should be altered with renal impairment. Give a loading dose followed by a 25–50% dose reduction administered at the same interval or normal dose with prolonged interval. Dose every 48–72 h instead of q24 h with significant renal impairment. Monitor plasma concentrations after the third dose and adjust dose so that trough concentrations are <2 µg/mL.

Administration

Hydrate animals and get baseline renal panel prior to administration. Tobramycin for injection as a dry powder is reconstituted with 30 mL of sterile water for injection to provide 40 mg/mL solution. The pre-mix solution or pharmacy bulk packs should only be used for IV injections. Once diluted into a parenteral admixture it is stable for 48 h at room temperature or refrigerated. The tobramycin dose is diluted in a minimum of 50 mL (50–100 mL) of normal saline for IV infusion. The appropriate dose of tobramycin should be withdrawn from the 10 mg or 40 mg/mL vial and injected directly for IM or SC administration.

Electrolyte contents

Not significant.

Storage/stability

The injectable solution, powder for dilution, and ophthalmic products are stored at room temperature. The reconstituted injectable solution is stable for 24 h at room temperature and 96 h when refrigerated.

Adverse reactions

>10%
Diarrhea, vomiting, and injection site reactions (SC, IM doses) reported in dogs and cats. Renal toxicity is common at doses >3 mg/kg/day in dogs/cats. Nephrotoxicity is polyuric, increased fractional electrolyte excretion, glycosuria, tubular casts, and may progress to oliguria. Acute tubular necrosis manifested by increases in serum creatinine and BUN. Typically reversible if maintain good urine output.

1–10%
Ototoxicity, high frequency hearing loss after prolonged therapy, may be irreversible. Neurotoxicity to the eighth cranial nerve. Vestibular injury and bilateral irreversible damage is related to the amount of drug given and duration of treatment. Cats may have vestibular toxicity (ataxia, impaired righting) several days prior to renal toxicity.

Other species
Hypotension, rash, eosinophilia, tremor, arthralgia, dyspnea, weakness, hypersensitivity reactions, drug fever, and anemia.

Drug interactions

In humans, concurrent use with renal toxic drugs (amphotericin B, iron, calcium channel blockers, cisplatin, NSAIDs, vancomycin, and polymyxin) may increase renal side effects. Neuromuscular blocking drugs may prolong or increase risk of neuromuscular toxicities. Loop diuretics may increase nephrotoxicity and ototoxicity. Beta-lactam antibiotics are synergistic against some types of bacteria. Beta-lactams inactivate aminoglycosides *in vitro* in serum samples, which may result in falsely decreased aminoglycoside concentrations. Aminoglycoside assays must be assessed immediately after collection.

Monitoring

Establish baseline renal function then monitor serum creatinine, urine output, urinalysis (casts). If possible, monitor peak and trough tobramycin concentrations.

Draw blood from alternative lumen or peripheral stick to avoid falsely high concentrations from central catheters. Both initial and periodic peak and trough levels should be obtained in patients with renal dysfunction or in serious infections. For serious infections, peak serum concentrations (30 min after a 30 min IV infusion) should be in the range of 6–10 µg/mL and trough concentrations (30 min prior to the next dose) should be 0.5–2 µg/mL. Peak concentrations following IM or SC dosing should be drawn at 1 h after dosing.

Overdose

Maintain good urine output, polyionic electrolyte fluid therapy >3 weeks may be required to reverse renal damage. Oliguria is a poor prognostic sign. Edrophonium, neostigmine, calcium chloride, or calcium gluconate may be used to reverse muscle paralysis. Hemodialysis is typically not required, but can remove 30% of the dose.

Diagnostic test interference

Beta-lactams and cephalosporins may decrease measured serum concentrations *in vitro*.

Mechanism

Bactericidal aminoglycoside. Inhibit protein synthesis in susceptible bacteria by binding to the 30s and 50s ribosomal subunits. This results in a defective bacterial cell membrane.

Pharmacology/kinetics

Absorption
Tobramycin is not absorbed orally. It is very well absorbed following IM and SC administration (>99% in cats).

Distribution
Tobramycin is widely distributed into most fluids and tissues with high concentrations found in the kidney, bronchial secretions, peritoneal, synovial, and abscess fluid. Protein binding in dog serum is <30%.

CNS penetration
Tobramycin has very little penetration into the CSF, even with inflamed meninges.

Metabolism
Tobramycin is not metabolized in the liver and is primarily excreted as parent drug in the urine.

Half-life
The half-life in serum of dogs is between 1–3.1 h depending on the route administered. Tissue binding may be much longer.

Pregnancy risk factor

Category C: Tobramycin crosses the placenta and has been reported in fetal fluids and tissues. Although the drug does not appear to be teratogenic, it has been reported to cause both renal and ototoxicity in human infants born to mothers receiving the drug.

Lactation
Tobramycin is excreted into milk in low concentrations. It is not absorbed well after oral administration, but may still cause modification of bowel flora in nursing animals.

Reference

Greene, C., Hartmann, K., *et al.* (2006) Antimicrobial drug formulary. Appendix 8. In: *Infectious Disease of the Dog and Cat.* Greene, C. (ed.), Elsevier, St. Louis, MO, pp. 1186–1333.

Further reading

Engle, J.E., Abt, A.B., Schneck, D.W., *et al.* (1979) Netilmicin and tobramycin. Comparison of nephrotoxicity in dogs. *Invest Urol.*, **17(2)**, 98–102.

Jernigan, A.D., Hatch, R.C., and Wilson, R.C. (1988) Pharmacokinetics of tobramycin in cats. *Am J Vet Res.*, **49(5)**, 608–612.

Ling, G.V., Conzelman, G.M., Franti, C.E., *et al.* (1981) Urine concentrations of gentamycin, tobramycin, amikacin, and kanamycin after subcutaneous administration to healthy adult dogs. *Am J Vet Res.*, **42(10)**, 1792–1794.

Szwed, J.J., Luft, F.C., Black, H.R., *et al.* (1974) Comparison of the distribution of tobramycin and gentamicin in body fluids of dogs. *Antimicrob Agents Chemother.*, **5(5)**, 444–446.

Chapter 168: Tylosin

US Generic (Brand) Name: Tylosin tartrate (Tylan)
Availability: Veterinary approved – Tylosin injectable (50, 200 mg/mL × 100 mL vials), tylosin powder (2.5–2.7 g per teaspoon × 100 g tub)
Resistance Mechanisms: Altered bacterial 23s rRNA (nucleosides G748 and A2058)

Use

Primarily used in small animals for treatment of chronic diarrhea not responsive to other antibiotics. Active against gram positive aerobic bacteria, as well as *Clostridium*, *Bacteroides*, *Fusobacterium*, and *Camphylobacter*. Is also active against *Pasteurella multocida* and *Mycoplasma*. It is not active against *E. coli* or *Salmonella*. Tylosin has been used in dogs for prevention of tear staining.

Contraindications/warnings

Hypersensitivity to tylosin or other macrolides.

Dosage

Tylosin powder has 3 g of tylosin tartrate per teaspoon. There is 1.1 g of tylosin tartrate per 1 g of tylosin base powder.

Canine
Susceptible infections: 7–15 mg/kg PO q12–24 h or 8–11 mg/kg IM q12 h (Papich 2002).

Colitis: 12–20 mg/kg PO q8 h with food, if there is a response decrease the interval to q12 h and eventually to q24 h for maintenance therapy.

Feline
Susceptible infections: 7–15 mg/kg PO q12–24 h or 8–12 mg/kg IM q12 h (Papich 2002).

Dose adjustments

Doses should be reduced in severe hepatic impairment.

Administration

Do not administer injectable solution IV. IM injections are painful. Do not inject more than 5 mL into one IM site. Administer oral powder on food or place into a gelatin capsule to mask taste. A 20 mg/kg dose for a 20 kg dog is approximately one-eighth of a teaspoon. For small patients, accurate doses may be weighed and placed in a small clear test tube or other measuring device that is marked with a line for clients to dose.

Electrolyte contents

Not significant. The injectable solution does contain 50% propylene glycol.

Storage/stability

Store injectable solution and powder at room temperature, in tightly sealed containers, protected from sunlight. Discard injectable solution 30 days after opening. Do not admix injectable with other drugs or it may precipitate.

Adverse reactions

>10%
Pain at the injection site, nausea, and foaming/salivation following oral administration in cats and dogs.

1–10%
Diarrhea and anorexia reported in cats and dogs.

<1%
At high doses (200 mg/kg/day) nephrosis and pyelonephritis have been reported in dogs. At 800 mg/kg/day, significant vomiting, salivation, and diarrhea are reported in dogs.

Drug interactions

There are no well documented drug interactions for tylosin. Sucralfate may decrease absorption.

Monitoring

Monitor liver and renal function with prolonged therapy.

Overdose

Oral overdoses to dogs up to 800 mg/kg resulted in gastrointestinal side effects. The injectable solution may result in toxicities similar to other macrolides including nausea, vomiting, diarrhea, and Q-T prolongation. Gastrointestinal decontamination and supportive care should be administered. Hemodialysis would not be expected to remove the drug.

Diagnostic test interference

May alter urinary catecholamines by fluorimetric determination. May cause falsely elevated liver enzyme (ALT, AST) tests by colorimetric assays.

Mechanism

Bacteriostatic macrolide. It binds to the 50s ribosome resulting in inhibition of protein synthesis. It may also have immunomodulatory effects.

Pharmacology/kinetics

Absorption
Oral bioavailability in dogs is low. Increases with higher doses and length of treatment. After 30 days, an oral dose of 25mg/kg/day results in peak concentrations of 1.4–2.7 µg/mL in dogs.

Distribution
Tylosin is widely distributed into most tissues and fluids. In dogs, the plasma:tissue ratio was reported to be only 0.68. Highest concentrations are reported in the liver, kidney, muscles, and lungs.

CNS penetration
Protein binding is 30–47%. Penetration into the CNS is poor (<0.5 µg/g) in cows.

Metabolism
Tylosin is metabolized in the liver and eliminated primarily via the bile. In dogs, 13.7% of a dose is excreted into bile within 5 h of a dose.

Half-life
The half-life in dogs is 54 min.

Pregnancy risk factor

Category B: There is no evidence that tylosin causes teratogenic effects. However, exposure in late term pregnancy may cause side effects in neonatal animals. Low birth weights and delayed ossification have been reported in laboratory animals exposed during late term pregnancy.

Lactation
Tylosin is excreted into milk in high concentrations (milk:plasma ratio of 1–55.4) with systemic administration, but it is unknown following oral administration.

Reference

Papich, M.G. (2002) *Saunders Handbook of Veterinary Drugs*. 2nd edn. Winkel, A. (ed.), W.B. Saunders Company, Philadelphia, pp. 678–679.

Further reading

Kilpinen, S., Spillman, T., Syria, P., *et al.* (2011) Effect of tylosin on dogs with suspected tylosin-resistant diarrhea: a placebo-controlled randomized, double blinded, prospective trial. *Acta Vet Scand.*, **53(1)**, 26–28.

VanLeeuwen, F. (1991) Tylosin. In: *Toxicological evaluation of certain veterinary drug residues in food. Thirty-eighth meeting of the Joint FAO/WHO Expert Committee on Food Additives (JE CFA).* WHO Food Additives, Series 29. International Program on Chemical Safety, WHO, Geneva, pp. 139–163.

Weisel, M.K., Powers, T.E., and Baggott, J.D. (1977) A pharmacokinetics analysis of tylosin in the normal dog. *Am J Vet Res.*, **38**, 273–275.

Westermarck, E., Frias, R., and Skrzypczak, T. (2005) Effect of diet and tylosin on chronic diarrhea in beagles. *J Vet Intern Med.*, **19(6)**, 822–827.

Chapter 169: Unasyn

US Generic (Brand) Name: Ampicillin/sulbactam (Unasyn, Unasyn Add-Vantage)
Availability: Human approved – Sterile powder for injection; ampicillin/sulbactam (1 g/0.5 g, 2 g/1 g, 10 g/5 g), Unasyn add-Vantage (1.5, 3.0 g)
Resistance Mechanisms: Altered bacterial penicillin binding proteins and beta lactamase (TEM-1) production, increased drug efflux (AdeB)

Use

Treatment of serious infections involving the respiratory tract, skin, reproductive tract, intra-abdominal, liver, cholangitis, pancreatitis, peritonitis, and abscesses. Active against *Acinetobacter* spp., *Bacteriodes* spp., *Prevotella* spp., *Pasteurella multocida*, *Proteus*, *Klebsiella*, and *Enterococcus faecalis*. Unasyn has similar coverage to ampicillin but also covers organisms that carry beta lactamases (*S. aureus*, *S. pseudintermedius*, *E. coli*, and anaerobes). Sulbactam is a beta lactamase inhibitor similar to clavulanate, but less active against gram negative beta-lactamases. Unasyn is not active against *Pseudomonas* spp.

Contraindications/warnings

Hypersensitivity to penicillins, cephalosporins, and sulbactam. Avoid use in patients with history of allergic reactions due to hypersensitivity reactions or atopic patients. Reduce dose in renal impairment.

Dosage

Dose according to the ampicillin fraction.

Feline/canine
Susceptible infections: 10–20 mg/kg IV or IM q8 h. Use higher doses for gram negative infections (Papich 2002).

Dose adjustments

The dosing frequency of Unasyn should be adjusted in patients with renal impairment according to the degree of impairment. Administer q12 h in moderate renal failure or q24 h in severe renal failure.

Administration

For intravenous injections, dilute the 1.5 or 3.0 gram vials with 3.2 or 6.4 mL, respectively, of sterile water for injection (or for intramuscular injections: 0.5% or 2% lidocaine) to make a 375 mg/mL solution. This contains 250 mg/mL of ampicillin and 125 mg/mL of sulbactam. Administer the appropriate dose deep into a large muscle within one hour after reconstitution. For intravenous administration, withdraw the appropriate dose and dilute immediately with a compatible intravenous solution (LRS, 0.9% NaCl, 5% dextrose and 0.45% NaCl) to yield a 3–45 mg/mL concentration (2–30 mg/mL ampicillin and 1–15 mg/mL sulbactam). Add-Vantage vials are reconstituted with 0.9% sodium chloride provided by the manufacturer. IV injections should be administered over 10–15 min to avoid seizures and IV infusions should be administered over 15–30 min.

Electrolyte contents

Each 1.5 g of Unasyn (1 g of ampicillin and 0.5 g of sulbactam) contains 5 mEq (115 mg) of sodium.

Storage/stability

Store at room temperature or cooler. Do not reconstitute with dextrose, which can hydrolyze Unasyn. After reconstitution with sterile water or lidocaine the product is only stable for one hour. Stability is concentration dependent so that further dilution improves stability. If diluted in 0.9% sodium chloride to 45 mg/mL (30 mg/mL of ampicillin and 15 mg/mL of sulbactam) it is stable for 8 h at room temperature or 48 h refrigerated. Solutions containing 30 mg/mL are stable refrigerated for 72 h.

Adverse reactions

>10%
Pain at the injection site, thrombophlebitis, and diarrhea have been reported in dogs

1–10%
Nausea, vomiting, allergic reactions (serum sickness, urticaria, angioedema, and bronchospasm) have been reported in dogs.

Other Species
Colitis, ataxia, neuromuscular hyperirritability, convulsions, penicillin encephalopathy, anemia, hemolytic anemia, elevated liver enzymes, eosinophilia, thrombocytopenia, granulocytopenia, and nephritis have been reported.

Drug interactions

Unasyn chemically inactivates aminoglycosides, so these cannot be intermixed. Tetracyclines may decrease the antibacterial effects of Unasyn. Unasyn may decrease the hormonal effects of estrogens (Incurin). Check specific references for drug compatibility. Many drugs cannot be admixed with Unyasyn (e.g., ondansetron and aminoglycosides).

Monitoring

With prolonged use, monitor CBC, renal, and hepatic function.

Overdose

Symptoms may include, seizures, neuromuscular hypersensitivity, electrolyte imbalance with sodium/potassium. Doses up to 3000 mg/kg have not demonstrated significant toxicity in cats and dogs. Hemodialysis can remove up to 35% of ampicillin and 45% of sulbactam in 4 h. Diazepam may be used for seizure control.

Diagnostic test interference

Ampicillin interferes with urinary glucose determination using Clinitest, but does not affect glucose oxidase tests (Clinistix and Tes-Tape).

Mechanism

Bactericidal aminopenicillin. Inhibits bacterial cell wall synthesis by binding to one or more penicillin binding proteins. This inhibits transpeptidation affecting peptidoglycan synthesis of bacterial cell walls. Sulbactam irreversibly binds beta lactamases that inactivate the beta lactam ring of ampicillin. This improves synergy against beta lactamase producing organisms.

Pharmacology/kinetics

Absorption
Sulbactam sodium is not orally absorbed and must be given intravenously or intramuscularly. An ester linked formulation is orally absorbed, but is not available in the USA.

Distribution
Both ampicillin and sulbactam are widely distributed in tissues, reaching 50–100% of serum concentrations. Highest concentrations in dogs are reported in the kidney and liver. It also reaches high concentrations in bronchial wall, alveolar fluid, pericardium, prostate, bile, ovaries, gallbladder, intestinal mucosa, and blister fluid. Concentrations within tissues are approximately equal, but are more variable for sulbactam and dependent on the degree of inflammation.

CNS penetration
Ampicillin and sulbactam only have minimal penetration across the blood brain barrier. Concentrations are increased with inflammation but are not considered therapeutic.

Metabolism
Both drugs are excreted primarily via renal excretion with 75–90% of the drug excreted as parent drug in urine within 8 h. Only small amounts are found in feces. Protein binding is 15–28% for ampicillin and 38% for sulbactam in humans.

Half-life
The half-life in dogs is 0.98 h for ampicillin and 0.76 h for sulbactam.

Pregnancy risk factor

Category B: No evidence of teratogenic effects in mice, rats, or rabbits at 10× the human dose. Unasyn has been noted to decrease estradiol concentrations and decrease uterine tone in pregnant human patients. Unasyn should only be used in pregnancy if the benefits outweigh the risks.

Lactation
Ampicillin and sulbactam are both excreted into milk and may alter bowel flora in nursing animals.

Reference

Papich, M.G. (2002) *Saunders Handbook of Veterinary Drugs*. 2nd edn. Winkel, A. (ed.), W.B. Saunders Company, Philadelphia, pp. 35–36.

Further reading

English, A.R., Girad, D., and Haskell, S.L. (1984) Pharmacokinetics of sultamicillin in mice, rats and dogs. *Antimicrob Agent. Chemo.*, **25(5)**, 599–602.

Greene, C., Hartmann, K., *et al.* (2006) Antimicrobial drug formulary. Appendix 8. In: *Infectious Disease of the Dog and Cat*. Greene, C. (ed.), Elsevier, St. Louis, MO, pp. 1186–1333.

Liu, C.X., Wang, J.R., and Lu, Y.L. (1990) Pharmacokinetics of sulbactam and ampicillin in mice and in dogs. *Yae Xue Xue.*, **25(6)**, 406–411.

Chapter 170: Vancomycin

US Generic (Brand) Name: Vanomycin (Vancocin)
Availability: Human approved – Vancomycin oral capsules (125, 250 mg: *not absorbed orally*), vancomycin sterile injectable (500 mg, 1 g), vancomycin injectable pharmacy bulk package (5, 10 g), vancomycin in dextrose injectable (frozen 5 mg/mL: 500 mg)
Resistance Mechanisms: Altered bacterial target enzymes (van A, van B, van C)

Use

Restrict use for organisms that are resistant to all other alternative antibiotics. Used for severe infections due to resistant gram positive organisms. Active against *Enterococcus* spp., *Rhodococcus* spp., *Staphylococcus* spp. (including methicillin resistant), *Streptococcus* spp., (drug resistant), *Corynebacterium*, and *Bacillus* spp. Not active against gram negative *Bacilli*, *Mycobacteria*, or fungi. Vancomycin can be given orally for treatment of Staphylococcal enterocolitis and *C. difficile*-associated diarrhea. Oral capsules/solutions are used to eradicate

Clostridium difficile or *Staphylococcus* enterocolitis. Vancomycin may also be used for catheter related infections when catheters cannot be removed.

Contraindications/warnings

Hypersensitivity to vancomycin. Use with caution in patients with renal failure. Vancomycin is not absorbed orally and cannot be used for systemic infections when given orally. Avoid concomitant use with other drugs that are nephrotoxic, ototoxic, or may cause neutropenia. Avoid rapid bolus infusions that may cause hypotension, shock, or cardiac arrest.

Dosage

Do not infuse rapidly, give as an infusion over 1 h.

Canine
Susceptible infections: 15 mg/kg IV q6–8 h (Papich 2002).

C. difficile colitis: 40 mg/kg PO divided q6–8 h for 7–10 days. The total daily dosage should not exceed 2 g (Extrapolated from human pediatrics).

Feline
Susceptible infections: 12–15 mg/kg IV q8 h (Papich 2002).

Dose adjustments

Dose adjustment should be made in renal impairment. Give the normal dose for a loading dose, then double the interval in moderate renal failure or for severe renal failure, base on vancomycin levels. Geriatric patients should have a reduced dose and should be monitored carefully.

Administration

Oral capsules are only given for *C. difficile* or *Staphylococcus* enterocolitis and cannot be used for systemic infections. Oral solutions can be compounded using the sterile injectable solution (25 mg/mL) (see Stability). Vancomycin is extremely irritating to tissues and should not be given IM or SC. The IV injectable vials (500, 750, 1 g) are diluted with 10, 15, and 20 mL of sterile water for injection, respectively. This results in solutions containing 50 mg/mL. This must be further diluted with 100, 150, or 200 mL of D5W or 0.9% sodium chloride, respectively. The dose can then be infused over a period of 1 h. The rate should not exceed 10 mg/min. Infusion sites should be rotated due to thrombophlebitis. Vancomycin may also be used for catheter infections where catheters cannot be removed. An IV solution of 2 mg/mL in D5W can be prepared and 3–5 mL can be infused into the catheter port as a flush solution in place of hep-lock flush. Do not admix with heparin.

Electrolyte contents

Not significant.

Storage/stability

Oral capsules and undiluted sterile powder for IV injection are stored at room temperature. Frozen solutions in dextrose should be used after thawing and not be re-frozen. Intravenous injectable solution reconstituted with sterile water for injection is stable for 14 days in the refrigerator. Following further dilution in D5W the product can be stored refrigerated for 14 days. Do not admix with other drugs (heparin, phenobarbital). Oral solutions (25 mg/mL) made with the injectable solution can be made with ora-sweet and water (1:1) in amber plastic vials and stored refrigerated for up to 75 days.

Adverse reactions

>10%
Nausea, vomiting, hypotension, and bradycardia with rapid infusions in dogs.

1–10%
Pruritus, eosinophilia, elevated BUN, and Scr reported in dogs.

Other species
Thrombophlebitis, fever, neutropenia, interstitial nephritis, ototoxicity, renal failure, thrombocytopenia, vasculitis, and rash reported in other mammals. With oral therapy in humans, the most common adverse reactions are nausea (17%), abdominal pain (15%), and hypokalemia (13%).

Drug interactions

In humans, renal toxic and ototoxic drugs (aminoglycosides, amphotericin B, bacitracin, cisplatin, colistin, and polymyxin B) will increase renal/ototoxicity of vancomycin. Synergistic with aminoglycosides, although renal toxic potential must be considered. Anesthetic drugs may increase infusion reactions (hypotension and pruritus). Alkaline solutions will precipitate the drug.

Monitoring

Get the baseline renal function. Then monitor renal function, ototoxicity, urinalysis, WBCs, and serum concentrations. Peak concentrations should be 25–40 µg/mL and troughs should be 5–12 µg/mL. Therapeutic range is between 10–30 µg/mL. Obtain drug concentrations after the third dose. Peaks are drawn 1 h after the end of infusion and troughs are drawn just before the next dose. Concentrations >80 µg/mL are considered toxic in humans. Renal and ototoxicity may still occur with prolonged oral therapy, monitor closely.

Overdose

Ototoxicity, nephrotoxicity may occur. The LD_{50} in dogs is 292 mg/kg. Supportive care is required. Peritoneal filtration and hemofiltration can reduce serum concentrations significantly. Hemodialysis can only remove 25% of the dose.

Diagnostic test interference

No data reported.

Mechanism

Bactericidal glycopeptide. Inhibits bacterial cell wall synthesis by blocking glycopeptides polymerization, inhibiting cell wall biosynthesis.

Pharmacology/kinetics

Absorption
Poor oral absorption (<5%), so cannot be used for systemic infections. Oral absorption may be increased with patients that have colitis or have renal failure. Clinically significant plasma concentrations may occur in some patients with chronic oral doses. IM, SC injections are erratically absorbed and are irritating to tissues.

Distribution
Vancomycin is widely distributed into most tissues and fluids. High concentrations are achieved in pleural, pericardial, ascetic, and synovial fluids. Protein binding in dogs is 55%.

CNS penetration
CSF penetration is low (18%) and is improved with inflammation (20–48% of serum concentration) but may not be therapeutic. In humans, intrathecal administration of 1–5 mg/mL (diluted with 0.9 % sodium chloride-preservative free) 5–10 mg/day is used to achieve therapeutic concentrations in neonates.

Metabolism
Vancomycin does not appear to be substantially metabolized and is excreted primarily via renal excretion (25–49% in 24 h in dogs) with small amounts excreted via bile. Oral administration produces high fecal concentrations.

Half-life
The half-life in healthy dogs is 104–137 min. With renal impairment, striking accumulations may occur with extended half-lives.

Pregnancy risk factor

Category C: Vancomycin crosses the placenta and does not appear teratogenic. It has caused bradycardia and ototoxicity in human infants exposed in third trimester pregnancy.

Lactation
Vancomycin is excreted into milk. Concentrations are equal to maternal plasma concentrations. Although vancomycin is poorly absorbed orally, it may alter gastric flora in nursing animals.

Reference

Papich, M.G. (2002) *Saunders Handbook of Veterinary Drugs*. 2nd edn. Winkel, A. (ed.), W.B. Saunders Company, Philadelphia, pp. 684–685.

Further reading

Ensom, M.H. (2010) Stability of vancomycin 25 mg/ml in Orasweet and water in unit-dose cups and plastic bottles at 4 degrees C and 25 degrees C. *Can J Hops Pharm.*, **63(5)**, 366–372.
Jackson, M.W, Panciera, D.L., and Hartmann, F. (1994) Administration of vancomycin for treatment of ascending bacterial cholangitis in a cat. *J Am Vet Assoc.*, **204(4)**, 602–605.
Zaghlol, H.A. and Brown, S.A. (1988) Single- and multiple-dose pharmacokinetics of intravenously administered vancomycin in dogs. *Am J Vet Res.*, **49(9)**, 1637–1640.

Chapter 171: Zosyn

> **US Generic (Brand) Name:** Piperacillin sodium and tazobactam sodium (Zosyn)
> **Availability:** Human approved – Zosyn sterile powder for IV Injection; piperacillin/tazobactam (2 g/0.25 g, 3 g/0.375 g, 4 g/0.5 g, 36 g/4.5 g), frozen pre-mix; piperacillin/tazobactam (40 g/5 g in 2% dextrose)
> **Resistance Mechanisms:** Altered bacterial penicillin binding proteins, increased beta-lactamases (Class B, C, and D)

Use

Used in small animals for severe infections involving the respiratory tract, skin and soft tissue, bone and joint, intra-abdominal, septicemia, and gynecologic infections. Piperacillin sodium in combination with tazobactam expands activity of piperacillin to include beta-lactamase producing strains of *S. aureus*, *Bacteriodes*, *Prevotella*, and gram negative bacteria (*E. coli*, *Acinetobacter baumanii*, *Klebsiella*, *Pseudomonas*) as well as gram positive bacteria. Coverage is similar to Timentin but has greater coverage for *Enterococcus faecalis* and *Klebsiella*.

Contraindications/warnings

Hypersensitivity to beta-lactamase inhibitors and penicillins. In patients with renal failure, modify dose to the degree of renal impairment. Use with caution in patients with pre-existing electrolyte imbalances or cardiac failure due to high sodium load.

Dosage

Dosing is generally based on the piperacillin component.

Canine/feline
Susceptible infections: 50 mg/kg IV or IM q4–6 h for 5–7 days (Greene *et al.*, 2006).

Dose Adjustments

Dosage adjustments are required in renal failure. The dosing frequency should be reduced to q8–12 h for moderate to severe renal impairment.

Administration

Zosyn vials containing 2.25, 3.375, or 4.5 g should be reconstituted with 10, 15, or 20 mL, respectively, of compatible diluents. Compatible diluents include 0.9% sodium chloride, sterile water for injection, 5% dextrose, bacteriostatic water, or saline for injection. The reconstituted solution should be further diluted to the desired volume (50–150 mL). This can include 0.9% sodium chloride or sterile water for injection (max of 50 mL), 5% dextrose injection, and 6% dextran in 0.9% sodium chloride. Only use LRS on Zosyn vials containing EDTA. Do not admix with other drugs, blood products, or albumin. IV infusion should be administered over 30 min.

Electrolyte contents

Each vial of the sterile powder contains 2.79 mEq (64 mg) of sodium per gram.

Storage/stability

Store vials at room temperature until reconstituted. After reconstitution vials can be stored at room temperature for 24 h or refrigerated for 7 days. Do not freeze. The pre-mix frozen solution should be stored frozen. Once thawed at room temperature they should be used within 24 h. If thawed in the refrigerator, they are stable for 14 days.

Adverse reactions

>10%
Nausea and diarrhea reported in dogs.

1–10%
Vomiting, agitation, pain, and hairloss with IM injections reported in dogs.

<1%
At high chronic doses, decreased platelets, decreased total protein, decreased cholesterol, and serum triglycerides and elevated liver enzymes have been reported in dogs.

Other species
Hypertension, hypotension, constipation, insomnia, fever, rash, pruritus, diarrhea, dyspepsia, rhinitis, serum sickness, bronchospasms, confusion, edema, colitis, eosinophilia, neutropenia, positive Coomb's test, prolonged PT, PTT, elevations in liver enzymes, and elevated creatinine.

Drug interactions

Aminoglycosides are synergistic with Zosyn but the two are not physically compatible and should be administered separately. Aminoglycoside induced renal impairment may also require dose reductions of Zosyn. Use of Zosyn with heparin, oral anticoagulants, or other agents affecting blood coagulation may result in bleeding and should be monitored frequently. Piperacillin may prolong the effect of neuromuscular blockers (vecuronium).

Monitoring

Monitor for hypersensitivity, with prolonged use monitor CBC, electrolytes, and liver /renal function.

Overdose

Symptoms in dogs receiving large doses (400 mg/kg/day) result in liver toxicity. Diarrhea, vomiting, electrolyte imbalance, and neurotoxicity may also occur. Supportive care may be the only treatment required. Hemodialysis removes 30–40% of a dose of piperacillin/tazobactam.

Diagnostic test interference

May interfere with urine glucose analysis if using the Clinitest. May cause false positive *Aspergillus* EIA tests.

Mechanism

Bactericidal extended spectrum penicillin with beta-lactamase inhibitor. Inhibits bacterial cell wall synthesis by binding to penicillin binding proteins resulting in inhibition of transpeptidation and bacterial cell wall autolysis. Tazobactam binds to beta-lactamases that inactivate piperacillin. Used together, the spectrum of activity is extended to cover beta-lactamase producing organisms.

Pharmacology/kinetics

Absorption
Piperacillin is poorly absorbed from the gastrointestinal tract and should be given intravenously. Following IM doses, in humans, the piperacillin bioavailability is 71% and 84% for tazobactam.

Distribution
Both piperacillin and tazobactam are widely distributed into tissues and bodily fluids. High concentrations are found in lung, mucosa, gallbladder, uterus, ovary, interstitial fluid, and bile. Protein binding in dogs is 26–33% for piperacillin and 31–32% for tazobactam.

CNS penetration
CNS penetration is poor and considered erratic.

Metabolism
Piperacillin is minimally metabolized in the liver to a minor desethyl piperacillin metabolite. Tazobactam is also minimally metabolized to an inactive metabolite. Both are primarily excreted unchanged into urine as parent drug. In dogs, piperacillin decreases tazobactam urinary excretion. Small amounts of both drugs are eliminated via bile.

Half-life
The half-life of piperacillin and tazobactam in dogs is reported to be similar to that in people (0.7–1.2 h).

Pregnancy risk factor

Category B: Piperacillin penetrates across the placenta (fetal: maternal ratios of 0.17). No teratogenic or toxic effects have been reported in laboratory animals or humans exposed to piperacillin during pregnancy.

Lactation
Piperacillin is excreted into milk in low concentrations, but is not absorbed well orally so has limited side effects in nursing animals.

Reference

Greene, C., Hartmann, K., *et al.* (2006) Antimicrobial drug formulary. Appendix 8. In: *Infectious Disease of the Dog and Cat*. Greene, C. (ed.), Elsevier, St. Louis, MO, pp. 1186–1333.

Further reading

Hayashi, T., Yada, H., Blair, M., *et al.* (1994) A six month intravenous repeated dose toxicity study of tazobactam/piperacillin and tazobactam in dogs. *J Toxicol Sci.*, **19(2)**, 177–197.

Komuro, M., Maeda, T., Kakuo, H., *et al.* (1994) Inhibition of the renal excretion of tazobactam by piperacillin. *J Antimicrob Chemother.*, **34(4)**, 555–564.

Miyamoto, M., Sudo, T., Kuyama, T., *et al.* (1990) Assessment of antimicrobial penetration into the pancreatic juice of dogs. *Nihon Geka Hokan.*, **59(3)**, 205–210.

Sykes, J.E. and Papich, M.G. (2013) Antibacterial drugs. Ch. 8. In: *Canine and Feline Infectious Diseases*, Sykes, J.E. (ed.), Elsevier, St. Louis, MO. pp. 66–86.

Tables Antibiotic Sensitivities

The tables reflect clinical efficacy and incorporate *in vitro* sensitivities, *in vivo* efficacy, and potential resistance.

Definitions: MS = Methicillin sensitive, MR = Methicillin resistance, A*-C* = Drug is only effective in combination with another drug (see text on organisms).

Drug selections:

Category A = Drug of choice for sensitive organisms based on *in vitro* sensitivity and *in vivo* efficacy.

Category B = Drug is a good clinical alternative but may be more expensive or have more side effects then drugs in Category A.

Category C = Drug may be an alternative if the organism is sensitive and the animal tolerates the drug.

Category D = Drug is typically very effective, but should be restricted for human use or to animals with infections that demonstrate high resistance to all other antibiotic choices.

		Gram Positives										
	A. Clinically recommended B. Clinical alternative C. Usually sensitive D. Sensitive but reserved for highly resistant organisms	Staphylococcus aureus (MS)	Staphylococcus aureus (MR)	Staphylococcus pseudintermedius (MS)	Staphylococcus pseudintermedius (MR)	Staphylococcus (Coag.Neg) (MS)	Staphylococcus (Coag.Neg) (MR)	Streptococcus canis	Streptococcus bovis	Corynebacterium sp.	Enterococcus faecalis	Enterococcus faecium
Penicillin	Amoxicillin	B		B		B		A	B		A	A
	Ampicillin							A	B		A	
	Penicillin G	A		A		A		A	A		B	
	Piperacillin							B	B		B	C
	Ticarcillin							C	C			
Penicillin Related	Amoxicillin/Clavulanate	A		A		B		A	A		A	C
	Ampicillin/Sulbactam	C		C		B		C	C		B	C
	Ticarcillin/Clavulanate	C		C		B		C	C			C
	Imipenem/Cilastatin	D		D		D		D	D		D	D
	Meropenem	D		D		D		D	D		D	
	Piperacillin/Tazobactam	B		C		C		C	C			C
Other Antibiotics	Chloramphenicol	C	B	C	B	C		C	C	A	C	B
	Clindamycin	A	A	B	A	C		C	C	C		
	Co-trimoxazole	B	B	B	B	C	B	C	C			
	Linezolid	D	D	D	D	D	D	D	D		D	D
	Metronidazole											
	Tetracyclines	A	C	A	C	C		C	C	A	C	C
	Vancomycin	D	D	D	D	D	D	D	D	D	D	D
UTI agents	Nitrofurantoin										B	C

	A. Clinically recommended B. Clinical alternative C. Usually sensitive D. Sensitive but reserved for highly resistant organisms	Staphylococcus aureus (MS)	Staphylococcus aureus (MR)	Staphylococcus pseudintermedius (MS)	Staphylococcus pseudintermedius (MR)	Staphylococcus (Coag.Neg) (MS)	Staphylococcus (Coag.Neg) (MR)	Streptococcus canis	Streptococcus bovis	Corynebacterium sp.	Enterococcus faecalis	Enterococcus faecium
								Gram Positives				
1st Gen	Cefadroxil	B		B		B		C	C			
1st Gen	Cefazolin	A		A		A		A	B			
1st Gen	Cephalexin	B		B		B		B	B			
2nd Gen	Cefaclor	C		C		C		C	C			
2nd Gen	Cefoxitin	B		B		C		C	C			
2nd Gen	Cefuroxime	B		B		C						
3rd Gen	Cefdinir											
3rd Gen	Cefixime											
3rd Gen	Cefotaxime	A		A		A		C	C			
3rd Gen	Cefovecin							B				
3rd Gen	Cefpodoxime	C		C		C		B	C			
3rd Gen	Ceftazidime	C		C		C		C	C			
3rd Gen	Ceftiofur							B				
3rd Gen	Ceftriaxone	A		A		C		C	C		C	C
4th Gen	Cefipime	A	C	A	C	B		C	C			
Aminoglyc-osides	Amikacin	B*	B*	B*	B*	B*	A*	C	C	C	C*	C
Aminoglyc-osides	Gentamicin	C*	B*	C*	B*	C*	B*	C	C		C*	B
Aminoglyc-osides	Tobramycin	C*	B*	C*	B*	C*	B*	C				
Macro-liddes	Azithromycin	B		B		B			A			
Macro-liddes	Clarithromycin	B	B	B	B	B	B		A			
Macro-liddes	Erythromycin	B	B	B	B	B	B		A			
Quinolones	Ciprofloxacin	C	C	C	C	C	C	C	C		C	C
Quinolones	Enrofloxacin	B	C	B	C	C	C		C	C		
Quinolones	Marbofloxacin	B	C	B	C	C	C		C			
Quinolones	Orbifloxacin	B	C	B	C	C	C		C			
Quinolones	Pradofloxacin	B	C	B	C							

| | | Gram Negative Aerobes | | | | | | | | |
| | | Enteric Bacilli | | | | | | | | |
	A. Clinically recommended B. Clinical alternative C. Usually sensitive D. Sensitive but reserved for highly resistant organisms	Yersinia enterolitica	Shigella sp.	Serratia sp.	Salmonella sp.	Proteus sp.	Klebsiella pneumoniae	Escherichia coli	Enterobacter sp.	Citrobacter sp.
Penicillin	Amoxicillin				C	C		C		
	Ampicillin		A		B	C		C		
	Penicillin G									
	Piperacillin			A		C	B	C	B	A
	Ticarcillin			A		C	C	C	B	A
Penicillin Related	Amoxicillin/Clavulanate				B	C	C	A	A	B
	Ampicillin/Sulbactam		C		C	C	B	B	B	B
	Ticarcillin/Clavulanate			A	C	C	B	C	B	A
	Imipenem/Cilastatin			D	D	D	D	D	D	D
	Meropenem		D	D	D	D	D	D	D	D
	Piperacillin/Tazobactam		C	A	C	B	B	C	A	A
Other Antibiotics	Chloramphenicol	B	C		B			C	B	
	Clindamycin									
	Co-trimoxazole	B	B	C	B		C	B	C	C
	Linezolid									
	Metronidazole									
	Tetracyclines	A	C			C		C		
	Vancomycin									
UTI Agents	Nitrofurantoin						C	C	C	C

		Gram Negative Aerobes								
		Enteric Bacilli								
	A. Clinically recommended B. Clinical alternative C. Usually sensitive D. Sensitive but reserved for highly resistant organisms	*Yersinia enterolitica*	*Shigella* sp.	*Serratia* sp.	*Salmonella* sp.	*Proteus* sp.	*Klebsiella pneumoniae*	*Escherichia coli*	*Enterobacter* sp.	*Citrobacter* sp.
1st Gen	Cefadroxil					B	B	B		
	Cefazolin					B	A	B		
	Cephalexin					B	A	B		
2nd Gen	Cefaclor					C	B	C		
	Cefoxitin			C		C	A	C		
	Cefuroxime	C	C			C	B	C		
3rd Gen	Cefdinir			C	C	C	C	C	C	C
	Cefixime		C	C	B	C	B	C		
	Cefotaxime	B	B	A	A	A	B	C	A	A
	Cefovecin						C	C		C
	Cefpodoxime					C	A	B		
	Ceftazidime		B	A		A	A	A	A	A
	Ceftiofur			C	C	C	C	C		
	Ceftriaxone	B	B	A	B	A	A	A	A	A
4th Gen	Cefipime			C	C	C	B		B	
Aminoglyc-osides	Amikacin	A		C		C	C	B	C	C
	Gentamicin	A	C	C	C	C	C	B	C	C
	Tobramycin	A		C	C	C	C	C	C	C
Macro-liddes	Azithromycin									
	Clarithromycin									
	Erythromycin									
Quinolones	Ciprofloxacin	C	B	C	B	B	C	B	C	C
	Enrofloxacin	C	B	C	B	B	C	B	C	B
	Marbofloxacin	C	B	C	B	B	C	B	C	B
	Orbifloxacin	C	B	C	B	B	C	B	C	B
	Pradofloxacin					B	C	B		

Chapter 171: Zosyn **217**

		Stenotrophonomas maltophilia	Pseudomonas sp.	Pasteurella multocida	Francisella tularensis	Campylobacter jejuni	Brucella sp.	Bordetella sp.	Acinetobacter sp.
	Gram-Negative Aerobes								
	Other Bacilli								
A. Clinically recommended									
B. Clinical alternative									
C. Usually sensitive									
D. Sensitive but reserved for highly resistant organisms									
Penicillin	Amoxicillin			A				C	
	Ampicillin			C		C		C	
	Penicillin G			A					
	Piperacillin			C					C
	Ticarcillin			C					C
Penicillin Related	Amoxicillin/Clavulanate			A				B	C
	Ampicillin/Sulbactam			B				B	C
	Ticarcillin/Clavulanate	B	A	C					A
	Imipenem/Cilastatin		D	D					D
	Meropenem		D	D		D		D	D
	Piperacillin/Tazobactam		A	C				B	A
Other Antibiotics	Chloramphenicol	C		C	A	C	B		
	Clindamycin					C			
	Co-trimoxazole	A		C			C	B	
	Linezolid								
	Metronidazole								
	Tetracyclines		C	B	B	A	A*	A	
	Vancomycin								
UTI Agents	Nitrofurantoin								

| | | Gram-negative Aerobes | | | | | | | |
| | | Other Bacilli | | | | | | | |
	A. Clinically recommended B. Clinical alternative C. Usually sensitive D. Sensitive but reserved for highly resistant organisms	Stenotrophomonas maltophilia	Pseudomonas sp.	Pasteurella multocida	Francisella tularensis	Campylobacter jejuni	Brucella sp.	Bordetella sp.	Acinetobacter sp.
1st Gen	Cefadroxil							B	
	Cefazolin							B	
	Cephalexin							B	
2nd Gen	Cefaclor								
	Cefoxitin			C	C			C	
	Cefuroxime			C					
3rd Gen	Cefdinir								
	Cefixime								C
	Cefotaxime	C		C	C				A
	Cefovecin								C
	Cefpodoxime								
	Ceftazidime	C	A		C				A
	Ceftiofur								C
	Ceftriaxone	C		C	C				A
4th Gen	Cefipime		C						C
Aminoglyc-osides	Amikacin	C	B		A	C	A*	C	C
	Gentamicin	C	B		A	C	A*	C	C
	Tobramycin	C	A			C	A*	C	C
Macrolides	Azithromycin			C		A	C	B	
	Clarithromycin			C		A	C	C	
	Erythromycin			C		A	C	C	
Quinolones	Ciprofloxacin	B	A	B	C	C		C	C
	Enrofloxacin	B	A	B	B	B	B*	B	C
	Marbofloxacin	B	B	B	B	B	B*	B	C
	Orbifloxacin	B	B	B	B	B	B*	B	
	Pradofloxacin								

	A. Clinically recommended B. Clinical alternative C. Usually sensitive D. Sensitive but reserved for highly resistant organisms	Others						Anaerobes			
		Actinomyces	Leptospira sp.	Borrelia burgdorferi	Rickettsia sp.	Mycoplasma sp.	Chlamydia sp.	Bacteriodes sp.	Sterptococcus anaerobes	Clostridium perfringens	Clostridium difficile
Penicillin	Amoxicillin	B		B				C	C	C	
	Ampicillin	A	C	B				C	C	C	
	Penicillin G	A	B	B				C	A	A	
	Piperacillin								C	C	
	Ticarcillin	C							C	C	
Penicillin Related	Amoxicillin/Clavulanate	B					B	B	C	C	
	Ampicillin/Sulbactam	B						B	C	C	
	Ticarcillin/Clavulanate	B						B	C	C	
	Imipenem/Cilastatin	D						D	D	D	
	Meropenem	D						D	D	D	
	Piperacillin/Tazobactam	C						C	C	C	
Other Antibiotics	Chloramphenicol				B			C	C	C	C
	Clindamycin	B						A	B	B	
	Co-trimoxazole								B		
	Linezolid										
	Metronidazole								A	C	A	A
	Tetracyclines	B	A	A	A	A	A	C	C	C	
	Vancomycin								D		D
UTI agents	Nitrofurantoin										

	A. Clinically recommended B. Clinical alternative C. Usually sensitive D. Sensitive but reserved for highly resistant organisms	Others						Anaerobes		
		Actinomyces	Leptospira sp.	Borrelia burgdorferi	Rickettsia sp.	Mycoplasma sp.	Chlamydia sp.	Bacteriodes sp.	Sterptococcus anaerobes	Clostridium perfringens	Clostridium difficile
1st Gen	Cefadroxil								B		
	Cefazolin								B		
	Cephalexin								B		
2nd Gen	Cefaclor										
	Cefoxitin	B						B	C	C	
	Cefuroxime		A	A					C	C	
3rd Gen	Cefdinir										
	Cefixime										
	Cefotaxime		B	B					C	C	
	Cefovecin										
	Cefpodoxime										
	Ceftazidime									C	
	Ceftiofur										
	Ceftriaxone		B	B					C		
4th Gen	Cefipime										
Aminoglyc-osides	Amikacin										
	Gentamicin								C		
	Tobramycin										
Macro-liddes	Azithromycin		C			C				C	
	Clarithromycin		C			C				C	
	Erythromycin	C	C			C				C	
Quinolones	Ciprofloxacin				C	C	C				
	Enrofloxacin		C			B	B	B			
	Marbofloxacin		C			B	B	B			
	Orbifloxacin		C			B	B	B			
	Pradofloxacin					A	B	C			

SECTION E

Antifungal Agents

Chapter 172: Amphotericin B

US Generic (Brand) Name: Amphotericin B conventional (Fungizone, Amphocin), Ampho-B cholesteryl sulfate complex (Amphotec), Ampho-B Lipid complex (Abelcet), Liposomal amphotericin B (AmBisome)
Availability: Human Approved – Fungizone, Amphocin (50 mg IV), Amphotec (50, 100 mg IV), Abelcet (5 mg/mL IV), AmBisome (50 mg IV)
Resistance Mechanisms: Altered membrane composition, upregulation of ATP-binding cassette transporters, upregulation of metabolic pathways

Use

Primarily used for invasive, life threatening fungal infections caused by *Aspergillus* and other mold species, *Blastomyces, Candida, Coccidioides, Cryptococcus, Histoplasma,* and *Sporotrix*. Has also been used for Leishmaniasis in dogs and may be useful for amebic meningoencephalitis (*Naegleria fowleri*) and neutropenic fever in patients refractory to antibiotics. Although renal toxicity limits the use of conventional amphotericin B, the newer lipid complex and encapsulated formulations have significantly reduced renal toxicity (8–10-fold) and permit much larger cumulative doses to be administered. Liposomal amphotericin B has improved efficacy, reduced renal toxicity, and increased penetration into the CNS. It is considered the drug of choice in severe infections involving the CNS. It is often combined with itraconazole, voriconazole, flucytosine (cats only), or terbinafine for improved efficacy, depending on the organism.

Contraindications/warnings

Contraindicated in significant renal impairment. Hypersensitivity reactions, including anaphylactic reactions may occur with initial doses. Sodium depletion may further predispose animals to renal toxicity.

Dosage

Beware of 10-fold differences in doses between conventional amphotericin B and liposome encapsulated amphotericin B. Substitution of conventional amphotericin B at liposomal amphotericin B doses has led to death in human patients. If CNS or ocular involvement, liposomal encapsulated amphotericin B should be combined with fluconazole or voriconazole in dogs or flucytocine or fluconazole in cats due to their increased penetration into these sites.

Dogs

Conventional (standard) amphotericin B desoxycholate (Fungizone, Amphocin): Severe systemic infections (Aspergillus, Histoplasmosis, Cryptococcus): Dilute quantity of stock solution to 0.25 mg/kg in 250–500 mL of dextrose 5% in water. Administer IV over 4–6 h. If tolerated, administer 0.5 mg/kg IV three times a week (Monday, Wednesday, Friday) until the cumulative dose is given (Greene 2006). Reported cumulative doses for *Aspergillus* are 9–12 mg/kg and for *Histoplasmosis* are 7.5–8.5 mg/kg.

Conservative treatment of Cryptococcus: Administer 0.5–0.8 mg/kg SC 2–3 times per week. Dilute dose in 0.45% saline with 2.5% dextrose (500 mL for dogs <20 kg or 1000 mL for dogs >20 kg). Treat until a cumulative dose of 8–26 mg/kg is reached. Final concentration must be <20 mg/L or it may cause tissue irritation and/or

Drug Therapy for Infectious Diseases of the Dog and Cat, First Edition. Valerie J. Wiebe.
© 2015 John Wiley & Sons, Inc. Published 2015 by John Wiley & Sons, Inc.

abscesses. Concurrent oral therapy should be administered at the start of amphotericin B.

Intralesional for Sporothrix: Typically a 50 mg vial is diluted with 5 mL of 2% lidocaine and 5 mL of distilled water to make a 5 mg/mL solution. Administration of 0.5–1.5 mL can be given intralesionally once a week to every other week.

Amphotericin B lipid coimplex (Abelcet): Caution: Only use high doses for lipid complex/encapsulated amphotericin B or toxicity will occur.

Severe systemic infections: Administer a dose of 1–2.5 mg/kg/day IV three times a week (Monday, Wednesday, Friday) until a cumulative dose of 12 mg/kg is reached. Infuse over 1–2 h (Greene 2006).

Liposome encapsulated amphotericin B (AmBisome): Systemic Mycoses: Administer 1–2.5 mg/kg IV over 1–2 h three times a week until a cumulative dose of 12 mg/kg is reached. Concurrent oral therapy should be administered at the start of amphotericin B (Greene 2006).

Leishmaniasis: Administer 3–3.3 mg/kg/day IV q72–96 h, until a total dose of 15 mg/kg is reached (Greene 2006).

Cats
Conventional (standard) amphotericin B (Fungizone, Amphocin): Severe systemic infections (Aspirgillus/ Histoplasmosis/ Blastomycosis/Cryptococcus): Administer 0.15–0.4 mg/kg IV in 30 mL D$_5$W over 30–60 min. Administer three times a week until a total dose of 2–4 mg/kg (*Histoplasmosis/Blastomycosis*) or 4–6 mg/kg (*Aspergillus, Cryptococcus*) is achieved or the BUN is >50 mg/dL, then decrease to 0.15–0.25 mg/kg IV once a month as maintenance (Greene 2006). Give with itraconazole 5 mg/kg PO q12 h for susceptible infections (*Aspergillus, Histoplasmosis,* or *Blastomycosis*) until remission. For *Cryptococcus* infections involving the CNS, flucytosine 125–250 mg/day PO in 2–4 divided doses should be administered acutely at the initiation of amphotericin B (2 weeks), followed by maintenance therapy with oral fluconazole.

Conservative treatment of Cryptococcus: Administer 0.5–0.8 mg/kg SC 2–3 times per week. Dilute dose in 0.45% saline with 2.5% dextrose (400 mL). Treat until a cumulative dose of 8–26 mg/kg is reached. Final concentration must be <20 mg/L or it may cause tissue irritation, abscesses. Concurrent oral therapy (flucytocine, fluconazole) should be administered at the start of amphotericin B.

Amphotericin B lipid complex (Abelcet): Cryptococcus: Administer 1 mg/kg IV over 1–2 h three times a week until a cumulative dose of 12 mgs/kg is reached. Give with flucytosine 125–250 mg/day in 2–4 divided doses.

Dose adjustments

Doses of conventional amphotericin B should be reduced by 50% or the interval prolonged to every third or fourth day in patients developing mild to moderate renal dysfunction. Liposomal amphotericin B should be used in place of conventional amphotericin B to prevent further renal toxicity.

Administration

Pretreatment (30 min prior) with antihistamines and glucosteroids (dexamethasone 0.1 mg/kg IV) is recommended to avoid hypersensitivity reactions. Hydration and sodium loading with 0.9% normal saline prior to amphotericin B administration may help prevent renal toxicity. Reconstitute amphotericin B powder with preservative free sterile water (10 mL) to a concentration of 5 mg/mL. Further dilute (1:50) in dextrose 5% in water to a concentration of 0.1 mg/mL prior to infusion. IV infusions require an in-line filter (>1 μm). Test doses of amphotericin B (0.1/kg/day) can be infused over 30–60 min. IV infusions are given slowly over 1–6 h depending on the dose. Doses should be infused using a separate line, if this cannot be done, flush line extensively with dextrose 5% in water prior to administration. Rapid infusion may cause hypotension, hypokalemia, arrhythmias, and shock. Amphotericin B lipid complex (Abelcet concentrate 100 mg/20 mL) should be shaken gently until there is no evidence of yellow sediment, withdraw dose and filter (using a 5 μm filter) prior to dilution. Dilute with dextrose 5% in water to a final concentration of 1 mg/mL prior to infusion. The infusion rate should be 2.5 mg/kg/h. The infusion container should be shaken every 2 h during infusion. Liposome encapsulated amphotericin B (AmBisome) must be diluted with 12 mL of sterile water to provide a 4 mg/mL solution. Withdraw the appropriate dose and use the 5 μm disposable filter to inject into the appropriate volume of dextrose 5% in water to make a final concentration of 0.2–2 mg/mL. This should be infused over 2 h. For subcutaneous administration, dilute conventional amphotericin B dose in 0.45% saline with 2.5% dextrose prior to administration. See previous section for intralesional administration.

Electrolyte contents

Not significant.

Storage/stability

Conventional amphotericin B powder should be stored refrigerated and protected from light. Once reconstituted, the 5 mg/mL amphotericin B solution should be kept in the dark and remains stable for 24 h at room temperature, or 1 week in the refrigerator. Admixtures (1:50) can be stored at room temperature for 24 h or refrigerated for 48 h. Anecdotal information suggests that the 5 mg/mL concentrate in sterile water can be drawn up using aseptic technique into aliquots and frozen at −20°C for up to 1 month. Amphotericin B lipid complex (Abelcet) single use vials are stored refrigerated, protected from light. Dilute solutions are stable for up to 15 h when refrigerated and an additional 6 h at room temperature. For AmBisome, package instructions should be followed exactly. Infusion must be done within 6 h of dilution.

Adverse reactions

>10%
Dose limiting nephrotoxicity (at doses >6 mg/kg), azotemia, renal tubular acidosis, and renal failure are noted in cats and dogs. Cats appear more sensitive to renal toxicity.

1–10%
Hypersensitivity reactions, respiratory distress, hypotension, hypertension, anorexia, vomiting, nausea, urinary retention, and anemia have been reported in dogs and cats. Sterile abscesses, local tissue irritation, and calcinosis cutis have been reported in cats and dogs following subcutaneous administration.

Other species
Anuria, acute liver failure, seizures, leucopenia, thrombocytopenia, thrombophlebitis, hypokalemia, and hypomagnesemia have been reported.

Drug interactions

In humans, drug interactions have included: increased nephrotoxicity with other nephrotoxic agents and hypokalemia if administered with other potassium depleting drugs (e.g., furosemide and thiazides), neuromuscular blockers, steroids, or digoxin. Amphotericin B preparations are not compatible with most drugs and electrolytes and should not be mixed, diluted with or given via the same IV line unless suggested in the package insert.

Monitoring

BUN, creatinine, CBC, liver function tests, electrolytes, and temperature.

Overdose

Clinical signs of overdose may include renal dysfunction, anemia, thrombocytopenia, granulocytopenia, cardiac arrest, fever, nausea, and vomiting. Inadvertent administration of standard amphotericin B (Fungizone) at lipsomal encapsulated amphotericin B (AmBisome) doses in humans has resulted in cardiac arrhythmias, anemia, acute renal failure, and death. Supportive care including fluids and mannitol may reduce renal toxicity. Amphotericin B is not removed by dialysis. Plasmapheresis has been used successfully in human overdoses.

Diagnostic test interference

None noted.

Mechanism

Binds to ergosterol altering fungal cell wall permeability.

Pharmacology/kinetics

Absorption
Amphotericin B is poorly absorbed from the gastrointestinal tract. Effective systemic treatment requires IV or SC administration.

Distribution
Amphotericin B is rapidly distributed into tissues and is 90% bound to plasma proteins. It only achieves minimal concentrations in most fluid compartments (pleural, synovial, amniotic, and aqueous humor). The lipid complex is sequestered by the reticular endothelial system (RES) and concentrates in liver, bone marrow, and spleen. Higher doses can be achieved with lipid preparations due to less free drug binding to renal tubules resulting in toxicity.

CNS penetration
CSF penetration of conventional amphotericin B is low (1–3%). This is improved with liposome encapsulated amphotericin B due to increased lipophilicity. However,

the use of lipid complex formulations (Amphotec, Abelcet) does not appear as effective as either the encapsulated or conventional forms of amphotericin B for CNS infections. Intrathecal doses are required to achieve cidal levels of amphotericin B in the CSF.

Metabolism

Conventional amphotericin B is excreted unchanged in the urine of dogs (25%) with another 40% excreted into feces. This suggests that metabolism plays a minor role in the elimination of amphotericin B.

Half-life

The half-life of elimination of conventional amphotericin B in dogs is 44–47 h.

Pregnancy risk factor

Category B: Amphotericin B crosses the placenta readily. High cord blood to placenta ratios of 0.68–1.0 are noted, but have not been associated with congenital defects in humans or animals. Amphotericin B may be safer than other systemic antifungal agents during pregnancy.

Lactation

Liposomal amphotericin B administered to rats had no detectable concentrations in milk. It is poorly absorbed orally and would not be expected to achieve high systemic concentrations in nursing animals.

Reference

Greene, C.E. (2006) Histoplasmosis. In: *Infectious Disease of the Dog and Cat*. 3rd edn., Greene, C. (ed.), Elsevier, St. Louis, MO, pp. 577–584.

Further reading

Foy, D.S. and Trepanier, L.A. (2010) Antifungal treatment of small animal veterinary patients. *Vet Clin Small Animal.*, **40**, 1171–1188.

Hodge,s R.D., Legendre, A.M., Adams, L.G., *et al.* (1994) Itraconazole for the treatment of histoplasmosis in cats. *J Vet Intern Med.*, **8(6)**, 409–413.

Kim, H., Loebenberg, D., Marco, A., *et al.* (1984) Comparative pharmacokinetics of Sch 28191 and amphotericin B in mice, rats, dogs and cynomologus monkeys. *Antimicrob Agents and Chemother.*, **26(4)**, 446–449.

Legendre, A.M. (1989) Systemic mycotic infections. In: *The Cat: Diseases and Clinical Management, Vol. 1*. Sherding, R.G. (ed.), Churchill Livingstone, New York, pp. 427–457.

Macy, D.W. (1987) Fungal diseases: Dog, cat. In: *The Bristol Handbook of Antimicrobial Therapy*. Johnston, D.E. (ed.), Veterinary Learning Systems, Evansville, pp. 152–157.

Malik, R., Craig, A.J., Wigney, D.I., *et al.* (1996) Combination chemotherapy of canine and feline cryptococcosis using subcutaneous administered amphotericin B. *Aust Vet J.*, **73(4)**, 124–128.

Noxon, J.O. (1989) Systemic antifungal therapy. In: *Current Veterinary Therapy X: Small Animal Practice*. Kirk, R.W. (ed.), W.B. Saunders, Philadelphia, pp. 1101–1108.

Taboada, J. (1999) How I treat pythiosis. *Proceedings: The North American Veterinary Conference*, Orlando.

Taboada, J. (2000) Systemic mycosis: *Textbook of Veterinary Internal Medicine: Diseases of the Dog and Cat, Vol. 1*, Ettinger, S. and Feldman, E. (eds.), W.B. Saunders, Philadelphia, pp. 453–476.

Chapter 173: Caspofungin

US Generic (Brand) Name: Caspofungin (Cancidas)
Availability: Human Approved – Sterile injectable powder (50, 70 mg)
Resistance Mechanisms: Mutations in the *FKS1* gene resulting in altered target (serine 645 position in Fks1p with substitutions of proline, tyrosine, and phenylalanine)

Use

Invasive, severe, resistant, systemic infections due to *Aspergillus* and *Candida* or in patients unable to tolerate azoles or amphotericin B. In humans, it has fewer adverse effects than amphotericin B and may be synergistic with it in certain infections. Caspofungin has fungicidal activity against a variety of *Candida* (*C. albicans, C. tropicalis, C. glabrata, C. dubliniensis, C. lusitaniae*). Both *C. krusei* and *C. parapsilosis* are less susceptible. Caspofungin has variable activity against *Aspergillus, Histoplasma, Blastomyces, Coccidioides, Sporothrix*, dematiaceous fungi, and several rare molds, such as *Alternaria, Curvularia, Scedosporium, Acremonium, Bipolaris*, and *Trichoderma*. It has some activity against *Lagenidium* and *Pythium*, but is generally not active against *Cryptococcus, Trichosporon, Zygomyces*, and *Dermatophytes*.

Contraindications/warnings

Caspofungin is contraindicated in patients with known hypersensitivity to echinocandins, those treated with other hepatotoxic drugs, or those with severe liver impairment. Do not use in patients that are dehydrated.

Caspofungin causes histamine release with rapid infusions. Evaluate drug interactions, avoid admixture with other drugs and diluents not recommended by the manufacturer.

Dosage

Not well defined in cats and dogs. Large, intermittent doses (every other day or 3 times/week) are efficacious in humans. Loading doses are required.

Canine/feline
Documented dose: 0.5–2 mg/kg IV q24 h (administered over 1 h) for an average duration of 1 month (Koch *et al.*, 2012). Doses up to 5 mg/kg IV are tolerated in healthy dogs.

Dose adjustments

In humans, no dose adjustments are suggested in renal impairment. It is recommended that doses be reduced by 30% in patients with moderate hepatic impairment. Increased doses (20%) may be necessary in obese patients.

Administration

Removed from the refrigerator just prior to use and equilibrated to room temperature. Pretreatment with antihistamines or glucocorticoids are advised. Reconstitute with 10.8 mL of diluent (0.9% saline, sterile water for injection-USP, or bacteriostatic water for injection). Once diluted, the reconstituted vial will contain either 7.2 mg/mL (70 mg vial) or 5.2 mg/mL. Mix gently and remove the appropriate dose. Further dilute in 250 mL of saline (0.9%, 0.45%) or lactated ringers solution. The drug should be administered by slow IV infusion over 1 h. Rapid infusions have resulted in a higher incidence of allergic reactions.

Electrolyte contents

Not significant.

Storage/stability

The lyophilized powder must be stored refrigerated. Once diluted, it is only stable for one hour at 25°C. Following further dilution, it should be used within 24 h if stored at room temperature or within 48 h if stored in the refrigerator (2–8°C).

Adverse reactions

In dogs
Swollen muzzle, edema, pruritus, eosinophilia, tachycardia, and hypotension have been noted in dogs receiving rapid infusions.

>10%
In humans, nausea, vomiting, diarrhea, fever, allergic reactions (swollen face, edema, pruritus, and eosinophilia), tachycardia, and hypotension have been noted (related to rapid infusions).

1–10%
In humans, cough, hepatotoxicity, rashes, anaphylaxis, decreased hematocrit, and urticarial reactions.

<1%
In humans, hypokalemia, nephrotoxicity, arrhythmias, mucosal inflammation, convulsions, tremors, and pancreatitis have been reported rarely.

Drug interactions

In humans, dexamethasone, rifampin, phenytoin all decrease caspofungin plasma concentrations. Cyclosporin increases caspofungin plasma concentrations and increase the chance of hepatoxicity. Amphotericin B is synergistic with caspofungin.

Monitoring

Monitor for hypersensitivity reactions, elevations in liver enzymes, hypo/hypertension, hypokalemia, and diarrhea.

Overdose

Overdoses should be treated with supportive care. Overdoses of up to 400 mg/day have been tolerated in humans. The drug is not removed by dialysis.

Diagnostic test interference

None noted.

Mechanism

A fungicidal echinocandin. Caspofungin inhibits synthesis of 1,3-beta-glycan linkages in fungal cell walls. These are predominant in the cell walls of *Candida* and *Aspergillus* spp.

Pharmacology/kinetics

Absorption
Oral absorption is poor (<0.2%), and the drug is irritating to mucosal membranes.

Distribution
Caspofungin is highly protein bound (>97%) and does not achieve significant concentrations in CNS or vitreous humor in the absence of inflammation. Distribution into tissues may take days to reach maximum concentrations. It is widely distributed into liver, kidneys, large intestine, and nasal sinuses.

CNS penetration
Caspofungin has limited penetration into CSF but has been efficacious in human CNS aspergillosis.

Metabolism
Caspofungin undergoes spontaneous degradation and further metabolism involving peptide hydrolysis and N-acetylation. Less than 3% is excreted as active parent drug acutely in urine after a single dose, but 42% is excreted in urine and 29% is excreted in feces over a 12-day period due to high protein binding in tissues.

Half-life
Unknown in dogs and cats. The $T_{1/2}$ in rats and monkeys is variable (4–8 h) and is dose and schedule dependent. In humans, there is a polyphasic decline in plasma concentrations, with half-lives of 9–11 h and 45 h. Distribution rather than excretion dictates plasma clearance. Chronic dosing can result in drug accumulation and extended half-life.

Pregnancy risk factor

Category C: Caspofungin has been associated with incomplete ossification of the skull, torso, talus/calcaneus, and increased resorption in rats and rabbits. It is contraindicated in pregnant animals.

Lactation
Caspofungin has been detected in the milk of lactating rats. It is not absorbed well orally, so nursing animals should not have significant exposure to caspofungin.

Reference

Koch, S., Torres, S., and Plumb, D. (2012) *Canine and Feline Dermatology Handbook. Section 1: Systemic Drugs*. Wiley-Blackwell, Ames, Iowa, pp. 23–24.

Further reading

Eschenauer, G., DePestel, D.D., and Carver, P. (2007) Comparison of echinocandin antifungals. *Ther Clin Risk Manag.*, **3(1)**, 71–97.

Gumbo, T. (2007) Impact of pharmacodynamics and pharmacokinetics on ecinocandin dosing strategies. *Current Opin Inf Dis.*, **20(6)**, 587–591.

Said, T., Nampoory, M., Nair, M., *et al.* (2005) Safety of caspofungin for treating invasive nasal sinus aspergillosis in a kidney transplant recipient. *Transplantation Proceed.*, **37(7)**, 3038–3040.

Chapter 174: Clotrimazole

US Generic (Brand) Name: Clotrimazole (Lotrimin, Lotrisone, Cruex, Otomax otic, DVMAX otic, Vetrmax otic, etc.)
Availability: Human and Veterinary Approved – Multiple topical 1% sprays/solutions (10, 30 mL), 1% creams and lotions (15, 30, 45 g), multiple combination products with antibiotics (gentamycin) or steroids (betamethasone, mometasone), and USP grade chemical
Resistance Mechanisms: Overexpression of efflux pump genes including *CDR1* and *CDR2*

Use

Clotrimazole is a broad spectrum antifungal agent that is active against *Dermatophytes* such as *Trichophyton* and *Microsporum* and yeasts such as *Malassezia* and *Candida*. It is fungistatic against *Aspergillus* spp. Clotrimazole should not be used to treat systemic disease. It is primarily used in topical combination products for *Malassezia* infections of the ears and skin or as sole topical therapy as a compounded 1% solution in polyethylene glycol for treatment of sinonasal *Aspergillus* and *Candida* lower urinary tract infections.

Contraindications/warnings

Contraindicated in patients with known hypersensitivity to clotrimazole or azoles. Do not administer intranasally to patients if the cribriform plate is not intact as determined by advanced imaging. Avoid use in or around the eyes. Products containing propylene glycol and isopropyl alcohol produce local irritation when applied to mucous membranes and should not be used for intranasal infusions.

Dosage

Canine

Sinonasal Aspergillosis: Treatment consists of a bilateral infusion of a 1% clotrimazole solution (1 g clotrimazole powder (USP)/100 mL polyethylene glycol (USP). Animals are anesthetized and fungal plaques are debrided endoscopically. After occluding the nasopharynx with a retroflexed Foley catheter and packing the pharynx with laparotomy sponges, clotrimazole 1% (30 mL: small dogs and 60 mL: large dogs) is then infused through catheters into the nasal cavity and frontal sinuses over a 1-h period. The head is rotated every 15 min to assure penetration to all sites. Trephination of the frontal sinuses may be required in order to facilitate treatment. Repeat treatments may be necessary if plaques persist on follow-up rhinoscopic evaluation at monthly intervals.

Otitis Externa (Malassezia): Administer topical preparations according to the manufacturer's instructions. Typically a small amount (4–8 drops or up to 1 mL) is administered q12–24 h for 2–4 weeks. Limit extended use of combination products that contain glucocorticoids.

Feline

Sinonasal Aspergillosis: Administer 1% clotrimazole in polyethylene glycol (PEG) intranasally over 1 h while the patient is under anesthesia following rhinoscopy and debridement of fungal plaques. Topical clotrimazole is not effective as a sole therapy for sino-orbital aspergillosis in cats. Itraconazole or posaconazole oral therapy should be considered.

Dose adjustments

No dose adjustments are necessary in hepatic or renal impairment.

Administration

For topical application, owners should be instructed to wear gloves and wash hands afterwards. The animal should not be permitted to lick, bite, or chew area for 30 min after application. Warn the owner about potential for iatrogenic hyperadrenocorticism with prolonged use of combinations that contains glucocorticoids. For intranasal infusions see detailed instructions prior to use (Mathews *et al.*, 1998, Sykes 2013).

Electrolyte contents

Not significant.

Storage/stability

Storage of all commercial topical creams, solutions, or lotions is at room temperature between 2–30°C. Clotrimazole 1% solution for nasal instillation should be made in a sterile environment just prior to use.

Adverse reactions

>10%

Highly irritating to skin and mucus membranes. Topical application can result in erythema, edema, swelling, epistaxis, upper airway obstruction, and severe pharyngitis in some patients after intranasal infusions in dogs and cats.

1–10%

Gastrointestinal irritation (nausea, vomiting, salivation, and diarrhea) have been reported in animals licking off topical medication. Head tilt and ataxia may occur with otic preparations if the tympanic membrane is not intact.

<1%

With a breach in the cribiform plate, significant CNS levels may be achieved during intranasal installation to result in significant CNS toxicity.

Drug interactions

Not significant with topical therapy.

Monitoring

Animals treated with intranasal clotrimazole infusions should be monitored closely for severe epistaxis or respiratory difficulty for at least 12 h after recovery from anesthesia. Follow-up rhinoscopic exams are recommended to evaluated treatment success/failure for patients with sinonasal aspergillosis. Serologic testing for anti-*Aspergillus* antibodies does not appear to correlate with treatment outcome.

Overdose

A significant amount must be ingested orally for acute toxicity (CNS depression, cortical encephalopathy, and liver impairment) to occur. Due to limited absorption orally and via topical administration an overdose would be unlikely. The oral LD_{50} in dogs is >2000 mg/kg and in cats is >1000 mg/kg. If large amounts are consumed orally, induce vomiting and apply supportive care. Monitor liver function.

Diagnostic test interference

Prolonged use of combination otic products that contain glucocorticoids may induce serum alkaline phosphatase activity and alter endocrine test results secondary to alteration of the hypothalamic-pituitary-adrenal axis.

Mechanism

Inhibits the biosynthesis of ergosterol in the fungal cell wall.

Pharmacology/kinetics

Absorption
Clotrimazole has poor oral absorption in dogs. Bioavailability is only 4.9% following a 5 mg/kg oral dose. Absorption of 1% solution/creams is also minimal with no detectable plasma concentrations at 48 h after administration. Following intra-nasal administration systemic absorption is minimal.

Distribution
Following oral administration (5 mg/kg) in dogs, for the small amount of drug that is absorbed, there is a significant first-pass effect with 90% of the absorbed dose being metabolized before reaching the systemic circulation. Plasma protein binding is 50%.

CNS penetration
CNS penetration is poor unless the cribiform plate is not intact.

Metabolism
Absorbed clotrimazole is rapidly metabolized in the liver to inactive metabolites that are eliminated via bile. Less than 10% is excreted via urine in 24 h.

Half-life
The half-life is 4.6 h in dogs receiving oral doses of 5 mg/kg.

Pregnancy risk factor

Category B (topical) or Category C (oral/systemic): Large oral doses (100 mg/kg) given to rats has resulted in embryotoxicity but not teratogenic effects. It would be contraindicated in pregnancy.

Lactation
Little is known about excretion into milk but its limited oral bioavailability suggest that the risks to nursing animals would be minimal.

References

Mathews, K.G., Davidson, A.P., Koblik, P.D., *et al.* (1998) Comparison of topical administration of clotrimazole through surgically placed versus nonsurgically placed catheters for treatment of nasal aspergillosis in dogs: 60 cases (1990–1996). *J Am Vet Med Assoc.*, **213(4)**, 501–506.

Sykes, J.E. (2013) Aspergillosis. In: *Canine and Feline Infectious Diseases*, Sykes, J.E. (ed.), Elsevier, St. Louis, MO. pp. 633–648.

Further reading

Caulkett, N., Lew, L., and Fries, C. (1997) Upper airway obstruction and prolonged recovery from anesthesia following intranasal clotrimazole administration. *J Am Anim Hosp Assoc.*, **33(3)**, 264–267.

Conte, L., Ramis, J., Mis, R., *et al.* (1992) Pharmacokinetic study of 14 C-flutrimazole after oral and intravenous administration in dogs. Comparison with clotrimazole. *Arzneimitleforsch.*, **42(6)**, 854–858.

Furrow, E. and Groman, R.P. (2009) Intranasal infusion of clotrimazole for the treatment of nasal aspergillosis in two cats. *J Am Vet Med Assoc.*, **235(10)**, 1188–1193.

Mathews, K., Linder, K., Davidson, G., *et al.* (2009) Assessment of clotrimazole gels for in vitro stability and *in vivo* retention in the front sinus of dogs. *Amer J Vet Research.*, **70(5)**, 640–647.

Pomrantz, J.S. and Johnson, L.R. (2010) Repeated rhinoscopic and serologic assessment of intranasally administered clotrimazole for the treatment of nasal aspergillosis in dogs. *J Am Vet Med Assoc.*, **236(7)**, 757–762.

Chapter 175: Enilconazole

US Generic (Brand) Name: Enilconazole (Imaverol)
Availability: Veterinary Approved – Imaverol 10% concentrate (not in the USA), enilconazole USP chemical grade powder
Resistance Mechanisms: Overexpression of efflux pump genes including *CDR1, CDR2*

Use

Enilconazole has been used topically as a treatment for dermatophytes and as an environmental spray for cages, bedding, stalls, and equipment. It is used as an alternative to clotrimazole for treatment of sinonasal aspergillosis in dogs. It is often used in patients that have failed oral azole treatment or clotrimazole instillation. This procedure is not recommended unless performed by a highly trained individual.

Contraindications/warnings

Contraindicated in patients with hypersensitivity to azoles or in those that do not have an intact cribriform plate. Use of EPA chemicals (e.g., Imaverol and Clinafarm) off-label is illegal. Cats may also be more sensitive to enilconazole's irritant/allergenic properties.

Dosage

Canine/feline

Sinonasal Aspergillosis: Treatment consists of a bilateral infusion of 1–2% enilconazole solution. Animals are anesthetized and fungal plaques are debrided endoscopically. After occluding the nasopharynx with a retroflexed Foley catheter and packing the pharynx with laparotomy sponges, enilconazole 1% (30 mL: small dogs and 60 mL: large dogs) is then infused through catheters into the nasal cavity and frontal sinuses over a 1-h period. The head is rotated every 15 min to assure penetration to all sites. Trephination of the frontal sinuses may be required in order to facilitate treatment. Repeat treatments may be necessary if plaques persist on follow-up rhinoscopic evaluation at monthly intervals.

Dose adjustments

No adjustments are needed for topical therapy.

Administration

Clinafarm EC has historically been used off-label as a topical dip for dogs with dermatophytosis as well as intranasally for dogs with sinonasal aspergillosis. It has currently been removed from the market. Imaverol, remains available but has not demonstrated equal efficacy when administered intranasally. Enilconazole USP chemical can be mixed with propylene glycol to make a 1% solution. For intranasal infusions see detailed instructions prior to use (Sykes 2013).

Electrolyte contents

Not significant.

Storage/stability

Store at room temperature (<30°C). Freezing should be avoided. Compounding of enilconazole powder in polyethylene glycol should be performed just prior to administration due to lack of stability data.

Adverse reactions

>10%

In dogs, pharyngitis, edema, and prolonged recovery are reported with the use of vehicles containing alcohol and propylene glycol given intranasally. Transient post-operative subcutaneous emphysema, inappetence, and ptyalism are reported following intranasal administration with surgically placed catheters. In cats, hypersalivation, nausea, vomiting, and anorexia are reported following topical use.

1–10%

Weight loss, idiopathic muscle weakness, and elevated serum alanine aminotransferase concentrations have been reported in cats following topical therapy.

<1%

Severe complications leading to euthanasia in dogs have included neurological signs compatible with cortical encephalopathy and suppurative meningitis when enilconazole has been administered intranasally in dogs without an intact cribriform plate.

Other species

Hepatic changes (centri-lobular swelling, fatty changes, and vacuoles), vomiting, tremors, muscle incoordination, and decreased blood pressure when enilconazole was given orally at >20 mg/kg.

Drug interactions

Not significant with topical therapy.

Monitoring

Monitor efficacy/side effects if using intranasal installation.

Overdose

Oral bioavailability is poor, so unless very large amounts are ingested orally, toxicity should be minimal. Signs of acute toxicity may involve nausea, vomiting, diarrhea, and elevated liver enzymes. Supportive care including induction of vomiting and activated charcoal may be indicated.

Diagnostic test interference

None reported.

Mechanism

Inhibits ergosterol synthesis by fungi and disrupts the fungal cell wall.

Pharmacology/kinetics

Absorption

Enilconazole is rapidly absorbed orally in dogs, but due to a very high first pass metabolism bioavailability is very low (1.4%). Transdermal absorption is also very low (<5%).

Distribution

Enilconazole concentrations in plasma are insignificant following topical, oral and intranasal administration. The highest concentrations noted are in the liver, kidney, muscles, and fat.

CNS penetration

CNS penetration is extremely low with no detectable concentrations following chronic administration to rats.

Metabolism

Enilconazole undergoes extensive first pass metabolism into at least 35 metabolites following oral administration. Large species differences in metabolism are noted.

Half-life

The half-life of the parent drug in dogs is approximately 1 h.

Pregnancy risk factor

Category B: No teratogenic effects have been reported in laboratory animals, but an increase in gestational time, a decrease in live pups, and a greater number of stillbirths were noted in rats and rabbits at high oral doses (80 mg/kg). Risks would have to be weighed with benefits in pregnant animals.

Lactation

Only minor amounts (0.1%) are excreted into goat/cow milk after topical dosing. Due to poor oral bioavailability and minimal absorption following topical administration to dogs or cats, risks to nursing animals would be considered very low.

Reference

Sykes, J.E. (2013) Aspergillosis. In: *Canine and Feline Infectious Diseases*, Sykes, J.E. (ed.), Elsevier, St. Louis, MO. pp. 633–648.

Further reading

Committee for Veterinary Medicinal Products (1998) *Econazole summary report*. The European Agency for the Evolution of Medicinal Products, Veterinary Medicine Evaluation Unit. Sept. 1998. EMEA/MRL/496/98-Final.

Hnilica, K.A. and Medleau, L. (2002) Evaluation of topically applied enilconazole for the treatment of dermatophytes in a Persian cattery. *Vet Derm.*, **13(1)**, 23–28.

Pomrantz, J.S. and Johnson, L.R. (2010) Repeated rhinoscopic and serologic assessment of intranasally administered clotrimazole for the treatment of nasal aspergillosis in dogs. *J Am Vet Med Assoc.*, **236(7)**, 757–762.

Sharman, M., Lenard, Z., Hosgood, G., *et al.* (2012) Clotrimazole and enilconazole distribution within the frontal sinuses and nasal cavity of nine dogs with sinonasal aspergillosis. *J Small Animal Practice.*, **53(3)**, 162–167.

Sharp, N., Sullivan, M., Harvey, C., and Webb, T. (1993) Treatment of canine nasal aspergillosis with enilconazole. *J Vet Intern Med.*, **7(1)**, 40–43.

Zonderland, J., Stork, C., Saunders, J., *et al.* (2002) Intranasal infusion of enilconazole for treatment of sinonasal aspergillosis in dogs. *J Am Vet Med Assoc.*, **221(10)**, 1421–1425.

Chapter 176: Fluconazole

US Generic (Brand Name): Fluconazole (Diflucan)
Availability: Human Approved – Tablets (50, 100, 150, 200 mg), powder for oral suspension (10 mg/mL, 40 mg/mL), sterile injection (2 mg/mL × 100 mL, 200 mL)
Resistance Mechanisms: Increased levels of expression of the *ERG11* gene, increasing enzymes in ergosterol biosynthesis, overexpression of efflux pump genes including *CDR1*, *CDR2*, and *MDR1*

Use

Fluconazole is the drug of choice for susceptible superficial or systemic mycosis including those that involve the CNS, urinary tract, and eye. Fluconazole has similar antifungal activity as itraconazole with the exception that it lacks activity against most molds including *Aspergillus*, and has limited activity against *Microsporum canis* and the yeast *Malassezia*. It has activity against *Blastomyces*, *Candida*, *Coccidioides*, and *Histoplasma*, although activity may be lower than for other azoles such as itraconazole. Due to its superb penetration across the blood-brain barrier it is often the preferred azole for infections involving the CNS. It has been used successfully to treat dogs that develop hepatotoxicity as a result of itraconazole therapy.

Contraindications/warnings

Avoid in patients with significant hepatic impairment or known hypersensitivity to azoles. Use cautiously in patients taking other hepatotoxic drugs.

Dosage

For severe infections, a loading dose (2× the maintenance dose for 2–3 days) can be given to reach therapeutic concentrations rapidly. Treatment should continue at least 30 days after resolution of clinical signs.

Canine
Systemic Mycosis (Blastomycosis, Cryptococcosis, Coccidioidomycosis, Candidiasis): 5–10 mg/kg PO, IV q12–24 h); the high end of the dose range is recommended for treatment of cryptococcosis and coccidioidomycosis (Greene *et al.*, 2006).

Feline
Cryptococcus: Most cats respond to a 50 mg (total dose) PO q24 h (Greene *et al.*, 2006). For CNS, intraocular or multisystemic infections higher doses (50–100 mg/cat PO or IV q12 h) may be required.

Dose adjustments

For animals receiving chronic doses with significant renal impairment, administer a loading dose Day 1: then give 50% of the recommended dose or administer every 48 h rather than 24 h.

Administration

The oral tablets and suspension may be given with food. Parenteral fluconazole (200 mg/100 mL) is formulated in sodium chloride. It should be given as an intravenous infusion over 1–2 h. Do not exceed 200 mg/h.

Electrolyte contents

The sterile injectable solution contains 9 mg sodium chloride (equivalent to 0.154 mmol sodium) per mL.

Storage/stability

Tablets are stored at room temperature. The injectable should be stored at 5–25°C, avoid freezing. The powder for oral suspension should be stored at room temperature and after reconstitution can be stored at room temperature for up to 14 days.

Adverse reactions

>10%
Diarrhea, inappetence, and vomiting are common at high doses in dogs and cats.

1–10%
Elevated liver enzyme activities (especially serum ALT activity) that may decrease or normalize following dose reduction and hepatotoxicity (idiosyncratic and dose dependent) has also been reported in both species.

Other species
Lethargy, ataxia, jaundice, rash, hypokalemia, thrombocytopenia, anemia, neutropenia, anaphylaxis, erythema multiforme, exfoliative cutaneous reactions, and QT prolongation have all been reported.

Drug interactions

Fluconazole's activity may be reduced when administered concurrently with rifampin, cimetidine, and amphotericin-B. Fluconazole may increase the plasma concentrations and toxicity of vincristine, vinblastine, cyclophosphamide, sulfonylureas, tricyclic antidepressants, theophylline, quinidine, NSAIDs, benzodiazepines, fentanyl, cyclosporine, corticosteroids, and cisapride. Fluconazole's effects on the QT interval may be increased by other drugs affecting the QT interval (macrolides and cisapride).

Monitoring

Establish baseline liver values and monitor liver enzyme (AST, ALT, and alkaline phosphatase) activities monthly during treatment. Monitor patient for signs of hepatotoxicity (vomiting, diarrhea, and anorexia). Monitor serum potassium and renal function with chronic use.

Overdose

Clinical signs of overdose in rats and mice treated with doses >1000 mg/kg have included decreased lacrimation, salivation, respiratory depression, urinary incontinence, and cyanosis. Provide supportive care, gastrointestinal decontamination, and hemodialysis if available (3 h removes 50% of drug).

Diagnostic test interference

None noted.

Mechanism

First generation triazole. Inhibits fungal lanosterol 14-alpha demethylase, leading to ergosterol depletion, and accumulation of toxic sterols in the fungal cell membrane.

Pharmacology/kinetics

Absorption
Fluconazole is well absorbed from the gastrointestinal tract of fasted animals (>90% oral bioavailability). It does not rely on gastric acidity or the presence of food in the stomach to be absorbed. Peak absorption occurs at 1.3 h in cats and 4 h after oral administration in dogs.

Distribution
Fluconazole differs from the other azoles in its extent of protein binding. It is only 11% protein bound in most species and is widely distributed throughout tissues including aqueous humor and bronchial tissues.

CNS penetration
Due to low protein binding it penetrates easily (>70%) into the CSF.

Metabolism
Fluconazole is eliminated primarily via the kidneys and active drug is found in high concentrations in urine.

Half-life
The half-life of fluconazole is long (24 h) in cats. In dogs, it is 15 h after a single oral dose. A loading dose is recommended for severe infections.

Pregnancy risk factor

Category C: Teratogenic effects have been noted with first trimester exposure in humans. It is generally not recommended in pregnancy unless the benefits outweigh the risks.

Lactation

Fluconazole is excreted in high concentrations in milk, and chronic exposure may predispose nursing animals to adverse effects including hepatotoxicity.

Reference

Greene, C., Hartmann, K., *et al.* (2006) Antimicrobial drug formulary. Appendix 8. In: *Infectious Disease of the Dog and Cat.* Greene, C. (ed.), Elsevier, St. Louis, MO, pp. 1186–1333.

Further reading

Foy, D.S. and Trepanier, L.A. (2010) Antifungal treatment of small animal veterinary patients. *Vet Clin Small Anim.*, **40**, 1171–1188.

Papich, M.G., Heit, M.C., and Riviere, J.E. (2001) Antifungal and antiviral drugs. In: *Veterinary Pharmacology and Therapeutics*, 8th edn, Adams, H.R. (ed.), Iowa State University Press, Ames, pp. 918–946.

Taboada, J. (2000) Systemic Mycosis. *Textbook of Veterinary Internal Medicine. Diseases of the Dog and Cat. Vol. 1.* Ettinger, S. and Feldman, E. (eds), W.B. Saunders, Philadelphia, pp. 453–476.

Vaden, S.L., Heit, M.C., Hawkins, E.C., *et al.* (1997) Fluconazole in cats: pharmacokinetics following intravenous and oral administration and penetration into cerebrospinal fluid, aqueous humor and pulmonary epithelial lining fluid. *J Vet Pharmacol Ther.*, **20(3)**, 181–186.

Chapter 177: Flucytosine

US Generic (Brand) Name: Flucytosine, 5-FC, 5-flurocytosine (Ancobon, Ancotil)
Availability: Human Approved – Oral capsules (250, 500 mg), sterile injectable (10 mg/mL), compounded oral suspension (10 mg/mL)
Resistance Mechanisms: Inactivation of the *FCY2* (cytosine permease), *FCY1* (cytosine deaminase), and FUR1 (uracil phosphoribosyltransferase) genes

Use

Flucytosine must not be used as monotherapy in life-threatening fungal infections due to relatively weak antifungal effects and rapid development of resistance during treatment. Instead it is used in combination with amphotericin B and/or azole antifungals such as fluconazole or itraconazole. Flucytosine is primarily used in the treatment of systemic fungal infections of cats due to *Cryptococcus* and *Candida*. It also has activity against *Aspergillus* spp. Although it is currently expensive, flucytosine in combination with amphotericin B is currently the treatment of choice for cats with cryptococcosis. It is not recommended in dogs due to potential dermal toxicity.

Contraindications/warnings

Contraindicated in canine patients or patients hypersensitive to flucytosine. Use with extreme caution in patients with significant renal and liver impairment or with bone marrow suppression. Caution when combined with nephrotoxic drugs (amphotericin B, aminoglycosides, etc.). Animals with azotemia are at high risk of developing bone marrow toxicity.

Dosage

Feline

Administer 25–50 mg/kg PO, IV q6 h or 50–65 mg/kg PO q8 h. Amphotericin B or an azole must be given in combination. Treatment is often long term (1–9 months). (Greene and Watson 1989, Malik and Krockenberger, 2006, Koch *et al.*, 2012).

Dose adjustments

For patients with severe renal impairment, administer the dose every 24 h, for patients with mild to moderate renal impairment adjust frequency to q12–16 h rather than q6–8 h. Monitor plasma concentrations if possible.

Administration

The injectable form should be diluted with saline (250 mL) to contain 2.5 g (10 mg/mL). The solution is not compatible with other drugs including amphotericin B. The infusion should be given over 20–40 min. The oral capsules should be administered with food and the dose may be given over a 15 min period to prevent nausea.

Electrolyte contents

Ancotil injection contains 3.16 mg per mL of sodium.

Storage/stability

Flucytosine capsules should be protected from light and stored at room temperature. A stable compounded suspension (10 mg/mL) can be made using the commercial capsules. Use (4) × 250 mg (or 2 × 500 mg) capsules triturated in a mortar with a small amount of Ora-plus. Transfer the product to an 8 oz oral, amber plastic vial. Use small amounts of Ora-Plus to rinse the mortar several times and transfer into the amber vial (qs to the 50 mL line). Add Ora-Sweet to make a final volume of 100 mL (10 mg/mL). Shake well and refrigerate for up to 60 days.

Adverse reactions

Serum levels in excess of 100 μg/mL are associated with a higher incidence of adverse effects. Periodic measurements of serum levels are recommended for patients with renal damage.

>10%

Nausea, vomiting, anorexia, and diarrhea are commonly reported in cats and dogs. Cutaneous lesions (depigmentation, ulceration, exudation, crust formation) develop in almost all dogs within 20 days of commencing flucytosine and may take up to 2 months to resolve.

1–10%

Bone marrow suppression has occurred in dogs and cats (more severe in immunocompromised animals), and elevated liver enzymes reported in cats and dogs.

Other species

Elevated BUN, serum creatinine, crystaluria, malaise, inappetence, oral ulcers, hepatotoxicity, severe drug reactions (anaphylaxis, fever, erythema, edema), photosensitivity reactions of skin, toxic epidermal necrosis, aberrant behavior, seizures, ataxia, neuropathy, and sedation.

Drug interactions

Other nephrotoxic drugs (amphotericin B, aminoglycosides, vancomycin, etc.) may increase serum concentrations of flucytocine resulting in bone marrow toxicity. Drugs that cause myelosuppression or hepatotoxicity should be avoided in patients treated with flucytosine if possible. Co-administration with aluminum hydroxide or magnesium hydroxide may delay the absorption of flucytosine.

Monitoring

Therapeutic concentrations in plasma are between 25–100 μg/mL. Trough concentrations should be determined just prior to dosing and peaks should be obtained 2 h after dosing. Concentrations greater than 100 μg/mL may result in bone marrow toxicity. Monitor the CBC on a weekly basis during treatment. Obtain renal panel just prior to doses of amphotericin B when flucytosine is used in conjunction. Consider monitoring of liver enzyme activities monthly.

Overdose

Clinical signs may include bone marrow suppression, gastrointestinal irritation, and liver and kidney dysfunction. Vigorous hydration and hemodialysis may be helpful to remove the drug particularly when impaired renal function is present.

Diagnostic test interference

Flucytosine causes markedly false elevations in serum creatinine when using an Ektachem analyzer.

Mechanism

Penetrates into the fungal cell wall where it is converted into fluorouracil. The fluorouracil competes with uracil eventually inhibiting fungal RNA and protein synthesis.

Pharmacology/kinetics

Absorption
Flucytosine oral absorption is not well understood in cats. It is well absorbed orally (75–90%) in humans. Administration with meals slows the absorption but does not change the amount absorbed.

Distribution
The drug readily distributes into CSF, aqueous humor, joints, peritoneal fluid, and bronchial secretions.

CNS penetration
Protein binding is minimal (2–4%) with very high concentrations being achieved in the CSF (>70%).

Metabolism
Metabolism of flucytosine is minimal, it is primarily excreted unchanged in urine (90%) of most species including dogs, with only trace amounts excreted in feces. Urinary metabolites account for only 5% of drug in dogs.

Half-life
The half-life in veterinary patients is not well studied. In humans, it is highly variable and dependent on renal function. With normal renal function it is 3–4 h, but up to 85 h with severe renal disease.

Pregnancy risk factor

Category C: Teratogenicity has been demonstrated in rats. It is contraindicated in pregnancy.

Lactation
Penetration into milk is unknown, but the risks of toxicity would outweigh the benefits.

References

Greene, C. and Watson, A. (2006) Antimicrobial drug formulary. In: *Infectious Disease of the Dog and Cat*. 3rd edn, Greene, C. (ed.), Elsevier, St. Louis, MO, pp. 790–919.

Koch, S.N., Torres, S.M., and Plumb, D.C. (2012) *Canine and Feline Dermatology Drug Handbook*. Wiley Publishers, Ames, Iowa, p. 92.

Malik, R. and Krockenberger, M. (2006) Cryptococcus. In: *Infectious Disease of the Dog and Cat*. 3rd edn, Greene, C. (ed.), Elsevier, St. Louis, MO, pp. 584–598.

Further reading

Allen, L.V. and Erickson, M.A. (1996) Stability of acetazolamide, allopurinol, azathioprine, clonazepam and flucytosine in extemporaneously compounded oral liquids. *Am J Health Sys, Phar.*, **53(16)**, 1944–1950.

Malik, R., Medeiros, C., and Love, D.N. (1996) Suspected drug eruption in seven dogs during administration of flucytosine. *Aust Vet J.*, **74(4)**, 285–288.

Vermes, A., Guchelaar, H.J., and Dankert, J. (2000) Flucytosine: a review of its pharmacology, clinical indications, pharmacokinetics, toxicity and drug interactions. *J Antimicrob. Chemother.*, **46(2)**, 171–179.

Chapter 178: Itraconazole

US Generic (Brand) Name: Itraconazole (Sporanox)
Availability: Human Approved – Itraconazole oral capsules (100 mg), oral solution 10 mg/mL, sterile injection kit (10 mg/mL): variable availability
Resistance Mechanisms: Increased levels of expression of the *ERG11* gene, enzymes in the ergosterol biosynthetic, overexpression of efflux pump genes including *CDR1*, *CDR2*, and *MDR1*

Use

Treatment of a variety of systemic and superficial fungal infections including blastomycosis, histoplasmosis, coccidioidomycosis, cryptococcosis, sporothrichosis, zygomycosis, phaeohyphomycosis, hyalohypomycosis, aspergillosis, dermatophytosis, candidiasis, and *Malassezia dermatitis*. Some *Pythium* infections may also be controlled with itraconazole. Itraconazole is considered the drug of choice for treatment of sporotrichosis in dogs and cats and is preferred over fluconazole for treatment of blastomycosis, histoplasmosis, and mold infections.

Contraindications/warnings

Avoid if known hypersensitivity to azoles or significant hepatic dysfunction. Avoid use of the oral solution or injectable solution in renal failure due to accumulation of the hydroxypropyl-beta-cyclodextrin additive. The solution and capsules are not interchangeable due to the increased absorption of the solution.

Dosage

Dogs
Mycosis: A loading dose of twice the maintenance dose may be required in severe disease to establish therapeutic concentrations rapidly. Then give 5–10 mg/kg/day PO q24 h (Davidson and Mathews 2000, Legendre and Toal 2000, Taboada 2000).

Pythiosis/Aspergillus: 10 mg/kg PO q24 h in combination with terbinafine for non-resectable pythiosis and disseminated aspergillosis.

Cats
Mycosis: Give a loading dose (2× maintenance dose); then 3 mg/kg PO q24 h (oral commercial solution) or 5–10 mg/kg PO q24 h (commercial capsules) (Legendre and Toal 2000, Taboada 2000).

Dose adjustments

Not necessary in renal failure. Dose reduction may be required with significant elevations in liver enzyme activities.

Administration

All capsules must be given with an acidic food and the oral solution must be given on an empty stomach for adequate absorption. Some veterinarians suggest a dose decrease by 25–50% when switching from the capsules to the oral solution. Treatment should be given for at least 30 days beyond the resolution of clinical signs. Avoid use of compounded medications which may be unstable or may not be absorbed orally. Intravenous injection solution comes as a kit with ampules that should be diluted in 0.9% sodium chloride provided with a filtered infusion set. Infusion must be over 1 h.

Electrolyte contents

Electrolyte concentration negligible. The oral solution contains hydroxypropyl-B-cyclodextrin (400 mg/mL). The injectable solution contains hydroxyl-B-cyclodextrin and propylene glycol.

Storage/stability

Oral capsules and solution should be stored at room temperature, protected from UV light, moisture, and freezing. If available, the injectable powder once diluted should be stored refrigerated or at room temperature for up to 48 h.

Adverse reactions

>10%
Nausea, vomiting, anorexia, weight loss, and elevated liver enzyme activities (dose related). Slight increases in ALT are not indicative of hepatotoxicosis. Discontinue until enzymes normalize, may be followed by reinitiation at a lower dose.

1–10%
Hepatotoxicosis (idiosyncratic). This is often associated with anorexia, lethargy, and jaundice and may be serious enough to discontinue therapy. Ulcerative skin lesions have been reported in 7% of dogs receiving itraconazole at 10 mg/kg/day.

Other species
Negative inotropic effects on the heart, ventricular tachycardia, rash, pruritus, lethargy, fever, hypertriglyceridemia, adrenal suppression, hypokalemia, myelosuppression, and albuminuria.

Drug interactions

Absorption requires gastric acidity, so antacids, histamine blockers, proton pump inhibitors, and sucralfate should not be administered concomitantly. P450 enzyme inducers (phenobarbital, rifampin) may decrease serum levels of itraconazole, decreasing efficacy. Rifampin should not be co-administered with itraconazole due to its hepatotoxic effects. Itraconazole is a P450 inhibitor that may increase the plasma concentrations and toxicity of cyclosporine, digoxin, sulfonylureas, amlodipine, benzodiazepines, cisapride, glucocorticoids, vincristine, vinblastine, and clarithromycin.

Monitoring

Baseline liver function tests (AST, ALT, Alkaline phosphatase), potassium, and renal function. Monitor liver enzymes monthly during treatment; particularly evaluate drug interactions with limited creatinine clearance.

Overdose

Overdoses are typically not life threatening. May require GI decontamination, antacids to reduce absorption, and supportive care. Dialysis is not effective.

Diagnostic test interference

None noted.

Mechanism

Azole antifungal drug. Fungistatic or cidal depending on organism. Inhibits fungal lanosterol 14-alpha demethylase, leading to ergosterol depletion, accumulation of toxic sterols in the fungal cell membrane.

Pharmacology/kinetics

Absorption
Variable, dependent on species and formulation. In dogs, bioavailability is >90% when capsules given with acidic food, but only 40% in fasted dogs. Generic capsules have demonstrated an increased AUC (104.2%) over brand name capsules in dogs. In cats, the bioavailability of the commercial oral solution is 70% on an empty stomach. The commercial oral solution is generally better absorbed than the capsules. Note: Oral capsules contain protective film coated beads and the oral solution contains a hydroxypropyl-beta-cyclodextrin carrier that facilitates absorption. Compounded preparations made from bulk drug lack stability and absorption and their use is typically associated with treatment failure. Plasma concentrations can be monitored to document absorption.

Distribution
Itraconazole is highly protein bound (99%), and accumulates in skin, liver, fat, stratum corneum, and adrenal medulla.

CNS penetration
Itraconazole has poor penetration into the CNS (<10%), but clinically is reported to be effective in some cases of CNS disease (cryptococcal meningoencephalitis in cats).

Metabolism
Itraconazole undergoes extensive metabolism in the liver to a variety of metabolites. The major metabolite (hydroxyitraconazole) has activity similar to the parent drug. Elimination is primarily via biliary secretion with <1% eliminated through the urinary tract.

Half-life
After single doses in cats and dogs, the half-life is 28–30 h. Oxidative pathways may become saturated with chronic dosing causing accumulation of drug.

Pregnancy risk factor

Category C: Dose related embryotoxicity, teratogenicity, skeletal, and tooth defects are reported in rats and mice. It is contraindicated in pregnancy.

Lactation
Itraconazole crosses into milk and may cause side effects in nursing animals. It is not considered safe in nursing animals.

References

Davidson, A. and Mathews, K. (2000) CVT Update: Therapy for nasal aspergillosis. *Kirk's Current Veterinary Therapy: XIII Small Animal Practice*. Bonagura, J. (ed.), W.B. Saunders, Philadelphia, pp. 315–317.

Legendre, A. and Toal, R. (2000) Diagnosis and treatment of fungal diseases of the respiratory system. *Kirk's Current Veterinary Therapy: XIII Small Animal Practice*. Bonagura, J. (ed.), W.B. Saunders, Philadelphia, pp. 815–819.

Taboada J. (2000) Systemic mycosis. *Textbook of Veterinary Internal Medicine. Diseases of the Dog and Cat. Vol. 1.* Ettinger, S. and Feldman, E. (eds). W.B. Saunders, Philadelphia, pp. 453–476.

Further reading

Booth, D.M., Herring, I., Calvin, J., *et al.* (1997) Itraconazole disposition after single oral and intravenous and multiple oral dosing in healthy cats. *Am J Res.*, **58(8)**, 872–877.

Negre, A, Bensignor E, *et al.* (2009) Evidence based veterinary dermatology: a systematic review of interventions for *Malassezia* dermatitis in dogs. *Veterinary Dermatology*, **20(1)**, 1–12.

Papich, M.G., Heit, M.C., and Riviere, J.E. (2001) Antifungal and antiviral drugs. In: *Veterinary Pharmacology and Therapeutics*, 8th edn, Adams, H.R. (ed.), Iowa State University Press, Ames, pp. 918–946.

VanCauteren, H., Heykants, J., DeCoster, R., *et al.* (1987) Itraconazole: pharmacologic studies in animals and humans. *Rev Infect Dis.*, **9(Suppl 1)**, S43–S46.

Chapter 179: Ketoconazole

US Generic (Brand) Name: Ketoconazole (Nizoral, Ketochlor)
Availability: Human Approved – Ketoconazole tablets (200 mg), Nizoral shampoo 1%, 2%, Ketoconazole cream 2%. Veterinary Approved – Ketoconazole shampoo and combinations (Ketoconazole/ chlorhexidine)
Resistance Mechanisms: Increased levels of expression of the ERG11 gene, enzymes in the ergosterol

Use

Historically used to treat a variety of systemic mycosis in dogs and cats, but lost favor owing to a higher rate of adverse effects. Currently used topically for superficial mycosis, and to increase the plasma concentrations of cyclosporine via P450 inhibition, although the later practice is controversial due to the increased likelihood of adverse effects and possible selection for azole-resistant fungi.

Contraindications/warnings

Avoid with known hypersensitivity to azoles or significant hepatic dysfunction. Avoid in animals with thrombocytopenia. Avoid use in cats if alternatives are available. Avoid in breeding animals due to effects on fertility and teratogenicity. Monitor liver enzymes, potential drug interactions. Fatal drug interactions may result from ketoconazole drug interactions.

Dosage

Dogs
Susceptible infections: 10–15 mg/kg PO q12 h (Sykes and Papich 2013).

Cats
Susceptible infections: 5–10 mg/kg PO q12 h (Sykes and Papich 2013).

Dose adjustments

Not necessary in renal failure. Dose reduction may be required with significant elevations in liver enzymes.

Administration

Give oral preparations with an acidic food (fruit juice, cola). Give ketoconazole at least 1 h prior or 2 h after antacids, proton pump inhibitors or H_2 blockers. Follow manufacturer's recommendations for various shampoos.

Electrolyte contents

Not significant.

Storage/stability

Tablets, shampoos, creams can be stored at room temperature, protected from light and moisture. An oral liquid suspension (20 mg/mL) can be made using the 200 mg commercial tablets. Pulverize 12 × 200 mg tablets into fine powder in a mortar. Add 40 mL of Ora-Plus in small portions with thorough mixing. Transfer contents into an amber oral dispensing bottle. Measure out 80 mL of Ora-Sweet and add small proportions to the mortar to transfer remaining drug into the amber oral dispensing bottle. Add a sufficient quantity to a final volume of 120 mL. This is stable for 60 days (>95%) refrigerated and protected from light.

Adverse reactions

>10%
Nausea (7%), vomiting (7%), anorexia (5%), and weight loss (dose related in cats/dogs). All adverse reactions are more prevalent in cats. Elevated liver enzyme activities (ALT) occur in at least 5–10% of dogs/ cats and are dose dependent. Slight increases are not indicative of hepatotoxicosis.

1–10%
Hepatotoxicosis (idiosyncratic) is often associated with lethargy, anorexia, and icterus and may be serious enough to discontinue therapy.

<1%
Skin reactions (erythema, pruritus), lightening of hair coat, alopecia, decreased testosterone levels in dogs, and depressed serum cortisol (with high doses: 30 mg/kg) in dogs with hyperadrenocorticism, thrombocytopenia,

immunosuppression (T-lymphocyte suppression), and cataract formation has been noted after long-term administration (15 months) to dogs.

Drug interactions

Absorption requires gastric acidity, so antacids, histamine blockers, proton pump inhibitors, and sucralfate should not be administered concomitantly. P450 enzyme inducers (phenobarbital, rifampin) and macrolides (azithromycin, erythromycin, and clarithromycin) may decrease serum levels of ketoconazole. Rifampin should not be co-administered with ketoconazole due to its hepatotoxic effects. Ketoconazole is a P450 inhibitor that may increase the plasma concentrations and toxicity of amitriptylline, cyclosporine, digoxin, sulfonylureas, amlodipine, benzodiazepine, cisapride, glucocorticoids, cyclophosphamide, fentanyl, ivermectin, vincristine, verapamil, vinblastine, quinidine, and theophylline. Death, ventricular tachycardia, and torsade de pointes noted in humans taking ketoconazole in combination with cisapride, terfenadine, astemizole, and macrolides.

Monitoring

Baseline and periodic liver function tests (AST, ALT, and alkaline phosphatase), potassium, and renal function tests.

Overdose

Overdoses are typically not life threatening. May require gastrointestinal decontamination, antacids to reduce absorption, and supportive care. Dialysis is not effective. Hepatoxicity is caused by an oxidative metabolite, and is reversed by glutathione experimentally.

Diagnostic test interference

Can alter serum cortisol levels acutely as well as adrenal function tests.

Mechanism

Considered a fungistatic imidazole. Inhibits fungal lanosterol 14-alpha-demethylase, leading to ergosterol depletion, and accumulation of toxic sterols in the fungal cell membrane.

Pharmacology/kinetics

Absorption
Highly variable oral absorption in dogs; may be increased with acidic foods. Gastric acid suppression may decrease absorption. Peak serum concentrations occur in (1.1–45.6 μg/mL) between 1–4.25 h after dosing dogs.

Distribution
Highly protein bound (>98%), good distribution into joints, bile, liver, lungs, kidneys, tendons, skin, and soft tissues. Poor penetration into CNS, anterior chamber of eye, and prostate.

CNS penetration
Poor penetration (<10% serum concentrations in humans).

Metabolism
Metabolized primarily in the liver into inactive metabolites. Excreted via the bile, only 2–4% of active parent drug is excreted into urine.

Half-life
In dogs, the half-life is 1–6 h (average 2.7 h), no information is available in cats.

Pregnancy risk factor

Category C: Can cause still births and mummified fetuses in dogs. Cleft palates and digital anomalies have been seen in rodents. It is considered contraindicated in pregnancy.

Lactation
Ketoconazole is excreted in high concentrations in milk, and its use in lactating animals is not recommended.

Reference

Sykes, J.E. and Papich, M.G. (2013) Antibacterial drugs. Ch. 8. In: *Canine and Feline Infectious Diseases*, Sykes, J.E. (ed.), Elsevier, St. Louis, MO. pp. 66–86.

Further reading

Allen, L.V. and Erickson, M.A. (1996) Stability of ketoconazole, metolazone, metronidazole, procainamide hydrochloride, and spironolactone in extemporaneous compounded oral liquids. *Am J Health Systems Pharm.*, **53(17)**, 2073–2078.

Foy, D.S. and Trepanier, L.A. (2010) Antifungal treatment of small animal veterinary patients. *Vet Clin Small Anim.*, **40**, 1171–1188.

Frank, L. (2000) Dermatophytosis. *Kirk's Current Veterinary Therapy.; XIII Small Animal Practice*. Bonagura, J. (ed.), W.B. Saunders, Philadelphia, pp. 577–580.

Greene, C.E., O'Neal K.G., *et al.* (1984) Antimicrobial chemotherapy: *Clinical microbiology and infectious diseases of the dog and cat*. Greene, C. (ed.), W.B. Saunders, Philadelphia, pp. 144–188.

Greene, C., Hartmann, K., *et al.* (2006) Antimicrobial drug formulary. Appendix 8. In: *Infectious Disease of the Dog and Cat*. Greene, C. (ed.), Elsevier, St. Louis, MO, pp. 1186–1333.

McAnulty, J.F. and Lensmeyer, G.L. (1999) The effects of ketoconazole on the pharmacokinetics of cyclosporine A in cats. *Vet Surg.*, **28(6)**, 448–455.

Papich, M.G., Heit, M.C., and Riviere, J.E. (2001) Antifungal and antiviral drugs. In: *Veterinary Pharmacology and Therapeutics*, 8th edn, Adams, H.R. (ed.), Iowa State University Press, Ames, pp. 918–946.

Taboada, J. (2000) Systemic mycosis. In: *Textbook of Veterinary Internal Medicine. Diseases of the dog and Cat. Vol. 1*. Ettinger, S and Feldman, E. (eds), W.B. Saunders, Philadelphia, pp. 453–476.

Chapter 180: Posaconazole

US Generic (Brand) Name: Posaconazole (Noxafil)
Availability: Human Approved – Noxafil extend release tablets (100 mg), oral suspension (40 mg/mL × 123 mL), Noxafil injection (18 mg/mL × 16.7 mL), Veterinary Approved – Posatex otic suspension (posaconazole 1 mg/orbifloxacin 10 mg/mometasone 1 mg per gram suspension (7.5, 15, 30 g bottle)
Resistance Mechanisms: Single amino acid change in the *cyp51A* gene and an alteration in the gene's promoter region

Use

Has similar activity to other azoles, but more active against *Aspergillus* spp., *Fusarium* spp., and *Zygomycetes* spp. Used for invasive infections caused by susceptible organisms that are not susceptible to other azoles. Posaconazole is also used topically as an otic preparation in dogs. The otic suspension is indicated for the treatment of otitis externa in dogs associated with susceptible strains of yeast (*Malassezia pachydermatitis*). It also contains orbifloxacin to cover bacteria (coagulase positive *Staphylococci*, *Pseudomonas aeruginosa*, *Enterococcus*) and mometasone as an anti-inflammatory.

Contraindications/warnings

Avoid with known hypersensitivity to azoles. Correct underlying electrolyte imbalances (K, Mg, Ca) prior to systemic administration. Use with caution in patients with pro-arrhythmic conditions, pre-existing liver impairment, drugs that inhibit P450 (CYP) isoenzymes.

Do not use otic drops with known tympanic perforation. Do not use otic preparation long term due to systemic absorption of glucocorticoid component and signs of iatrogenic hyperadrenaocorticism.

Dosage

Dogs
Disseminated mycosis: 5–10 mg/kg PO q12–24 h (Nomeir *et al.*, 2000, Armentano *et al.*, 2013).

Otitis externa: Instill 4 drops q24 h into ear canals for dogs weighing 13.6 kg/30 lbs and 8 drops q24 h for dogs weighing >13.6 kg/30 lbs. Therapy should continue for 7 days.

Cats
Disseminated mycosis: 5 mg/kg q24 h PO (McLellan *et al.*, 2006).

Dose adjustment

No dose adjusting is required in mild to moderate renal or hepatic failure. Monitor patients closely for adverse effects with severe renal impairment.

Administration

The white cherry flavored immediate release (40 mg/mL) suspension is palatable to cats and can be easily dosed. Patients should be given the dose on a full stomach (within 20 min of a meal). Fatty or acidic meals improve absorption, but care should be taken when advising due to potential predisposition to pancreatitis. The extend release tablets have not been studied in dogs, but are better absorbed on an empty stomach in humans than the suspension. In human patients, dividing the daily dose and giving it q6 h can increase absorption. Shake otic suspension before administering. Four drops of otic suspension delivers 1 mg orbifloxacin, 0.1 mg mometasone, and 0.1 mg of posaconazole. The intravenous solution (16.7 mL) must be brought to room temperature and the entire 150 mL must be diluted with 5% dextrose in water or sodium chloride 0.9%. The dose should be infused IV over 90 min.

Electrolyte contents

Not significant.

Storage/stability

The oral suspension should be stored at room temperature and comes in a glass vial that has a three-year shelf life. Once opened it is good for only 4 weeks. It should be kept from freezing. The otic suspension is stored at room temperature. The single dose sterile vials can be stored in the refrigerator for 24 h.

Adverse reactions

>10%
Erythema noted in dogs receiving the otic suspension (due to vehicle).

1–10%
Aural pain, swelling, and heat noted in dogs receiving the otic preparation. An increase in serum cortisol concentration after ACTH stimulation was noted in dogs receiving high doses of the otic preparation (30–40% mometasone absorption transdermally).

<1%
Hearing loss has been reported rarely in dogs receiving the otic preparation. Erythema and pruritus of the pinna with superficial excoriation of the skin from self-trauma has been reported in a cat receiving oral posaconale. At doses >40 mg/kg, cardiac changes were noted in dogs (increased Q-T intervals, reversal of T-waves).

Other species
Nausea, vomiting, pyrexia, hyperbilirubinemia, electrolyte imbalance, anorexia, malaise, neutropenia, prolonged Q-T interval, rash, tremors, ataxia, adrenal suppression, thrombocytopenia, coagulopathy, anorexia, eosinophilia, lymphadenopathy, and leucopenia have been reported.

Drug interactions

Drugs that are metabolized by P450 (CYP) will have significantly elevated plasma concentrations (cyclosporine, midazolam, vinca alkaloids). Reduce cyclosporine dosages by 25% if initiating posaconazole therapy. Concomitant use with drugs that prolong the Q-T interval (quinidine, macrolides, cisapride, etc.) may lead to torsades de pointes. Inhibitors or inducers of P-glycoproteins may increase or decrease posaconazole concentrations (increased calcium channel blocker concentrations). Phenobarbital, H_2 antagonists, proton pump inhibitors, and metoclopramide decreases the plasma concentrations of posaconazole (20–50%) in humans.

Monitoring

Liver enzyme activities should be monitored monthly. Monitoring serum posaconazole concentrations has also been suggested because of the variability in absorption.

Overdose

Accidental overdoses have occurred in humans with no adverse reactions noted that differed from those seen at lower doses. Posaconazole is not removed by dialysis.

Diagnostic test interference

None noted.

Mechanism

A fungistatic triazole. Blocks the synthesis of fungal ergosterol via inhibition of the fungal enzyme lanosterol 14-alpha-demethylase.

Pharmacology/kinetics

Absorption
Posaconazole has limited oral absorption in dogs (27% with food). Posaconazole absorption is increased four-fold in the presence of food. Maximum absorption occurs in 3 h with a peak concentration of 3.5 μg/mL. It is significantly decreased when administered with proton pump inhibitors or H-2 antagonists (20–30%). Transdermal absorption was between 3–4% of all three components of the otic preparation within 24 h after application.

Distribution
Posaconazole has extensive extracellular distribution and penetration into tissues.

CNS penetration
Posaconazole has limited penetration into the CSF, but may increase with inflammation. CSF concentrations have achieved 47% of plasma concentrations in human patients with significant inflammation.

Metabolism

Posaconazole is metabolized in the liver to a number of inactive metabolites, which become glucuronidated. Limited glucuronidation in cats may be an issue, but the drug has been well tolerated in this species. The majority of the parent drug following transdermal application is eliminated in urine with up to 70–90% of polar metabolites being excreted in feces.

Half-life

The half-life in dogs is 7 h following a 10 mg/kg dose.

Pregnancy risk factor

Category C: It has caused skeletal malformations, dystocias, decreased litter size, and postnatal viability in rats and mice. This may be due to altered steroidogenesis. It is contraindicated in pregnancy.

Lactation

Posaconazole is excreted into milk: only use if the benefit outweighs the risk in lactating animals.

References

Armentano, R.A., Cooke, K.L., and Wickes, B.L. (2013) Disseminated mycotic infections caused by *Westerdykella* species in a German Shepherd dog. *JAVMA*, **242(3)**, 381–387.

McLellan, G.J., Aquino, S.M., Mason, D.R., *et al.* (2006) Use of posaconazole in the management of invasive orbital *aspergillus* in a cat. *J Am Anim Hosp Assoc.*, **42(4)**, 302–307.

Nomeir, A.A., Kuman, P., Hilbert, M.J., *et al.* (2000) Pharmacokinetics of SCH 56592, a new azole broad-spectrum antifungal agent, in mice, rats, rabbits, dogs and cynomolgus monkeys. *Antimicrob Agents Chemother.*, **44(3)**, 727–731.

Further reading

European Medicines Agency (2006) Posaconazole SP. *European Public Assessment Report (EPAR)* Available at: http://www.ema.europa.eu/docs/en_GB/document_library/EPAR_-_Summary_for_the_public/human/000611/Wc500056313.pdf. Accessed February 9, 2015.

Krockenberger, M.B. (2010) Localized *Microsphaeropsis arundinis* infection of the subcutis of a cat. *J Feline Med Surg.*, **12(3)**, 231–236.

Wray, J.D., Sparkes, A.H., and Johnson, E.M. (2008) Infection of the subcutis of the nose in a cat caused by *Mucor species*: Successful treatment using posaconazole. *J Feline Med Surg.*, **10(5)**, 523–527.

Chapter 181: Terbinafine

US Generic (Brand) Name: Terbinafine (Lamisil)
Availability: Human Approved – Terbinafine tablets 250 mg, topical cream 1% (OTC), topical gel 1%, extemporaneous compounded oral suspension (25 mg/mL)
Resistance Mechanisms: Single base pair exchanges in the ERG1 gene coding for squalene epoxidase, the target of terbinafine

Use

Treatment of dermatophytosis and *Malassezia* infections. Terbinafine has also been used with triazoles to treat systemic mycoses such as aspergillosis and pythiosis.

Contraindications/warnings

Contraindicated if allergic to terbinafine or pre-existing liver or renal failure. Hepatotoxicity may occur in patients with or without pre-existing liver disease. Discontinue for symptoms or signs of hepatobiliary dysfunction, cholestatic hepatitis or skin hypersensitivity.

Dosage

Canine

Dermatophytic infections: 30 mg/kg PO q day × 21 days or once daily for 2 consecutive days per week × 6 doses (Berger *et al.*, 2012).

Pythiosis: 5–10 mg/kg PO q24 h with itraconazole 10 mg/kg PO q12 h (Thieman *et al.*, 2011).

Feline

Dermatophytic infections: 30–40 mg/kg PO q24 h (Kotnik 2002).

Dose adjustments

In patients with moderate to severe renal impairment or with hepatic dysfunction the clearance of the drug is decreased by about 50%, so doses should be reduced by 50%.

Administration

Administer with food.

Electrolyte contents

Not significant.

Storage/stability

Store tablets at room temperature, protect from light. A stable suspension can be made in Ora-Sweet: Ora-Plus (1:1) at a concentration of 25 mg/mL. Store at room temperature or refrigerated for 42 days.

Adverse reactions

> 10%
Facial pruritus, urticaria in 2/10 cats 7–14 days after treatment, vomiting in 8–40% of cats (dose related).

1–10%
Gastrointestinal upset, salivation, diarrhea, and decreased appetite noted in 2/20 dogs has been reported. Elevated liver enzyme activities (ALT: 2.3×) reported in 1/20 dogs and excessive panting in 1/20 dogs has been reported.

<1%
Ocular lens changes and retinal changes reported in dogs. Skin rashes reported rarely in cats and dogs.

Other species
Alopecia, depression, anxiety, ataxia, paresthesia, myelosuppression, autoimmune disorders, erythema multiforme, urticarial, lupus erythematosus, and taste disturbance (both acute and chronic) is reported in humans and can be severe.

Drug interactions

In humans, terbinafine inhibits P450 liver enzymes that may increase the plasma concentrations of tricyclic antidepressants, selective serotonin reuptake inhibitors (fluoxetine), MAO inhibitors (amitraz, selegiline), beta-blockers, and antiarrhythmics (flecainide). Terbinafine increases the clearance of cyclosporine by 15%. Terbinafine clearance is increased 100% by rifampin and decreased 33% by cimetidine.

Monitoring

Get baseline liver function tests, monitor for changes in liver function. Monitor for ocular lens changes, retinal changes or neutropenia and/or pancytopenia.

Overdose

Pre-clinical data suggest doses of 100 mg/kg orally given to dogs may result in hepatotoxic and nephrotoxic effects. Doses up to 200 mg/kg × 26 weeks have been administered to dogs which resulted in gastrointestinal toxicity and hepatotoxicity in 75% of dogs. Doses of 60 mg/kg have been determined to be the no-toxic-effect level. Symptoms of overdose may include nausea, vomiting, abdominal pain, ataxia, frequent urination, and elevated liver enzymes. Accidental ingestion of the entire tube of terbinafine (OTC) only contains 300 mg of terbinafine.

Diagnostic test interference

None noted.

Mechanism

Terbinafine hydrochloride is an allylamine antifungal that blocks the fungal biosynthesis of ergosterol. It is fungicidal against many dermatophytes but is fungistatic against yeasts.

Pharmacology/kinetics

Absorption
Oral absorption is variable in animals with only 21–41% bioavailability noted in fasted healthy cats. An increase in the total amount of drug absorbed may be noted when administered with food.

Distribution
Terbinafine rapidly diffuses from the bloodstream into the dermis and epidermis. It is highly protein bound (99%) and is highly lipophilic. The drug concentrates in hair follicles, skin, nails, adipose tissue, and stratum corneum. Cats receiving 34–35 mg/kg/day × 14 days maintain therapeutic plasma concentrations up to 5 weeks.

CNS penetration
Terbinafine does not obtain fungicidal concentrations in the CNS.

Metabolism
Prior to elimination, terbinafine undergoes extensive metabolism in the liver to multiple inactive metabolites in dogs. Approximately 70% of the dose is eliminated in urine.

Half-life
The half-life of terbinafine in dogs is reported to be 8.6 h after oral doses of 30 mg/kg/day.

Pregnancy risk factor

Category B: No evidence of fetal harm or altered fertility with oral doses up to 9–12 times the maximum human dose in rats and rabbits. It is generally considered safe in pregnancy.

Lactation

Terbinafine concentrates in human milk (7:1 milk:plasma ratio) and should not be given to lactating animals unless the benefits outweigh the risks.

References

Berger, D.J., Lewis, T.P., Schick, A.E., *et al.* (2012) Comparison of once daily versus twice weekly terbinafine administration for the treatment of canine *Malassezia* dermatitis: A pilot study. *Vet Derm.*, **23(5)**, 418–420.

Thieman, K.M., Kirkby, K.A., Flynn-Lurie, A., *et al.* (2011) Diagnosis and treatment of truncal cutaneous pythiosis in a dog. *J Am Vet Med Assoc.*, **239(2)**, 1232–1235.

Kotnik, T. (2002) Drug efficacy of terbinafine hydrochloride (Lamisil) during oral treatment of cats, experimentally infected with *Microsporum canis*. *J Vet Medicine. Infectious Diseases and Veterinary Public Health.*, **49**, 120–122.

Further reading

Abdel-Rahman, S.M. and Nahata, M.C. (1999) Stability of terbinafine HCL in an extemporaneous prepared oral suspension at 25 and 4 degrees C. *Am J Health Syst Pharm.*, **56(3)**, 243–245.

Balda, A. and Larson, C. (2009). Evaluation of Terbinafine Hair concentration in Persian cats with dermatophytosis and healthy carriers of *Microsporium canis* treated with pulse or continuous therapy. *Proceedings WSAVA*. Accessed via: Veterinary Information Network. http://goo.gl/v5oxW.

Foust, A. and Marsella, R. (2007) Evaluation of persistence of terbinafine in the hair of normal cats after 14 days of daily therapy. *Vet Derm.*, **18(4)**, 246–251.

Machard, B., Misslin, P., and Lemaire, M. (1989) Influence of plasma protein binding on the brain uptake of an antifungal agent, terbinafine in rats. *J Pharm Pharmacol.*, **41**, 700–704.

Sorenson, K.N., Sobel, R.A., Clemons, K.V., *et al.* (2000) Comparative efficacies of terbinafine and fluconazole in treatment of experimental coccidioidal meningitis in a rabbit model. *Antimicrob Agents Chemother.*, **44(11)**, 3087–3091.

Williams, M.M., Davis, E.G., and Kukanich, B. (2011) Pharmacokinetics of oral terbinafine and greyhound dogs. *J Vet Pharmacol Ther.*, **34(3)**, 232–237.

Chapter 182: Voriconazole

US Generic (Brand) Name: Voriconazole (Vfend)
Availability: Human Approved – Voriconazole tablets (50, 200 mg), powder for oral suspension (40 mg/mL), sterile IV injectable (voriconazole 200 mg with 3200 mg of sulfobutyl ether beta-cyclodextrin sodium), compounded ophthalmic solution 1%
Resistance Mechanisms: Single amino acid change in the *cyp51A* gene and an alteration in the gene's promoter region

Use

Voriconazole is fungistatic against *Candida* and *Cryptococcus* and fungicidal against *Aspergillus* spp. It also has activity against other molds such as *Fusarium* spp., *Scedosporium* spp., and *Cladophialophora* spp. Due to its excellent CNS penetration, it is also used in CNS fungal infections caused by susceptible organisms. It is active against some protozoa, including *Acanthamoeba* spp., which cause disseminated infections in dogs and keratitis in feline patients. The sterile compounded 1% ophthalmic solution has been effective for treatment of fungal keratitis.

Contraindications/warnings

Contraindicated if hypersensitive to azoles and in severe hepatic dysfunction. Monitor liver enzyme activities monthly. Use with caution in patients with proarrhythmic conditions and patients concurrently taking drugs that may interact with voriconazole (rifampin, long acting barbiturates). Avoid intravenous drug in patients with renal impairment due to accumulation of the sulfobutyl ether beta-cyclodextrin (SBECD) in the vehicle.

Dosage

Dogs
Systemic Mycosis: 4 mg/kg PO q12 h (Graupmann-Kuzma and Valentine 2008, Bentley *et al.*, 2011).

Keratomycosis: Voriconazole 1% ophthalmic solution (Compounded). Instill 1–2 drops every 1–4 h in the affected eye(s) (Puckett *et al.*, 2012).

Cats

Systemic Mycosis: 5–13 mg/kg q24 h or 5 mg/kg IV q12 h have been administered to cats, but have resulted in significant neurotoxicity (Smith and Hoffman 2010). Rate limiting glucuronidation of voriconazole in cats suggest that lower doses (4 mg/kg q48 or q72 h PO) may achieve optimal concentrations (1–4 μg/mL) with less toxicity.

Keratomycosis: Voriconazole 1% ophthalmic solution (Compounded). Instill 1–2 drops every 1–4 h in the affected eye(s) (Puckett *et al.*, 2012).

Dose adjustments

Voriconazole stimulates its own metabolism in dogs, which may result in subtherapeutic concentrations during chronic dosing. Doses must be adjusted based on drug tolerance and if possible plasma concentrations. The maintenance dose in mild to moderate hepatic disease should be reduced by approximately 50%.

Administration

The film coated tablets or oral suspension should be administered on an empty stomach either 1 h prior or 2 h after a meal. To dilute the pediatric suspension to 40 mg/mL; Add 46 mL of water to the 45 g oral powder and shake well. This provides a usable volume of 70 mL. The intravenous powder for reconstitution should be diluted with 19 mL of sterile water (USP). This makes a 10 mg/mL solution, which needs further dilution to a concentration of 0.5 to 5 mg/mL. The calculated dose should be given over 1–2 h at a maximum rate of 3 mg/kg/h. Dilution should only be done with recommended vehicles. Note: The IV solution contains an excipient (SBECD: 160 mg/mL) reported to cause vacuolation in renal tubular cells, urinary tract, and hepatocytes of dogs. SBECD is not metabolized, it is excreted renally and may accumulate in animals with renal impairment. Voriconazole ophthalmic 1% solution can be made by aseptically adding 19 mL of sterile water to the 200 mg vial of injectable voriconazole and filtering the solution with a 0.2 μm-pore size filter syringe into a sterile dropper.

Electrolyte contents

Not significant.

Storage/stability

Voriconazole tablets, oral suspension, and powder for injection should be stored at room temperature until the manufacturer's expiration date. Following reconstitution, the orange flavored suspension is good for 14 days at room temperature. The reconstituted intravenous solution should be used immediately or stored in the refrigerator for no longer than 24 h. The aseptically compounded 1% ophthalmic suspension is stable for 14 days under refrigeration.

Adverse reactions

>30%
CNS toxicity (ataxia), paraplegia, mydriasis, decreased papillary light and menace responses, arrhythmias, and hypokalemia, especially in cats (which may be dose related). Miosis occurs in cats at lower doses (4 mg/kg).

>10%
Nausea, vomiting, anorexia, and visual disturbances (dose related). Visual changes in dogs appear to be reversible with the primary target being the retina.

1–10%
Elevated liver enzymes (ALT, AST) in dogs that may decrease or normalize following dose reduction. Oral chronic dosing in dogs (6–12 months) at 12 mg/kg resulted in hepatotoxicity (idiosyncratic and dose dependent). Prolonged Q-T interval changes and cardiac arrhythmias have been noted with very high doses (7×) in dogs.

Other species
Approximately 30% of humans develop severe CNS toxicity with trough concentrations >5.5 μg/mL. Nausea, vomiting, anorexia, visual disturbances, elevated liver enzymes, hepatotoxicosis, prolonged Q-T interval changes, and cardiac arrhythmias are reported. Rare adverse reactions in humans include: rash, serious cutaneous reactions, photosensitivity reactions, hypokalemia, and infusion reactions.

Drug interactions

In humans, voriconazole is a CYP2C9 enzyme inducer. Decreased effects of voriconazole are seen with rifampin, cimetidine and phenobarbital. Voriconazole may increase the plasma concentrations or toxicity of cyclosporine, amlodipine, diltiazem, verapamil, prednisolone, omeprazole, vincristine, vinblastine, cyclophosphamide, sulfonylureas, tricyclic antidepressants, theophylline, NSAIDs, benzodiazepines, fentanyl, methadone, and cisapride.

Monitoring

Get baseline liver, renal and electrolyte values prior to initiating therapy. Correct any electrolyte imbalances prior to starting treatment. Monitor liver enzymes monthly during treatment. Animals should be monitored for signs of hepatotoxicosis (lethargy, anorexia, vomiting, and diarrhea) or neurologic/ophthalmic signs (optic neuritis and papilledema).

Overdose

Dog toxicity studies demonstrated hepatotoxicosis, kidney, and adrenal toxicity at 24 mg/kg × 30 days. Anemia may also occur. In cats, neurologic signs and arrhythmias are likely. Gastrointestinal decontamination and supportive care are warranted. Voriconazole can be hemodialyzed with a clearance of 121 mL/min. The sulfabutyl ether beta-cyclodextrin sodium (SBECD) vehicle in the IV formulation is relatively toxic to animals but can also be hemodialyzed with a clearance of 55 mL/min.

Diagnostic test interference

None noted.

Mechanism

Voriconazole is a triazole that can be fungistatic or fungicidal depending on the organism. It inhibits fungal lanosterol 14-alpha demethylase, leading to ergosterol depletion, and accumulation of toxic sterols in the fungal cell membrane. It also inhibits 24-methylene dehydrolanosterol demethylation in molds such as *Aspergillus* spp.

Pharmacology/kinetics

Absorption
Complete absorption occurs in dogs receiving oral voriconazole with a Cmax of 6.5 µg/mL at 3 hours after a single 6 mg/kg dose. Food may affect absorption so both the suspension and tablets should be given on an empty stomach.

Distribution
Voriconazole is extensively distributed throughout the tissues. It penetrates into the brain, kidney, heart, lung, CSF, and bone. Plasma protein binding varies from 45–67% in animals.

CNS penetration
Voriconazole penetrates the CNS and is effective for treatment of CNS infections. In animals the CSF:plasma ratio is (0.68–1.3).

Metabolism
In dogs, voriconazole is metabolized in the liver to an N-oxide metabolite. Another major pathway involves hydroxylation followed by glucuronide conjugation. The primary route of excretion (55–87%) in dogs is via urine, with only 5% being active drug. Another 7–37% is excreted in the feces. Metabolism has not been evaluated in cats but due to their limited ability to glucuronidate, it is likely that saturation of metabolic clearance may occur. Autoinduction of metabolism is noted in dogs and most other species.

Half-life
In dogs, the half-life is 4.5 h. In cats the half-life after oral administration is 80–90 h.

Pregnancy risk factor

Category D: Studies in rats and rabbits demonstrate cleft palates, reduced ossification, hydroureter, hydronephrosis, and embryo mortality. Do not administer to pregnant animals.

Lactation
Voriconazole penetrates into milk in quantities sufficient to expose fetuses to significant amounts of drug. It is contraindicated in nursing animals.

References

Bentley, R.T., Faissler, D., and Sutherland-Smith, J. (2011) Successful management of an intracranial phaeohyphomycotic fungal granuloma in a dog. *JAVMA*, **239(4)**, 480–485.

Graupmann-Kuzma, A. and Valentine, B.A. (2008) Coccidioidomycosis in dogs and cats: A review. *J Amer Animal Hospital Assoc.*, **44(5)**, 2008.

Puckett, J.D., Allbaugh, R.A., and Rankin, A.J. (2012) Treatment of dematiaceous fungal keratitis in a dog. *J Am Vet Med Assoc.*, **240(9)**, 1104–1108.

Smith, L.N. and Hoffman, S.B. (2010) A case series of unilateral orbital aspergillosis in three cats and treatment with voriconazole. *Veterin Ophthalmol.*, **13(3)**, 190–203.

Further reading

Dupuis, A., Tournie, N., LeMoal, G., *et al.* (2009) Preparation and stability of voriconazole eye drop solution. *Antimic. Agents and Chem.*, **53(2)**, 798–799.

Papich, M.G., Heit, M.C., and Riviere, J.E. (2001) Antifungal and antiviral drugs. In: *Veterinary Pharmacology and Therapeutics*. Adams, H.R. (ed.), 8th edn, Iowa State University Press, Ames, pp. 918–946.

Roffey, S.J., Cole, S., Comby, D., *et al.* (2003) The disposition of voriconazole in mouse, rat, rabbit, guinea pig, dog, and human. *Drug Metabol Disposit.*, **31(6)**, 731–741.

Quimby, J.M., Hoffman, S.B., Duke, J., *et al.* (2010) Adverse neurologic events associated with voriconazole use in 3 cats. *J Vet Intern Med.*, **24(2)**, 647–649.

SECTION F

Antiparasitic Agents

Chapter 183: Albendazole

US Generic (Brand) Name: Albendazole (Albenza, Valbazen)
Availability: Human Approved – Albendazole tablets (200 mg), Veterinary Approved – Albendazole oral paste 30% (205 g), albendazole suspension 113.6 mg/mL (500, 1000, 5000 mL)

Use

Albendazole is typically used for the treatment of tissue and CNS infections due to larval forms of cestodes (*Echinococcus* spp.), and *Ascaris* spp. in large animals. In small animals, it is used to treat *Filaroides* (lung worm), *Giardia* spp., and trematodes (*Paragonimus kellicotti*-liver fluke). Albendazole is active against hookworms (*Ancylostoma* spp.), whipworms (*Strongyloides* spp.), *Toxocara* spp., *Capillaria* spp., and *Microsporidia*. Due to its superb penetration into the CNS and cystic fluid, it is the drug of choice for infections in these sites. Prolonged use is limited due to risks of bone marrow toxicity.

Contraindications/warnings

Hypersensitivity to benzimidazoles. Avoid use in pregnant or lactating animals or animals with severe liver impairment.

Dosage

Canine
Capillaria plica: 50 mg/kg PO q12 h × 10–14 days (Brown and Barsanti 1989).

Paragonimus kellicotti: 25 mg/kg PO q 12 h × 14 days (Reinemeyer 1995).

Filaroides hirthi/Oslerus osleri: 25 mg/kg PO q12 h × 5 days; Repeat in 2 weeks (Reinemeyer 1995).

Giardia: 25 mg/kg PO q12 h for 4 doses (Barr *et al.*, 1993).

Feline
Paragonimus kellicotti: 25 mg/kg PO q12 h × 14 days (Reinemeyer 1995).

Platynosum/Opisthorchiidae: 50 mg/kg PO q24 h until negative stools (Fann 2001).

Dose adjustments

Albendazole should be avoided in severe hepatic impairment. Doses should be reduced (25–50%) in moderate impairment or with extrahepatic obstruction in relationship to the degree of impairment.

Administration

Albendazole absorption is improved five-fold when given with a fatty meal. Oral tablets may be crushed, chewed or added to food.

Electrolyte contents

Not significant.

Storage/stability

Tablets, paste, and solution are all stored at room temperature.

Adverse reactions

>10%
Anorexia and depression reported in cats and dogs.

Drug Therapy for Infectious Diseases of the Dog and Cat, First Edition. Valerie J. Wiebe.
© 2015 John Wiley & Sons, Inc. Published 2015 by John Wiley & Sons, Inc.

1–10%

Elevated liver enzymes, nausea, vomiting, and diarrhea reported in dogs and cats.

<1%

Neutropenia and aplastic anemia reported in dogs and cats mostly with prolonged therapy (>5 days).

Other species

Alopecia, rash, urticaria, leucopenia, granulocytopenia, pancytopenia, thrombocytopenia, elevated liver enzymes, and ataxia are reported.

Drug interactions

In humans, cimetidine, dexamethasone, praziquantel, and fatty foods all increase the plasma concentrations and half-life of albendazole, which may be an advantage due to its limited bioavailability. Phenobarbital and phenytoin decrease plasma concentrations of albendazole.

Monitoring

Get baseline CBC and liver panel and monitor every 2 weeks if on prolonged therapy. Discontinue drug if liver enzyme values exceed two-fold or CBC demonstrates bone marrow suppression.

Overdose

Anorexia, neutropenia, and weight loss reported in cats receiving high doses. Gastrointestinal lavage and supportive care should be instituted.

Diagnostic test interference

None reported.

Mechanism

Binds microtubules in the intestine and tegmental cells of intestinal helminthes and larvae. Results in glycogen depletion, altered glucose uptake, cholinesterase secretion, and decreased ATP production resulting in death.

Pharmacology/kinetics

Absorption

Albendazole has limited oral absorption but is better absorbed and reaches higher plasma concentrations than fenbendazole.

Distribution

Following absorption, albendazole is rapidly metabolized to active and inactive metabolites, which are well distributed into tissues and fluids. Active metabolites are measured in urine, bile, liver, cyst walls, cyst fluid, and CSF.

CNS penetration

Albendazole and its active metabolites readily penetrate (2–10%) into the CNS.

Metabolism

Albendazole undergoes extensive first pass metabolism in the liver with both active (albendazole sulfoxide) and inactive metabolites being excreted primarily into urine.

Half-life

Due to the rapid conversion of albendazole to its metabolites, it is rapidly eliminated from plasma. The half-life of the sulfoxide and sulfone metabolites in dogs is 1–3 h.

Pregnancy risk factor

Category C: Albendazole has been demonstrated to be embryotoxic and teratogenic in laboratory animals (rats, mice, and sheep) and should not be used during pregnancy.

Lactation

Albendazole sulfoxide is the primary metabolite excreted into milk (1.5% of a maternal dose). Due to the poor oral absorption of albendazole and its metabolites, it would not be expected to have significant effects in nursing animals.

References

Barr, S.C., Bowman, D.D., Heller, R.L., *et al.* (1993) Efficacy of albendazole against giardiasis in dogs. *Am J Vet Res.*, **54(6)**, 926–928.

Brown, S.A. and Barsanti, J.A. (1989) Diseases of the bladder and urethra. *Textbook of Veterinary Internal Medicine. Vol. 2.* Ettinger, S.J. (ed.), W.B. Saunders Company, Philadelphia, pp. 2108–2141.

Fann, T.M. (2001) Hepatic infections. In: *Feline Internal Medicine Secretes.* Lappin MR Ed., Elsevier, St. Louis, MO, p. 132.

Reinemeyer, C. (1995) Parasites of the respiratory system. *Kirk's Current Veterinary Therapy XII.* Bonagura, J. (ed.), W.B. Saunders Company, Philadelphia, pp. 895–898.

Further reading

Dib, A., Palma, S., Suarez, G., *et al.* (2010) Albendazole sulphoxide kinetic disposition with different formulations in dogs. *J Vet Pharmacol Therap.*, **34**, 136–141.

Gokbulut, C., Bilgili, A., Hanedan, B., *et al.* (2007) Comparative plasma disposition of fenbendazole, oxfendazole and albendazole in dogs. *Vet Parasitol.*, **148(3–4)**, 279–287.

Schipper, H.G., Koopmans, R.P., Nagg, J., *et al.* (2000) Effect of dose increase or cimetidine co-administration on albendazole bioavailability. *Am J Trop Med.*, **63(5)**, 270–273.

Chapter 184: Atovaquone

US Generic (Brand) Name: Atovaquone (Mepron), Atovaquone/proquanil (Malarone)
Availability: Human Approved – Atovaquone oral suspension (750 mg/5 mL × 210 mL), or combination product Atovaquone/proquanil oral tablets (62.5 mg/25 mg, 250 mg/100 mg)

Use

Atovaquone is active against *Babesia* spp. (*B. canis vogeli*, *B. canis canis*, *B. canis rossi*, *B. gibsoni*, *B. conradae*, *B. microti-like*, *B. felis*, *B. cati*, *B. leo*) commonly found in dogs and cats. It is often used in combination with azithromycin. Treatment failures have occurred clinically in dogs infected with *B. conradae*. Treatment is typically reserved for patients that are symptomatic. Coinfection with other tick transmitted organisms (*Erlichiosis*, *Anaplasmosis*) may necessitate additional drug therapy. Atovaquone may also be effective in the treatment of *Pneumocystis* spp., *Toxoplasmosis* and *Cytauxzoon felis*. In humans, proquanil is combined with atovaquone due to resistance although it is not as well tolerated in canine and feline patients.

Contraindications/warnings

Contraindicated if hypersensitive to atovaquone. Avoid use in patients that cannot take with food or that have impaired gastrointestinal absorption syndromes (irritable bowel disease, chronic diarrhea, and malabsorption syndrome). Caution in patients with severe liver impairment.

Dosage

Canine
Babesiosis: 13.3 mg/kg PO q8 h with azithromycin 10 mg/kg PO q24 h × 10 days (Sykes and Papich 2013).

Pneumocystosis: 15 mg/kg PO q24 h × 21 days (Greene *et al.*, 2006).

Feline
Babesiosis: 13.3 mg/kg PO q8 h with azithromycin 10 mg/kg PO q24 h × 10 days (Sykes and Papich 2013).

Cytauxzoonosis: 15 mg/kg PO q8 h and azithromycin PO q24 h × 10 days (Sykes and Papich 2013).

Dose adjustments

Decrease dose in severe liver and renal impairment.

Administration

Administer oral doses with food. High fat meals may significantly increase absorption. Shake the oral suspension well before administering.

Electrolyte contents

Not significant.

Storage/stability

The suspension should be stored at room temperature, protected from light.

Adverse reactions

>10%
Few side effects are reported with atovaquone as a single agent in cats and dogs. Nausea has been reported in dogs. Severe vomiting may occur in dogs when combined with proguanil.

1–10%
Ataxia, itching, and hypersensitivity reactions reported in dogs.

<1%
In dogs, fibrovascular proliferation in the right atrium, pyelonephritis, bone marrow hypocellularity, lymphoid atrophy, and gastritis/enteritis were observed with proguanil at a dose of 12 mg/kg/day for 6 months. Bile duct hyperplasia, gall bladder mucosal atrophy, and interstitial pneumonia was observed in dogs treated with proguanil at a dose of 4 mg/kg/day for 6 months. Adverse heart, lung, liver, kidney, and gall bladder effects observed in dogs were not reversible.

Other species

Fever, rashes, weakness, elevated liver enzymes, elevated BUN/Scr, anemia, neutropenia, leukopenia, hypoglycemia, hyponatremia, anxiety, and insomnia. Significantly more side effects are noted with the proquanil containing product.

Drug interactions

In humans, atovaquone may increase the plasma concentrations of drugs that are highly protein bound. Rifampin decreases atovaquone plasma concentrations by >50%. Metaclopramide and tetracycline decrease atovaquone plasma concentrations.

Monitoring

Get baseline liver panel and monitor closely. Monitor efficacy, if no improvement consider co-infection with *Erlichia* or *Anaplasma*.

Overdose

Large overdoses of atovaquone have occurred in humans (31,500 mg) with few side effects. Nausea, vomiting and diarrhea may occur with high doses. Supportive care and gastrointestinal lavage are recommended with ingestion of extremely high doses.

Diagnostic test interference

None noted.

Mechanism

Atovaquone is an antiprotozoal, hydroxynaphthoquinone derivative that selectively inhibits mitochondrial electron transport which results in inhibition of pyrimidine synthesis.

Pharmacology/kinetics

Absorption
Oral absorption of atovaquone is erratic and highly variable in dogs. Two peak concentrations (5.2–6.5 µg/mL) occur in dogs (first occurs at 1.5–3 h and second at 24–72 h). Bioavailability is only 25–50% in humans and dose escalation does not appear to increase absorption. Food, particularly high fat meals, increases oral absorption at least 2–3-fold.

Distribution
The drug is highly protein bound (>99%) and may have long, residual tissue binding but does not appear to accumulate over time. The volume of distribution varies with the weight of the animal so that an increase in weight shows a direct increase in volume of distribution.

CNS penetration
In dogs penetration across the blood/brain barrier is minimal: 1%.

Metabolism
Atovaquone undergoes extensive entrohepatic recirculation. It is primarily excreted unchanged in feces (>94%).

Half-life
The half-life of elimination in dogs is long (1–3 days).

Pregnancy risk factor

Category C: Teratogenic effects have not been noted in laboratory animals. Maternal and embrotoxic effects (decreased weights, fetal resorption, and loss) have been reported in rabbits. Use during pregnancy should be weighed against risks and administration in early pregnancy should be avoided.

Lactation
Atovaquone is excreted into rat milk in significant concentrations (30% of plasma concentrations). Use with caution in lactating animals.

References

Greene, C., Chandler, F.M., Lobetti, R., et al. (2006) Pneumocystosis. In: *Infectious Disease of the Dog and Cat.* Greene, C. (ed.), Elsevier, St. Louis, MO, pp. 651–658.

Sykes, J.E. and Papich, M.G. (2013) Antiprotozoal drugs. Ch. 10. In: *Canine and Feline Infectious Diseases*, Sykes, J.E. (ed.), Elsevier, St. Louis, MO. pp. 97–104.

Further reading

Birkenheuer, A., Levy, M., and Breitschwerdt, E. (2004) Efficacy of combined atovaquone and azithromycin for therapy of chronic *Babesia gibsoni* (Asian genotype) infections in dogs. *J Vet Intern Med.*, **18(4)**, 494–498.

Birkenheuer, A. (2013) Babesiosis. Ch. 75. In: *Canine and Feline Infectious Diseases*, Sykes, J.E. (ed.), Elsevier, St. Louis, MO. pp. 727–738.

DiCicco, M.F., Downey, M.E., Beeler, E., *et al.* (2012) Re-emergence of *Babesia conradae* and effective treatment of infected dogs with atovaquone and azithromycin. *Vet Parasitol.*, **187(1–2)**, 23–27.

Matsuu, A., Koshida, Y., Kawahara, M., *et al.* (2004) Efficacy of atovaquone against *Babesia gibsoni in vivo* and *in vitro*. *Vet Parasitol.*, **124(1–2)**, 9–18.

Chapter 185: Fenbendazole

US Generic (Brand) Name: Fenbendazole (Panacur, Panacur granules, Panacur plus, Safeguard)
Availability: Veterinary Approved – Panacur granules 222 mg/g (0.18 oz, 1, 2, 4 g, and 1 lb), fenbendazole suspension 10% (92 g/32 oz) and 100 mg/mL (500 mL), multiple equine/bovine pastes, medicated feeds, pellets, and so on. Combination products for dogs: Panacur plus soft chews containing fenbendazole, ivermectin, praziquantel (small: 2.16 g and large: 5.4 g)

Use

Fenbendazole is used commonly in cats and dogs for a variety of intestinal parasite infections. It is labeled for use in small animals for roundworm, hookworm, whipworm, and tapeworms. It is active against adult forms of *Ancylostoma caninum*, *Capillaria aerophilia*, *Filaroides hirthi*, *Paragonimus kellicotti*, *Taenia pisiformis*, *Toxocara canis*, *T. leonine*, and *Unicinaria stenocephala*. It is often used in cats for a variety of infections including lungworms, flukes, and helminth infections. It is commonly given to cats and dogs for the treatment of *Giardia* infections. However, large doses are required and failure rates may be as high as 50%.

Contraindications/warnings

Hypersensitivity to benzimidazoles. Do not use in combination with bromsalan flukicides. Avoid prolonged use in patients with moderate to severe liver impairment.

Dosage

Canine
Ascaris, whipworms, hookworms, tapeworms: 50 mg/kg q24 h PO × 3 days (Hoest package insert).

Giardia: 50 mg/kg/day PO × 3–7 days (Zajac *et al.*, 1998).

Capillaria, Paragonimus kellicott, Eucoleus boehm, Filaroides: 50 mg/kg q24 h PO × 10–14 days (Reinemeyer 1995).

Transmammary T. canis and A. caninum: Transplacental transmission 50 mg/kg PO from the 40th day of gestation to the 14th day postpartum (Burke and Roberson 1983).

Feline
Ascaris, Hookworms, Strongyloides, Tapeworms: 50 mg/kg PO q24 h × 5 days (Dimski 1989).

Giardia: 50 mg/kg q24 h × 3–7 days (Gruffydd-Jones *et al.*, 2013).

Lungworms (Aelurostrongylus abstrusus): 20 mg/kg q24 h × 5 days, repeat after 5 days (Reinemeyer 1995).

Capillaria aerophilis, Paragonimus kellicotti: 50 mg/kg q24 h PO × 10–14 days (Reinemeyer 1995).

Dose adjustments

Dose adjustments may be required in severe liver impairment.

Administration

Fenbendazole granules and oral suspension can be administered mixed in food.

Electrolyte contents

Not significant.

Storage/stability

Store granules and suspension at room temperature, protected from light, and in a tightly sealed container.

Adverse reactions

>10%
Few side effects at common doses 50–250 mg/kg q24 h × 6 days.

1–10%
Salivation, vomiting, and diarrhea reported in dogs and cats.

<1%
At high doses or with prolonged therapy, fatty degeneration of the liver, nodular appearance of the gastric mucosa, lymph follicle proliferation, focal encephalomalacia, cerebrum perivascular inflammation, satellitosis, and neuronophagia were observed in the cerebra of dogs

given 125 mg/kg q24 h and hyperplasia and congestion of the mesenteric lymph nodes were noted in dogs administered 8 to 20 mg/kg q24 h × 30 days.

Other species

Elevated alkaline phosphatase and SGOT, enlargement or cyst formation in lymph nodes, liver masses, cyst formation in the liver, liver hypertrophy and hyperplasia, hepatocellular cytoplasmic vacuolation, bile duct proliferation, biliary cyst formation, and nodular hepatocellular hyperplasia have been reported.

Drug interactions

Do not use in combination with bromsalan flukicides.

Monitoring

Monitor liver function with high doses and prolonged therapy.

Overdose

Very large doses have been administered to laboratory animals (100×) with few acute side effects. Acute side effects in dogs and cats may include nausea, vomiting, and the potential for hypersensitivity reactions to a high burden of dying parasites (steroids could be indicated in this case). Treatment may not be required and would be supportive if required.

Diagnostic test interference

None noted.

Mechanism

Binds microtubules in the intestine and tegmental cells of intestinal helminthes and larvae. Results in glycogen depletion, altered glucose uptake, cholinesterase secretion, decreased ATP production, and death.

Pharmacology/kinetics

Absorption

Absorption in dogs is limited (<20%) following oral dosing. Maximum serum concentrations reported in dogs after a 10 mg/kg PO dose is 0.4 µg/mL at 24 h.

Distribution

Fenbendazole metabolites are widely distributed into tissues. High concentrations can be found in the liver, kidney, fat, and muscle.

CNS penetration

Fenbendazole penetrates into the CNS but percentages are unknown.

Metabolism

Fenbendazole is rapidly metabolized in the liver of dogs to oxfendazole, oxfendazole sulfone, and p-OH-oxfendazole. Greater than 90% of fenbendazole and its active metabolites are excreted in feces and only 7% is excreted in urine after oral dosing.

Half-life

The plasma elimination half-life in dogs is 15 h.

Pregnancy risk factor

Fenbendazole is considered safe for use in pregnancy and has been used prophylactically to reduce prenatal and lactogenic infections (*Toxocara canis, Ancylostoma*) in pregnant canines starting the fortieth (40th) day of gestation through the fourteenth (14th) day post-partum. Doses of 50 mg/kg q24 h PO were considered safe and decreased *Ascaris* populations by 89% and hookworms by 99% in pups.

Lactation

Fenbendazole is poorly excreted into milk, but its more soluble metabolites (sulfoxide and sulfone) are excreted into milk in low concentrations. Due to the low oral absorption and high index of safety of fenbendazole, the drug is considered safe during lactation.

References

Burke, T.M. and Roberson, E.L. (1983) Fenbendazole treatment of pregnant bitches to reduce prenatal and lactogenic infections of *Toxocara canis* and *Ancylostoma caninum* in pups. *J Am Vet Med Assoc.*, **183(9)**, 987–990.

Dimski, D.S. (1989) Helminth and noncoccidial protozoan parasites of the gastrointestinal tract. In: *The Cat: Diseases and Clinical Management. Vol. 1.* Sherding, R.G. (ed.), Churchill Livingstone, New York, pp. 459–477.

Gruffydd-Jones, T., Addie, D., Belak, S., *et al.* (2013) Giardiasis in cats; ABCD guidelines on prevention and management. *J Feline Med Surg.*, **15(7)**, 650–652.

Reinemeyer, C. (1995) Parasites of the respiratory system. *Kirk's Current Veterinary Therapy XII.* Bonagura, J (ed.), W.B. Saunders Company, Philadelphia, pp. 895–898.

Zajac, A.M., LaBranche, T.P., Donoghue, A.R., *et al.* (1998) Efficacy of fenbendazole in the treatment of experimental *Giardia* infection in dogs. *Am J Vet Res.*, **59(1)**, 61–63.

Further reading

Goldenthal, E.I. (1978) *Six-month oral toxicity study in dogs.* Unpublished report, International Research and development corporation, Mattawan, MI, USA. Submitted to WHO by Hoeschst AG, Frankfurt am Main, Germany.

Kramer and Schultes (1974). *A subchronic tolerance trial (90 days) with HOE 881 in dogs.* Hoecst-Roussel unpublished report. Submitted to WHO by Hoechst–Roussel unpublished report. Submitted to WHO by Hoechst AG, Frankfurt am Main, Germany.

Chapter 186: Fipronil

US Generic (Brand) Name: Fipronil (Frontline, Frontline Plus, Topspot, Fiprogaurd, PetArmor, Combat)
Availability: Veterinary Approved – Fipronil 9.7% (Frontline Topspot) (kittens/cats: 50 mL × 3, 6 doses), (puppies/dogs: 50 mL × 3, 6 doses), fipronil 9.8% (Frontline Plus) (kittens/cats with (S)-methoprene 11.8%: 50 mL × 3, 6 doses), For: puppies/dogs with (S)-methoprene 8.8% (11–22 lb = 0.67 mL, 23–44 lb = 1.34 mL, 45–88 lb = 2.68 mL and 89–132 lb = 4.02 mL)

Use

Fipronil is labeled in small animals for the treatment of fleas, ticks, chewing lice, and sarcoptic mites. Fipronil works directly on the adult insects. In combination with the growth regulator (S)-methoprene found in Frontline Plus, the combination works on all stages (eggs, larvae, nymph, pupae, and adult) of insects. It is specifically labeled for ticks including the brown dog tick (*R. sanguineues*), American dog tick (*D. variabilis*), Lone star tick (*A. americanum*), and deer ticks (*I. scapularis*). It is also used off label for the treatment of *Cheyletiellosis*, *Otocariosis*, and chigger infestations.

Contraindications/warnings

Fipronil should not be used on animals with hypersensitivity to fipronil or in animals <8 weeks of age. Avoid use on damaged epidermis due to potential for increased absorption. Use caution on animals used for breeding, showing, or competition due to potential for application site reactions. Fipronil may degrade into products more or equally toxic to mammals. Avoid contact with skin, eyes, or clothing when applying. Avoid contact with application area until dry. Fipronil is categorized as a Group C (possible human) carcinogen. It has been shown to cause an increase in thyroid follicular cell tumors in rats, which may be specific to this species. Gloves should be worn when applying. Fipronil is an ecological toxin that is highly toxic to wildlife (fish, birds, bees, crustaceans, rabbits, lizards, and zooplankton). Avoid use around water sources and aquatic species. Extreme care should be taken to limit environmental contamination.

Dosage

Canine
Fleas/ticks/chewing lice: Apply appropriate size per weight topically (0.0305 mL/lb) once monthly (Merial package insert).

Otoacariosis (ear mites): Apply two drops of Fipronil 10% solution (Frontline Spot-On) into both ears and the remaining product between the shoulder blades once; then repeat in 30 days (Curtis 2004).

Feline
Fleas/ticks/chewing lice: Apply appropriate size per weight topically (0.0305 mL/lb) once monthly (Merial package insert).

Otoacariosis (ear mites): Apply two drops of Fipronil 10% solution (Frontline Spot-On) into both ears and the remaining product between the shoulder blades once, then repeat in 30 days (Curtis 2004).

Dose adjustments

Dosing should potentially be reduced in severely debilitated or aged animals.

Administration

Apply topically only. Wear gloves when applying. Lift and remove the plastic tab to expose foil backing, then peel away the foil or cut with scissors. Hold upright with foil side toward you and snap applicator tip. Part hair between shoulder blades. Place applicator tip just above skin and squeeze. Apply entire contents in a single spot. Do not apply on top of the hair coat. Avoid contact with treated area until dry. Avoid bathing for 48 h after application.

Electrolyte contents

Not significant.

Storage/stability

Store at room temperature away from heat or open flames. Do not contaminate water, food, or feed by storage and disposal. Store out of the reach of children and animals.

Adverse reactions

>10%
Local irritation at application site (erythema, irritation, puritus, and coat discoloration) in cats and dogs. Alopecia in cats and hot spots in dogs.

1–10%
Neurologic side effects reported in cats and dogs with high doses or if oral ingestion from grooming. Lethargy, inappetence, salivation, and vomiting reported in cats. Ataxia, lethargy, biting, aggression, vomiting, and diarrhea reported in dogs.

Other species
Long-term exposure reported to cause thyroid tumors in rats, although this is thought to be species specific. When administered IV, IP, inhaled, or with high doses in feed it is reported to have significant side effects in most species (rats, mice, dogs, cats, rabbits, humans, etc.) including increased excitability, seizures, head twitching, facial clonus, altered gait, tremors, irritability, death, altered thyroid hormones, increased liver and thyroid mass, and kidney effects.

Drug interactions

Fipronil increases hepatic metabolism and excretion of thyroid hormones in laboratory animals. It affects P450 liver enzymes and is expected to interact with ketoconazole, diazepam, and testosterone.

Monitoring

Monitor for neurologic toxicity and with long term use, monitor liver function.

Overdose

In dogs, oral doses of 20 mg/kg/day produce inappetence 1–2 days after ingestion and neurotoxicity starting at 5–13 days after ingestion. Less than 5% of a topical dose is absorbed in dogs and cats, with 3.3% remaining on skin. Grooming in cats can increase the risk of toxicity. For dermal overdoses, wash animal with soap and water to expedite hydrolysis and remove residues from skin/hair. If ingested orally, gastric lavage with activated charcoal is indicated. Overdoses are treated with supportive care and diazepam for seizures if required. Phenobarbital or propofol may be useful for prolonged seizures.

Diagnostic test interference

None noted.

Mechanism

Broad spectrum insecticide that disrupts the insects central nervous system by blocking the passage of chloride ions through the GABA receptor and glutamine-gated chloride channels. Results in hyperexcitation of insects nerves/muscles. The selectivity of fipronil for arthropod and insect GABA chloride channels is 59 times that of mammals. Fipronil targets adult insects while (S)-methoprene effects juvenile growth hormone slowing development during metamorphosis and larval development. It concentrates in adult ovaries resulting in sterile egg production.

Pharmacology/kinetics

Absorption
Fipronil is applied topically and gets absorbed within 48 h into sebaceous glands. From here, it is slowly released via follicular ducts. It is not detected in dermis or adipose tissue. Less than 5% of fipronil and its active metabolites are absorbed transdermally. Following oral exposure fipronil is well absorbed.

Distribution
The manufacturer states that fibronil spreads from the point of application rapidly covering the entire animal and localizing in the hair on the surface of the skin and in the superficial skin layers and sebaceous glands of dogs and cats. After oral ingestion, fipronil concentrates in the stomach, fat, and adrenal glands. Low levels are also found in the liver, pancreas, thyroid, and ovaries.

CNS penetration
Fipronil crosses readily into the CSF if administered systemically. Topical application is not expected to result in significant CSF concentrations.

Metabolism
In dogs and cats, fipronil is primarily metabolized to fipronil sulfone. Hydrolysis occurs more rapidly on hot or basic skin (pH >7). The drug is also photodegraded

to desulfinylfipronil. Metabolites have 10-fold more toxicity to mammals then the parent drug. Toxicity in mammals is therefore related to the conversion of the parent drug to it more stable and less selective active metabolites. The fipronil parent drug and metabolites are excreted primarily in feces (45–75%) with a small amount in urine (5–25%).

Half-life

The half-life following ingestion or systemic administration is long (2–8 days) in most species. Following topical administration to cats and dogs, radiolabeled fipronil can still be measured in the epithelial layers and hair for up to 2 months. Residue peak concentrations are reported at 24 h (589 ppm) and decline steadily to 448 ppm at 8 days. The parent compound has a half-life of 34 days in loamy soil.

Pregnancy risk factor

The manufacturer states that fipronil is safe in breeding and pregnant animals. There have been no reports of teratogenic effects in dogs and cats. However, high doses (26 mg/kg/day) can reduce fertility, delay development, decrease litter size, decrease body weight, and cause fetal mortality in rat pups.

Lactation

The manufacturer states that fipronil is safe in lactating animals. It is excreted into breast milk (1–5%) in goats following oral exposure in feed. Topical application would not result in significant concentrations in milk. However, exposure to residues on maternal skin may be more significant.

Reference

Curtis, C.F. (2004) Current trends in the treatment of *Sarcoptes*, *Cheyletiella* and *Otodectes* mite infestations in dogs and cats. *Vet Dermatol.*, **15(2)**, 108–114.

Further reading

Birckel, P., Cochet, P., Benard, P., *et al.* (1996) Cutaneous distribution of 14-C-Fipronil in the dog and in the cat following a Spot-On administration. *Third World Congress of Veterinary Dermatology*, Edinburgh, Scotland.

US Environmental Protection Agency. (2000) Fipronil: *Third Reevaluation: Report of the Hazardous Identification Assessment Review Committee*. HED Doc No 014400: Health Effects Division, US Government Printing Office, Washington D.C., pp. 1–24.

Federal Register. (2005) *Fipronil; Notice of filing a pesticide petition to establish a tolerance for a certain pesticide chemical in or on food.* August 24, **70(163)**, 49599–49607.

Ohi, M., Dalsenter, P., Andrade, A., *et al.* (2004) Reproductive adverse effects of fipronil in Wister rats. *Toxicol Lett.*, **146(2)**, 121–127.

Zhao, X., Yeh, J., Salgado, V., *et al.* (2005) Sulfone metabolite of fipronil blocks gamma-aminobutyric acid and glutamine-activated chloride channels in mammalian and insect neurons. *J Pharmacol Exp Ther.*, **314(1)**, 363–373.

Chapter 187: Imidacloprid

US Generic (Brand) Name: Imidacloprid (Advantage, Advantage II, Advantage Multi, Advantics)
Availability: Veterinary Approved – Imidacloprid topical (Advantage: 9.1% (w/w) (kittens < 9 Lbs, cats >9 lbs), (dogs <10 lbs, 11–20 lbs, 21–55 lbs, >55 lbs × 4 or 6 packs) or with pyriproxyfen (0.46%) (Advantage II), or with moxidectin (10–25 mg/mL) (Advantage Multi) or with pyrethrin (44%)/ pyriproxyfen (0.44%) (Advantix) (for dogs only)

Use

Imidacloprid is used as a systemic insecticide in the treatment of domestic pets to control fleas and lice. It is a rapid acting once a month topical treatment. Imidacloprid kills fleas within 12 h. Reinfesting fleas are killed within 2 h with protection against further flea infestation lasting for up to four (4) weeks. Preexisting pupae in the environment may continue to emerge for six (6) weeks or longer depending upon the climatic conditions. Larval flea stages in the pet's surroundings are killed following contact.

Contraindications/warnings

Hypersensitivity to imidacloprid. Do not administer to kittens/cats <8 weeks of age or on puppies <7 weeks of age. Avoid use on damaged epidermis. Avoid use around water sources and aquatic species. Imidacloprid is highly toxic to bees and wildlife and care should be taken to limit environmental contamination.

Dosage

Canine

Fleas: Dosed at 7.5–10 mg/kg topically once monthly (Bayer Package Insert); May be administered q7 days for severe infestations. Do not administer more often than every 7 days. Return to monthly treatment after flea control is attained.

Feline

Fleas/Cheyletiellosis: Dosed at 7.5–10 mg/kg topically once monthly (Bayer Package Insert). May be administered every 7 days for severe infestations. Do not administer more often than every 7 days. Return to monthly treatment after flea control is attained.

Dose adjustments

Dosing should be reduced in severely debilitated or aged animals.

Administration

Hold applicator tube in an upright position. Pull cap off tube. Turn the cap around and place other end of cap back on tube. Twist cap to break seal, then remove cap from tube. Part the hair on the neck at the base of the skull until the skin is visible. Place the tip of the tube on the skin and squeeze the tube to expel the entire contents of the tube directly on the skin. The product is bitter tasting and salivation may occur for a short time if a cat licks the product immediately after treatment. Advantage is waterproof and remains effective following a shampoo treatment, swimming or after exposure to rain or sunlight.

Electrolyte contents

Not significant.

Storage/stability

Store in a cool, dry place. Do not contaminate water, food, or feed by storage or disposal.

Adverse reactions

>10%

Severe reactions are rarely seen. Lethargy and vomiting may be seen. Cats may have salivation, hyperactivity, and tremors if ingested orally.

1–10%

Decreased appetite and diarrhea

<1%

Fever, nervousness, salivation, incoordination, trembling, seizures, and increased heart rate, reported in dogs/cats.

Other species

In humans, side effects include above in addition to cough, palpitation, stomach ache, muscle spasms, weakness, and bradycardia. The primary effects of longer term, low-dose exposure to imidacloprid are on the liver, thyroid, body weight, testes, thymus, bone marrow, pancreatitis, and cardiovascular and hematological systems.

Drug interactions

Do not use imidacloprid with any other insecticides or flea medications.

Monitoring

Monitor for signs of nicotinic side effects (gastrointestinal, neurologic, cardiac, etc.).

Overdose

In mammals, acute high-dose oral exposure to imidacloprid results in mortality and transient cholinergic effects (dizziness, drowsiness, apathy, locomotor effects, labored breathing, and emesis). In dogs, the LD_{50} is 450 mg/kg of body weight. Gastrointestinal lavage with charcoal may reduce exposure. Supportive care with atropine, pralidoxime, propranolol, and furosemide may be required.

Diagnostic test interference

None noted.

Mechanism

Imidacloprid is a chloronicotinyl, neonicotinoid that binds nicotinic receptors, leading to the accumulation of acetylcholine, resulting in the insect's paralysis, and eventually death.

Pharmacology/kinetics

Absorption

Following topical application the drug remains primarily on the body surface with minimal amounts being absorbed across the skin. It is absorbed rapidly and completely following oral ingestion.

Distribution

Imidacloprid localizes in the lipid layer of the skin surface, which spreads not only over the surface of the skin but also onto the hair. Fleas do not need to bite a treated animal to be exposed to imidacloprid. It is absorbed across their intersegmental membranes. A small amount is absorbed across the skin of cats and dogs where it is distributed into most fluids and tissues.

CNS penetration

Due to the weak nature of the interaction with mammalian nicotinergic receptors and the postulated poor penetration through the blood-brain barrier in mammals, imidacloprid has minimal effects on mammalian CNS at normal doses.

Metabolism

Imidacloprid is metabolized in the liver to 6-chloronicotinic acid, an active metabolite. The metabolite is conjugated with glycine and is eliminated or reduced to guanidine. The majority of the drug is eliminated via urine (70–80%).

Half-Life

After topical application of the product, imidacloprid is rapidly distributed over the animal's skin within one day of application. It can be detected on the body surface throughout the 28 day treatment interval. Approximately 96% of the total dose is eliminated in 48 h.

Pregnancy risk factor

Dermal application to pregnant bitches at three times the dose at 2–4 weeks apart did not result in any teratogenic effects. However, low- to mid-dose oral exposures have been associated with reproductive toxicity, developmental retardation, and neurobehavioral deficits in rats and rabbits. Benefits should be weighed against the risks.

Lactation

Imidacloprid would be expected to penetrate into milk. Dermal application to lactating bitches at three times the dose at 2, 3, or 4 weeks apart did not result in any side effects on lactating pups at various stages of lactation.

Further reading

Allen, T.R., Frei, T., Luetkemeier, H., *et al.* (1992) *52-week oral toxicity (feeding) study with NTN 33893 technical in the dog.* Unpublished report from Research & Consulting Company AG, report No. R 4856, dated 19 October 1989, GLP, amendment No. R 4856A, dated 3 March 1992. Submitted to WHO by Bayer AG, Mannheim, Germany.

Arther, R.G., Cunningham, J., Dorn, H., *et al.* (1997) Efficacy of imidacloprid for removal and control of fleas (*Ctenocephalides felis*) on dogs. *Am J Vet Res.,* **58(8)**, 848–850.

Becker, H., Vogel, W., and Terrier, C. (1988) *Embryotoxicity study (including teratogenicity) with NTN 33893 technical in the rabbit.* Unpublished report from Research & Consulting Company AG, report No. R 4583, dated 24 November 1988, GLP. Submitted to WHO by Bayer AG, Mannheim, Germany.

Everett, R., Cunningham, J., Arther, R., *et al.* (2000) Comparative evaluation of the speed of flea kill of imidacloprid and selamectin on dogs. *Vet Ther.,* **1(4)**, 229–234.

Mehlhorn, H., Mencke. N., and Hansen, O. (1999) Effects of imidacloprid on adult and larval stages of the flea *Ctenocephalides felis* after *in vivo* and *in vitro* application: a light- and electron-microscopy study. *Parasitol Res.,* **85**, 625–637.

Tomizawa, M. and Casida, J. (2005) Neonicotinoid insecticide toxicology: mechanisms of selective action. *Ann Rev Pharmacol Toxicol.,* **45**, 247–268.

Chapter 188: Imidocarb Dipropionate

US Generic (Brand) Name: Imidocarb (Imizol)
Availability: Veterinary Labeled – Imidocarb dipropinate sterile Injection (120 mg/mL × 10 mL) for IM or SC administration

Use

Imidocarb is used in the treatment of *Babesia* spp., Ehrlichiosis, and Hepatozonosis in dogs and Cytauxzoonosis in cats. It is typically very effective for the treatment of large *Babesia* spp. but much less effective against some of the smaller species such as *B. felis*.

Contraindications/warnings

Hypersensitivity to imidocarb. Use with caution in dogs with impaired liver/renal or pulmonary function. Pretreatment of young animals with glycopyrolate and atropine is advised, particularly in debilitated animals. Do not use in combination with other cholinesterase inhibitors.

Dosage

Canine

Babesia: 6.6 mg/kg IM or SC × 1, repeat dose in 2 weeks (Intervet Package Insert).

Ehrlichiosis: 5 mg/kg SC, repeat in 2 weeks. Give with doxycycline 10 mg/kg q24h × 28 days (Sainz *et al.*, 2000).

Hepatozoonosis: 5 mg/kg IM or SC every 14 days until hepatozoonosis is cleared (Baneth 2011).

Feline

Cytauxzoon felis: 5 mg/kg IM × 1; repeat in 14 days (Greene *et al.*, 2006).

Ehrlichiosis/Anaplasmosis: 5 mg/kg IM q14 days × 2–4 treatments (Baneth 2011).

Dose adjustments

Imidocarb dose adjustments are not established but due to its high renal excretion a reduction in dose by 25–50% is suggested in renal failure.

Administration

Pretreat with atropine or glycopyrrolate prior to administration. Inject IM or SC. Do not give IV. Supportive care including isotonic fluids, subcutaneous heparin may be required for animals that develop dehydration or disseminated intravascular coagulation post treatment.

Electrolyte contents

Not significant.

Storage/stability

Store at room temperature, protected from light.

Adverse reactions

>10%
Pain during injection, salivation, and vomiting reported in dogs and cats.

1–10%
Diarrhea, restlessness, weight loss, and injection site reactions reported in dogs and cats.

<1%
Respiratory distress (pulmonary congestion), tachycardia, panting, weakness, edema, profuse diarrhea, eosinophilia, ataxia, and severe renal tubular/hepatic necrosis in dogs, increased bilirubin, and enlarged spleen reported rarely in dogs, mainly at high doses.

Other Species

Increased incidence of tumors was observed in rats given imidocarb.

Drug interactions

Do not use cholinesterase inhibiting drugs such as pesticides and flea/tick collars, and so on while using imidocarb.

Monitoring

Monitor for side effects and administer atropine/glycopyrrolate if needed. Get baseline liver and kidney panel and monitor for signs/symptoms of impairment.

Overdose

Low therapeutic index. At 1.5 times the dose (9.9 mg/kg) dogs developed vomiting, weakness, salivation, liver, kidney, and pulmonary adverse reactions. Treatment is supportive with muscarinic agents, atropine, glycopyrrolate, IV fluids, analgesics, and transfusions if necessary.

Diagnostic test interference

Increases in creatinine kinase have been reported when imidocarb is injected IM.

Mechanism

Imidocarb binds to nucleic acids (DNA) of susceptible organisms resulting in denaturation and inhibition of replication and cellular repair. It may interfere with polyamine synthesis and function.

Pharmacology/kinetics

Absorption
Imidocarb is rapidly absorbed after IM and SC dosing. No oral absorption information is available.

Distribution
Imidocarb is rapidly distributed into fluids and tissues after administration. The volume of distribution is equal to or greater than total body fluid. It concentrates in liver and renal tissues.

CNS penetration

Imidocarb readily penetrates into the CSF, with high concentrations detected in all regions of the central nervous system.

Metabolism

Imidocarb is metabolized in the liver and excreted by the kidney by glomerular filtration and tubular reabsorption.

Half-life

The half-life in dogs is 207 min with 80% of the drug cleared in 8 h. Prolonged tissue concentrations in liver and kidneys are noted that may last up to months.

Pregnancy risk factor

Imidocarb crosses into the placenta in high concentrations. At very high dosages administered to rats and mice, no teratogenic effects were noted, but there was a decrease in the weights of offspring and number of live offspring. Doses up to 14 mg/kg did not appear to be teratogenic in dogs.

Lactation

Imidocarb is excreted into milk in high concentrations. Milk concentrations may exceed plasma concentrations in some species (sheep and goats). The risk of toxicity in lactating animals may not be worth the risk.

References

Baneth, G. (2011) Perspectives on canine and feline hepatozoonosis. *Vet Parasitol.*, **181(1)**, 3–11.

Greene, C.E., Meinkoth, J., and Kocan, A.A. (2006) Cytauxzoonosis. In: *Infectious Disease of the Dog and Cat*. Greene, C. (ed.), 3rd edn. Elsevier, St. Louis, MO, pp. 716–722.

Sainz, A., Tesouro, M.A., Amusategui, I., *et al.* (2000) Prospective comparative study of 3 treatment protocols using doxycycline or imidocarb dipropionate in dogs with naturally occurring ehrlichiosis. *J Vet Intern Med.*, **14(2)**, 134–139.

Further reading

Abdullah, A.S. and Baggot, J.D. (1983) Pharmacokinetics of imidocarb in normal dogs and goats. *J Vet Pharmacol Ther.*, **6(3)**, 195–199.

Abdullah, A.S., Sheikh-Omar, A.R., Baggot, D.J., *et al.* (1984) Adverse effects of imidocarb dipropionate (Imizol) in dogs. *Vet Res Commun.*, **8(1)**, 55–59.

Cohn, L.A., Birkenheuer, A.J., Brunker, J.D., *et al.* (2011) Efficacy of atovaquone and azithromycin or imidocarb dipropionate in cats with acute cytauxzoonosis. *J Vet Intern Med.*, **25(1)**, 55–60.

Eddlestone, S.M., Neer T.M., Gaunt, S.D., *et al.* (2006) Failure of imidocarb dipropionate to clear experimentally induced *Ehrlichia canis* infection in dogs. *J Vet Intern Med.*, **20(4)**, 840–844.

Greene, C.E., Latimer K., Hopper, E., *et al.* (1999) Administration of diminazene aceturate or imidocarb dipropionate for treatment of cytauxzoonosis in cats. *J Am Vet Med Assoc.*, **215**, 497–500.

Kuttler, K.L. (1980) Pharmacotherapeutics of drugs used in treatment of anaplasmosis and babesiosis. *J Amer Vet Med Assoc.*, **176**, 1103–1108.

Lappin, M.R., Brewer, M., and Radecki, S. (2002) Effects of imidocarb dipropionate in cats with chronic haemobartonellosis. *Vet Ther.*, **3(2)**, 144–149.

Solano-Gallego, L. and Baneth, G. (2011) Babesiosis in dogs and cats-expanding parasitogical and clinical spectra. *Vet Parasitol.*, **181(1)**, 48–60.

Chapter 189: Ivermectin

US Generic (Brand) Name: Ivermectin (Ivomec, Ultramectrin, Eqvalan, Heartgard, Heartgard Plus, Heartgard Plus Chews, Panacur Plus, Stromectol)
Availability: Human Approved – Ivermectin oral tablets (3 mg), Veterinary Approved – Heartgard oral tablets and chew tablets (dogs: 68, 136, 272 µg tabs × 6 and cats: 55 and 165 µg × 6), ivermectin sterile injectable 1% (10 mg/mL × 50, 200, 500 mL), variety of injectable liquids, oral pastes, and topical drenches labeled for large animals. Combination products: Panacur plus soft chews containing: Fenbendazole/ivermectin/praziquantel (small dog: 454 mg/27 µg/23 mg, large dog: 1.134 g/68 µg/57 mg), Heartgard plus chews (ivermectin/pyrantel) 68 µg/57 mg, 136 µg/114 mg, 272 µg/228 mg)

Use

Used in small animals for a variety of parasitic infections including roundworms, strongloides, hookworms, filariasis, whipworms, lice, and mites. Has also been the drug of choice for demodectic and sarcoptic mange treatment in dogs. Commonly used for prevention of heartworm (*D. immitis*) infection. It is currently recommended in the treatment of active heartworm disease in combination with doxycycline prior to melarsomine treatment. Ivermectin is cidal against *D. immitis* larval stages 3, 4, and early 5 and static against microfilaria and adults. It is inactive against liver flukes and tapeworms due to their lack of GABA neurotransmitter receptors.

Contraindications/warnings

Contraindicated in patients hypersensitive to ivermectin. Avoid use in patients with compromised blood-brain barrier disorders (meningitis), seizures or in breeds (Australian shepherds, collies, long-haired whippets, and shelties) with a predilection toward mutation of the ABCB1–1Δ gene. Do not use large animal pastes or drenches on cats or dogs. Avoid use in animals >6 weeks of age.

Dosage

Canine

Heartworm prophylaxis: Ivermectin 6–12 µg/kg PO q month (Knight 2000).

Active heartworm infection: Stabilize animal, restrict exercise, then:

Day 0; Begin prednisone 0.5 mg/kg PO q12 h × 7 days; then 0.5 mg/kg PO q 12 h × 7 days; then 0.5 mg/kg q48 h × 14 days.

Day 1: Ivermectin 6–14 µg/kg PO q 30 days continuously plus doxycycline 10 mg/kg PO q12 h × 4 weeks.

Day 60: Give first melarsomine injection 2.5 mg/kg IM with cage rest.

Day 90: second melarsomine injection 2.5 mg/kg IM, cage rest.

Day 91: Administer third melarsomine injection 2.5 mg/kg IM, cage rest. Continue exercise restriction for 6–8 weeks.

Day 120: Test for presence of microfilariae, if positive, repeat doxycycline × 30 days and retest in 4 weeks. Continue heartworm preventative and retest on *Day 271*. (Current American Heartworm Society recommendations: info@heartwormsociety.org).

Active heartworm infection: For animals where arsenical therapy is contraindicated: Restrict exercise, start ivermectin 6–14 µg/kg PO q30 days continuously plus doxycycline 10 mg/kg PO q12 h × 4 week cycles repeated every 3–4 months. An antigen test should be performed q6 months; continue combination treatment until two consecutive negative tests are obtained (Current American Heartworm Society recommendations: info@heartwormsociety.org).

Eucoleus boehmi/Capillaria: Ivermectin 0.2 mg/kg PO × 1 (Reinmeyer 1995)

Oslerus osleri: Ivermectin 0.4 mg/kg SC × 1 (Reinmeyer 1995)

Demodicosis: Titrate up slowly observing for side effects. *Day 1:* 0.05 mg/kg (50 µg/kg), *Day 2–7:* give: 0.12 mg/kg/day (120 µg/kg); *Day 8–10:* 0.20 mg/kg (200 µg/kg); *Day 11–On:* Increase dose by 0.1 mg/kg each week until a max of 0.6 mg/kg (600 µg/kg) is reached. Continue for 2 months past negative scrapings (3–7 months). Discontinue if signs of toxicity (Mueller 2011).

Sarcoptic Mange/Lice: Ivermectin 0.2–0.4 mg/kg PO or SC at 14 day intervals (Scheidt *et al.,* 1984).

Feline

Heartworm prophylaxis: Ivermectin 0.024 mg/kg (24 µg/kg) PO q30–45 days.

Aelurostrongylus abstrusus: Ivermectin 0.4 mg/kg SC once (Reinemeyer 1995).

Ear Mites: Ivermectin 0.6 mg/kg SC × 2 doses (14 days apart).

Dose adjustments

Dose adjustments may be required in severe liver failure.

Administration

Confirm that the animal is hydrated prior to administering. Ivermectin tablets should be taken with water. The sterile cattle injectable (Ivomec) 10 mg/mL (1%) can be given orally or SC in cats and dogs.

Electrolyte contents

Not significant.

Storage/stability

Store tablets and solutions at room temperature, protected from light. The injectable 1% solution is poorly soluble in water but can be mixed with vegetable oil or other oil for diluting very small doses.

Adverse reactions

>10%
Diarrhea and vomiting are reported in dogs and cats.

1–10%
Anorexia and decreased activity are reported in dogs and cats.

<1%
Hypersensitivity reactions are reported rarely. High doses in dogs (>1000 µg/kg) or moderate doses (120 µg/kg) in ABCB1–1Δ mutant dog breeds may result in mydriasis,

decreased weight, salivation, tremors, ataxia, and dehydration. At >5000 μg/kg, side effects may include absence of pupillary response, sedation, paralysis, paresis, recumbancy, coma, and death. In kittens, high doses (>110 μg/kg) or in adult cats (>750 μg/kg), ataxia, disorientation, agitation, vocalization, mydriasis, tremors, blindness, decreased pupillary light reflexes, head pressing, and decreased oculomotor menace reflex may occur.

Drug interactions

Barbiturates and benzodiazepines may increase side effects when combined with ivermectin. Amiodarone, carvedilol, clarithromycin, cyclosporine, erythromycin, itraconazole, ketoconazole, quinidine, and verapamil may inhibit P-gylcoprotein and increase toxicity of ivermectin. Inducers of P-glycoprotein (clotrimazole, phenothiazines, rifampin, and St. John's wort) may decrease ivermectin concentrations.

Monitoring

Observe breeds with likelihood of ABCB1–1Δ for up to 8 h after administering for signs of toxicity. Repeat stool examinations or skin scrapings to confirm clearance of parasites. Repeat heartworm test yearly and prior to administration of large doses of ivermectin for demodicosis.

Overdose

Symptoms may include mydriasis, ataxia, vomiting, tachycardia, lethargy, and seizures and may appear 8–10 h after administration. Emesis and/or gastrointestinal lavage should be done as soon as possible. Additional purgatives, parenteral fluids, electrolytes, pressor agents, and respiratory support may be required. Most animals should begin to improve neurologically within 2–5 days, but may take weeks for complete recovery.

Diagnostic test interference

False negative heartworm tests are unlikely since the antibody tests measure antigen to the adult female *D. immitis* oviduct.

Mechanism

Ivermectin binds selectively to glutamine-gated-chloride ion channels (GABA) in invertebrate nerve cells. This leads to an increased permeability of parasitic nerve and muscle cells to chloride ions with subsequent hyperpolarization and death of susceptible parasites.

Pharmacology/kinetics

Absorption
Oral absorption of ivermectin is >95% in dogs, but is reported to be less in cats. High fat meals may increase oral absorption.

Distribution
Ivermectin is distributed throughout tissues and is concentrated in the liver and adipose tissue.

CNS penetration
Only low concentrations of ivermectin penetrate the CSF (<1%). Levels are regulated by P-glycoprotein so that much higher CSF levels are noted in animals with the ABCB1–1Δ mutation.

Metabolism
Ivermectin is metabolized in the liver of cats and dogs and is primarily excreted via feces.

Half-life
The half-life of ivermectin in dogs is 2 days.

Pregnancy risk factor

Category C: Ivermectin did not demonstrate any teratogenic or embryotoxic effects in pregnant dogs receiving 500 μg/kg oral doses at 5, 15, 25, and 35 days of gestation. Teratogenic effects (cleft palate, clubbed forepaws) and embryotoxic effects were seen in rabbits, rats, and mice with repeat dosing at or near maternotoxic doses. Benefits should be weighed against the risks in pregnancy.

Lactation
Ivermectin is excreted into milk in low concentrations. Very large doses may expose nursing animals to significant concentrations and side effects.

References

Knight, D. (1995) Guidelines for diagnosis and management of heartworm (*Dirofilaria immitis*) infection. In: *Kirk's Current Veterinary Therapy XII*. Bonagura, J. (ed.), W.B. Saunders Company, Philadelphia, pp. 879–887.

Mueller, R.S. (2011) Evidence-based treatment of canine demodicosis. *Tierarz Praxis Klein.*, **6**, 419–424.

Reinemeyer, C. (1995) Parasites of the respiratory system. In: *Kirk's Current Veterinary Therapy XII*. Bonagura, J. (ed.), W.B. Saunders Company, Philadelphia, pp. 895–898.

Scheidt, V.J., Medleau, L., Seward, R.L., *et al.* (1984) An evaluation of ivermectin in the treatment of sarcoptic mange in dogs. *Am J Vet Res.*, **45(6)**, 1201–1202.

Further reading

Bauer, T.G. (1988) Pulmonary parenchymal disorders. In: *Handbook of Small Animal Practice.* Morgan, R.V. (ed.), Churchill Livingstone, New York, pp. 185–193.

Clarke, D., Lee, J., Murphy, L., *et al.* (2011) Use of intravenous emulsion to treat ivermectin toxicosis in a Border collie. *J Am Vet Med Assoc.*, **239(10)**, 1328–1333.

Kittleson, M. (2006) Heartworm infection and disease (Dirofilariasis). Ch. 23: In: *Small Animal Cardiology.* 2nd edn, Mosby, St. Louis, MO, pp. 370–401.

Chapter 190: Lufenuron

US Generic (Brand) Name: (Program, Lufenuron with Capstar, Sentinel)
Availability: Veterinary Approved – Lufenuron oral suspension (Program for Cats) 135 mg, 270 mg × 6 tubes, flavored tablets (Program) Dogs: 45, 90, 204.9, 409.8 mg and cats: 90, 204.9 mg, sterile long acting injectable for cats (100 mg/mL) 0.4 mL × 10 syringes, lufenuron/nitenpyram oral tablets (Program Flavored tabs and Capstar Flea Management Program), lufenuron/nitenpyram(mg/mg) Dogs: 45/11.4, 90/11.4, 204.9/11.4, 204.9/57, 409.8/57 tabs. Cats: 90/11.4, 204.9/11.4 tabs, milbemycin/lufenuron/nitenpyram oral tablets (Sentinel flavor tabs with Capstar) Milbemycin/lufenuron (mg each)/nitenpyram (mg) dogs: 46/11.4, 115/11.4, 230/57, 460/57 and cats: 90/11.4, 204.9/11.4 tabs

Use

Lufenuron is an ectoparasiticide that is used to control fleas in dogs and cats 6 weeks of age or older. It is not active against ticks and does not kill adult fleas. It specifically acts on the developing eggs by inhibiting chitin synthesis. It is not effective as sole therapy or in multianimal households unless combined with other therapies that target adult fleas. It shows activity *in vitro* against some fungal species and *E. caniculi* but is not considered effective as a sole agent. Its primary use has been in combination therapy with adulticide activity against fleas (Sentinel and Program with Capstar).

Contraindications/warnings

Hypersensitivity to lufenuron. Do not use injectable feline product in dogs. Do not use on animals <4 weeks of age. Read the manufacturer's contraindications on combination treatments.

Dosage

Canine

Flea prevention: Dose orally once monthly according to the manufacturer's label (Program: Novartis). For dogs up to 10 lbs (45 mg), 21–45 lbs (204.9 mg), 46–90 lbs (409.8 mg), > 90 lbs (give the appropriate combination/weight).

Dermatophytosis: 50–100 mg/kg PO q2 weeks × 2 doses then once monthly until culture negative (Mantousek 2003).

Feline

Flea prevention: Dose orally once monthly according to the manufacturer's label (Program-Novartis). For cats up to 6 lbs (90 mg), 7–15 lbs (204.9 mg), >15 lbs (give the appropriate combination/weight).

Dermatophytosis: 50–100 mg/kg PO q2 weeks × 2 doses then once monthly until culture negative (Mantousek 2003).

Dose adjustments

None noted.

Administration

Administer oral tablets with food to increase absorption. Do not split tablets. Should be used every 30 days. If dosed within two hours of vomiting, re-dosing is recommended. Injectable should be given every 6 months. Injectable takes 2–3 weeks to reach effective levels. For optimum control of flea populations, begin treatment early in the season.

Electrolyte contents

Not significant.

Storage/stability

Store tablets, suspension or injectable at room temperature. Do not reuse already opened packages. Maintain in the manufacturer's packaging.

Adverse reactions

>10%

Very few reactions reported as a single agent. Vomiting and lethargy have been reported in dogs/cats.

1–10%

Diarrhea and anorexia, reported in dogs/cats. Pruritus and local injection reactions reported in cats.

<1%

Dyspnea, reddened skin, and urticaria reported in dogs/cats.

Drug interactions

None reported.

Monitoring

Efficacy.

Overdose

Very high doses (30×) given to growing pups and cats (17×) have not demonstrated any toxicity. If toxic effects are noted, treat with supportive care.

Diagnostic test interference

None noted.

Mechanism

A chitin synthesis inhibitor that specifically targets chitin polymerization and deposition resulting in inhibition of flea egg development.

Pharmacology/kinetics

Absorption

Poorly absorbed orally, particularly on an empty stomach. Approximately 40% is absorbed with the remaining being climinated in feces/bile.

Distribution

Following oral administration, lufenuron is rapidly distributed via the blood to the adipose tissue (2 h). It is constantly released from adipose tissues for up to 1 month.

CNS penetration

Lufenuron has poor CNS penetration.

Metabolism

Lufenron does not undergo significant metabolism. The majority of drug that is absorbed is eliminated as parent drug into urine.

Half-life

Lufenuron is slowly released from fat with a half-life between 15–50 days.

Pregnancy risk factor

Neither fetal or neonatal toxicity has been reported in animals using monotherapy with lufenuron.

Lactation

Lufenuron is excreted into milk. However, it is considered safe in lactating animals due to its low toxicity profile.

Reference

Mantousek, J. (2003) Infectious skin diseases. *Handbook of Small Animal Practice*, 4th edn. Morgan, R., Bright, R., and Swartout, M. (eds), W.B. Saunders Company, Philadelphia, pp. 842–857.

Further reading

Ben-Ziony, Y. and Arzi, B. (2000) Use of lufenuron for treating fungal infections of dogs and cats: 297 cases (1997–1999) *JAVMA*, **217(10)**, 1510–1513.

DeBoer, D.J., Moriella, K.A., Blum, J.L., *et al.* (2003) Effects of lufenuron treatment in cats on the establishment and course of *Microsporum canis* infection following exposure to infected cats. *J Am Vet Med Assoc.*, **222(9)**, 1216–1220.

Miller, P.F., Peters, B.A., and Hort, C.A. (2001) Comparison of lufenuron and nitenpyram versus imidacloprid for integrated flea control. *Vet Ther.*, **2(4)**, 285–292.

Chapter 191: Meglumine Antimoniate

US Generic (Brand) Name: Meglumine antimoniate (Glucantime, Glucantim)

Availability: Human Approved – Not available in the USA commercially. Available as Glucantime or Glucantim in Europe and South America. Sterile ampules (81 mg/mL × 5 mL) may be available through the CDC, imported or purchased via Compounding Pharmacies. Contact the CDC for sources of drug, at www.cdc.gov/ncidod/srp/drugs/drugs-service.html

Use

Meglumine antimoniate is a pentavalent antimonial drug used for Leishmaniasis. It is used as a primary agent in the treatment of visceral Leishmaniasis in humans and dogs caused by: *L. donovani, L. donovani donovani, L. infantum,* and *L. chagasi.* It is also used for the treatment of cutaneous Leishmaniasis caused by *L. tropica, L. major, L. amazonensis, L. braziliensis, L. guyanensis, L. mexicana, L. panamensis,* and *L. peruviana.* It is currently used alone or in combination with allopurinol for the treatment of canine Leishmaniasis. Used alone, recurrence is common. The drug has also been combined with topical imiquimod 5%, topical or intralesional rhGM-CSF, oral pentoxifylline, and paromomycin to improve cure rates and reduce meglumine treatment cycles in humans, but this has yet to be examined in dogs. Availability, toxicity, and cost may limit the use of this drug.

Contraindications/warnings

Avoid use in animals hypersensitive to meglumine antimoniate. Do not use in animals with significant cardiac, renal, or hepatic impairment due to increased risk of toxicity. Avoid use of drugs that are renal toxic or that can prolong the Q-T interval.

Dosage

Canine

Leshmaniasis: 75–100 mg/kg 24 h SC × 1–2 months in combination with allopurinol 10 mg/kg PO q12 h × 6–12 months (Solano-Gallego *et al.*, 2009).

Dose adjustments

Dose adjustments are required in moderate renal impairment (25%). Meglumine should not be used in moderate to severe renal impairment.

Administration

Determine species by PCR if possible. Not all species are sensitive to meglumine. Resistance may occur with *L. infantum.* Get baseline CBC, renal, liver, and cardiac values. Hydrate and correct any electrolyte imbalances. Administered by SC injection. Monitor closely for any adverse reactions.

Electrolyte contents

Not significant.

Storage/stability

Ampules should be stored at room temperature and protected from light and freezing.

Adverse reactions

>10%

Apathy, anorexia, and pain at injection site reported in dogs.

1–10%

Vomiting, diarrhea, and renal tubular damage (without clinical signs of renal failure) reported in dogs.

<1%

Acute tubular necrosis and apoptosis reported in dogs.

Other species

Lethargy, anorexia, pneumonia, nausea, urticaria, fever, vomiting, arthralgias, pancreatic enzyme abnormalities, neutropenia, thrombocytopenia, QT prolongation, ventricular extrasystoles, ventricular tachycardia, hepatotoxicity, and nephrotoxicity reported in humans. Acute tubular necrosis followed by death also reported.

Drug interactions

Avoid use of drugs that are nephrotoxic (aminoglycosides, amphotericin-B) or that can prolong the Q-T interval (macrolides, tricyclic antidepressants, quinidine, procainamide, etc.) when administering meglumine.

Monitoring

Monitor renal function closely. Monitor urine concentrating capacity and for presence of casts in urine. Renal tubular necrosis may occur without clinical signs. Monitor CBC, liver function, serum lipase, and amylase.

Overdose

May result in vomiting, diarrhea, lethargy, and renal damage. Supportive care and careful monitoring of renal function are indicated.

Diagnostic test interference

None noted.

Mechanism

Inhibition of enzymes involved in the glycolytic and fatty acid oxidation pathway of parasites.

Pharmacology/kinetics

Absorption
Following SC injection, rapid absorption occurs with bioavailability in dogs of >99%. Maximum concentrations are reported within 3–5 h.

Distribution
The drug is readily distributed throughout tissue and fluids. It concentrates in skin, liver, spleen, lymph nodes, kidneys, adrenals, bones, skeletal muscles, heart, and skin.

CNS penetration
Meglumine does not penetrate into the CNS in significant concentrations (200 mg/g).

Metabolism
Meglumine antimoniate is converted inside cells from the pentavalent form to the trivalent form. Greater than 80% of the pentavalent antimony is excreted into urine within 9 h. The majority of drug is eliminated by glomerular filtration.

Half-life
The half-life in dogs after SC injection is 121 min with the majority of drug being eliminated by 18 h after injection. A slow terminal elimination of the trivalent antimony occurs with a much longer half-life (76 h).

Pregnancy risk factor

Causes teratogenic and embryotoxic effects in pregnant rats at high doses. A single report in a 4-year-old dog receiving meglumine during pregnancy demonstrated loss of four pups just after birth and survival of two healthy pups. Vertical transmission of Leishmaniasis to all pups was prevented by meglumine antimoniate (PCR negative).

Lactation
It is not known if meglumine antimoniate penetrates into milk. Similar antimonials have been reported to pass into milk in low concentrations, suggesting that low levels would be present. Benefits should be weighed against risks.

Reference

Solano-Gallego, L., Koutinas, A., Miro, G., *et al.* (2009) Directions for the diagnosis, clinical staging, treatment and prevention of canine Leishmaniasis. *Vet Parasitol.*, **165**, 1–18.

Further reading

Almeida, O.L. and Santos, J.B. (2011) Advances in the treatment of cutaneous Leishmaniasis in the new world in the last ten years: a systematic literature review. *An Bras Dermatol.*, **86(3)**, 497–506.

Bianciardi, P., Brovida, C., Valente, M., *et al.* (2009) Administration of miltesine and meglumine antimoniate in healthy dogs: clinicopathological evaluation of the impact on the kidneys. *Toxicol Pathol.*, **37(6)**, 770–775.

Friedrich, K., Vieira, F.A., Porrozzi, R., *et al.* (2012) Disposition of antimony in rhesus monkeys infected with *Leishmania braziliensis* and treated with meglumine antimoniate. *J Toxicol Environ Health.*, **75(2)**, 63–75.

Mateo, M., Maynard, L., Vischer, C., *et al.* (2009) Comparative study on the short term efficacy and adverse effects of miltefosine and meglumine antimoniate in dogs with natural leishmaniosis. *Parasitol Res.*, **105(1)**, 155–162.

Slappendel, R.J. and Teske, W. (1997) The effect of intravenous or subcutaneous administration of meglumine antimonite (Glucantime) in dogs with leishmaniasis. A randomized clinical trial. *Vet Q.*, **19(1)**, 10–13.

Spada, E., Proverbio, D., Groppetti, D., *et al.* (2011) First report of the use of meglumine antimoniate for treatment of canine leishmaniasis in a pregnant dog. *J Am Anim Hosp Assoc.*, **47(1)**, 67–71.

Valladares, J.E., Riera, C., Alberola, J., *et al.* (1998) Pharmacokinetics of meglumine antimoniate after administration of a multiple dose in dogs experimentally infected with *Leishmania infantum*. *Vet Parasitol.*, **75(1)**, 33–40.

Chapter 192: Melarsomine

US Generic (Brand) Name: Melarsomine (Immiticide) **Availability:** Veterinary Approved – Melarsomine powder for injection (50 mg/vial: 25 mg/mL) (Immiticide)

Use

Melarsomine dihydrochloride is an organic arsenical agent. Melarsomine is indicated in the treatment of heartworm infection caused by immature (4-month-old, fifth-stage larvae, L5, to mature adult infections of *D. immitis* in dogs with stabilized Class 1, 2, and 3 heartworm infections). Melarsomine has not been shown to have significant activity against worms <4 months old. Therefore, a three-dose protocol (first dose followed after one month with two subsequent doses 24 h apart) is now considered optimal in order to decrease side effects and obtain 98% efficacy (Heartworm Society at www.heartwormsociety.org). Furthermore, classification of dogs into Class 1–3 was not shown to be a good indicator of treatment efficacy or prognosis, so Classes (1–3) are now treated equally.

Contraindications/warnings

Hypersensitivity to melarsomine. Do not use in Class 4 (caval syndrome) disease. For severe infections, surgical removal of adult worms from the right atrium and venae cavae with subsequent stabilization of the patient are required prior to treatment with melarsomine. Caution in dogs >8 years due to increased risk of inappetence, lethargy, and vomiting. Do not use in cats due to extreme toxicity.

Dosage

To determine the most current recommendations for treating adult heartworm infection see the Heartworm Society website (www.heartwormsociety.org). All dogs should be observed during treatment and for 24 h after the last injection.

Canine
Class 1–3: Dogs should be stabilized prior to treatment. Give 2.5 mg/kg deep IM injection × 1 dose as directed. After 1 month, give 2.5 mg/kg deep IM injection q24 hours × 2 doses. Alternate sides for injection.

Dose adjustments

Dose reductions have not been studied in renal or hepatic failure. Dogs older than 8 years of age may need dose reductions (10–25%) due to an increased risk of side effects.

Administration

Reconstitute the powder with sterile water for injection (2 mL) to make a 25 mg/mL solution. Melarsomine should be administered by deep IM injection (NOT IV) into the lumbar (epaxial) muscles only at the level of the third to fifth lumbar vertebrae (L3–L5), with special care taken to avoid superficial injection or leakage into superficial tissues. For dogs <10 kg, a 23-gauge, 1-inch needle should be used. A 22-gauge, 1½-inch needle should be used for dogs weighing more than 10 kg. Total doses exceeding a volume of 5 mL may be divided and administered in two sites, the second site approximately

two lumbar vertebrae cranial to the initial site. Exercise restriction, based on the severity of the heartworm disease, is generally recommended for 4–6 weeks following treatment to help prevent thromboembolism.

Electrolyte contents

Not significant.

Storage/stability

Store the undiluted powder at room temperature. After reconstitution, melarsomine retains its potency for 24 h if refrigerated, stored upright, and protected from light. The reconstituted solution should not be frozen.

Adverse reactions

Adverse reactions observed after treatment with melarsomine may be directly attributable to the medication or may be secondary to worm death or the underlying heartworm disease process.

>10%
Anorexia, inappetence (13%), coughing, gagging (22.2%), injection site reaction (32%), lethargy, and depression (15.4%) reported in dogs.

1–10%
Gastrointestinal effects (diarrhea and vomiting), hypersalivation, pyrexia, and respiratory effects (dyspnea, hemoptysis, panting, and pulmonary congestion) reported in dogs.

<1%
Other side effects reported in dogs include: anemia, disseminated intravascular coagulation, fatigue, bloody diarrhea, colitis, gingivitis, hemoglobinemia, icterus, elevated liver enzymes, leukocytosis, ataxia, convulsions, disorientation, restlessness, pancreatitis, bronchitis, pneumonia, tachypnea, tracheobronchitis, wheezing, polydipsia/polyuria, discolored urine, hematuria, inappropriate urination, low urine specific gravity, pyuria, weight loss, alopecia, altered hair color and coat character, rare reports of paresis, paralysis, coma, and death.

Drug interactions

Drugs that may have adverse effects similar to those of melarsomine (e.g., depression, lethargy, inappetence, etc.) should be avoided to prevent synergistic side effects. The efficacy of melarsomine may be reduced by coadministration with dimercaprol.

Monitoring

Monitor temperature, respiratory rate, and effort (pyrexia, dyspnea, and cough may be signs of pulmonary thromboembolism) for up to 24 h after the injection. Repeat heartworm antigen test (treatment successful if there is conversion to a negative antigen test 4 months after treatment).

Overdose

Melarsomine has a low margin of safety. Single doses of 7.5 mg/kg (3× labeled dose) can result in cyanosis, diarrhea, vomiting, ataxia, tremor, dyspnea, panting, tachycardia, pulmonary inflammation, edema, and death. With doses of 5 mg/kg (2× dose) diarrhea, fever, panting, restlessness, salivation, and vomiting occur. Severe injection site reactions that involve extension of the inflammation from the injection site into the abdominal cavity, causing intra-abdominal adhesions have occurred with twice the dose. Treatment includes a Dimercaprol injection. (BAL in Oil Ampules Akorn, San Clemente, California, at 1–800–223–9851). Give 3 mg/kg IM within 3 hours, repeat dose once or twice, 3 h apart. Length of treatment is dependent on response.

Diagnostic test interference

Serum liver enzymes may go up significantly even in healthy dogs receiving the labeled dose. SGOT may go up seven-fold, ALT (2×) and CK may go up 25-fold within 8 h, returning to normal within 72 h.

Mechanism

The effects of trivalent arsenicals on heartworms have not been completely defined but include alterations in glucose uptake and metabolism, inhibition of glutathione reductase, and alterations of the structure and function of the parasite's intestinal epithelium.

Pharmacology/kinetics

Absorption

Rapidly absorbed after intramuscular administration. With intramuscular administration, the absorption half-life is 2.6 min. Peak plasma concentrations occur within 11 min.

Distribution

Melarsomine is highly distributed throughout body tissues and fluids, including the CNS.

CNS penetration

Melarsomine penetrates into the CNS in a dose dependent manner in immature mice where the blood brain barrier may not be mature.

Metabolism

Melarsomine is metabolized in the liver to various arsenic species. Metabolites and the parent compound are eliminated in the bile and urine.

Half-life

The elimination half-life in dogs is 3 h.

Pregnancy risk factor

Melarsomine has not been tested in pregnant dogs. However arsenical compounds that are similar have been shown to cause significant embryo toxicity and teratogenicity (skeletal, neural abnormalities and weight loss) in mice. The drug is contraindicated in pregnancy.

Lactation

Arsenical compounds have been evaluated in lactating mice. Very low concentrations penetrate into milk and may have adverse side effects (neurologic) in growing pups.

Further reading

Hettlich, B.F., Ryan, K., Bergman, R.L., *et al.* (2003) Neurologic complications after melarsomine dihydrochloride treatment for *Dirofilaria immitis* in three dogs. *J Am Vet Med Assoc.*, **15**; **223(10)**, 1456–1461.

Hill, D.S., Wlodarczyk, B.J., and Finnell, R.H. (2008) Reproductive consequences of oral arsenate exposure during pregnancy in a mouse model. *Birth Defects Res B Dev Reprod Toxicol.*, **83(1)**, 40–47.

McTier, T.L., McCall, J.W., Dzimianski, M.T., *et al.* (1994) Use of melarsomine dihydrochloride (RM 340) for adulticidal treatment of dogs with naturally acquired infections of *Dirofilaria immitis* and for clinical prophylaxis during reexposure for 1 year. *Vet Parasitol.*, **55(3)**, 221–233.

Jin, Y., Wang, G., Zhao, F., *et al.* (2010) Distribution of speciated arsenicals in mice exposed to arsenite in the early life. *Ecotoxicol Environ Saf.*, **73(6)**, 1323–1326.

Jin, Y., Xi, S., Li, X., *et al.* (2006) Arsenic speciation transported through the placenta from mother mice to their newborn pups. *Environ Res.*, **101(3)**, 349–355.

Chapter 193: Miltefosine

US Generic (Brand) Name: Miltefosine (Milteforan)
Availability: Human Approved – Miltefosine oral capsules (10, 50 mg caps) (Impavido), not available in the USA commercially. Veterinary Approved – Miltefosine oral solution 20 mg/mL (30, 50, 90 mL) (Milteforan). Not available in the USA commercially. May be available through the CDC, imported or purchased via Compounding Pharmacies. Contact the CDC at: www.cdc.gov/ncidod/srp/drugs/drugs-service.html

Use

Miltefosine is an afntfhmanial drug that has been used for its anineoplastic, antiviral, and immunomodulatory activities. More recently it has been used in place of meglumine antimoniate for Leishmaniasis due to its reduced renal toxicity in dogs. It is currently used alone or in combination with allopurinol for the treatment of canine Leishmaniasis. Used alone, recurrence is common and efficacy is similar to monotherapy with meglumine antimoniate. Miltefosine is used for the treatment of cutaneous Leishmaniasis caused by *L infantum*, *L. tropica*, *L. major*, *L. amazonensis*, *L. braziliensis*, *L. guyanensis*, *L. mexicana*, *L. panamensis*, and *L. peruviana*. Miltefosine has also been proven effective for the treatment of disseminated *Acanthamoeba* and *Acanthamoeba keratitis*. Availability and cost may limit the use of this drug.

Contraindications/warnings

Avoid in patients allergic to miltefosine. Do not use in breeding, pregnant, or lactating animals. Avoid using in combination with other hepatotoxic drugs. Avoid in patients with severe hepatic or renal impairment. Immunocompromised patients may require longer dosing. Patients with prior autoimmune disease may have exacerbations.

Dosage

Canine
Leishmaniasis: Miltefosine 2 mg/kg/day PO with food × 28 days (Virbac Package Insert). Dose on exact weight. Do not underdose. Can administer with allopurinol (10 mg/kg/day PO) for 28 days, and then with allopurinol alone, at the same dosage, for 12 months (Manna *et al.*, 2009).

Acanthamoebia: Miltefosine 2 mg/kg/day PO with food × 28 days (Virbac Package Insert).

Dose adjustments

Although minor dose adjustment may be required in severe liver impairment, reduction of doses may increase the risk of treatment failure.

Administration

Personal protective equipment consisting of gloves and glasses should be worn when handling. The product should not be administered by pregnant women, by women intending to become pregnant or whose pregnancy status is unknown. Do not allow treated dogs to lick persons immediately after intake of the medication. Do not drink, eat, or smoke when administering the product. Administer orally with food. Shake oral suspension well prior to dosing. The oral product should be poured onto the food, the full meal or one part of the meal, once a day for 28 days. It is crucial to comply with the treatment duration (28 days) to ensure the efficacy of the product.

Electrolyte contents

Not significant.

Storage/stability

Store at room temperature protected from light and freezing.

Adverse reactions

>10%
Nausea, vomiting (16%), and diarrhea (12%) reported in dogs.

1–10%
Elevated liver enzymes, anorexia, elevated serum creatinine, and BUN reported in dogs.

<1%
Nephrotoxicity, hepatotoxicity reported rarely in dogs.

Drug interactions

No drug interactions reported.

Monitoring

Get baseline liver and renal panel. Monitor liver enzymes, BUN, and Scr.

Overdose

Overdose symptoms may include nausea, vomiting, diarrhea, and elevated liver enzymes. Uncontrolled vomiting was noted in an overdose study in dogs at twice the recommended dose. Administration of an antiemetic and supportive care are recommended.

Diagnostic test interference

None reported.

Mechanism

Miltefosine is an alkylphosphocholine. Its exact mechanism as an antileishmanial drug remains unknown. Preliminary studies in *L. mexicana* promastigotes show an association between the efficacy of miltefosine and perturbation of ether-phospholipid metabolism, glycosylphosphatidylinositol anchor biosynthesis, and signal transduction within the parasite.

Pharmacology/kinetics

Absorption
Following oral administration in dogs the bioavailability is >94% with peak levels occurring between 4–48 h.

Distribution
Miltefosine is widely distributed into body tissues and fluids. The highest accumulation of drug is reported in the liver, lungs, kidneys, and spleen.

CNS penetration
Miltefosine penetrates into the CSF and achieves clinically significant concentrations.

Metabolism
In dogs, very little first pass metabolism occurs. The drug undergoes a slow breakdown in the liver into choline and choline-containing metabolites. Elimination is via biliary excretion in dogs with the majority of drug excreted into feces. Renal clearance is negligible (0.03%).

Half-life
The half-life in dogs is 153 h (6.3 days). Steady state concentrations are not achieved for 3–4 weeks.

Pregnancy risk factor

Studies with rats and rabbits demonstrated embryotoxic, fetotoxic, and teratogenic effects following multiple subtherapeutic doses of miltefosine (1.2 mg/kg). Miltefsine is contraindicated in pregnancy.

Lactation
Miltefosine has not been studied in lactating animals but would be expected to penetrate into milk and is not considered safe for lactating animals.

Reference

Manna, L, Vitale, F, Reale, S, *et al.* (2009) Study of efficacy of miltefosine and allopurinol in dogs with Leishmaniasis. *Vet J.*, **182**(3), 441–445.

Further reading

Mateo, M., Maynard, L., Vischer, C., *et al.* (2009) Comparative study on the short term efficacy and adverse effects of miltefosine and meglumine antimoniate in dogs with natural leishmaniosis. *Parasitol Res.*, **105**(1), 155–162.

Mohebali, M., Fotouhi, A., Hooshmand, B., *et al.* (2007) Comparison of miltefosine and meglumine antimonite for the treatment of zoonotic cutaneous leishmaniasis (ZCL) by a randomized clinical trial in *Iran. Acta Trop.*, **103**(1), 33–40.

Oliva, G., Foglia Manzillo, V., and Pagano, A. (2004) Canine Leishmaniasis: evolution of the chemotherapeutic protocols. *Parasitoloogia*, **46**(1–2), 231–234.

Soto, J. and Berman, J. (2007) Treatment of new world cutaneous leishmaniasis with miltefosine. *Acta Trop.*, **103**(1), 33–40.

Woerly, V., Maynard, L., Sanquer, A., *et al.* (2009) Clinical efficacy and tolerance of miltefosine in the treatment of canine leishmaniosis. *Parasitol Res.*, **105**(2), 463–469.

Chapter 194: Milbemycin Oxime

US Generic (Brand) Name: Milbemycin oxime (Interceptor, Milbemax, Sentinel, Trifexis)
Availability: Veterinary Approved – Milbemycin oral tablets (Interceptor) (2.3, 5.75, 11.5 23 mg), Milbemycin flavored tabs with lufenuron (Sentinel) 2.3/46 mg, 5.75/115 mg, 11.5/230 mg, 23/460 mg, Milbemycin with Spinosad chew tabs (Trifexis) 2.3/140 mg, 4.5/270 mg, 9.3/560 mg, 13.5/810 mg, 27/1620 mg), Milbemycin with Praziquantel (Milbemax) tablets (Cats: 16/40 mg, Kittens: 4/10 mg, Dogs: 12.5/125 mg, Puppies: 21.5/25 mg)

Use

Milbemycin oxime is used primarily in the prevention of heartworm (*D. immitis*) infection in cats and dogs. It is not believed to be as effective as ivermectin but may be safer in breeds with mutation of the ABCB1–1Δ gene. It is also active against hookworms, roundworms, and whipworms. It may be used as a miticide in the treatment of demodicosis. Milbemycin oxime alone is ineffective against tapeworms, flukes, fleas, ticks, lice, mosquitoes, and flies.

Contraindications/warnings

Hypersensitivity to milbemycin. Avoid use in patients with compromised blood-brain barrier disorders (meningitis), seizures, or in breeds (Australian shepherds, collies, long-haired whippets, and Shelties) with a predilection toward mutation of the ABCB1–1Δ gene. Avoid use in dogs <4 weeks of age or <2 lbs, or in kittens <6 weeks or <1.5 lbs.

Dosage

See manufacturer's guidelines for combination product dosing.

Canine
Heartworm Prophylaxis/Endoparasites: Give 0.5 mg/kg PO once monthly (Novartis: Interceptor Label).

Demodicosis: Start at 0.5 mg/kg q24 h and work up to 2 mg/kg q24 h PO × 2–4 months or 1 mg/kg q24 h until a clinical cure is observed, followed by 3 mg/kg PO per week until negative scrapings (Papich 2002).

Sarcoptic mange: 2 mg/kg PO q7 days × 3–5 weeks (Papich 2002).

Cheyletiellosis: 2 mg/kg PO q7 days × 3 doses (Papich 2002).

Nasal mites: 0.5–1.0 mg/kg body weight PO q7 days × 3 weeks (Gunnarsson *et al.*, 1999).

Feline
Heartworm Prophylaxis/Endoparasites: Give 2.0 mg/kg PO once monthly (Novartis: Interceptor Label).

Dose adjustments

Dose adjustments (25–50%) may be required in severe liver failure.

Administration

Monitor heartworm status prior to administration. Administer tablets once monthly. Give tablets with food for maximum effectiveness. If vomiting occurs within an hour of administration, redose with another full dose. Wash hands after administering.

Electrolyte contents

Not significant.

Storage/stability

Store at room temperature in tightly closed container, protected from light.

Adverse reactions

>10%
Diarrhea, vomiting, and salivation are reported in dogs and cats.

1–10%
Anorexia, drooling, decreased activity, and lethargy are reported in dogs and cats. Dermatitis and reddening of the skin/ears reported in dogs with Trifexis.

<1%
Muscle tremors and ataxia are reported rarely in dogs and cats at standard doses. At high doses or in ABCB1–1Δ mutant dog breeds side effects may include: tremors, ataxia, mydriasis, decreased weight, dehydration, sedation, agitation, vocalization, paralysis, paresis, recumbency, coma, and death.

Drug interactions

Barbiturates, benzodiazepines may increase side effects when combined with milbemycin. Amiodarone, carvedilol, clarithromycin, cyclosporine, erythromycin, itraconazole, ketoconazole, quinidine, and verapamil may inhibit P-gylcoprotein and increase toxicity of milbemycin. Inducers of P-glycoprotein (phenothiazines, rifampin, St. John's wort) may decrease milbemycin concentrations.

Monitoring

Observe breeds with likelihood of ABCB1–1Δ for up to 8 h after administering for signs of toxicity. Repeat stool examinations to confirm clearance of parasites. Repeat heartworm test yearly and prior to administration of large doses of milbemycin for demodicosis.

Overdose

Symptoms may include mydriasis, ataxia, vomiting, tachycardia, lethargy, and seizures. Symptoms appear 8–10 h after administration. Emesis and/or gastrointestinal lavage should be done as soon as possible. Additional purgatives, parenteral fluids, electrolytes, pressor agents, and respiratory support may be required. Most animals should begin to improve neurologically within 2–5 days, but may take weeks for complete recovery.

Diagnostic test interference

False negative heartworm tests are unlikely since the antibody tests measure antigen to the adult female *D. immitis* oviduct.

Mechanism

Milbemycin binds selectively to glutamine-gated-chloride ion channels (GABA) in invertebrate nerve cells. This leads to an increased permeability of parasitic nerve and muscle cells to chloride ions with subsequent hyperpolarization and death of susceptible parasites.

Pharmacology/kinetics

Absorption
Milbemycin is well absorbed orally (80%). It is rapidly absorbed in about 2–4 h.

Distribution
Milbemycin is widely distributed into tissues and fluids. It concentrates in liver, kidney, testes, adrenal, pancreas, lymph nodes, heart, and fat.

CNS penetration
Milbemycin readily penetrates into CSF. Dogs with the ABCB1–1Δ gene mutation receiving 1–22 mg/kg/day demonstrate milbemycin accumulation and neurotoxicty.

Metabolism
Milbemycin is primarily metabolized in the liver. It is extensively metabolized by hydroxylation with most metabolites excreted via feces and a small amount via urine.

Half-life
Milbemycin has a half-life of 1–4 days in dogs.

Pregnancy risk factor

Milbemycin has been administered at three times the daily dose to pregnant dogs throughout pregnancy. No teratogenic effects or other adverse effects were noted. In queens treated with milbemycin and praziquantel throughout pregnancy at the highest recommended dose once weekly, no adverse effects were reported in the queen or the kittens. It is considered safe in pregnant animals.

Lactation
Milbemycin is excreted into milk. Puppies administered very high oral doses (19×) only demonstrated temporary toxicity with reversal of symptoms within 2 days. It is considered safe if administered during lactation.

References

Gunnarsson, L.K., Moller, L.C., Einarsson, A.M., *et al.* (1999) Clinical efficacy of milbemycin oxime in the treatment of nasal mite infection in dogs. *J Am Animal Hosp Assoc.*, **35(1)**, 81–84.
Papich, M.G. (2002) *Saunders Handbook of Veterinary Drugs.* 2nd edn. Winkel, A. (ed.), W.B. Saunders Company, Philadelphia, pp. 438–439.

Further reading

Barber, J.L., Snook, T., *et al.* (2009) ABCB1–1 Δ (MDR1–1 Delta) genotype is associated with adverse reactions in dogs treated with milbemycin oxime for generalized demodicosis. *Vet Derm.*, **20(2)**, 111–114.
Kitagawa, H., Sasaki, Y., Kumasaka, J., *et al.* (1993) Clinical and laboratory changes following administration of milbemycin oxime in heartworm-free and heartworm-infected dogs. *Am J Vet Res.*, **54(4)**, 520–526.
Schenker, R., Cody, R., Strehlau, G., *et al.* (2005) Repeat dose tolerance of a combination of milbemycin oxime and praziquantel in breeding and lactating queens. *Intern J Appl Res Vet Med.*, **3(4)**, 360–366.

Chapter 195: Moxidectin

US Generic (Brand) Name: (Advantage Multi, Cydectin, Proheart)
Availability: Veterinary Approved – Moxidectin (10 mg/mL) and imidacloprid (100 mg/mL) topical solution (Advantage Multi) for cats (3 × 0.23 mL, 6 × 0.4 mL, 6 × 0.8 mL tubes) or moxidectin 25 mg/mL and imidacloprid 100 mg/mL) for dogs (6 × 0.4 mL, 6 × 1 mL, 6 × 2.5 mL, 6 × 4 mL tubes), moxidectin sterile injection (Cydectin) (10 mg/mL × 200 mL, 500 mL), moxidectin 10% sustained release (microspheres) injection (ProHeart 6) 598 mg/vial

Use

Moxidectin is used alone or in combination with other drugs for the prevention of heartworm disease caused by *D. immitis*. It is also indicated for the treatment of existing larval and adult hookworm (*A. caninum, U. stenocephala*) infections. Moxidectin is also used in combination with imidacloprid (Advantage Multi) as a topical once a month treatment in animals to prevent heartworm, control fleas, and kill intestinal parasites. Imidacloprid covers gastrointestinal worms such as roundworms (*T. canis, T. leonina*), hookworms (*A. caninum, U. stenocephala*), and whipworms (*T. vulpis*).

Contraindications/warnings

Hypersensitivity to avermectins. Avoid application onto abraded skin. Use caution in patients with compromised blood-brain barrier disorders, seizures, or in breeds (Australian shepherds, collies, long-haired whippets, and shelties) with a predilection toward mutation of the ABCB1–1Δ gene. Do not use in heartworm positive animals or those with microfilaria. Do not use on dogs <7 weeks or <3 lbs. ProHeart 6 should be administered with caution in dogs with pre-existing allergic disease, including food allergy, atopy, and flea allergy dermatitis. Do not administer Proheart 6 to animals <6 months of age, at a frequency of less than 6 months in time, or at the same time as vaccinations. Do not administer to dogs who are sick, debilitated, underweight, or who have a history of weight loss.

Dosage

Canine
Heartworm prevention: Administer Advantage Multi topically once a month (recommended dose is 10 mg/kg imidacloprid with 2.5 mg/kg moxidectin) as per

manufacturer's guidelines. Administer Proheart 6 (0.05 mL/kg = 0.17 mg moxidectin/kg or 0.0773 mg/lb) SC q6 months.

Demodicosis: Start at 100 µg/kg (0.1 mg/kg) PO q24 h and increase as tolerated to 400 µg/kg (0.4 mg/kg) PO q24 h until clinical cure is observed and there are two negative skin scrapings 1 month apart. The injectable (Cydectin) can be used orally or can be injected at 0.25 mg/kg SC q7 days × 3 doses. Base dose on accurate, current weight.

Feline
Heartworm prevention: Administer Advantage Multi topically once a month (recommended dose is 10 mg/kg imidacloprid with 1.0 mg/kg moxidectin) as per manufacturer's guidelines.

Aelurostrongylosis abstrusus: Administer Advantage Multi topically once monthly for 1–3 treatments (Conboy 2009).

Dose adjustments

Dose adjustments (25–50%) may be required in severe liver failure.

Administration

Confirm that the dog is heartworm negative prior to administration. To administer topical treatments, open tube, part the hair between the shoulder blades, and apply onto skin. For dogs <20 lbs, apply entire contents to the spot between the shoulder blades; for dogs 20 lbs and over, apply on three or four spots along the upper back in an area the dog will not be able to lick. Do not let the dog lick itself and the owner should not touch the area until the product dries (approximately 30 min after application). The injectable Cydectin solution (10 mg/mL) has been administered off-label for demodicosis. To administer Proheart 6, the two-part sustained release product must be mixed at least 30 min prior to use. ProHeart 6 consists of two separate vials: one vial contains 10% moxidectin sterile microspheres and the second vial contains a specifically formulated sterile vehicle for constitution with the microspheres. No other diluent should be used. Each mL of reconstituted drug product contains 3.4 mg moxidectin. Swirl vial gently before every use. Withdraw 0.05 mL of suspension/kg body weight into an appropriately sized syringe fitted with an 18 G or 20 G hypodermic needle. Dose promptly after drawing into dosing syringe. If administration is delayed, gently roll the dosing syringe prior to injection to maintain a uniform suspension. Inject the product subcutaneously in the left or right side of the dorsum of the neck cranial to the scapula. No more than 3 mL should be administered in a single site. The location(s) of each injection (left or right side) should be noted so that prior injection sites can be identified and the next injection can be administered on the opposite side.

Electrolyte contents

Not significant.

Storage/stability

Store Advantage Multi at room temperature in the manufacturer's packaging. Cydectin injectable is stored at room temperature, protected from light. Proheart 6 Injectable can be stored at room temperature, protected from light. After reconstitution, it is stable for 4 weeks in the refrigerator.

Adverse reactions

>10%
Damp, stiff, or greasy hair, white deposit on the hair, mild erythema, and localized pruritus reported in dogs.

1–10%
Diarrhea, bloody stools, vomiting, anorexia, lethargy, coughing, hyperkeratosis, ocular discharge, and nasal discharge reported in dogs

<1%
Other side effects reported in dogs include: weakness, depression, unsteadiness, salivation, poor appetite, lethargy, weakness, restlessness, agitation, disorientation, ataxia, muscle tremors, seizures, elevated liver enzymes, hypoproteinemia, hyperbilirubinemia, hepatopathy, elevated BUN, elevated creatinine, hematuria, polydipsia, polyuria, elevated body temperature, panting, labored breathing, acute pulmonary edema, hives, rash, leukocytosis, anemia, thrombocytopenia, swollen face and ears, anaphylaxis, alopecia, hot spots, local discomfort, and discoloration of the hair at the application site. Dogs with clinically significant weight loss (>10%) are more likely to experience severe adverse reactions. Accidental oral ingestion in dogs causes salivation, vomiting, muscle tremor, seizures, mydriasis, ataxia, lethargy, disorientation, agitation, and poor appetite. In cats treated topically with imidacloprid/moxidectin for dogs, side effects included application site and skin reactions, vomiting, lethargy, agitation, and neurologic signs. Following administration

of Proheart 6 anaphylactic reactions have resulted in liver disease and death. These reactions were felt to be related to the microsphere vehicle, which has been reformulated to potentially improve its safety.

Drug interactions

Barbiturates, benzodiazepines may increase side effects. Amiodarone, carvedilol, clarithromycin, cyclosporine, erythromycin, itraconazole, ketoconazole, quinidine, and verapamil may inhibit P-gylcoprotein and increase toxicity of moxidectin. Inducers of P-glycoprotein (clotrimazole, phenothiazines, rifampin, St. John's wort) may decrease moxidectin concentrations.

Monitoring

Observe breeds with likelihood of ABCB1–1Δ for up to 8 h after administering for signs of toxicity. Repeat stool and skin scraping examinations to confirm clearance of parasites. Repeat heartworm test yearly and prior to administration of large doses.

Overdose

Symptoms may include mydriasis, ataxia, vomiting, tachycardia, lethargy, and seizures and may appear 8–10 h after administration. Emesis and/or gastrointestinal lavage should be done as soon as possible. Intravenous fat emulsions have been used to treat avermectin toxicities. Additional purgatives, parenteral fluids, electrolytes, pressor agents, and respiratory support may be required. Most animals should begin to improve neurologically within 2–5 days, but may take weeks for complete recovery.

Diagnostic test interference

False negative heartworm tests are unlikely since the antibody tests measure antigen to the adult female *D. immitis* oviduct.

Mechanism

Moxidectin binds selectively to glutamine-gated-chloride ion channels (GABA) in invertebrate nerve cells. This leads to an increased permeability of parasitic nerve and muscle cells to chloride ions with subsequent hyperpolarization and death of susceptible parasites.

Pharmacology/kinetics

Absorption
Following injection with ProHeart 6, peak moxidectin blood levels will be observed approximately 7–14 days after treatment. At the end of the 6 month dosing interval, residual drug concentrations are negligible.

Distribution
Extensively distributed into tissues where it is stored in fat and other tissues. Residue tissue concentrations are greater than plasma concentrations with very prolonged tissue half-lives.

CNS penetration
Moxidectin readily penetrates into the CNS with concentrations being comparable to ivermectin, but appears to demonstrate a much lower neurotoxic potential than ivermectin.

Metabolism
Moxidectin has very limited metabolism in most species. Minor metabolites (mono- and di-hydroxylated moxidectin) are noted in dogs. The majority of drug is excreted unchanged in feces.

Half-life
Very prolonged half-life compared to other macrocyclic lactones. Following oral ingestion the half-life is 8 days in dogs. Following SC injection the half-life is 35 days.

Pregnancy risk factor

Teratogenic effects have not been seen in dogs or cats exposed to moxidectin during pregnancy. However, embryotoxicity has been noted in laboratory animals (mice and rats) fed moxidectin containing diets (0, 25, 50, 125 mg/kg) during pregnancy. In rats given high doses, there was evidence of both materno- and fetotoxicity, as shown by increased incidences of cleft palate and wavy or incompletely ossified ribs.

Lactation
Moxidectin is excreted into milk and may have adverse effects on nursing animals. Reduced weight gain, decrease in the number of live pups and death during lactation were noted in laboratory animals.

Reference

Conboy, G. (2009) Helminth parasites of the canine and feline respiratory tract. *Vet Clin North Amer Small Animal Pract.*, **39**(6), 1109–1113.

Further reading

Barton, W. and Rulli, R.D. (2000) *Final report of a three year study with moxidectin canine SR injectable.* Fort Dodge Animal Health Report Number GASD 07–21.00.

Janco, C. and Geyer, J. (2013) Moxidectin has a lower neurotoxic potential but comparable brain penetration in P-glycoprotein-deficient CF-1 mice compared to ivermectin. *J Vet Pharmacol Ther.*, **36**(3), 275–284.

Schulze, G.E. (1991) One-year dietary toxicity study in purebred beagle dogs with AC 301.423. Study conducted by Hazeleton Washington, Inc. Vienna, VA. HWA Study 362–2000. American Cyanamid Protocol Number 971–88–175.

Schroeder, R.E. (1991) *A three generation (two-litters) reproduction study with AC 301,423 to rats.* Study conducted by Bio-dynamics Inc., East Millstone, New Jersey, USA. Project ID# 88–3388. American Cyanamid Protocol number 971–88–176.

Vanapalli, A.M., Hung, Y.P., Fleckenstein, L., *et al.* (2002) Pharmacokinetics and dose proportionality of oral moxidectin in beagle dogs. *Biopharm Drug Dispos.*, **23**, 263–272.

Chapter 196: Nitazoxanide

US Generic (Brand) Name: Nitazoxanide (Alinia)
Availability: Human Approved – Nitazoxanide oral tablets 500 mg, oral powder for suspension 20 mg/mL (60 mL) (Alinia)

Use

Nitazoxanide is an antiprotozoal prodrug used off label in small animals for *Cryptosporidium parvum, Isospora, Entamoeba,* and *Giardia lamblia.* It has been studied in cats co-infected with *Cryptosporidium* spp. and *T. foetus* where it reduced shedding of organisms but did not eliminate the infections. It is also active against *Ascaris, Ancylostoma, Trichuris, Taenia, Helicobacter, Campylobacter jejuni,* and some anaerobic bacteria. Recent studies have also shown efficacy against canine influenza virus (CIV) *in vitro* and other human viruses (H1N1 and Hepatitis B/C).

Contraindications/warnings

Hypersensitivity to nitazoxanide. Caution in geriatric patients who may be more pre-disposed to side effects. While no studies have been done in hepatic, biliary, or renal disease, caution should be taken in these patients.

Dosage

Canine

Cestodes: 100 mg/kg q24 h PO × 1 (Euzeby *et al.*, 1980).

Giardia: 25 mg/kg PO q12 h × 5 days (Anecdotal-efficacy unknown).

Cryptosporidium: 100 mg/animal PO q12 h × 3 days (Sykes and Papich 2013).

Feline

Cestodes: 100 mg/kg q24 h PO × 1 (Euzeby *et al.*, 1980).

Giardia: 25 mg/kg PO q12 h × 5 days (Anecdotal-efficacy unknown).

Cryptosporidium: 100 mg/animal PO q12 h × 3 days (Sykes and Papich 2013).

Dose adjustments

Dose adjustment in liver or renal impairment has not been studied.

Administration

Mix the oral powder for suspension with 48 mL of water, shake well, and store at room temperature. The suspension has better oral absorption than the tablets. Administer with food to minimize gastrointestinal adverse reactions and increase absorption.

Electrolyte contents

Not significant. The oral suspension contains 1.48 g of sucrose per 5 mL.

Storage/stability

Nitazoxide is stored at room temperature. The oral solution is stable for 7 days once mixed.

Adverse reactions

>10%

Salivation, vomiting, and diarrhea reported in dogs.

1–10%

Anorexia seen in dogs. Dark, foul smelling stools in cats.

Other species

Side effects in humans and other mammals have included: yellow discoloration of sclera, fever, chills, dizziness, insomnia, tremor, discolored urine, dysuria, increased SGPT, anemia, leukocytosis, rash, pruritus, epistaxis, tachycardia, syncope, hypertension, myalgia, leg cramps, and spontaneous bone fracture.

Drug interactions

None noted. Other highly protein bound drugs may have altered binding.

Monitoring

Monitor efficacy, hydration, electrolytes, CBC, serum albumin, and protein.

Overdose

Overdoses may cause salivation, vomiting, lethargy, diarrhea, increased liver, and spleen weight. The oral LD_{50} in cats and dogs is 10 g/kg. Supportive care and gastrointestinal decontamination may be required for very large overdoses.

Diagnostic test interference

None noted.

Mechanism

Nitazoxanide is believed to inhibit pyruvate ferredoxin oxidoreductase. This enzyme is involved in electron transfer reactions essential to anaerobic and protozoal energy metabolism.

Pharmacology/kinetics

Absorption

Nitazoxanide is well absorbed after oral administration. The suspension has better oral absorption than the tablet in humans. It is not found in the bloodstream due to rapid metabolism via hydrolysis.

Distribution

Nitazoxanide is a prodrug that is highly protein bound (>90%) and rapidly converted into active metabolites. Tissue and fluid distribution of metabolites is unknown in cats and dogs to date.

CNS penetration

Nitazoxanide penetrates into the CSF in concentrations that are therapeutic for most targeted organisms (0.1 μg/ml).

Metabolism

Nitazoxanide is rapidly metabolized in the liver to two active metabolites; tizoxanide and tizoxanide glucuronide. The metabolites are excreted in urine (26%), bile, and feces (46%) in dogs.

Half-life

No data was noted in cats/dogs. The half-life of nitazoxanide in humans is only 6 min due to the fact that it is a prodrug and rapidly metabolized.

Pregnancy risk factor

Category B: Nitazoxanide has not shown evidence of teratogenic effects or maternal toxicity in laboratory animals.

Lactation

Low levels of the active metabolite, tizoxanide, have been reported in human milk. It is unlikely that lactating animals would have significant concentrations in milk to be harmful to lactating animals.

References

Euzeby, J., Prom Tep, S., and Rossignol, J.F. (1980) Study of the anthelmintic properties of nitazoxanide in dog, cat and sheep. *Revue de Medecine Veterinaire*, **131**(10), 687–696

Sykes, J.E. and Papich, M.G. (2013) Antiprotozoal drugs. Ch. 10. In: *Canine and Feline Infectious Diseases*, Sykes, J.E. (ed.), Elsevier, St. Louis, MO. pp. 97–110.

Further reading

Anderson, V.R. and Curran, M.P. (2007) Nitazoxanide: a review of its use in the treatment of gastrointestinal infections. *Drugs*, **67**(13), 1947–1967.

Ashton, L.V., Callan, R.L., Rao, S., *et al.* (2010) *In vitro* susceptibility of canine influenza A (H3N8) virus to nitazoxanide and tizoxanide. *Vet Med Int.*, Aug **12**, p. ii: 891010. doi: 10.4061/2010/891010.

Gookin, J.L. Levy, M.G., Law, J.M., *et al.* (2001) Experimental infection of cats with *Tritrichomonas foetus*. *AJVR*, **62**, 1690–1697.

Murphy, J.R. and Friedmann, J.C. (1985) Pre-clinical toxicology of nitazoxanide-a new antiparasitic compound. *J Appl Toxicol.*, **5**, 49–52.

Rossignol, J.F. (2009) Thiazolides: A new class of antiviral drugs. *Expert Opin Drug Metab Toxicol.*, **5**, 667–674.

Stockis, A., DeBruyn, S., Gengler, C., *et al.* (2002) Nitazoxanide pharmacokinetics and tolerability in man during seven days dosing with 0.5 g and 1 g twice daily. *Int J Clin Pharmacol Ther.*, **4**, 221–2217.

Chapter 197: Nitenpyram

US Generic (Brand) Name: Nitenpyram (Capstar, Program Flavored tablets with Capstar, Capstar flea management system for dogs/cats, Sentinel Flavored tablets and Capstar)
Availability: Veterinary Approved – Nitenpyram tablets (Capstar) (11.4, 57 mg), Program flavored tablets with Capstar, Capstar flea management system for dogs/cats, Sentinel flavored tablets and Capstar

Use

Used in the treatment of small animals as a flea adulticide. It actively kills fleas within 30 min but has no effects on eggs, larvae, or immature fleas. Typically combined with other products, such as lufenuron, to target egg and larvae viability and milbemycin, to target heartworm and other endo/ectoparasites. Anecdotally used rectally and topically. Used off label for the treatment of fly strike. Aids in killing blowfly and screwworm fly maggots in wounds. Although thought to be highly specific for insect nicotinic receptors and very safe for mammals, post marketing experience suggests that nicotinic side effects do occur rarely in mammals.

Contraindications/warnings

Hypersensitivity to nitenpyram. Caution in animals <2 lbs, <4 weeks in age or poor body condition due to increased risk of neurologic signs/death. Caution in animals with CNS disease and/or seizures. Avoid environmental contamination; highly toxic to bees and other beneficial insects.

Dosage

Typically dosed at 1 mg/kg q24 h PO unless in combination therapy with lufenuron (Program) where it is given once monthly.

Canine

Fleas: For 2–25 lbs: Give 11.4 mg tablet PO q24 h or 25–125 lbs: Give 57 mg tablet PO q24 h (give either 1–2 times weekly or once daily) (Package Insert).

Myiasis (Screwworm/Blow fly maggots): Give 1.4–4.4 mg/kg PO q6 h × 2 doses (Zhang *et al.*, 2010).

Feline

Fleas: For 2–25 lbs: Give 11.4 mg tablet PO q day (Package Insert).

Myiasis (Screwworm/Blow fly maggots): Give 11.4 mg tablet PO q 24 h × 1–2 days.

Dose adjustments

Dose reductions (25–50%) may be required in patients with severe renal or hepatic impairment.

Administration

Administer orally with food to induce bile flow and help dissolve chemical. All animals in a household need to be treated at the same time or reinfection will occur. May be administered once daily for severe flea infestation/flea allergy. Anecdotally has been administered rectally as a tab, or as a suspension made in water for acute control of fleas or maggots. It has also been administered directly onto maggot infested wounds.

Electrolyte contents

Not significant.

Storage/stability

Store at room temperature, protected from light, and in manufacturer's packaging.

Adverse reactions

>10%

Three- to five-fold increase in itching and grooming directly after administration due to hyperactivity of dying fleas. Hyperactivity, vomiting, panting, and lethargy reported in dogs/cats.

1–10%

Vocalization, decreased appetite, diarrhea, and urticaria reported in dogs and cats.

<1%

Fever, nervousness, salivation, incoordination, trembling, seizures, increased heart rate, and red skin reported in dogs/cats.

Other species

Nicotinic side effects demonstrated as above in addition to: fatigue, tremors, fever, cough, palpitation, stomach ache, muscle spasms, weakness, tachycardia, and bradycardia.

Drug interactions

None identified to date in animals. Caution with any other insecticides or flea medications.

Monitoring

Monitor for signs of nicotinic side effects (gastrointestinal, neurotoxic, fever, and cardiac).

Overdose

Gastrointestinal lavage for acute high oral doses. Supportive care including treatment for seizures if needed.

Diagnostic test interference

None noted.

Mechanism

Rapid acting adulticide for insects. First generation neonicotinoid that is an agonist to insect-specific nicotinic actylcholine receptors in post-synaptic membranes. Binds to receptors causing nicotinic poisoning (rigidity, paralysis and death).

Pharmacology/kinetics

Absorption

Nitenpyram is rapidly absorbed from the gastrointestinal tract (<90 min) with bioavailability of >99%. Efficacy (>90% decreased flea counts) is seen in cats at 6 h and dogs at 4 h.

Distribution

Highly lipophilic, distributed through tissues and fluids.

CNS penetration

Penetrates into the CNS readily.

Metabolism

Nitenptram is rapidly metabolized in the liver of cats and dogs by hydroxylation followed by conjugation. It is excreted primarily via the urine (>90%) within 48 h. A 6-chloronicotinic acid metabolite was the primary metabolite found in urine.

Half-life

The half-life in dogs is 2.8 h and is 7.7 h in cats.

Pregnancy risk factor

Birth defects and fetal/neonatal loss have been reported after treatment of pregnant animals. It is contraindicated during pregnancy.

Lactation

Nitenpyram is highly lipophilic and is excreted readily into milk. Newborn puppies and kittens (neonates) have been reported to die following administration of nitenpyram to the mother during lactation. It is contra-indicated during lactation.

Reference

Zhang, J., Liu, J., Qin, X.W., *et al.* (2010) Analysis of time-and concentration-mortality relationship of nitenpyram against different larval stages of *Nilaparvata lugens (Hemiptera: Delphacidae)*. *J Econ Entomol.*, **103**(5), 1665–1669.

Further reading

Correia, T.R., Scotta, F.B., Verocaia, G.G., *et al.* (2010) Larvicidal efficacy of nitenpyram on the treatment of myiasis caused by Cochliomyia hominivorax (Diptera: Calliphoridae) in dogs. *Vet Parasitol.*, **173(1–2)**, 169–172.

Rust, M.K., Waggoner, M.M., Hinkle, N.C., *et al.* (2003) Efficacy and longevity of nitenpyram against adult cat fleas (Siphonaptera: Pulicidae). *J Med Entomol.*, **40**, 678–681.

Schenker, R., Tinembart, O., Humbert-Droz, E., *et al.* (2003) Comparative speed of kill between nitenpyram, fibronil, imida-cloprid, selamectin and cythioate against adult Ctenocephalides felis (Bouche) on cats and dogs. *Vet Parasitol.*, **112**, 249–254.

Taira, K., Aoyama, Y., Kawakami, T., *et al.* (2011) Detection of chloropyridinyl neonicotinoid insecticide metabolite 6-chlo-ronicotinic acid in the urine: six cases with subacute nicotinic symptoms. *Chudoku Kenkyu.*, **24(3)**, 222–230.

Tomizawa, M. and Casida, J.E. (2003) Selective toxicity of neonicotinoids attributable to specificity of insect and mam-malian nicotinic receptors. *Annu Rev Entomol.*, **48**, 339–364.

Chapter 198: Ponazuril (Toltrazuril Sulfone)

US Generic (Brand) Name: Ponazuril (Marquis)
Availability: Veterinary Approved – Ponazuril paste 15% (Marquis) 150 mg/g × 127 g tubes × 4. Single tubes may be available from www.agri-med.com

Use

Ponazuril is a triazine antiprotozoal (anticoccidial) labeled for horses for use on Equine Protozoal Myeloencephalitis (*Sarcocystis neurona*). Ponazuril is active against several genera of the phylum *Apicomplexa*. It is active against *Toxoplasma gondii*, *Isospora* spp., *Eimeria* spp., and *Neospora caninum*. Ponazuril is also active in the treatment of *Cystoisospora ohioensis* infections in puppies. It is not active against *Cryptosporidium* spp. It shows some efficacy against *Hepatozoon americanum* in dogs but may not clear the infection if used alone. Ponazuril is an active metabolite of toltrazuril; the alternate chemical name for ponazuril is toltrazuril sulfone. The drug is not labeled for use in small animals, but it is commonly used by kennels and shelters for the treatment of coccidia. While not a standard treatment, a compounded version of ponazuril made from the commercial Marquis paste is frequently used.

Contraindications/warnings

Avoid use in animals allergic to ponazuril. Use with cau-tion in animals with pre-existing seizures. Although its safety is not documented in pregnancy and lactation and it is considered contraindicated, ponazuril has been be used to prevent neonatal transmission of *Neospora* in pregnant dogs with good outcome.

Dosage

Canine/feline

Coccidiosis/Isospora spp.: 20–50 mg/kg q 24 h PO × 2–5 days (Sykes and Papich 2013).

Neosporosis: 7.5–15 mg/kg q24 h × 28 days (Greene *et al.*, 2006).

Toxoplasmosis: 20 mg/kg PO q12 h × 4 weeks (Lappin 2013).

Dose adjustments

None noted to date.

Administration

Dilute 1 tube of paste (127 g paste × 150 mg ponazuril/ 1 g paste = 19.05 g ponazuril/tube) in 21 mL of water or other carrier (Val Syrup) (total volume = 141 mL) to make a 135 mg/mL solution. Stir well. Note: 127 g paste = 120 mL paste. Administer 1 mL/10 lbs (30 mg/ kg) orally.

Electrolyte contents

Not significant.

Storage/stability

Store at room temperature in the manufacturer's packaging or a light proof container. There is no stability data on diluted drug to date.

Adverse reactions

>10%
Mild gastro-intestinal upset, vomiting, and diarrhea reported in dogs and cats.

1–10%
Keratoconjunctivitis sicca (KCS) has been reported in some dogs, particularly in breeds with a predisposition to KCS. Sporadic inappetence, weight loss, and moderate edema in the uterine epithelium reported in dogs.

<1%
High doses (200–5000 ppm over 13 weeks) to dogs resulted in decreased weight gain, hematologic effects, and decreased food consumption.

Other species
Allergic reactions (blisters and wheals), diarrhea, mild colic, skin rashes, hives, seizures, and uterine edema have been reported in horses.

Drug interactions

Dogs with myasthenia gravis receiving pyridostigmine may experience extreme weakness if these two drugs are combined.

Monitoring

Monitor efficacy, weight loss, and CBC.

Overdose

Under research conditions, a 10-fold overdose of ponazuril repeated for 3 days caused no adverse effects on beagle puppies. The NOEL for dogs is reported to be 200 ppm.

Diagnostic test interference

None noted.

Mechanism

Ponazuril is a triazinetrione anti-protozoal drug. It is a coccidiocidal drug that is active against the plastid body of the parasite.

Pharmacology/kinetics

Absorption
Ponazuril has limited oral absorption in horses (54%). No data was noted in small animals. Absorption is increased (71%) after oral administration in horses if administered in DMSO or corn oil.

Distribution
Ponazuril is readily distributed throughout body tissues and fluids including the CSF.

CNS penetration
Ponazuril readily penetrates into the CSF. In horses, a 5 mg/kg orally results in CSF concentrations >0.1 µg/mL after Day 7 of treatment.

Metabolism
Ponazuril is metabolized in the liver, but its route of elimination has not been studied in small animals.

Half-life
The half-life in most species studied is >50 h.

Pregnancy risk factor

Ponazuril crosses the placental barrier. In rats and rabbits, maternal and fetal toxicity was noted at high doses (>30 mg/kg). Ponazuril may be used to prevent neonatal transmission of *Neospora* in pregnant dogs, but its safety has not been proven.

Lactation

The safe use of ponazuril in lactating animals has not been evaluated. Due to its lipophilicity it is expected to be excreted into breast milk.

References

Greene, C., Hartmann, K., *et al.* (2006) Antimicrobial drug formulary. Appendix 8. In: *Infectious Disease of the Dog and Cat.* Greene, C. (ed.), Elsevier, St. Louis, MO, pp. 1186–1333.

Lappin, M.R. (2013) Toxoplasmosis. Ch. 72. In: *Canine and Feline Infectious Diseases*, Sykes, J.E. (ed.), Elsevier, St. Louis, MO. pp. 693–701.

Marquis (Ponazuril) (2004) *EPM Paste*, MSDS Number R37641, Bayer Animal Healthcare LLC, Shawnee, KS, 2004.

Sykes, J.E. and Papich, M.G. (2013) Antiprotozoal drugs. Ch. 10. In: *Canine and Feline Infectious Diseases*, Sykes, J.E. (ed.), Elsevier, St. Louis, MO. pp. 97–104.

Further reading

Darius, A.K., Mehlorn, H., and Heydorn, A.O. (2004) Effects of toltrazuril and ponazuril on the fine structure and multiplication of tachyzoites of the NC-1 strain of *Neospora caninum* (a synonym of *Hammondia heydorni*) in cell culture. *Parasitol Res.*, **92(6)**, 453–458.

Gottstein, B., Eperon, S., Dai, W.J., *et al.* (2001) Efficacy of toltrazuril and ponazuril against experimental *Neospora caninum* infection in mice. *Parasitol Res.*, **87(1)**, 43–48.

Gottstein, B., Razmi, G.R., Ammann, P., *et al.* (2005) Toltrazuril treatment to control diaplacental *Neospora caninum* transmission in experimentally infected pregnant mice. *Parasitol.*, **130(1)**, 41–48.

Chapter 199: Praziquantel

US Generic (Brand) Name: Praziquantel (Biltricide, Droncit, Drontal, Drontal-Plus, Virbantel Chews, Panacur Plus Chews)
Availability: Human Approved – Praziquantel film coated tablets (600 mg). Veterinary Approved – Praziquantel tablets (feline: 23 mg), (canine: 34 mg), sterile injectable 56.8 mg/mL (10, 50 ml), combination products: Drontal: praziquantel/pyrantel pamoate (cats: 13.6 mg/54.3 mg, 18.2 mg/72.6 mg, 27.2 mg/108.6 mg. Panacur plus soft chews: praziquantel/ivermectin/fenbendazole, multiple other combinations (pastes, gels, etc.) for equine patients

Use

Praziquantel is active against Cestodes (tapeworms) and flukes (*Paragonimus*). In dogs it is active against *Dipylidium caninum, Echinococcus multiocularis*, and *E. granulosus* and *Taenia pisiformis*. In cats, it is useful for *Dipylidium caninum* and *Taenia taeniaeformis*. Also active against *Alaria* spp. in dogs and *Spirometra mansonoides* in cats.

Contraindications/warnings

Hypersensitivity to praziquantel. Use with caution in patients with hepatic impairment. Contraindicated in puppies <4 weeks and kittens <6 weeks of age. Use with caution in patients with cardiac irregularities or with prior seizures.

Dosage

Canine
Cestodes: Praziquantel injectable (56.8 mg/mL) IM or SC × 1 (<5 lbs = 0.3 mL, 6–10 lbs = 0.5 mL, 11–25 lbs = 1 mL, >25 lbs = 0.2 mL/5 lbs) (3 mL = maximum) or oral tablets < 5 lbs = 1/2 tablet, 6–10 lbs = 1 tablet, 11–15 lbs = 1.5 tablets, 16–30 lbs = 2 tablets, 31–45 lbs = 3 tablets, 46–60 lbs = 4 tablets, >60 lbs = 5 tablets (Maximum) (Bayer package insert).

Taenia/Echinococcus/Dipylidium caninum/ mesocestoides: 5 mg/kg PO or SC × 1 (Tuzer *et al.*, 2010).

Diphyllobothrium/Sparganum spp.: 7.5 mg/kg PO q24 h × 2 days (Roberson 1988).

Paragonimus kellicotti: 23–25 mg/kg PO q8 h × 3 days (Reinemeyer 1995).

Feline
Cestodes: Praziquantel injectable (56.8 mg/mL) IM or SC × 1 (<5 lbs = 0.2 mL, 5–10 lbs = 0.4 mL, >10 lbs = 0.6 mL (max) or oral tablets (23 mgs): <4 lbs = 1/2 tablet, 5–11 lbs = 1 tablet, >11 lbs = 1.5 tablets.

Taenia/Echinococcus/Dipylidium caninum/mesocestoides: 5 mg/kg PO or SC × 1 (Tuzer *et al.*, 2010).

Paragonimus kellicotti: 23–25 mg/kg PO q8 h × 3 days (Reinemeyer 1995).

Dose adjustments

Decrease dose (25–50%) in patients with severe hepatic impairment.

Administration

Administer tablets with water and food. Avoid letting animals chew tablets due to a bitter taste.

Electrolyte contents

Not significant.

Storage/stability

Both the injectable and oral tablets are stored at room temperature, protected from light.

Adverse reactions

>10%
Loss of appetite and pain at the injection site reported in cats and dogs.

1–10%
Vomiting, diarrhea, nausea, ataxia, and malaise at high doses, which is greater with the injectable. Salivation in cats.

<1%
Hypersensitivity (rashes, itching, and fever), elevated liver enzyme activities reported in dogs and cats.

Drug interactions

Avoid drugs that affect the activity of CYP isoenzymes. Dexamethasone, phenobarbital, phenytoin, and rifampin may decrease praziquantel concentrations. Cimetidine, erythromycin, itraconazole, and ketoconazole may increase concentrations of praziquantel.

Monitoring

Monitor efficacy, repeat stool examination.

Overdose

Ataxia, lethargy, and elevated liver enzyme activity may occur. The LD_{50} in dogs is 200 mg/kg. Gastrointestinal lavage with charcoal and cathartics along with supportive care are recommended.

Diagnostic test interference

None reported.

Mechanism

Increases cellular permeability to calcium, causing paralysis of worms, impairment of sucker function, and dislodgement of worms.

Pharmacology/kinetics

Absorption
Rapidly and almost completely absorbed following oral administration. Maximum absorption occurs at 0.5–1.5 h in dogs.

Distribution
Praziquantel is distributed throughout body fluids and tissues.

CNS penetration
Very good penetration into the CSF (14–20%).

Metabolism
Praziquantel is extensively metabolized in the liver by first pass metabolism. In dogs, the primary metabolite is 4-hydroxy-praziquantel. Praziquantel and its metabolites are primarily excreted in urine.

Half-life
The half-life in dogs is 3 h.

Pregnancy risk factor

Category B: Praziquantel has not demonstrated embryotoxic or teratogenic effects, but has demonstrated both mutagenic and carcinogenic activity, so it is not recommended during pregnancy unless the benefits outweigh the risks.

Lactation
Praziquantel is excreted into milk. Milk concentrations are approximately 25% of plasma concentrations. Due to the mutagenic/carcinogenic potential, it is not recommended in lactating animals.

References

Reinemeyer, C. (1995) Parasites of the respiratory system. In: *Kirk's Current Veterinary Therapy XII*. Bonagura, J. (ed.), W.B. Saunders Company, Philadelphia, pp. 895–898.

Roberson, E.L. (1988) Anticestodal and antitrematodal drugs. In: *Vet Pharmacology and Therapeutics*. Booth, N.H. and McDonald, L.E. (eds), Iowa State University Press, Ames, pp. 928–949.

Tuzer, E., Bilgin, Z., Oter, K., *et al.* (2010) Efficacy of praziquantel injectable solution against feline and canine tapeworms. *Turkiye Parazitol Derg.*, **34(1)**, 17–20.

Further reading

Eom, K.S., Kim, S.H., and Rim, H.J. (1988) Efficacy of praziquantel (Cesocide injection) in treatment of Cestode infections in domestic and laboratory animals. *Kisaengchun. Chapchi.*, **26(2)**, 121–126.

Chapter 200: Primaquine Phosphate

US Generic (Brand) Name: Primaquine phosphate
Availability: Human Approved – Primaquine phosphate oral tablets 26.3 mg (equivalent to 15 mg of primaquine base)

Use

Primaquine phosphate is an 8-amino-quinoline, a synthetic compound with potent antimalarial activity. It is labeled for human use only for the treatment of malaria. In small animals it is used off-label for the treatment of *Babesia felis* in cats. It is considered the drug of choice for cats with *Babesia felis*.

Contraindications/warnings

Hypersensitivity to primaquine. It is contraindicated in acutely ill patients, patients that may have a tendency to develop granulocytopenia and patients receiving drugs that are bone marrow suppressive.

Dosage

Base dose on primaquine base (15 mg base/26.3 mg tablets)

Feline
Babesiosis: 0.5 mg/kg (primaquine base) PO q24 h × 1–3 days (Birkenheuer 2013).

Dose adjustments

No data available for dose reduction. Due to the significant hepatic metabolism and renal excretion of this drug it is recommended to decrease doses (25–50%) in significant impairment.

Administration

Each tablet contains 26.3 mg of primaquine phosphate (equivalent to 15 mg of primaquine base). The dosage is customarily expressed in terms of the base. Give with meals to decrease gastrointestinal effects.

Electrolyte contents

Not significant.

Storage/stability

Tablets should be stored in a tight, light resistant container at room temperature.

Adverse reactions

>10%
Nausea and vomiting in cats.

1–10%
Methemoglobinemia reported in cats.

<1%
Elevated liver enzymes, hypoglycemia, degenerative changes in liver and kidneys, pneumonia, elevated haptoglobin, lymphoid depletion, methaemoglobinaemia, thrombocytopenia, and inflammatory and degenerative changes of striated muscle (including the myocardium, diaphragm, tongue, and skeletal muscle) in dogs.

Other species
Pruritus, arrhythmias, agranulocytosis, leukocytosis, leucopenia, shortness of breath, and skin discoloration (chocolate cyanosis).

Drug interactions

Drugs that cause bone marrow suppression (cyclosporine, chemotherapeutics, azithioprine, etc.) or those that can cause hemolytic effects (sulfonamides, quinidine, sulfonylureas, etc.) should be avoided.

Primaquine may decrease the plasma concentrations of tricyclic antidepressants, benzodiazepines, propranolol, and theophylline.

Monitoring

Periodic CBC and urinalysis: check for color changes (darkening).

Overdose

Symptoms may involve vomiting, cyanosis, methemoglobinemia, leucopenia, acute hemolytic anemia, and granulocytopenia. With chronic overdoses, ototoxicity, and retinopathy may also occur. Single doses in excess of 1 mg/kg are known to cause mortality in cats. Gastrointestinal decontamination and supportive care (fluids, blood transfusions, and methylene blue for methemoglobinemia if severe).

Diagnostic test interference

None reported.

Mechanism

The exact mechanism of action is not well understood. Primaquine is an 8-aminoquinoline. Primaquine disrupts parasite mitochondrial function and also binds to DNA. It eliminates tissue (exoerythrocytic) infections.

Pharmacology/kinetics

Absorption
Absorption following oral doses is >90% in most species studied.

Distribution
Primaquine is extensively distributed into fluids and tissues following oral ingestion.

CNS penetration
Primaquine is reported to readily penetrate into the CNS and achieves therapeutic levels.

Metabolism
Metabolism in cats and dogs has not been studied. In other species, primaquine is rapidly metabolized to inert carboxyprimaquine, which undergoes biotransformation to unknown metabolites that are probably more toxic than the parent compound. Less than 1% is excreted unchanged in urine.

Half-life
The half-life in cats is not known. In other species, the half-life of elimination is 4–7 h.

Pregnancy risk factor

Catagory C: Can cause hemolytic anemia in fetuses and is considered contraindicated during pregnancy.

Lactation
No information is available. However, it is expected that primaquine is excreted into milk due to its lipophilic properties. Due to its potential for toxicity in nursing animals it would be contraindicated.

Reference

Birkenheuer, A.J. (2013) Babesiosis. Ch. 75. In: *Canine and Feline Infectious Diseases*, Sykes, J.E. (ed.), Elsevier, St. Louis, MO. pp. 727–738.

Further reading

Ayoob, A.L., Prittie, J., and Hackner, S.G. (2010) Feline babesiosis. *J Vet Emerg Crit Care.*, **20(1)**, 90–97.

Jacobsona, L.S., Schoemana, T., and Lobetti, R.G. (2000) A survey of feline babesiosis in South Africa. *J South African Vet Ass.*, **71(4)**, 222–228.

Penzhorn, B.L., Lewis, B.D., Lopez-Rebollar, L.M., *et al.* (2000) Screening of five drugs for efficacy against *Babesia felis* in experimentally infected cats. *J S Afr Vet Assoc.*, **71(1)**, 53–57.

Potgieter, F.T. (1981) Chemotherapy of *Babesia felis* infection: efficacy of certain drugs. *J S Afr Vet Assoc.*, **52(4)**, 289–293.

Chapter 201: Pyrantel Pamoate

US Generic (Brand) Name: Pyrantel pamoate (Strongid-T, Nemex, Antiminth, Pin-Rid, Pin X, Reese's Pinworm medicine)
Availability: Human Approved – Oral capsule (180 mg = 62.5 mg base), oral liquid 50 mg/mL (30 mL), oral suspension 50 mg/mL (60 mL). Veterinary Approved – Pyrantel pamoate oral suspension for horses 50 mg/mL, pyrantel pamoate oral suspension 4.54 mg/mL (as base) for dogs (60, 120, 280, 473 mL), pyrantel pamoate tablets for dogs (227 and 113.5 mg-base). Multiple other products and combinations, Drontal, Virban Flavored Chews (praziquantel/pyrantel), Drontal Plus (praziquantel, pyrantel, febantel), Heartgard Plus and Tri-Heart Plus Chews (ivermectin/pyrantel).

Use

Pyrantel pamoate is commonly used in small animals for the treatment of roundworms (*T. canis*, *T. leona*), hookworms (*Ancylostoma caninum*), *U. stenocephala* and whipworms (*T. trichiura*). It is also effective against *Physaloptera* spp. in cats. Pyrantel is effective against mature and immature forms of susceptible helminths within the intestinal tract but not against migratory stages in the tissues or against ova. It is used commonly in kittens and puppies as young as 2–3 weeks of age.

Contraindications/warnings

Hypersensitivity to pyrantel pamoate. Caution in patients with severe liver impairment, anemic animals, or those with severe malnutrition. Do not use in pregnant animals.

Dosage

Canine

Susceptible parasites: 10 mg/kg PO (as base) for <5 lbs or 5 mg/kg PO (as base) for >5 lbs at 2, 3, 4, 6, 8, and 10 weeks of age and in lactating bitches at 2–3 week intervals after whelping (Pfizer package Insert).

Hookworms/Roundworms: 5 mg/kg PO once, repeat in 7–10 days with food (Papich 2002).

Feline

Ascarids, hookworms, Physaloptera: 5 mg/kg PO repeat in 14 days (Dimski 1989).

Ancylostoma tubaeformae/Toxocara cati: 20 mg/kg PO × 1 (Ridley *et al.*, 1991).

Dose adjustments

Doses should be reduced (25–50%) for patients with moderate to severe liver impairment.

Administration

Administer oral doses with or without food. Shake suspensions well before administering. For maximum control and prevention of reinfestation, it is recommended that puppies be treated at 2, 3, 4, 6, 8, and 10 weeks of age. Lactating bitches should be treated at 2–3 weeks after whelping. Adult dogs kept in heavily contaminated quarters should be treated at monthly intervals.

Electrolyte contents

Not significant.

Storage/stability

Store at room temperature, protected from light.

Adverse reactions

>10%

Pyrantel pamoate is extremely well tolerated with no or few side effects reported in many dog breeds, ages and conditions. Salivation, nausea, loss of appetite reported in dogs.

1–10%

Vomiting and diarrhea reported in dogs.

Other species

Elevated liver enzymes, drowsiness, insomnia, rash, and ataxia reported in other species. Worsening of preexisting myasthenia gravis in humans.

Drug interactions

Piperazine decreases the effects of pyrantel pamoate. Levamasole, morantel, diethylcarbamazine, and organophosphates increase the risk of side effects.

Monitoring

Repeat stool sample to confirm eradication of eggs/worms. Monitor liver enzymes for prolonged treatment.

Overdose

At doses of 100 mg/kg daily for 3 days in cats there were no side effects, a single dose of 230.6 mg/kg produced vomiting and diarrhea in 2/92 cats. The LD_{50} in dogs is >690 mg/kg, which is in excess of 138 times the recommended dosage. Symptoms may include nausea, vomiting, ataxia, diarrhea, and increased respiratory rates. Gastrointestinal decontamination and supportive care are recommended with extreme overdoses.

Diagnostic test interference

None noted.

Mechanism

The drug is a neuromuscular blocking agent that causes release of acetylcholine and inhibition of cholinesterase. This results in paralysis, which is followed by expulsion of worms.

Pharmacology/kinetics

Absorption
Pyrantel pamoate salt is poorly absorbed from the gastrointestinal tract of cats and dogs, and is active mainly against luminal organisms. Peak plasma levels are reached in 1–3 h.

Distribution
Due to the limited oral absorption, the majority of drug is retained in the intestine and passed out in the feces.

CNS penetration
No information was found on CNS penetration. Due to the CNS side effects noted, at least minimal drug is expected to penetrate.

Metabolism
Pyrantel pamoate undergoes extensive metabolism in dogs. The acidic metabolites are excreted in urine (40% in dogs). In most species, the majority of drug is excreted unchanged in feces (>50%) and only small amounts are excreted in urine.

Half-life
The half-life in most species is approximately 1.5–3 h.

Pregnancy risk factor

Category C: In mice a decrease in liter size, increase in gestation period and increase in stillborn births has been reported. Pyrantel is considered contraindicated in pregnancy.

Lactation
Pyrantel is poorly and incompletely absorbed from the gastrointestinal tract and resulting maternal serum concentrations are low (0.05 to 0.13 µg/mL). Therefore, it is unlikely that significant amounts of pyrantel would be excreted in milk. It is considered safe in lactating animals.

References

Dimski, D.S. (1989) Helminth and noncoccididal protozoan parasites of the gastrointestinal tract. *The Cat: Diseases and Clinical Management. Vol. 1*. Sherding, R.G. (ed.), Churchill Livingstone, New York, pp. 459–477.

Papich, M.G. (2002) *Saunders Handbook of Veterinary Drugs*. 2nd edn. Winkel, A. (ed.), W.B. Saunders Company, Philadelphia, pp. 572–573.

Ridley, R.K., Terhune, K.S., and Granstrom, D.E. (1991) The efficacy of pyrantel pamoate against ascarids and hookworms in cats. *Vet Res Commun.*, **15(1)**, 37–44.

Further reading

Clark, J.N., Pulliam, J.D., and Daurio, C.P. (1992) Safety study of a beef-based chewable tablet formulation of ivermectin and pyrantel pamoate in growing dogs, pups, and breeding adult dogs. *Am J Vet Res.*, **53(4)**, 608–612.

Dryden, M.W. and Ridley, R.K. (1999) Efficacy of fenbendazole granules and pyrantel pamoate suspension against *Toxocara canis* in greyhounds housed in contaminated runs. *Vet Parasitol.*, **82(4)**, 311–315.

Owaki, Y., Sakai, T., and Momiyama, H. (1989) Teratological studies on pyrantel pamoate in rats. *Catalog of Teratogenic Agents.* 6th edn, Johns Hopkins University Press, Baltimore, MD, p. 536.

Reinemeyer, C.R. and DeNovo, R.C. (1990) Evaluation of the efficacy and safety of two formulations of pyrantel pamoate in cats. *Am J Vet Res.*, **51(6)**, 932–934.

Chapter 202: Ronidazole

US Generic (Brand) Name: Ronidazole (no US Brand name. International Brands are Belga, Ronida, Ronizol, Turbosol, Trichocure, Trichorex)
Availability: Not available in the USA. Chemical powder is dangerous to manipulate outside a chemical hood. It is available from Compounding Pharmacies

Use

Ronidazole is an antiprotozoal agent used in veterinary medicine for the treatment of Histomoniasis and swine dysentery. In small animals, it is used for the treatment of *Tritrichomonas foetus* infection in cats.

Contraindications/warnings

Hypersensitivity reactions to ronidazole. Ronidazole is a potentially mutagenic, carcinogenic, and embryotoxic chemical. Avoid long term exposure to the chemical. Owners should wear gloves and understand the risks of exposure. Do not open capsules. Pregnant or lactating owners should not administer the drug or change the litter box while the cat is receiving the drug.

Dosage

Feline

Tritrichomonas foetus: 30 mg/kg PO q24 h × 14 days (Lappin 2013).

Dose adjustments

Not required in mild liver disease. Doses may need to be reduced (25–50%) in severe liver disease or in geriatric patients.

Administration

Owners should wear gloves when administering ronidazole and when cleaning the litter box during treatment. Feces should be double bagged. Capsules should not be opened. The drug is extremely bitter in taste and may be administered with food.

Electrolyte contents

Not significant.

Storage/stability

Store capsules at room temperature. Do not expose the capsules to light for prolonged periods of time.

Adverse reactions

>10%

Drowsiness, weakness, and loss of appetite reported in cats.

1–10%

Nausea, vomiting, and diarrhea reported in cats.

<1%

With high doses: ataxia, seizures, nystagmus, and decreased heart rate reported in cats.

Drug interactions

Ronidazole interactions not reported specifically. Similar to metronidazole it may cause increases in the effects of oral anticoagulants. Phenobarbital may decrease its half-life; cimetidine may increase serum concentrations and toxicity.

Monitoring

Get baseline CBC, total and differential leukocyte count, and liver enzymes.

Overdose

Symptoms may include nausea, vomiting, ataxia, seizures, neuropathy, mydriasis, nystagmus, and bradycardia. Gastrointestinal decontamination and supportive care may be required. Hemodialysis may remove 50–100% of a dose. Diazepam can be used for seizures.

Diagnostic test interference

Can alter ALT, AST, triglycerides, glucose, and LDH testing.

Mechanism

Ronidazole is bactericidal. It is a nitroimidazole that is reduced to a compound that interacts with DNA resulting in bacterial, protozoal DNA damage, and inhibition of protein synthesis.

Pharmacology/kinetics

Absorption
After oral administration to cats, absorption is rapid and complete (99.6%).

Distribution
Ronidazole is widely distributed into tissues and fluids. High concentrations are reported in brain, fat, heart, kidney, liver, lung, muscle, pancreas, skin, and spleen. Tissue residues may have prolonged concentrations compared to plasma levels.

CNS penetration
There is no data reported. Ronidazole is expected to have significant penetration into the CNS similar to metronidazole (43%: uninflamed, 100%: inflamed).

Metabolism
Extensively metabolized in the liver. Multiple metabolites have been noted in other species (2-hydroxymethyl, N-methylglycolamide, methylamine, and oxalic

acid). Ronidazole is excreted in the urine (30–36%) and feces (16–40%).

Half-life
The half-life in cats is 10.5 h following oral administration.

Pregnancy risk factor

Category C: Ronidazole is embryotoxic in mice, rats, and rabbits, and is carcinogenic in mice and rats. It is contraindicated in pregnancy.

Lactation
Ronidazole is excreted into milk and has been shown to be carcinogenic to a variety of animal species. It would be considered contraindicated in lactating animals.

Reference

Lappin, M.R. (2013) Trichomoniasis. Ch. 80. In: *Canine and Feline Infectious Diseases*, Sykes, J.E. (ed.), Elsevier, St. Louis, MO. pp. 779–784.

Further reading

Gookin, J.L., Copple, C.N., Papich, M.G., *et al.* (2006) Efficacy of ronidazole for treatment of feline *Tritrichomonas foetus* infection. *J Vet Intern Med.*, **20(3)**, 536–543.

LeVine, D.N., Papich, M.G., Gookin, J.L., *et al.* (2011) Ronidazole pharmacokinetics after intravenous and oral immediate-release capsule administration in healthy cats. *J Feline Med Surg.*, **13(4)**, 244–250.

Papich, M.G., Levine, D.N., Gookin, J.L., *et al.* (2013) Ronidazole pharmacokinetics in cats following delivery of a delayed release guar gum formulation. *J Vet Pharmacol Ther.*, **36(4)**, 399–407.

Chapter 203: Selamectin

US Generic (Brand) Name: Selamectin (Revolution)
Availability: Veterinary Approved – Selamectin topical solution (Revolution) 60 and 120 mg/mL. Cats: 15, 45 mg tubes) and Dogs: 15, 30, 60, 120, 240 mg tubes

Use

Selamectin is used in dogs to prevent heartworm, control fleas, mites, ticks, and ear mites. It is also indicated in the treatment of sarcoptic mange. In cats it is used to control fleas, prevent heartworm, control ear mites, and for the treatment of roundworm (*T. cati*) and hookworms (*A. tubaeforme*). Selamectin does not treat adult heartworms and does not clear microfilariae. It is active against *D. immitis* larval stages 3, 4 and early fifth. It kills adult fleas within 36 h but does not prevent existing pupae from emerging.

Contraindications/warnings

Hypersensitivity to selamectin or other avermectins. Use caution in patients with compromised blood-brain barrier disorders (meningitis), seizures or in breeds (Australian shepherds, collies, long-haired whippets, and Shelties) with a predilection toward mutation of the ABCB1–1Δ gene. Selmectin appears to be much safer than ivermectin in animals with mutation of ABCB1–1Δ gene. Use caution in debilitated, sick, or underweight animals.

Dosage

Canine/ feline
Heartworm prevention/ear mites/fleas: 6–12 mg/kg applied topically every 30 days (Papich 2002).

Sarcoptic Mange/Nasal mites: 6–12 mg/kg topically 30 days apart × 2 doses or at 2–3 week intervals (Papich 2002).

Dose adjustments

Dose adjustments (25–50%) may be required in severe liver failure.

Administration

Heartworm test prior to administration. Revolution is formulated to deliver 2.7 mg/lb (6 mg/kg) of body weight. Administer once monthly. Avoid contact with skin in humans, may cause hives, itching, and redness. Avoid application onto abraded skin. It is recommended for dogs >6 weeks of age and cats ≥8 weeks of age. Firmly press the cap down to puncture. Remove cap. Administer the entire contents of a single tube (unless

>130 lb, then 2 tubes are needed). Part hair on the back of the animal at the base of the neck in front of shoulder blades until skin is visible. Squeeze tube 3–4 times onto skin. Do not message into skin. Do not apply onto wet hair and do not bathe for 2 or more hours after application.

Electrolyte contents

Not significant. Vehicle contains isopropyl alcohol and butylated hydroxytoluene.

Storage/stability

Store at room temperature in manufacturer's packaging. Avoid storage next to heat, sparks, and open flames.

Adverse reactions

>10%
Stiff or clumping of hair, discoloration, and powdery residue, typically temporary in cats and dogs.

1–10%
Alopecia and inflammation at application site in cats.

<1%
Rarely nausea, lethargy, salivation, tachypnea, muscle tremors, diarrhea, vomiting, anorexia, pruritus, urticaria, and erythema in dogs and cats. With high doses, seizures, ataxia in cats and dogs reported. Oral administration of the topical formulation causes mild, intermittent, self-limiting salivation, and vomiting in cats. When administered to heartworm infected animals and animals of reproductive age, selamectin demonstrated no adverse effects.

Drug interactions

Barbiturates, benzodiazepines may increase side effects when combined with selamectin. Amiodarone, carvedilol, clarithromycin, cyclosporine, erythromycin, itraconazole, ketoconazole, quinidine, and verapamil may inhibit P-glycoprotein and increase toxicity of selamectin. Inducers of P-glycoprotein (clotrimazole, phenothiazines, rifampin, St. John's wort) may decrease selamectin concentrations.

Monitoring

Observe breeds with likelihood of ABCB1–1Δ for up to 8 h after administering for signs of toxicity. Repeat stool examinations to confirm clearance of worm burden. Repeat heartworm test yearly.

Overdose

Symptoms may include mydriasis, ataxia, vomiting, tachycardia, lethargy, and seizures and may appear 8–10 h after administration. Emesis and/or gastrointestinal lavage should be done as soon as possible. Additional purgatives, parenteral fluids, electrolytes, pressor agents, and respiratory support may be required. Most animals should begin to improve neurologically within 2–5 days, but may take weeks for complete recovery.

Diagnostic test interference

False negative heartworm tests are unlikely since the antibody tests measure antigen to the adult female *D. immitis* oviduct.

Mechanism

Selamectin binds selectively to glutamine-gated-chloride ion channels (GABA) in invertebrate nerve cells. This leads to an increased permeability of parasitic nerve and muscle cells to chloride ions with subsequent hyperpolarization and death of susceptible parasites.

Pharmacology/kinetics

Absorption
Selamectin is minimally absorbed via transdermal absorption in dogs (5%) but has much higher absorption in cats (75%). Peak absorption occurs in 3 days in dogs and within 15 h in cats. Grooming, resulting in oral ingestion of topically applied selamectin as well as a greater transdermal flux rate, may account for its high bioavailability in cats. Oral absorption of the topical formulation is >60% in cats and dogs.

Distribution
Selamectin is distributed into sebaceous glands, hair follicles, and basal layers of the epithelium. It is distributed into the blood stream and excreted into

the gastrointestinal tract where it is active against endo-parasites. Substantial amounts of circulating selamectin are deposited in the sebaceous glands which act as reservoirs to provide persistent activity against ectopar-asites mainly during the blood meal.

CNS penetration

Selamectin readily penetrates into CSF with brain:plasma ratios of 0.32 vs ivermectin 0.09. However, with ABCB1–1Δ mutations the ratios switch to 1.6 for selamectin versus 6.5 for ivermectin suggesting that selamectin may be the drug of choice in animals with these gene mutations.

Metabolism

Selamectin is metabolized in the liver of cats and dogs. Dogs have very little metabolism compared to cats and metabolic routes are different between species. Dogs excrete the parent drug into feces (40–64%), shed fur (40–64%), and urine (1–3%). Minor metabolites (hydroxylated and O-desmethylated) are found in small amounts in dog feces (<10%). In cats, selamectin is metabolized via oxidation into carboxylic acid metabolites. Parent drug (26–43%) and O-desmethyl glycoside (3%) are primarily excreted via feces (48–60%), with 1–3% excreted in urine.

Half-life

Half-life in dogs is 11 days and in cats is 8 days.

Pregnancy risk factor

Selamectin has been administered at 40 and 10 days before parturition and 10 and 40 days after parturi-tion to dams topically at a minimum unit dosage of 6 mg/kg with naturally acquired *T. canis* infections and experimentally induced *C. felis* infestations. Selamectin was safe and highly effective in the treatment, control, and prevention of adult *T. canis* infection and *C. felis* infestation affecting both the dams and their pups. It had no apparent teratogenic or fetotoxic effects.

Lactation

Selamectin is excreted into milk but appears to be safe in lactating pups. Following doses of 6 mg/kg to the dam during pregnancy, mean fecal egg counts in lactating pups were reduced by >96% on the twenty-fourth (24th) and thirty-fourth (34th) days after birth and the number of adult worms recovered from the gastrointes-tinal tract of pups from selamectin-treated dams was reduced by 98.2%.

Reference

Papich, M.G. (2002) *Saunders Handbook of Veterinary Drugs*. 2nd edn. Winkel, A. (ed.), W.B. Saunders Company, Philadelphia, pp. 593–594.

Further reading

Krautmann, M.J., Novotny, M.J., DeKeulenaer, K., *et al.* (2000) Safety of selamectin in cats. *Vet Parasitol.*, **91(3–4)**, 393–403.

Novotny, M.J., Krautmann, MJ, Ehrhart, J.C., *et al.* (2000) Safety of selamectin in dogs. *Vet Parasitol.*, **91(3–4)**, 377–391.

Payne-Johnson, M., Maitland, T.P., Sherington, J., *et al.* (2000) Efficacy of selamectin administered topically to pregnant and lactating female dogs in the treatment and prevention of adult roundworm (*Toxocara canis*) infections and flea (*Ctenocephalides felis felis*) infestations in the dams and their pups. *Vet Parasitol.*, **91(3–4)**, 347–358.

Chapter 204: Spinosid

US Generic (Brand) Name: Spinosad (Comfortis, Natroba Topical)

Availability: Veterinary Approved – Spinosad oral chew tablets 140, 270, 560, 810, and 1620 mg (Comfortis), spinosad in combination with melbe-mycin (Trifexis), Human Approved – Spinosad 0.9% topical suspension (120 mL)

Use

Spinosad is a pediculicide and is generally used as an insecticide in veterinary medicine. Spinosad is used orally to treat the adult cat flea (*C. felis*), in cats and dogs. Spinosad plus milbemycin (Trifexis) prevents heart-worm disease and treats and controls adult hookworm, roundworm, and whipworm infections. Trifexis is not effective against adult *D. immitis*.

Contraindications/warnings

Hypersensitivity to spinosad or animals with pork or soy allergies. Do not use in combination with high doses of ivermectin. Use caution in animals with poor body condition due to increased risk of neurologic signs and other side effects. Caution in animals with CNS disease and seizures. Avoid environmental contamination, highly toxic to bees and other beneficial insects. Comfortis tablets must not be used in dogs or cats <14 weeks of age.

Dosage

Accurate dosing is not possible in dogs weighing <1.3 kg and in cats weighing <1.2 kg. The use of the product in smaller dogs and cats is therefore not recommended.

Canine

Flea prevention and control: 30–60 mg/kg PO once a month with food (Comfortis: Lilly Manufacturer's Label).

Flea/Heartworm/Intestinal parasites: Spinosad 30 mg/kg PO with milbemycin oxime 0.5 mg/kg PO once a month (Trifexis) Elanco Manufacturer's Package insert).

Feline

Flea prevention and control: 50 mg/kg PO once a month with food. For cats over 24 lbs administer the appropriate combination of tablets (Comfortis: Lilly Manufacturer's Label).

Dose adjustments

Dose adjustments are not required in renal impairment, for severe liver impairment, monitor closely, and lower dose if side effects are apparent.

Administration

Spinosad/milbemycin is applied once monthly at intervals beginning within 1 month of the dog's first seasonal exposure and continuing until at least 3 months after the dog's last seasonal exposure to mosquitoes. Test for heartworm prior to administration of Trifexis. Treatment with fewer than 3 monthly doses after the last exposure to mosquitoes may not provide complete heartworm prevention. Flea treatment and prevention with spinosad alone (Comfortis) should start one month before fleas become active and continue monthly through the end of flea season. To minimize reinfestation, treat all animals in the household. The tablets should be given with food to prevent nausea. Spinosad is given orally once monthly and does not wash off with bathing or swimming. If vomiting occurs within 1 h of dosing, redose with a full dose.

Electrolyte contents

Not significant.

Storage/stability

Store at room temperature, protected from light.

Adverse reactions

>10%
Nausea and vomiting in cats and dogs (greater in puppies <14 weeks of age)

1–10%
Lethargy, decreased appetite, weight loss, and diarrhea in dogs and cats. Incoordination, ataxia and itching reported in dogs.

<1%
Trembling, excessive salivation, seizures, elevations in liver enzymes, and phospholipidosis (vacuolation) of the lymphoid tissues reported in dogs. In combination with ivermectin, the incidence of these side effects increased as well as excessive dilation of pupils, blindness, and disorientation. In combination with milbemycin (Trifexis), mild, transient hypersensitivity reactions manifested as labored respiration, vomiting, salivation, and lethargy, have been noted in some dogs treated with milbemycin oxime carrying a high number of circulating microfilariae. These reactions are presumably caused by release of protein from dead or dying microfilariae.

Drug interactions

Avoid use in combination with ivermectin. Spinosad has been shown to be a substrate for P-glycoprotein. Spinosad could interact with other P-glycoprotein substrates (digoxin, doxorubicin) and possibly enhance adverse reactions or decrease efficacy.

Monitoring

Baseline heartworm testing and yearly testing if using Trifexis. Get baseline liver panel and monitor yearly.

Overdose

Overdoses (3–5×) result in vomiting and nausea. Higher doses may result in seizures. With chronic overdosing, weight loss, elevations in ALT, and cytoplasmic vacuolations, in the liver, lung, and adrenal gland. Gastrointestinal decontamination and supportive care may be necessary. Diazepam can be used for seizure control.

Diagnostic test interference

None reported.

Mechanism

Spinosad is a non-antibacterial tetracyclic macrolide insecticide. Spinosad contains two major elements, spinosyn A and spinosyn D, derived from the naturally occurring bacterium, Saccharopolyspora spinosa. Spinosyn A resembles a GABA antagonist and acts similar to avermectin on insect neurons. It activates nicotinic acetylcholine receptors (nAChRs) in insects.

Pharmacology/kinetics

Absorption
Maximum oral absorption occurs at 5 h in dogs.

Distribution
Spinosad is readily distributed throughout tissues and fluids. High concentrations are reported in the liver, lung, kidney, thyroid, and plasma.

CNS penetration
Spinosad penetrates into the CNS in concentrations that potentiate ivermectin neurotoxicity in susceptible breeds.

Metabolism
Spinosad is metabolized in the liver by O- or N-demethylation. It then undergoes conjugation with glutathione. Conjugates are excreted in feces and urine.

Half-life
The half-life in dogs is 10 days.

Pregnancy risk factor

No teratogenic effects have been reported. However, dams exposed during pregnancy were reported to have greater vomiting than controls and pups had lower body weight, lethargy, dehydration, weakness, and a lower body temperature. Benefits should be weighed against risks in pregnancy.

Lactation

Spinosad is excreted in the milk of dogs. When a dose (1.5×) was given at 28 weeks gestation and at 24 h prior to parturition, mortality and morbidity were greatest in pups from dams with the highest spinosyn levels in milk. Milk concentrations were 2.2–3.5 times the plasma concentrations of the dam. It is not considered safe in lactating animals.

Further reading

Dunn, S.T., Hedges, L., Sampson, K.E., *et al.* (2011) Pharmacokinetic interaction of the antiparasitic agents ivermectin and spinosad in dogs. *Drug Metab Dispos.*, **39(5)**, 789–795.

Holstrom, S.D., Totten, M.L., Newhall, K.B., *et al.* (2012) Pharmacokinetics of spinosad and milbemycin oxime administered in combination and separately per os to dogs. *J Vet Pharmacol Ther.*, **35(4)**, 351–364.

Snyder, D.E. and Wiseman, S. (2012) Dose confirmation and non-interference evaluations of the oral efficacy of a combination of milbemycin oxime and spinosad against the dose limiting parasites, adult cat flea (*Ctenocephalides felis*) and hookworm (*Ancylostoma caninum*) in dogs. *Vet Parasitol.*, **184(2–4)**, 284–290.

Chapter 205: Sulfadimethoxine

US Generic (Brand) Name: Sulfadimethoxine (Albon, Di-Methox)
Availability: Veterinary Labeled Only – Tablets 125, 250, 500 mg, oral suspension 50 mg/mL × 2, 16 oz, sterile injectable 400 mg/mL × 100 mL

Use

Active against a variety of organisms including *Streptococcus* spp., *Staphylococcus* spp., *E. coli*, *Klebsiella*, *Enterobacter* spp., *Proteus*, *Aeromonas*, *Bordetella* spp., *Burkheria*, *Cyclospora*, *Isospora*, *Moraxella*, *Shigella*, *Stenotrophomonas*, and anaerobes. However, resistance develops rapidly in bacteria, so it is commonly combined with ormetoprim. It has been used in veterinary medicine to treat urinary tract, respiratory, and soft tissue infections. Currently used in small animals for the treatment of *Coccidia*.

Contraindications/warnings

Hypersensitivity to sulfas. Avoid in severe liver and renal impairment, anemia, dehydrated, malnourished, thyroid dysfunctional, animals with blood dyscrasias, or very young animals. Do not use in pregnant or lactating animals. Doberman pinchers are more susceptible to idiosyncratic sulfonamide toxicosis compared to other breeds. Slow acetylators (canines) at increased risk of toxicities. Avoid in animals (cats) with pre-existing urinary obstruction or urolithiasis.

Dosage

For bacterial infections: Length of treatment depends on the clinical response. Treatment should be continued until the animal is asymptomatic for 48 h. As an anti-protozoal, the length of treatment depends on the life cycle of the specific parasite, as well as environmental factors (multi-animal household, littermates, hygiene, etc.), and immune status.

Canine

Susceptible infections: 100 mg/kg PO loading dose; followed by 50 mg/kg PO q12 h (Papich 2002) or 55 mg/kg Loading dose IV or PO: followed by 27.5 mg/kg q24 h IV or PO (Pfizer package insert).

Isospora spp./*Coccidiosis:* 50–60 mg/kg PO q24 h × 5–20 days (Lappin 2013).

Feline

Susceptible infections: 100 mg/kg PO loading dose; followed by 50 mg/kg PO q12 h (Papich 2002) or 55 mg/kg Loading dose IV or PO: followed by 27.5 mg/kg q24 h IV or PO (Pfizer package insert).

Isospora spp./*Coccidiosis:* 50–60 mg/kg PO q24 h × 5–20 days (Lappin 2013).

Dose adjustments

Doses should be reduced (25–50%) in impaired renal function. The dose and/or frequency should be modified in response to the degree of renal impairment.

Administration

Animals must be well hydrated prior to and during drug therapy. The appropriate dose should be withdrawn and given IV. Albon oral suspension comes in a custard-flavored carrier, shake well prior to dosing. The tablets and oral suspension can be given with food.

Electrolyte contents

Not significant.

Storage/stability

Store tablets, oral solution and injectable solutions at room temperature, protected from light. The injectable may crystallize at cold temperatures; crystals will dissolve either by storing at room temperature for several days or by heating the vial in warm water. Crystallization and redissolution do not impair the efficacy of the product.

Adverse reactions

>10%

Keratoconjunctivitis sicca (up to 15% in small dogs <12 kg), nausea, vomiting, and anorexia reported in dogs. Anorexia reported in cats.

1–10%

Diarrhea, depression, fever, pruritus, and facial swelling reported in dogs. Leukopenia and anemia reported in cats.

<1%

Idiosyncratic toxicosis reported in dogs at 8–20 days after starting treatment (blood dyscrasias including anemia, leucopenia, and thrombocytopenia), fever, focal retinitis, lymphadenopathy, non-septic polyarthritis, polymyositis, and skin rash: greater in Doberman pinschers and with prior sulfa exposure). Samoyeds and miniature schnauzers may also have an increased risk of toxicities. Typically reversible 2–5 days after sulfa is discontinued. Non-regenerative anemia with high dose, long term (60–120 mg/kg q24 h) therapy. Iatrogenic hypothyroidism in dogs with high doses (25 mg/kg q12 h × 6 weeks), hemolytic/aplastic anemia, cutaneous drug eruptions, erythema multiforme, perforating folliculitis, fever, severe hepatitis, aggression, ataxia, thrombocytopenia, seizures, hyperexcitability, and polyuria/polydipsia.

Other species

Crystallization of acetylated sulfa metabolite in urine with aciduria or dehydration (potentially not in dogs due to low acetylation), nephritis, hyperkalemia, hyper/hypoglycemia, pancreatitis, fatal hepatitis, dermatologic reactions, and kernicterus in neonates.

Drug interactions

In humans, sulfas may increase the plasma concentrations/toxicity of bone marrow suppressants, dapsone, amantidine, sulfonylureas, digoxin, oral anticoagulants, and procainamide. Sulfas may decrease the efficacy of tricyclic antidepressants and cyclosporine. Hepatotoxic drugs may increase the risk of hepatotoxicity from sulfas. Thiazide diuretics may increase sulfa-induced thrombocytopenia and pyrimethamine may increase the risk of sulfa induced megaloblastic anemia. Sulfas may increase the risk of hyperkalemia from ACE inhibitors and may decrease the efficacy of live vaccines. Antacids maydecreasethe bioavailability of sulfadimethoxine.

Monitoring

Monitor CBC with platelets and Schirmer's tear test closely if on long term therapy. Monitor for signs/symptoms of allergic/autoimmune disease. Monitor serum potassium if on concurrent ACE inhibitors.

Overdose

Nausea, vomiting, hypoglycemia, seizures, and colitis may be seen. Delayed toxicity may include bone marrow suppression and hepatotoxicosis. Gastrointestinal decontamination /lavage, fluid therapy, and diazepam for seizures are advised. Anemia may be reversible with folinic acid (Leucovorin) supplementation. Hemodialysis only removes a small portion of the drug.

Diagnostic test interference

False positive urine glucose (Benedict's), elevated (10%) creatinine with Jaffe reaction, false positive urine protein, false positive urine urobilinogen test, Thyroid tests (T4 and thyrotropin stimulation) may be significantly reduced (no alteration in T3).

Mechanism

Bacteriostatic sulfonamide. Inhibits bacterial utilization of para-aminobenzoic acid (PABA) for folic acid synthesis. It inhibits dihydrofolic acid formation. Trimethoprim and ormetroprim inhibits dihydrofolic acid reduction to tetrahydrofolate resulting in dual inhibition of enzyme in the folic acid pathway.

Pharmacology/kinetics

Absorption
Sulfadimethoxazole is rapidly absorbed following oral doses in cats and dogs. The oral suspension has variable absorption in dogs 32.8% (22.5–80.0%).

Distribution
Sulfas are widely distributed throughout most tissues and fluids, including the middle ear, prostate, bile, aqueous humor, CSF, peritoneal fluid, synovial fluid, and urine. Protein binding in dogs is >75% and in cats is 87.5%.

CNS penetration
Penetration of sulfadimethoxine into the CSF is very limited (2.7%). However, sulfas can accumulate in CSF over time with repeat dosing.

Metabolism
Sulfas are metabolized in the liver/tissues in most species (cats, humans) to N-acetyl metabolites. These metabolites are then glucuronidated and excreted into urine where their poor solubility may be the cause of crystalluria. In dogs, acetylation is limited, so sulfas are primarily excreted (>60%) as the active parent compound. The parent drug is soluble in urine and less likely to precipitate out to cause crystalluria.

Half-life
The half-life of sulfadimethoxazole in dogs is 13.1 h. In cats, the half-life is 10.2 h.

Pregnancy risk factor

Category C–D: Sulfonamides cross the placenta and are reported to cause significant teratogenic effects in mice and rats (malformations, cleft palates). Fetal toxic effects are also reported in late term pregnancy. Sulfonamides are contraindicated in pregnancy.

Lactation
Sulfonamides are distributed into milk in small quantities (0.5–2%). It is considered contraindicated during nursing.

References

Lappin, M.R. (2013) Isoporiasis. Ch. 82. In: *Canine and Feline Infectious Diseases*, Sykes, J.E. (ed.), Elsevier, St. Louis, MO. pp. 793–796.

Papich, M.G. (2002) *Saunders Handbook of Veterinary Drugs*. 2nd edn. Winkel, A. (ed.), W.B. Saunders Company, Philadelphia, pp. 438–439.

Further reading

Baggot, J.D. (1977) Pharmacokinetics of sulfadimethoxine in cats. *Aust J Exp Biol Med Sci.*, **55(6)**, 663–670.

Baggott, J.D., Ludden, T.M., and Powers, T.E. (1976) The bioavailability, disposition kinetics and dosage of sulphadimethoxine in dogs. *Can J Comp Med.*, **40**, 310–317.

Ford, R.B. and Aronson, A.L. (1985) Antimicrobial drugs and infectious disease. *Handbook of Small Animal Therapeutics*. Davis, L.E. (ed.), Churchill Livingstone, New York, pp. 45–88.

Morgan, R.V. and Bachrach, A. (1982) Keratoconjunctivitis sicca associated with sulfonamide therapy in dogs. *J Am Vet Med Assoc.*, **180**, 432–434.

Weiss, D.J. and Klausner, J.S. (1990) Drug-associated aplastic anemia in dogs: eight cases (1984–1988). *J Am Vet Med Assoc.*, **196(3)**, 472–475.

Chapter 206: Tinidazole

US Generic (Brand) Name: Tinidazole (Tinamax, Fasigyn, Simplotan)
Availability: Human Approved – Oral tablets 250 and 500 mg. Compounded oral suspension (66.7 mg/mL)

Use

Tinidazole is an anti-parasitic drug used against protozoan infections. It is widely known throughout Europe and the developing world as a treatment for a variety of amoebic and parasitic infections. It is chemically similar to metronidazole and has similar side effects, but has a shorter treatment course. It is considered an alternative to metronidazole for infections from *Amoebae, Giardia,* and *Trichomonas.* Tinidazole may also be used to treat a variety of other bacterial infections and can be used for combination therapy for *H. pylori.*

Contraindications/warnings

Hypersensitivity to tinidazole or metronidazole. Do not use in pregnant animals. Reduce dose frequency with severe liver, renal, or CNS disease. Use with caution in patients with a history of blood dyscrasias or seizures.

Dosage

Canine
Anaerobic Infections: 15–25 mg/kg PO q12 h (Greene *et al.,* 2006).

Giardia: 44 mg/kg PO q24 h for 3 days (Lappin 2013).

Feline
Anaerobic Infections: 15 mg/kg IV q24 h for 7 days (Greene *et al.,* 2006).

Giardia: 30 mg/kg PO q24 h for 3 days (Lappin 2013).

Dose adjustments

Not required in mild liver disease. Reduce dose (25–50%) in severe liver disease. Reduced doses may be necessary in geriatric patients.

Administration

Tinidazole tablets are taken with food. A suspension can be compounded for more accurate dosing in small animals. A 66.7 mg/mL suspension can be made by crushing 4 × 500 mg tablets in a mortar. Pour 30 mL of cherry syrup into a graduate vial. Add a small amount of cherry syrup (10 mL) and mix until a uniform suspension is made then pour into an amber glass/plastic dispensing bottle. Use the remaining cherry syrup to rinse the mortar and carefully transfer the remaining drug residue into the amber pour top vial until the final volume equals 30 mL. Label and store at room temperature for up to 7 days. Shake the suspension well before dosing and given with food (Tindamax Package Insert: Mission Pharm).

Electrolyte contents

Not significant.

Storage/stability

Keep in a tightly closed container protected from light, at room temperature. Discard remaining liquid after 7 days.

Adverse reactions

>10%
Lethargy, bitter taste, nausea, salivation, and loss of appetite in cats and dogs.

1–10%
Itchiness, ataxia, depression, hepatotoxicity, vomiting, and diarrhea reported in cats and dogs.

<1%

Most toxicities are dose related. Neurotoxicity with large doses including; seizures (cats), recumbency, opisthotonus, positional nystagmus, and muscle spasms.

Other species

Sensory polyneuropathy, syncope, nervousness, transient leucopenia and neutropenia, thrombocytopenia, bone marrow aplasia, polyuria, red/brown urine, photosensitivity, and metallic taste.

Drug interactions

In humans, tinidazole increases the effects of oral anticoagulants, phenobarbital decreases the serum half-life of tinidazole, cimetidine increases tinidazole concentrations and toxicity. Cyclosporine and tacrolimus concentrations may increase plasma concentrations/toxicities. Tinidazole may increase fluorouracil associated toxicities.

Monitoring

CBC, get baseline total and differential leukocyte count, and liver enzymes.

Overdose

Symptoms may include nausea, vomiting, ataxia, seizures, and neuropathy. Mydriasis, nystagmus, and bradycardia may occur in dogs at high doses or with chronic dosing. Gastrointestinal decontamination and supportive care may be required. Hemodialysis removes 50–100% of a dose. Diazepam can be used for seizures.

Diagnostic test interference

Can alter ALT, AST, triglycerides, glucose, and LDH testing.

Mechanism

Bactericidal nitroimidazole. Tinidazole is reduced to a compound that interacts with DNA resulting in bacterial, protozoal DNA damage, and inhibition of protein synthesis. The nitro-group of tinidazole is reduced by cell extracts of *Trichomonas*. The free nitro-radical generated as a result of this reduction may be responsible for the antiprotozoal activity.

Pharmacology/kinetics

Absorption

Tinidazole is well absorbed (88–129%) after oral dosing.

Distribution

Tinidazole is widely distributed throughout body tissues and fluids. High concentrations are noted in the gastrointestinal and genital tract, the buccal cavity, and the CSF.

CNS penetration

Tinidazole readily penetrates into the CNS.

Metabolism

Little is known about the metabolic route of tinidazole in cats and dogs. In humans, metabolism primary occurs in the liver by oxidation, hydroxylation, and conjugation. The parent drug and a 2-hydroxymethyl metabolite are the primary components found in plasma. Protein binding is 12%. Tinidazole is excreted in the urine (20–25%) mainly as unchanged drug. Approximately 12% of the drug is excreted in the feces.

Half-life

The half-life in dogs is 4.4 h and in cats is 8.4 h.

Pregnancy risk factor

Category C: Tinidazole crosses the placenta and should not be used in the first trimester of pregnancy where the drug has been shown to be teratogenic.

Lactation

Tinidazole penetrates into milk and has been noted to be tumorigenic. The risks most likely outweigh the benefits in nursing animals.

References

Greene, C.E., Hartmann, K., *et al.* (2006) Antimicrobial drug formulary. Appendix 8. In: *Infectious Disease of the Dog and Cat.* Greene, C.E. (ed.), Elsevier, St. Louis, MO, pp. 1186–1333.

Lappin, M.R. (2013) Giardiasis. Ch. 79. In: *Canine and Feline Infectious Diseases*, Sykes, J.E. (ed.), Elsevier, St. Louis, MO. pp. 771–778.

Further reading

Coker, H.A., Essien, E.E., and Edoho, E.J. (1990) N-oxidation: a possible route of tinidazole metabolism in man. *Afr J Med Sci.*, **19(2)**, 111–114.

Gookin, J.L., Stauffer, S.H., Coccaro, M.R., *et al.* (2007) Efficacy of tinidazole for treatment of cats experimentally infected with *Tritrichomonas foetus*. *Amer J Vet Res.*, **68(10)**, 1085–1088.

Sarkiala, E., Jarvinen, A., Valttila, S., *et al.* (1991) Pharmacokinetics of tinidazole in dogs and cats. *J Vet Pharmacol Ther.*, **14(3)**, 257–262.

Wood, B.A., Faulkner, J.K., and Monro, A.M. (1982) The pharmacokinetics, metabolism and tissue distribution of tinidazole. *J Antimicrob Chemother.*, **10(Suppl A)**, 43–57.

SECTION G
Antiviral Agents

Chapter 207: Acyclovir

US Generic (Brand) Name: Acyclovir (Zovirax)
Availability: Human Approved – Acyclovir tablets 400, 800 mg; capsules 200 mg; oral suspension 200 mg/5 mL (473 mL), acyclovir sodium for sterile injection 50 mg/mL; sterile powder for injection 500, 1000 mg per vial (50 mg/mL after dilution); acyclovir topical ointment (50 mg/g × 15 g), cream (50 mg/g × 2 g), ophthalmic ointment (3% w/w × 4.5 g)
Resistance Mechanisms: Absent, reduced or altered viral thymidine kinase, altered viral DNA polymerase

Use

In humans, acyclovir is used in the treatment and prophylaxis of human recurrent mucosal and cutaneous herpes simplex (HSV-1 and HSV-2) infections, herpes simplex encephalitis, herpes zoster, and varicella-zoster infections. In small animals, it has been used to treat feline herpesvirus-1 (FHV-1) infections but is considered more toxic when given systemically and less effective than newer antiherpesviral drugs (cidofovir, famciclovir, etc.). Ophthalmic preparations are safer, but must be administered five times daily to be effective. It has also been used orally to treat puppies with canine herpesvirus (CHV-1) infections, although further research is needed.

Contraindications/warnings

Caution in animals with prior renal/hepatic impairment or neurologic impairment. Avoid concurrent use of other nephrotoxic drugs. Correct any dehydration/electrolyte imbalances prior to giving acyclovir.

Dosage

Dose on either lean body weight or total body weight. Base on the smaller of the two.

Feline
FHV-1 Infections: 10–25 mg/kg PO q12 h. Systemic use in cats should generally be avoided due to the potential for toxicity. Ophthalmic ointment 3% administered 5 × daily.

Canine
CHV-1 Infections: 20 mg/kg PO q6 h × 7 days.

Dose adjustments

Adjust dose in renal failure. In moderate impairment, increase the dose interval according to the degree of renal impairment (administer q24 h in cats or q12 h in dogs). In severe renal impairment (administer 50% of the dose q24 h in cats or q12 h in dogs).

Administration

Acyclovir tablets and capsules may be taken with or without food.

Electrolyte contents

Not significant.

Storage/stability

Store tablets, capsules, and oral suspension at room temperature, protected from light. Ophthalmic ointment maintains sterility for 28 days after opening. Extemporaneous

Drug Therapy for Infectious Diseases of the Dog and Cat, First Edition. Valerie J. Wiebe.
© 2015 John Wiley & Sons, Inc. Published 2015 by John Wiley & Sons, Inc.

suspensions made from tablets/capsules are not stable and should be made only just prior to dosing.

Adverse reactions

>10%
Anorexia and nausea in cats and dogs.

1–10%
Vomiting, lethargy, diarrhea, and ataxia in dogs and cats and tremors in cats.

<1%
Reversible leucopenia and mild non-regenerative anemia in cats at high doses (100 mg/kg). Swollen eye lids following ophthalmic administration in cats.

Other species
Seizures, confusion, agitation, insomnia, coma, rash, pruritus, photosensitivity, rashes, impaired renal function, elevated liver enzymes, hepatitis, edema, neutropenia, neutrophilia, anemia, hemolysis, hemoglobinemia, and thrombocytopenia, are reported.

Drug interactions

Avoid other drugs that are nephrotoxic (amphotericin B, furosemide, aminoglycosides, etc.) or those capable of causing neurologic signs (high dose beta-lactams, etc.).

Monitoring

Obtain baseline CBC, renal/liver panel, urinalysis. Then monitor every 2–3 weeks for chronic therapy.

Overdose

Generally lethargy, nausea, vomiting, and diarrhea occur at mildly elevated doses. Higher doses (>189 mg/kg in dogs) may result in seizures, azotemia, polyuria, polydipsia, or acute renal failure. Gastrointestinal decontamination (emesis, activated charcoal) if oral overdose of >150 mg/kg is recommended. Supportive care may include fluid therapy for diuresis and diazepam for seizures. Hemodialysis removes approximately 60% of a dose.

Diagnostic test interference

None noted.

Mechanism

Acyclovir is converted inside cells to acyclovir monophosphate and then further converted to acyclovir triphosphate by intracellular enzymes. Acyclovir triphosphate competes with deoxyguanosine triphosphate for viral DNA polymerase and is incorporated into the viral DNA. The result is inhibition of viral DNA synthesis and thus virus replication.

Pharmacology/kinetics

Absorption
Oral absorption is highly variable in dogs and cats and appears dose dependent. Bioavailability in cats is low. In dogs, peak plasma drug concentrations are reached within 2 h of dosing. Bioavailability in dogs is between 80 and 91%. At high doses (50 mg/kg) there is a declined to 52%, suggesting a saturable process.

Distribution
Acyclovir is widely distributed into body fluids and tissues. It is found in high concentrations in brain, kidney, saliva, lung, muscle, spleen, CSF, uterus, and vaginal mucosa.

Metabolism
Acyclovir metabolism in animals is not well known. In humans, it is metabolized to a limited extent by the liver. The majority of drug (95%) is excreted as unchanged parent compound via the kidneys. In renal failure, a buildup of neurotoxic metabolites can occur.

CNS penetration
In humans, penetration into the CSF is approximately 50% of plasma concentrations.

Half-life
The half-life in dogs is 2.2–3.6 h and in cats is 2.6 h.

Pregnancy risk factor

Category C: Acyclovir crosses the placenta. It has teratogenic effects in rats (head and tail anomalies), as well as maternal toxicity. It is contraindicated in pregnant animals.

Lactation
Acyclovir is excreted into milk at concentrations that can exceed maternal plasma concentrations. It is not considered safe in nursing animals.

Further reading

Davidson, A.P. (2013) Canine herpesvirus infection. Ch. 16. In: *Canine and Feline Infectious Diseases*, Sykes, J.E. (ed.), Elsevier, St. Louis, MO. pp. 166–169.

Krasny, H.C., deMiranda, P., Blum, M.R., *et al.* (1981) Pharmacokinetics and bioavailability of acyclovir in the dogs. *J Pharmacol Exp Ther.*, **216(2)**, 281–288.

Owens, J.G., Nasisse, M.P., Tadepalli, S.M., *et al.* (1996) Pharmacokinetics of acyclovir in the cat. *J Vet Pharmacol Ther.*, **19**, 488–490.

Papich, M.G. (2002) *Saunders Handbook of Veterinary Drugs*. 2nd edn. Winkel, A. (ed.), W.B. Saunders Company, Philadelphia, pp. 17–19.

Plumb, D.C. (2011) *Veterinary Drug Handbook*. 7th edn. Plumb, D.C. (ed.), Wiley-Blackwell, Ames Iowa, p. 16.

Richardson, J.A. (2000) Accidental ingestion of acyclovir in dogs: 105 reports. *Vet Hum Toxicol.*, **42(6)**, 370–371.

Weiss, R.C. (1989) Synergistic antiviral activities of acyclovir and recombinant human leukocyte (alpha) interferon on feline herpesvirus replication. *Am J Vet Res.*, **50(10)**, 1672–1677.

Williams, D.L., Robinson, J.C., Lay, E., *et al.* (2005) Efficacy of topical acyclovir for the treatment of feline keratitis: Results of a prospective clinical trial and data from *in vitro* investigations. *Vet Rec.*, **27(9)**, 254–257.

Chapter 208: Famciclovir

US Generic (Brand) Name: Famciclovir (Famvir)
Availability: Human Approved – Tablets 125, 250, and 500 mg
Resistance Mechanisms: Mutations in viral thymidine kinase and DNA polymerase genes

Use

In small animals, famciclovir is used primarily for treatment of feline herpesvirus-1 (FHV-1) infections. It is more effective and considerably less toxic than acyclovir. In humans, famciclovir is used for the treatment of acute *Herpes zoster* and recurrent *Herpes simplex* infections. Famciclovir is a prodrug that undergoes rapid biotransformation to the active compound penciclovir. Effective dosing and plasma concentrations remain controversial. Effective penciclovir concentrations are reported to be higher (3.5 µg/mL) for FHV-1 than human *Herpes* viruses.

Contraindications/warnings

Avoid concurrent administration of drugs that are nephrotoxic (amphotericin B, aminoglycosides, etc.) or drugs that are extensively excreted via active renal tubular secretion that may increase penciclovir concentrations. Correct dehydration and electrolyte imbalances prior to administering. Animal studies have demonstrated an increased incidence of carcinomas, mutagenic changes, and decreases in fertility with high doses.

Dosage

Dogs
Following a dose of 40 mg/kg, the peak concentration of penciclovir was 3.5 µg/mL suggesting that therapeutic concentrations might be achieved with this dosing. However, famciclovir has not been widely used to treat dogs with *Herpes* infections so exact dosing is unknown.

Cats
FHV-1 Infections: 40–90 mg/kg PO q8 h. Dose escalation does not result in proportional increases in plasma penciclovir concentrations due to rate limiting conversion of 6-deoxypenciclovir to penciclovir. Because of saturation of the metabolism of famciclovir to penciclovir, equivalent serum and tear penciclovir concentrations can be achieved in cats with 40 or 90 mg/kg PO q8 h of famciclovir, so 40 mg/kg may be equally efficacious.

Dose adjustments

Dose reductions are required in patients with significant renal and hepatic impairment. The dosing frequency should be reduced from q8 h to either q12 h or q24 h depending on the degree of impairment.

Administration

The tablets may be taken with or without food. Suspensions made from tablets taste bitter, so it is best to cut tablets as needed and administer directly or place into gel capsules.

Electrolyte contents

Not significant, does contain high amounts of lactose (27, 54, 107 mg/tab) in the 125, 250, and 500 mg tablets, respectively.

Storage/stability

Store tablets at room temperature, protected from light.

Adverse reactions

Famciclovir is generally well tolerated in cats and can be safely administered to kittens.

>10%
Lethargy reported in cats.

1–10%
Anorexia and polydipsia reported in cats.

Other species
Adverse reactions have included nausea, diarrhea, vomiting, pruritus, paresthesia, rigors, arthralgia, neutropenia, acute renal failure (primarily with pre-existing renal impairment), elevated sodium/potassium concentrations, abnormal leukocyte count, abdominal pain, and elevated liver enzymes.

Drug interactions

In humans, cimetidine and theophylline may increase the plasma concentrations/toxicity of penciclovir. Famciclovir can increase peak concentrations/toxicity of digoxin.

Monitoring

Obtain baseline CBC and serum renal/hepatic values. Monitor CBC periodically if on prolonged therapy.

Overdose

Doses up to 250 mg/kg have been well tolerated in dogs. High doses may result in lethargy, polyuria, polydipsia, nausea, vomiting, and diarrhea. Overdoses have the potential to result in seizures or acute renal failure. Gastrointestinal decontamination (emesis, activated charcoal) are recommended for oral overdoses. Supportive care should include fluid therapy (diuresis) and diazepam for seizures. Hemodialysis removes approximately 60% of a dose.

Diagnostic test interference

None reported.

Mechanism

Famciclovir is phosphorylated by viral thymidine kinase in virus-infected cells to a monophosphate form. This is converted to penciclovir triphosphate and competes with deoxyguanosine triphosphate to inhibit viral polymerases, resulting in inhibition of DNA synthesis and replication.

Pharmacology/kinetics

Absorption
In cats given oral doses of 40 and 90 mg/kg, peak concentrations (1.34 and 1.28 µg/mL) of penciclovir occurred at 2.8 and 3.0 h, respectively. Oral bioavailability was 12.5 and 7%, respectively, suggesting saturation of famciclovir metabolism at the higher dose. In dogs given an oral dose of 40 mg/kg, oral absorption was rapid and reached peak concentrations (3.5 µg/mL) in the plasma at 30 min.

Distribution
Penciclovir is extensively distributed into tissues. In cats, tear penciclovir concentrations following a 40 mg/kg oral dose exceeded the concentration shown to have *in vitro* efficacy against FHV-1 (0.304 µg/mL) in about half of the specimens collected.

Metabolism
Following oral administration to dogs, famciclovir undergoes extensive first pass metabolism to a 6-deoxy precursor of penciclovir. This is then converted to penciclovir and essentially no parent compound is recovered from plasma or urine. In dogs, extensive conversion of famciclovir to penciclovir occurs but is slow. Penciclovir is predominantly eliminated unchanged by the kidney with minor amounts excreted via feces.

CNS penetration
No information is currently available on famciclovir CNS penetration.

Half-life
The half-life of penciclovir in cats following oral administration is 4.2–4.8 h.

Pregnancy risk factor

Category B: Famciclovir was tested on embryo-fetal development in rats and rabbits at oral doses up to 1000 mg/kg/day. No adverse effects were observed on embryo-fetal development. No reports of teratogenic effects have been reported in humans. Famciclovir is thus considered safe in pregnancy as long as the benefits outweigh the risks.

Lactation
Famciclovir does penetrate into milk. However, due to its tumorigenic potential it is contraindicated in nursing animals.

Further reading

Filer, C.W., Ramji, J.V., Allen, G.D., *et al.* (1995) Metabolic and pharmacokinetic studies following oral administration of famciclovir to the rat and dog. *Xenobiotica.*, **25(5)**, 477–490.

Malik, R., Lessels, N.S., *et al.* (2009) Treatment of feline herpesvirus-1 associated disease in cats with famciclovir and related drugs. *J Feline Med Surg.*, **11(1)**, 40–48.

Thomasy, SM., Covert, J.C., Stanley, S.D., *et al.* (2012) Pharmacokinetics of famciclovir and penciclovir in tears following oral administration of famciclovir to cats: a pilot study. *Vet Ophthalmol.*, **15(5)**, 299–306.

Thomasy, S.M., Lim, C.C., Reilly, C.M., *et al.* (2011) Evaluation of orally administered famciclovir in cats experimentally infected with feline herpesvirus type-1. *Am J Vet Res.*, **72(1)**, 85–95.

Thomasy, S.M., Whittem, T., Bales, J.L., *et al.* (2012) Pharmacokinetics of penciclovir in healthy cats following oral administration of famciclovir or intravenous infusion of penciclovir. *Am J Vet Res.*, **73(7)**, 1092–1099.

Chapter 209: Cidofovir

US Generic (Brand) Name: Cidofovir (Vistide)
Availability: Human Approved – Sterile injectable (75 mg/mL × 5 mL), Compounded ophthalmic preparations containing 0.5% cidofovir are available through sterile compounding pharmacies
Resistance Mechanism: Mutation in viral DNA polymerase

Use

In small animals, cidofovir is used topically as an ophthalmic solution to treat cats with feline herpesvirus-1 (FHV-1) infections. In humans, cidofovir is primarily used intravenously to treat cytomegalovirus retinitis in patients with acquired immunodeficiency syndrome.

Contraindications/warnings

Known hypersensitivity to cidofovir, or other sulfa-containing medications. This medication is carcinogenic. Medication must be prepared in a Sterile Class 2 Laminar flow hood or greater. Wear gloves when applying medication, dispose of all expired medications according to carcinogenic protocols.

Dosage

Feline
FHV-1 Infections: One drop of 0.5% cidofovir in each eye q12 h for 10 days.

Dose adjustments

None required for topical use.

Administration

Wash hands thoroughly with soap and water. Remove the protective cap. Make sure that the eye drops are not cloudy. Avoid touching the dropper tip against the eye or anything else. Hold the dropper tip down at all times to prevent drops from flowing back into the bottle and contaminating the remaining contents. Do not wipe or rinse off dropper.

Electrolyte contents

Each vial for injection (5 mL) contains 2.5 mmol (57 mg) of sodium.

Storage/stability

Store compounded solution as recommended by the compounding pharmacy. Discard 2 weeks after opening to reduce the likelihood of bacterial contamination. Cidofovir is stable when diluted with 0.9% NaCl and stored for up to 6 months in glass or plastic at 4, −20, and −80°C.

Adverse reactions

1–10%
Unknown with topical use in cats. Observe for ocular irritation.

Other species
Local irritation and scarring of the nasolacrimal duct has been reported with topical administration of cidofovir to humans and rabbits with keratoconjunctivitis. With systemic use, adverse effects reported in humans include

gastrointestinal signs, neurologic signs, myelosuppression, renal dysfunction, hypotension, allergic skin reactions, electrolyte abnormalities, and ocular signs such as iritis, uveitis, and retinal detachment.

Drug interactions

When given topically it is wise to withhold other topical medications for 20–30 min before instilling other medications. Products that may interact with this drug when given systemically to humans have included: acyclovir, angiotensin-converting enzyme inhibitors, phenobarbital, benzodiazepines, famotidine, furosemide, nonsteroidal anti-inflammatory drugs, theophylline, and zidovudine.

Monitoring

Perform ocular examinations on a regular basis to assess for ocular irritation.

Overdose

Overdoses in humans have resulted in renal impairment and were treated with fluid therapy.

Diagnostic test interference

None reported.

Mechanism

Cidofovir is converted to cidofovir diphosphate, which is the active intracellular metabolite. This is a nucleotide analog, which selectively inhibits viral replication when it is incorporated into viral DNA.

Pharmacology/kinetics

Absorption
Cidofovir enters ocular epithelial cells after topical administration by fluid-phase endocytosis and is phosphorylated to cidofovir monophosphate and subsequently to cidofovir diphosphate.

Distribution
Cidofovir is widely distributed throughout tissues and total body water. Protein binding in all species studied (monkeys, rats, and rabbits) is low (<10%).

Metabolism
The major route of elimination of cidofovir in laboratory animals (rats, mice) is by renal excretion of unchanged drug.

CNS penetration
Cidofovir does not cross significantly into the CSF.

Half-life
Prolonged antiviral effects of cidofovir are related to the half-lives of its metabolites; cidofovir diphosphate persists inside cells with a half-life of 17–65 h and a cidofovir phosphate-choline adduct has a half-life of 87 h, suggesting a long tissue residence time for these active metabolites.

Pregnancy risk factor

Category C: Adenocarcinomas have been reported in animal studies with systemic administration. The manufacturer considers the drug contraindicated in pregnancy. However, it is unlikely that topical use of cidofovir would achieve significant concentrations systemically that could harm a fetus.

Lactation
It is unknown if cidofovir penetrates into milk. It is carcinogenic. However, it is unlikely that topical use of cidofovir would achieve concentrations systemically that would result in significant levels in milk.

Further reading

Fontenelle, J.P., Powell, C.C., Veir, J.K., *et al.* (2008) Effect of topical ophthalmic application of cidofovir on experimentally induced primary ocular feline herpesvirus-1 infection in cats. *Am J Vet Res.*, **69(2)**, 289–293.

Stiles, J., Gwin, W., and Pogranichniy, R. (2010) Stability of 0.5% cidofovir stored under various conditions for up to 6 months. *Vet Ophthalmol.*, **13(4)**, 275–277.

Chapter 210: Idoxuridine

US Generic (Brand) Name: Idoxuridine (Dendrid, Herplex, Stoxil)

Availability: Not commercially available in the USA. Sterile ophthalmic products must be obtained from a Sterile Compounding Pharmacy. Compounded strengths have included: Idoxuridine 0.5% ointment and 0.1% solution

Resistance Mechanism: Most likely altered viral thymidine kinase and DNA polymerase

Use

Idoxuridine is an antiviral drug that has been primarily used topically to treat feline herpesvirus-1 (FHV-1) ocular infections in cats. It is not used systemically because of toxicity. It is less expensive, but appears to be less efficacious than cidofovir and requires more frequent administration.

Contraindications/warnings

Hypersensitivity to idoxuridine or other iodine containing products.

Dosage

Feline

FHV-1 Infections: Instill 1–2 drops of the 0.1% solution into the affected eye(s) 5–6 times daily or administer a 0.5 mm/ ¼-inch strip of the 0.5% ointment into the affected eye (s) every 4 h during the day and once before bedtime. Therapy is continued for 3–4 days after healing is complete.

Dose adjustments

Not necessary for topical administration.

Administration

Wash hands thoroughly with soap and water. Remove the protective cap. Make sure that the eye drops are not cloudy. Avoid touching the dropper tip against the eye or anything else. Hold the dropper tip down at all times to prevent drops from flowing back into the bottle and contaminating the remaining contents. Do not wipe or rinse off dropper.

Electrolyte contents

Not significant.

Stability/storage

Store according to the directions of the sterile compounding pharmacy. Store ophthalmic solution at 2–8°C (36–46°F) in a tight, light-resistant container unless otherwise directed. The ointment should be stored at 2–15°C (36–59°F). Most sterile ophthalmic solutions should be discarded 14 days after opening. Decomposed

idoxuridine not only has reduced antiviral activity but also may be toxic.

Adverse reactions

1–10%
Local irritation and stinging reported in cats.

Other species
Blurred vision, photophobia, corneal clouding, and damage to corneal epithelium have been reported.

Drug interactions

Do not use glucocorticoid eye medications, vitamins, or eye products that contain boric acid while using idoxuridine. Avoid use of other eye drops during treatment since these may precipitate with idoxuridine.

Monitoring

Perform ocular examinations on a regular basis to assess for ocular irritation.

Overdose

If excessive medication is administered topically, flush the eye with water for several minutes. If the drops are ingested, administer plenty of fluid orally to dilute the medication. The ingestion of a whole bottle of idoxuridine ophthalmic is not expected to cause harm because of its extremely low oral bioavailability.

Diagnostic test interference

None reported.

Mechanism

Idoxuridine is a halogenated thymidine analog. It is incorporated into viral DNA during replication.

Pharmacology/kinetics

Absorption
Oral bioavailability is only 0.5%. After topical administration, idoxuridine penetrates the cornea poorly and therefore is ineffective in the treatment of iritis or deep stromal infections.

Pregnancy risk factor

Category C: Idoxuridine crosses the placenta. Fetal malformations in rabbits (including exophthalmos and clubbing of forelegs) and chromosomal aberrations in mice have been reported. However, due to the limited systemic absorption it is doubtful that sufficient drug could cross the placenta to cause fetal abnormalities.

Lactation

It is unknown if idoxuridine is distributed into milk. Due to its limited systemic absorption concentrations in milk would most likely be negligible.

Further reading

Bryan, G.M. (1980) Idoxuridine for feline keratitis. *J Am Vet Med Assoc.*, **177(7)**, 602.Maggs, D.J. and Clarke, H.E. (2004) *In vitro* efficacy of ganciclovir, cidofovir, penciclovir, foscarnet, idoxuridine, and acyclovir against feline herpesvirus type-1. *Am J Vet Res.*, **64(4)**, 399–403.

Maggs, D.J., Miller, P., and Ofri, R. (2013) Ocular pharmacology and therapeutics. Ch. 7. In: *Slatter's Fundamentals of Veterinary Ophthalmology*. 5th edn. Maggs, D.J. (ed.), Elsevier, St. Louis, MO, pp. 150–155.

Maxwell, E. (1963) Treatment of *herpes keratitis* with 5-iodo-2-deoxyuridine (IDU): a clinical evaluation of 1500 cases. *Am J Ophthalmol.*, **56**, 571–573.

Seth, A., Misra, A., and Umrigar, D. (2004) Topical liposomal gel of idoxuridine for the treatment of *herpes simplex*: Pharmaceutical and clinical implications. *Pharm Dev Technol.*, **9(3)**, 277–289.

Chapter 211: Oseltamivir

US Generic (Brand) Name: Oseltamivir (Tamiflu)
Availability: Human Approved – Oseltamivir phosphate capsules (30, 45, 75 mg), Oseltamivir oral suspension (6 mg/mL × 60 mL) and compounded oral suspension (6 mg/mL)
Resistance Mechanism: Point mutation in viral neuraminidase

Use

Oseltamivir is primarily indicated for the treatment of human influenza. In humans, it is used to treat uncomplicated acute (<2 days) infections. Resistance can develop rapidly and the overall efficacy in human medicine remains controversial. It is currently not recommended for treatment of canine influenza virus infections because it is only beneficial early in the course of illness (<48 h) and most dogs do not present to a veterinarian within this time frame. Widespread veterinary use could also contribute to resistance in humans. Oseltamivir has been reported to reduce disease severity in canine parvovirus infections, possibly as a result of its effect on the neuraminidases of secondary bacterial invaders, but further research is needed.

Contraindications/warnings

Contraindications include known hypersensitivity to oseltamivir. Caution is also recommended in humans with seizure disorders, diabetes mellitus, or cardiac arrhythmias.

Dosage

Dosing is extrapolated from human patients and may not reflect accurate antiviral plasma concentrations in dogs. Drug must be administered as soon as diagnosis is made and should be continued for 5 days (or up to 10 days for severe infections).

Canine

Canine parvovirus infections: 2.2 mg/kg PO q12 h for 5–10 days. Use for this purpose is controversial.

Dose adjustments

In humans with severe renal impairment, it is recommended that the dose be administered once daily rather than twice daily.

Administration

The drug should be administered with food to decrease gastrointestinal upset. The capsules can be given directly and should not be chewed due to the bitter taste. The oral commercial powder for suspension should be mixed with 55 mL of water. The resulting suspension is 6 mg/mL. A compounded oral suspension (6 mg/mL) can be made using 75 mg capsules in one of the following vehicles: Cherry Syrup (Humco), Ora-Sweet SF (sugar-free) (Paddock Laboratories), or simple syrup. Instructions for preparation can be found at www.tamiflu.com/hcp/resources/hcp_dosing_storage.jsp.

Electrolyte contents

Not significant. A bottle of oseltamivir oral suspension contains approximately 11 g sorbitol. This may cause diarrhea in some animals.

Storage/stability

The oral capsules and powder for oral suspension should be stored at room temperature. After reconstitution, the commercial suspension should be stored at room temperature for 10 days or refrigerated for up to 17 days. Do not freeze. The compounded suspension is stable for 5 weeks (35 days) when stored in a refrigerator at 2–8°C (36–46°F).

Adverse reactions

1–10%
Little is known about adverse effects in animals, but some dogs may exhibit gastrointestinal signs such as vomiting immediately after administration. In humans, nausea, vomiting, diarrhea abdominal pain, and headache are common.

<1%
Rare side effects in humans include hepatotoxicity, rash, anaphylaxis, Stevens–Johnson syndrome, toxic epidermal necrolysis, cardiac arrhythmias, seizure, confusion, exacerbation of diabetes mellitus, and colitis.

Drug interactions

There is no data on drug interactions in veterinary patients. The low protein binding of oseltamivir and oseltamivir carboxylate suggests that the probability of drug displacement interactions is low. In vitro studies demonstrate that neither oseltamivir nor oseltamivir carboxylate is a good substrate for P450 enzymes or for glucuronyl transferases.

Monitoring

No special monitoring recommendations.

Overdose

Overdoses in humans typically result in gastrointestinal signs such as vomiting and diarrhea. Supportive care and fluid replacement may be required.

Diagnostic test interference

None reported.

Mechanism

Oseltamivir is a neuraminidase inhibitor that is a competitive inhibitor of the activity of viral neuraminidase (NA) enzyme on sialic acid, found on glycoproteins on the surface of normal host cells. By blocking the activity of the enzyme, oseltamivir prevents new viral particles from being released by infected cells.

Pharmacology/kinetics

The pharmacokinetics of oseltamivir have not been studied in dogs and cats.

Absorption
Oseltamivir phosphate is readily absorbed after oral administration and is extensively converted to oseltamivir carboxylate. Approximately 75% of an oral dose reaches the systemic circulation as oseltamivir carboxylate in humans.

Distribution
Oseltamivir carboxylate is extensively distributed throughout body tissues and fluids. It is readily distributed into the upper and lower respiratory tract. Protein binding is only 3% in humans.

Metabolism
Little is known in dogs and cats. The prodrug oseltamivir is metabolized in the liver to its active metabolite. This predominantly occurs by hepatic esterases to oseltamivir carboxylate. Oseltamivir carboxylate is primarily (>90%) excreted via glomerular filtration and tubular secretion. Only minor amounts are excreted in the feces (<20%) in humans.

CNS penetration
Oseltamivir penetrates into the CSF, but in low concentrations. Oseltamivir CSF/plasma ratios of 2.1% were noted in humans and 3.5% for oseltamivir carboxylate.

Half-life
In humans, the half-life of the parent drug is only 1–2 h and the active carboxylate metabolite is 6–10 h.

Pregnancy risk factor

Category C: There is no evidence that oseltamivir is associated with adverse effects in the fetus. Risks must be weighed against benefits.

Lactation

Oseltamivir is excreted into milk in lactating rats. No toxicity was observed after repeated administration of up to 500 mg/kg to developing juvenile rats 7–21 days old. It is unlikely to cause significant effects on nursing animals.

Further reading

Bahar, F.G., Ohura, K., Ogihara, T., *et al.* (2012) Species difference of esterase expression and hydrolase activity in plasma. *J Pharm Sci.*, **101(10)**, 3979–3988.

Donner, B., Niranian, V., and Hoffman, G. (2010) Safety of oseltamivir in pregnancy: A review of preclinical and clinical data. *Drug Saf.*, **33(8)**, 631–642.

MacIntire, D.K. and Douglass, K. (2006) Treatment of parvoviral enteritis. *Proceedings of the Western Veterinary Conference*, 2006. Retrieved 2007-06-09, available online securely.

Savigny, M.R. and MacIntire, D.K. (2010) Use of oseltamivir in the treatment of canine parvoviral enteritis. *J Vet Emerg Crit Care*, **20(1)**, 132–142.

Chapter 212: Vidarabine

US Generic (Brand) Name: Vidarabine (Vira-A)
Availability: Human Approved – Vidarabine ophthalmic ointment 3% (3.5 g). Commercial availability is variable. It can be obtained from Sterile Compounding Pharmacies as a 3% ointment or 3% solution
Resistance Mechanism: Altered DNA viral polymerase

Use

Vidarabine is a topical antiherpesviral drug. In veterinary medicine, vidarabine is used topically to treat cats with feline herpesvirus-1 (FHV-1) infections. Both idoxuridine and vidarabine are better tolerated than trifluridine in cats. Vidarabine can also be used to treat idoxuridine resistant strains of FHV-1. In humans, vidarabine is used for the treatment of acute herpetic keratoconjunctivitis.

Contraindications/warnings

Known hypersensitivity to vidarabine.

Dosage

Feline

FHV-1 Infections: Instill 0.5–1 cm/1/4–1/2 inch strip into the affected eye(s) 5–6 times daily.

Dose adjustments

Not required for topical treatment.

Administration

Wash hands first; do not let the tube tip touch the eye. Rolling the ointment tube in your hands for a minute will make the ointment flow easier. Place 0.5–1 cm/1/4–1/2 inch of ointment into the eye by squeezing the tube gently. If you are using an eye drop or ointment in addition to this medication, apply the eye drops or ointment first and wait at least ten minutes before applying vidarabine.

Electrolyte contents

Not significant.

Storage/stability

Store at room temperature. Protect from freezing.

Adverse reactions

1–10%
Lacrimation, irritation reported in cats.

Other Species
Conjunctival injection, burning, irritation, superficial punctate keratitis, pain, photophobia, and sensitivity.

Drug interactions

Topical administration of glucocorticoids concurrently may cause glucocorticoid-induced glaucoma or cataract formation and progression of bacterial or viral infections.

Monitoring

Perform ocular examinations on a regular basis to assess for ocular irritation.

Overdose

The oral LD_{50} for vidarabine is greater than 5020 mg/kg in mice and rats. No significant effects should result from ingestion of the entire contents of a tube because of rapid deamination to arabinosyl hypoxanthine.

Diagnostic test interference

None reported.

Mechanism

Vidarabine interferes with the synthesis of viral DNA. It is a nucleoside analog and has to be phosphorylated to be active. This is a three step process in which vidarabine is sequentially phosphorylated by kinases to the triphosphate ara-ATP. When used as a substrate for viral DNA polymerase, ara-ATP competitively inhibits dATP leading to the formation of faulty DNA.

Pharmacology/kinetics

Absorption
Systemic absorption of vidarabine does not occur following ocular administration and swallowing lacrimal secretions. In laboratory animals, vidarabine is rapidly deaminated in the gastrointestinal tract to its metabolite.

Distribution
Because of the low solubility of vidaribine, trace amounts of vidaribine and its metabolite can be detected in the aqueous humor only if there is an epithelial defect in the cornea. If the cornea is normal, only trace amounts of the metabolite can be recovered from the aqueous humor.

Metabolism
Vidarabine is rapidly deaminated to arabinosylhypoxanthine (Ara-Hx), the principal metabolite. Ara-Hx also possesses *in vitro* antiviral activity, but this activity is less than that of vidarabine.

CNS penetration
Vidarabine is able to cross the blood-brain barrier when converted to its active metabolite (Ara-Hx).

Half-life
The half-life in humans is 1 h. The half-life of the active triphosphate metabolite (ara-ATP) is three times longer in HSV-infected cells compared with uninfected cells.

Pregnancy risk factor

Category C: When 10% vidarabine ointment was applied to 10% of the body surface during organogenesis it induced fetal abnormalities in rabbits. The possibility of embryonic or fetal damage in pregnant animals receiving 3% vidarabine ophthalmic ointment is remote.

Lactation
Topical administration during lactation is unlikely to produce plasma concentrations sufficient to be detected in milk.

Further reading

Maggs, D.J., Miller, P., and Ofri, R. (2013) Ocular pharmacology and therapeutics. Ch. 7. In: *Slatter's Fundamentals of Veterinary Ophthalmology*. 5th edn. Maggs, D.J. (ed.), St. Louis, MO, pp. 150–155.

Nasisse, M.P. (1989) *In vitro* susceptibility of feline herpesvirus-1 to vidarabine, idoxuridine, trifluridine, acyclovir, or bromovinyldeoxyuridine. *Am J Vet Res.*, **50(1)**, 158–160.

Stiles, J. (1995) Treatment of cats with ocular disease attributable to herpesvirus infection: 17 cases (1983–1993). *J Am Vet Med Assoc.*, **207(5)**, 599–603.

Sykes, J.E. and Papich, M.G. (2013) Antiviral and immunomodulary drugs. Ch. 7. In: *Canine and Feline Infectious Diseases*, Sykes, J.E. (ed.), Elsevier, St. Louis, MO, pp. 54–63.

Chapter 213: Zidovudine

US Generic (Brand) Name: Zidovudine (Retrovir)
Availability: Human Approved – Zidovudine capsules (100 mg), tablets (300 mg), oral syrup (10 mg/mL × 240 mL), sterile injection 10 mg/mL (20 mL)
Resistance Mechanisms: Mutation in viral reverse transcriptase

Use

Zidovudine has been used for the treatment of feline leukemia (FeLV) and immunodeficiency virus (FIV) infections. In FIV-infected cats, it can decrease viral load, improve stomatitis, and increase CD4/CD8 ratios. In cats infected with FeLV, it has limited benefit but may improve stomatitis, reduce antigenemia, and reduce the development of lymphoma.

Contraindications/warnings

Known hypersensitivity to zidovudine. Its use in cats with significant anemia or neutropenia is not recommended. Use with caution in renal/hepatic impairment. Dosage reduction is indicated in cats with severe renal impairment. Avoid use or use with extreme caution in animals with liver impairment.

Dosage

Feline
FeLV/FIV Infections: 5–15 mg/kg PO/SC q12 h.

Dose adjustments

Reduce frequency of administration to q24 h in renal failure.

Administration

Oral tablets or capsules should be given 30 min before or 1 h after a meal followed by at least 3–6 mL of water (to prevent esophageal irritation). If not tolerated administer with a non-fatty meal. Subcutaneous administration may be used in cats unable to take oral dosage forms. The injectable can be irritating when given SC. The commercial IV formulation is available in a 10 mg/mL solution. Remove the appropriate dose and further dilute (<4 mg/mL) with isotonic sodium chloride solution to prevent local irritation.

Electrolyte contents

Not significant.

Storage/stability

Store oral capsules, tablets, oral solution and injectable at room temperature, protected from light. Following dilution the intravenous solution is stable for 24 h at room temperature or 48 h if refrigerated.

Adverse reactions

>10%
Diarrhea and weakness in cats.

1–10%
Heinz bodies, anemia reported in cats treated with high doses. Anemia becomes evident with doses of 60 mg/kg starting at Day 4 and 30 mg/kg at Day 13.

<1%
Neutropenia has also been reported in cats at high doses (>30 mg/kg).

Other Species
Hepatotoxicity, cardiomyopathy, rash, confusion, weight loss, headache, dizziness, and myopathy are reported.

Drug interactions

In humans, drugs that inhibit hepatic glucuronidation such as cimetidine may decrease the elimination rate and increased the plasma concentrations/toxicity of zidovudine. Doxorubicin's effects may be antagonized by zidovudine. Myelosuppressive drugs may potentiate the adverse effects of zidovudine. Co-administration with nephrotoxic drugs (amphotericin-B, flucytosine, aminoglycosides) or azole antifungal drugs may increase the concentrations/toxicity of zidovudine.

Monitoring

Baseline CBC and serum biochemistry profile. Monitor CBC weekly for 4 weeks, then monthly.

Overdose

Acute clinical signs of overdose may include nausea, vomiting, diarrhea, fever, and ataxia. At 2–3 days, anemia and/or neutropenia may develop. Gastrointestinal decontamination and supportive care are recommended. Dialysis has little effect on the removal of parent drug, but does remove the major metabolites.

Diagnostic test interference

None noted.

Mechanism

Zidovudine works by selectively inhibiting the viral reverse transcriptase enzyme.

Pharmacology/kinetics

Absorption
Zidovudine is well absorbed following oral administration to cats, with oral bioavailability of 70–95%.

Distribution
Zidovudine is lipophilic and is widely distributed into tissues. Protein binding in humans is <38%.

Metabolism
In humans, zidovudine is rapidly metabolized via glucuronidation in the liver. Cellular enzymes convert zidovudine and its metabolites into the active triphosphate form. Zidovudine and its metabolites are primarily eliminated (60–95%) via glomerular filtration and tubular secretion. Little is known in animals.

CNS penetration

Zidovudine and its metabolites penetrate into the CNS. In humans, the CSF/plasma ratio is 0.6.

Half-life

Following oral administration of zidovudine the elimination half time is 1.5 h in cats. Cats appear to have slower clearance of zidovudine compared to other species.

Pregnancy risk factor

Category C: Zidovudine and its metabolites cross the placenta and have been used in human patients to reduce maternal-fetal transmission of HIV. Teratogenic effects are only seen at extremely high doses (3683 mg/kg) in laboratory animals (rats/mice). Here, the benefits (reduced maternal-fetal transmission of immunodeficiency viruses) may outweigh the risks of adverse effects.

Lactation

Zidovudine is excreted into milk with concentrations similar to serum concentrations. Due to the potential to cause bone marrow toxicity in nursing animals, the benefits of use in lactating animals may not outweigh the risks.

Further reading

Hart, S. and Nolte, I. (1995) Long-term treatment of diseased, FIV-seropositive field cats with azidothymidine (AZT). *Zentralbl Veterinarmed A.*, **42(6)**, 397–409.

Hascheck, W.M., Weigel, R.M., Scherba, G., *et al.* (1990) Zidovudine toxicity to cats infected with feline leukemia virus. *Fundam Appl Toxicol.*, **14(4)**, 765–775.

Hosie, M.J., Addie, D., Belak, S., *et al.* (2009) Feline immunodeficiency. ABCD guidelines on prevention and management. *J Feline Med Surg.*, **11(7)**, 575–584.

Sykes, J.E. and Papich, M.G. (2013) Antiviral and immunomodulary drugs. Ch. 7. In: *Canine and Feline Infectious Diseases*, Sykes, J.E. (ed.), Elsevier, St. Louis, MO. pp. 54–63.

Zhang, W., Mauldin, J.K., Schmiedt, C.W., *et al.* (2004) Pharmacokinetics of zidovudine in cats. *Am J Vet Res.*, **65(6)**, 835–840.

Index

Drug Therapy for Infectious Diseases of the Dog and Cat, First Edition. Valerie J. Wiebe.
© 2015 John Wiley & Sons, Inc. Published 2015 by John Wiley & Sons, Inc.